Pathology Case Reports

Beyond the Pearls

Volume Editors:

MONISHA BHANOTE, MD, FCAP, FASCP
Consultant Pathologist and Integrative Medicine Physician
Breast, Cytopathology, Bone & Soft Tissue Pathology Sub-specialty
Integrative and Lifestyle Medicine Sub-specialty
Jacksonville Beach, Florida

DAVID G. HICKS, MD
Professor and Director of IHC-ISH Laboratory and Chief of Breast Subspecialty Services
University of Rochester Medical Center
Rochester, New York

Series Editors:

RAJ DASGUPTA, MD, FACP, FCCP, FAASM
Assistant Professor of Clinical Medicine
Division of Pulmonary/Critical Care/Sleep Medicine
Associate Program Director of the Sleep Medicine Fellowship
Assistant Program Director of the Internal Medicine Residency
Keck School of Medicine of the University of Southern California
Los Angeles, California

R. MICHELLE KOOLAEE, DO, CCD
Assistant Professor of Clinical Medicine
Division of Rheumatology
Keck School of Medicine of the University of Southern California
Los Angeles, California

ELSEVIER

Elsevier
1600 John F. Kennedy Blvd.
Ste 1800
Philadelphia, PA 19103-2899

PATHOLOGY CASE REPORTS: BEYOND THE PEARLS ISBN: 978-0-323-75489-7

Library of Congress Control Number: 2020938289

Content Strategist: James T. Merritt
Content Development Manager: Meghan B. Andress
Publishing Services Manager: Deepthi Unni
Senior Project Manager: Manchu Mohan
Design Direction: Bridget Hoette

Printed in China

Last digit is the print number: 9 8 7 6 5 4 3 2 1

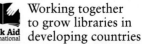

Pathology Case Reports Beyond the Pearls

DEDICATION

This book is dedicated to my Mom and Dad for their eternal support, continued motivation, and constant grounding during my medical career. - MB

To my lovely wife Patti—my best friend, soul mate, and golfing partner—and to our amazing children and grandchildren. I will forever be grateful to all of you for your love and support. - DGH

Michelle and I would like to dedicate this book to her father, Dr. Saeed Koolaee, who was diagnosed with a brain tumor called Glioblastoma Multiforme in August 2019. He could have easily given up to this horrible cancer; however, he continues to fight with dignity and courage despite the numerous challenges. I am honored to call him my father-in-law, whose shoes I could never fill. Your patients, friends, and family love you more than you will ever know. - RD & RMK

CONTRIBUTORS

Rana Ajabnoor, MBBS
Assistant Professor
Breast, Bone and Soft Tissue Pathologist
Department of Anatomical Pathology
King Abdulaziz University
Jeddah, Saudi Arabia

Phoenix D. Bell, MD, MS
Resident Physician
Department of Pathology and Laboratory Medicine
University of Rochester Medical Center
Rochester, New York, USA

Peter Chung, MD
Fellow Physician
Department of Pulmonary, Critical Care, and Sleep Medicine
University of Southern California
Los Angeles, California, USA

Lucas Cruz, MD
Fellow Physician
Department of Pulmonary and Critical Care Medicine
University of Southern California
Los Angeles, California, USA

Raj Dasgupta, MD, FACP, FCCP, FAASM
Assistant Professor of Clinical Medicine
Associate Program Director
Sleep Medicine Fellowship
Assistant Program Director
Internal Medicine Residency
Department of Medicine
Division of Pulmonary, Critical Care,
and Sleep Medicine
Keck School of Medicine of the University of Southern California
Los Angeles, California, USA

Daniel Faden, MD
Attending Surgeon
Division of Surgical Oncology
Department of Otolaryngology
Mass. Eye and Ear
Harvard Medical School
Boston, Massachusetts, USA

Lanisha Denise Fuller, MD
Resident Physician
Department of Pathology and Laboratory Medicine
Cleveland Clinic
Cleveland, Ohio, USA

Youssef Al Hmada, MD
Assistant Director of Anatomic Pathology
Assistant Professor of Pathology
Department of Pathology and Laboratory Medicine
University of Mississippi Medical Center
Jackson, Mississippi, USA

Aaron R. Huber, DO
Assistant Professor
Department of Pathology and Laboratory Medicine
University of Rochester Medical Center
Rochester, New York, USA

Phillip Huyett, MD
Clinical Instructor
Division of Sleep Medicine and Surgery
Massachusetts Eye and Ear Infirmary
Harvard Medical School
Boston, MA, USA

Anna-Karoline Israel, MD
Resident Physician
Department of Pathology and Laboratory Medicine
University of Rochester Medical Center
Rochester, New York, USA

Hasan Khatib, MD
Fellow Physician
Department of Pathology and Laboratory Medicine
University of Rochester Medical Center
Rochester, New York, USA

Mushal Noor, MBBS
Resident Physician
Department of Pathology and Laboratory Medicine
University of Rochester Medical Center
Rochester, New York, USA

Numbereye Numbere, MBBS
Resident Physician
Department of Pathology and Laboratory Medicine
University of Rochester Medical Center
Rochester, New York, USA

Anish R. Patel, MD
Fellow Physician
Department of Pulmonary, Critical Care, and Sleep Medicine
University of Southern California
Los Angeles, California, USA

Stefania A. Pirrotta, DO
Fellow Physician
Department of Pulmonary and Critical Care Medicine
University of Southern California
Los Angeles, California, USA

Jennifer J. Prutsman-Pfeiffer, PhD, PA(ASCP)^{CM}
Pathologists' Assistant
Department of Pathology and Laboratory Medicine
University of Rochester Medical Center
Rochester, New York, USA

Tatsiana Pukhalskaya, MD
Resident Physician
Department of Pathology and Laboratory Medicine
University of Rochester Medical Center
Rochester, New York, USA

Sahar Rabiei-Samani, MD
Fellow Physician
Department of Pulmonary, Critical Care, and Sleep Medicine
University of Southern California
Los Angeles, California, USA

Maria Cecilia D. Reyes, MD
Assistant Professor
Department of Pathology and Laboratory Medicine
University of Rochester Medical Center
Rochester, New York, USA

Cynthia Reyes Barron, MD
Resident Physician
Department of Pathology and Laboratory Medicine
University of Rochester Medical Center
Rochester, New York, USA

Linda Schiffhauer, MD
Associate Professor
Department of Pathology and Laboratory Medicine
University of Rochester Medical Center
Rochester, New York, USA

Julia Stiegler, MD
Resident Physician
Department of Dermatology
University of Rochester
Rochester, New York, USA

Bradley M. Turner, MD, MPH, MHA
Associate Professor
Department of Pathology and Laboratory Medicine
University of Rochester Medical Center
Rochester, New York, USA

Moises J. Velez, MD
Assistant Professor
Department of Pathology and Laboratory Medicine
University of Rochester
Rochester, New York, USA

SERIES EDITORS PREFACE

It is with great pleasure that we present to you our first book in the Case Reports: Beyond the Pearls series, *Pathology Case Reports: Beyond the Pearls*. Writing the "perfect" basic science review text has been a dream many years in the making. We envisioned a text that incorporates a United States Medical Licensing Examination (USMLE) Steps 1, 2, and 3 focus with up-to-date, evidence-based clinical medicine. We wanted the platform of the text to be drawn from a traditional theme that many of us are familiar with from medical school, the "case report" format. This book is geared toward medical students preparing for the USMLE Step 1 and COMLEX Level 1. Each case has been carefully chosen and covers scenarios and questions frequently encountered on the pathology basic science exam during medical school integrating both basic science and clinical pearls.

We would like to sincerely thank the many contributors who have helped to create this text. Their insightful work will be a valuable tool for medical students and physicians to gain an in-depth understanding of pathology. It should be noted that while a variety of clinical cases in pathology were selected for this book, it is not meant to substitute a comprehensive pathology reference.

We especially thank our volume editors, Dr. Bhanote and Dr. Hicks, for all of their hard work and dedication to this book. It was their vision and execution that helped in preparing this book. It was truly a pleasure to work with everyone associated with the book, and we look forward to our next project together.

Raj Dasgupta
R. Michelle Koolaee

VOLUME EDITORS PREFACE

This book was written to address the needs of medical students and residents preparing for their examinations. Successful exam completion is just one milestone for their medical career. The field of medicine is rapidly changing with new advances and breakthroughs happening on an almost daily basis. This rapid pace of change makes it challenging to remain current as a practicing physician. In consideration of pathology as the cornerstone of diagnosis and treatment for patients, having a solid foundation in pathology will help any doctor regardless of their final chosen specialty. Our goal was to present this material in an understandable and meaningful way to students and trainees who are trying to learn this content for the first time. We arranged cases by major organ systems and utilized a case-based format, which provided an ideal venue for presenting complex scientific and clinical information in the context of a particular patient. We have provided correlations with current advanced testing, including molecular analysis, and have carefully selected images for their illustrative purpose. We have included recent publications and references for those interested in reading more on specific topics.

On behalf of all the authors, we hope that this book will be a helpful resource for medical students and residents in not only completing their examinations but also providing them a pathology foundation for their medical career. Our hope is that the material will enrich their understanding of the field of medicine and the vital role that pathology plays in diagnosis and patient care. As we wistfully release our book out into the world, it is hard not to think about how nice it would have been if this content had been available to use when we were studying and trying to learn this material. This is probably the best possible reason for putting a book such as this together.

Monisha Bhanote
David G. Hicks

FOREWORD

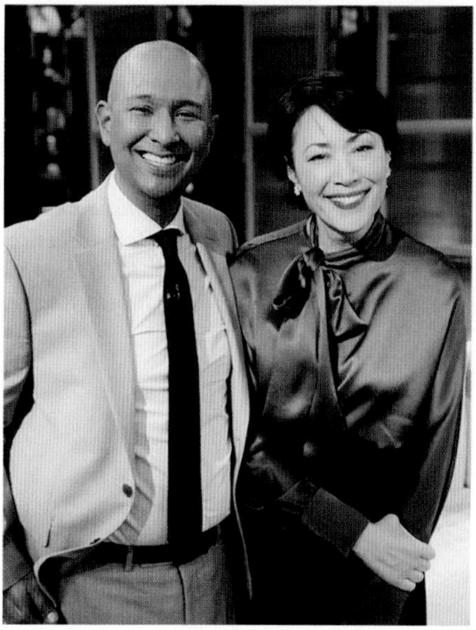

"Dr. Raj Dasgupta is the real deal: both a man of compassion, who cares deeply about easing human suffering and a highly capable physician, brilliant at solving even the most puzzling of medical cases. He is also a teacher who opens our minds and our hearts, and in this way, he makes us all better. I consider Dr. Dasgupta a true force for good."

—Ann Curry

ACKNOWLEDGMENTS

The preparation of a multi-authored book is a collaborative endeavor, and we are grateful to the Faculty and Trainees at the University of Rochester and University of Southern California for their enthusiasm during this project and the many wonderful and insightful chapters that they prepared. We are also grateful to Meghan Andress and Elsevier for all the help and support in preparation of this book.

Monisha Bhanote
David G. Hicks
Raj Dasgupta
R. Michelle Koolaee

CONTENTS

Introduction to Pathology/Primer

Linda Schiffhauer

OUTLINE

OBJECTIVES

By the end of this introduction the reader will be able to:

1) Describe the range of clinical practice in pathology
2) Recite how a specimen is processed Surgical Pathology and outline the different sections of a Surgical Pathology Report
3) List some common ancillary studies used for pathologic diagnosis and prognostication
4) Use the vocabulary of pathology and tumor biology to:
   a. communicate the principles of neoplasia and
   b. describe the morphologic characteristics of benign and malignant tumors
5) Describe basic mechanisms of inflammation

GOALS

The primary GOAL of this primer is to introduce the reader to basic concepts in pathology that will be used throughout the remainder of this book.

The Clinical Practice of Pathology

PATHOLOGY IS ...

The study of disease, the bridge between basic science and clinical medicine, and the medical specialty that reveals the scientific foundation of medical practice. There are four aspects for all disease processes: etiology (cause), pathogenesis (mechanism or sequence of events leading to disease), morphologic features (gross and microscopic), and clinical manifestations (the end result of the disease process, signs, symptoms, clinical course, and outcome).

TABLE 1 ■ **Areas of Clinical Practice in Pathology**

Clinical Pathology	Anatomic Pathology	Integrated
Blood bank/transfusion medicine	Autopsy Pathology (Medical/ Hospital and Forensic)	Aspiration techniques
Chemical Pathology	Surgical Pathology (subspecialties include: Bone, Breast, Cardiovascular, Dermatopathology, Endocrine, Gastrointestinal, Genitourinary, Gynecologic, Head and Neck, Hepatobiliary, Neuropathology, Ocular, Pediatric, Renal, Soft tissue, Thoracic)	Clinical Informatics
Coagulation	Cytopathology	Cytogenetics
		Hematopathology
Hematology	Histochemistry	Immunopathology
Urinalysis	Ultrastructural Pathology (Electron Microscopy)	Laboratory Management
Microbiology		Molecular Pathology
Toxicology		

THE PATHOLOGIST IS ...

A doctor who specializes in the diagnosis and management of diseases using laboratory methods. Pathologists practice as clinicians who render diagnoses, teachers who impart knowledge to others, and scientists who use the tools of laboratory science to advance the understanding of disease. Most pathologists practice in community hospitals where they play an important role and clinical decision making and continued medical education of physicians throughout the hospital. Pathologists can also be found practicing in medical schools and academic centers, military government agencies, research institutes, and pharmaceutical and biotechnical companies.

THE PRACTICE OF PATHOLOGY IS WIDE-RANGING

Pathologists can tailor their practice with varying degrees of clinical work, teaching, and research. Some pathologists are employed primarily in research and allocate their efforts to advancing the understanding of disease. Others devote the majority of their time to clinical practice. In clinical practice, anatomic pathologists can work in surgical pathology, cytopathology, and/or autopsy pathology to analyze gross and microscopic changes with their associated biochemical and genetic abnormalities caused by disease in tissues and cells removed by surgery, aspiration techniques, or at autopsy. In clinical practice, clinical pathologists test and handle body fluids in the areas of blood banking/transfusion medicine, chemistry, coagulation, hematology, immunology, and microbiology (Table 1). In both anatomic and clinical pathology, the pathologist plays a key role in consulting with other physicians and ensuring that the laboratory provides quality patient care. Indeed, the pathologist has long been considered the "doctor's doctor"; he or she is very often at the center of the clinical care team providing diagnoses and advising on the treatment and management of patients.

Surgical Pathology: Inside the Box

Surgical pathologists are responsible for rendering diagnoses on biopsies and surgically removed tissues. They play a central role in directing the management of patients as members of multidisciplinary teams in subspecialty practice. To many members of the healthcare team, however, surgical pathology is viewed as a "black box" —tissue goes in and, seemingly magically, diagnoses come out. However, understanding what happens within the lab is important to providing quality patient care.

HANDLING OF SURGICAL SPECIMENS

Once removed from a patient, a biopsy or surgical specimen is delivered to surgical pathology either "fresh" or "fixed" and given a unique **accession** number within the laboratory's information system (LIS). The LIS is a computer system dedicated to pathology that is separate and then integrated into electronic medical record systems. Since the specimen must be accompanied by a requisition for laboratory testing, and the majority of errors that lead to a delay in specimen processing are due to errors in the requisition, it is important for submitting physicians to review the requisition for legibility, accurate demographics, and pertinent clinical information before sending the specimen to surgical pathology. In order to ensure quality histopathology and accurate ancillary test results, the time between the removal of the tissue from the patient to the time it is placed in formalin (cold ischemic time) should be no more than 1 hour.

After accessioning, the specimen enters the surgical pathology **gross room** where pathologists, pathologist assistants, pathology residents, and/or biopsy technicians perform the gross examination. Specimens received "fresh" are best examined immediately to determine whether special procedures (such as culture, cytogenetics, electron microscopy, flow cytometry, molecular studies, photographs, radiographs, touch preparations, or tumor banking) other than routine gross and microscopic examination are necessary. If nothing special is indicated, the specimen is placed into a fixative (usually 10% buffered formalin) to prevent deterioration (autolysis) of the tissue.

For all specimens, a **gross examination** is performed and should be guided by the patient's clinical information. The process has been likened to the "physical examination" that is routinely performed on patients. Critical aspects include proper identification and orientation of the specimen, general inspection to identify normal and abnormal features, measuring dimensions and weights, and describing any abnormalities in detail to include the relationship of pathologic findings to normal tissue and specimen margins. Complete gross examination further includes dissection to reveal underlying abnormalities, documentation of important gross findings by photographs, and recording of all findings within the surgical pathology report. Once the gross examination is complete, specimens that require microscopic review are either submitted entirely, or "**trimmed**" to an optimal size for **histopathologic examination**.

In the **histology lab**, technical staff **process** the tissues submitted for microscopic review with the aid of automated specialized laboratory instruments. The most common "routine" histologic processing steps include: **fixation** (with formalin to prevent autolysis), **infiltration** (sequential dehydration to replace water in the tissue with paraffin), **embedding** (creating paraffin blocks by positioning tissues in a mold filled with hot paraffin followed by cooling), **sectioning** (cutting 4–5-micron-thick sections from the paraffin blocks on a microtome and placing the opaque tissue on microscopic slides), **staining** (coloring tissue on the slides with hematoxylin and eosin), and **mounting** (placing mounting media and a glass slide over the tissue).

Once the microscopic slides are created, **microscopic examination** is performed by the pathologist. The pathologist interprets the gross and microscopic findings, diagnoses are rendered, and the findings are communicated with the clinical team via the Surgical Pathology Report.

This routine H&E process is carried out on nearly all specimens that are submitted to the lab. Additional **ancillary studies** are available for specific purposes and include "special" stains, immunohistochemistry, and molecular techniques.

- **Special histologic stains** are histochemical techniques used when the routine H&E stain is insufficient for the visualization of specific elements within a specimen. Many hundreds of stains exist, but relatively few are used regularly in diagnostic practice (Table 2).

Text continues on p. 7

TABLE 2 ■ **Special Histologic Stains**

Special Stain	**To Visualize**	**Example**
PAS	Glycogen, neutral mucosubstances, basement membrane, fungi, parasites	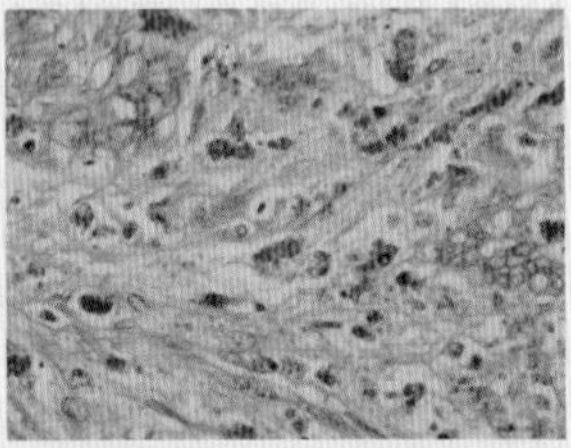
Brown and Brenn	Gram positive and negative bacteria	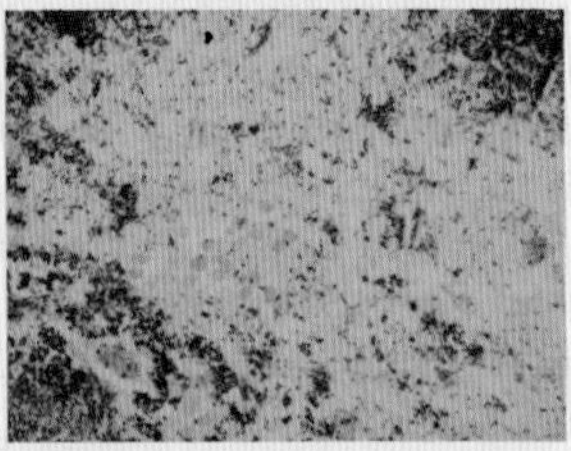
Ziehl-Neelsen	Acid fast bacteria	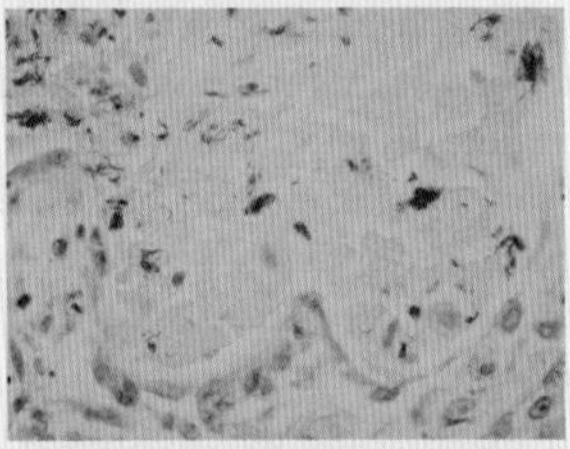
Grocott's silver	Fungi, pneumocystis	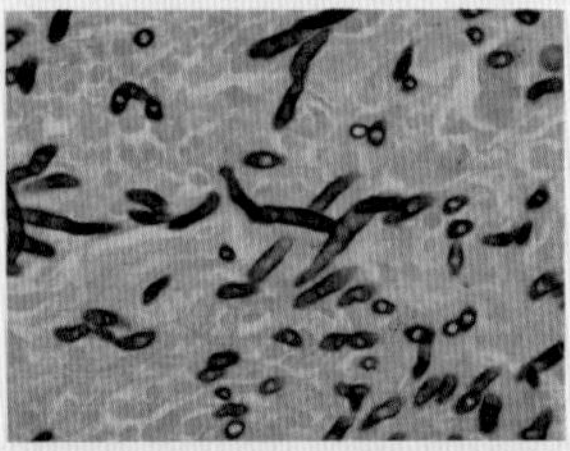
Dieterle/Warthin-Starry	Syphilis, Lyme disease	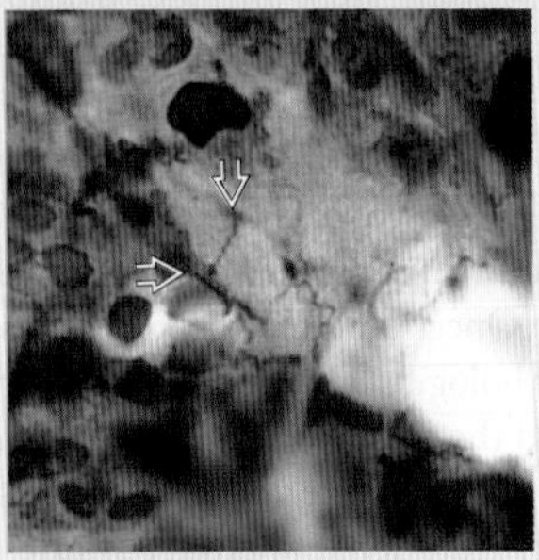

From *Diagnostic Pathology*. Copyright Elsevier.

TABLE 2 ■ **Special Histologic Stains—cont'd**

Special Stain	To Visualize	Example
Congo Red	Amyloid	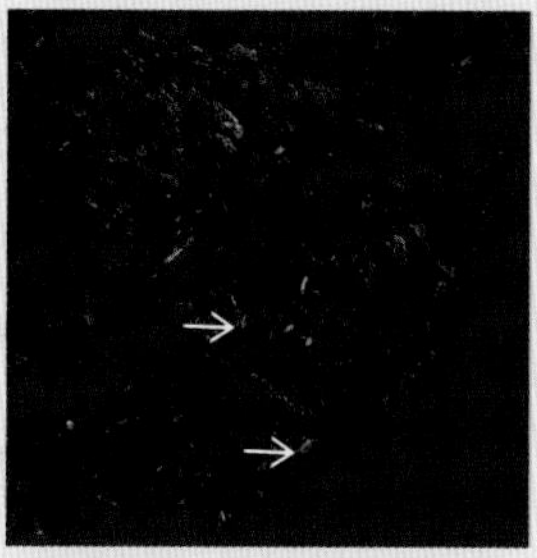 From *Diagnostic Pathology*. Copyright Elsevier.
Reticulin	Reticulin fibers and basement membrane	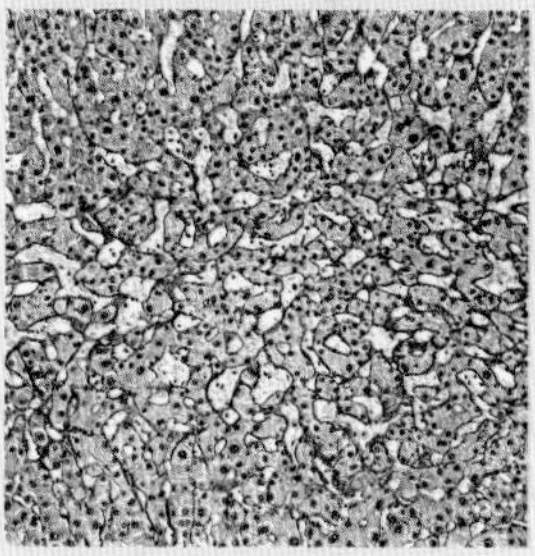 From *Diagnostic Pathology*. Copyright Elsevier.
Trichrome	Extracellular collagen	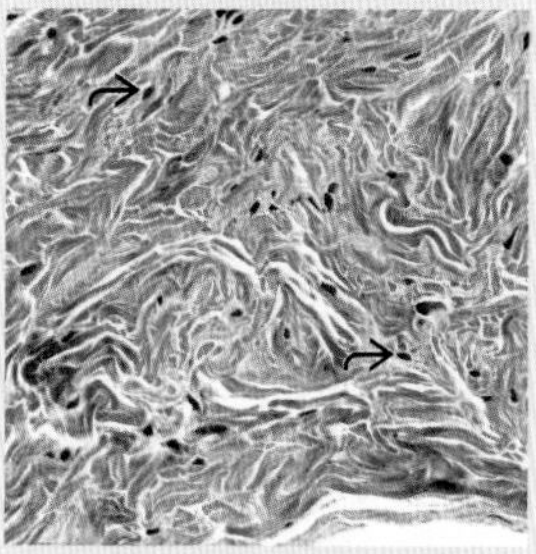 From *Diagnostic Pathology*. Copyright Elsevier.
Perls	Hemosiderin	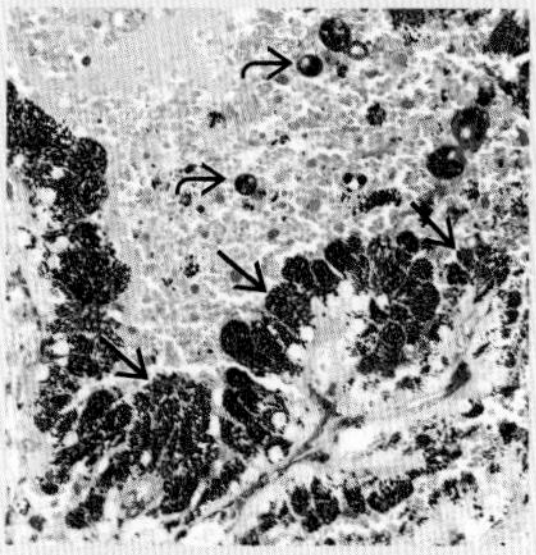 From *Diagnostic Pathology*. Copyright Elsevier.

Continued

TABLE 2 ■ **Special Histologic Stains—cont'd**

Special Stain	To Visualize	Example
Fontana-Masson	Melanin	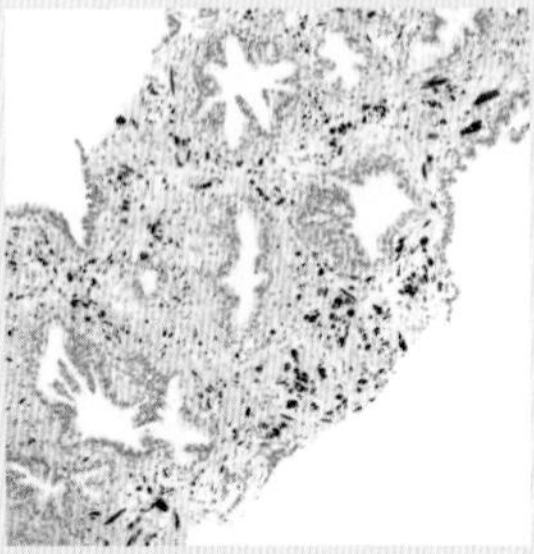 From *Diagnostic Pathology*. Copyright Elsevier.
Von kossa	Calcium	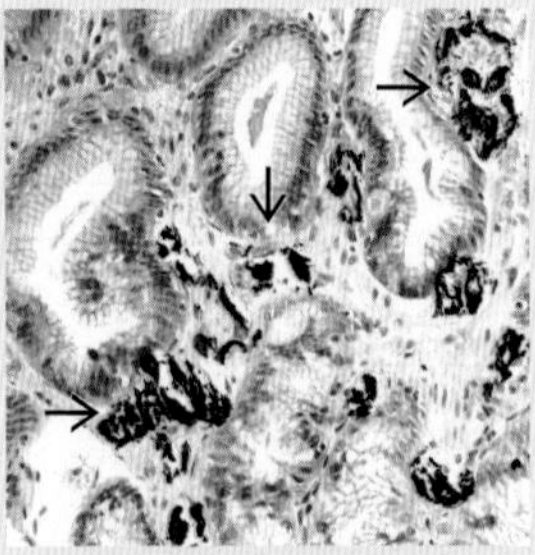 From *Diagnostic Pathology*. Copyright Elsevier.
Prussian blue	Iron	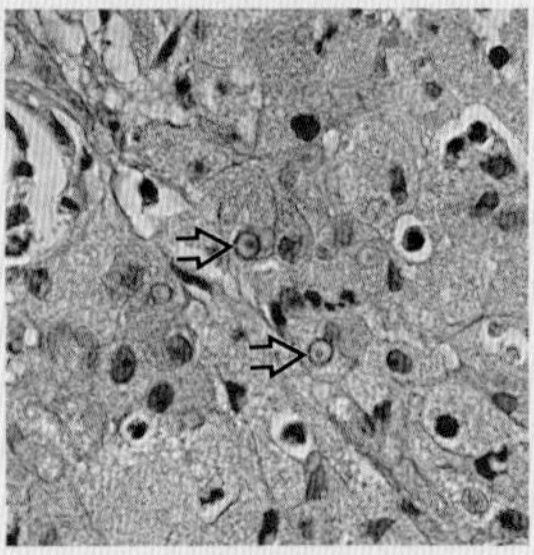 From *Diagnostic Pathology*. Copyright Elsevier.
Oil Red O	Neutral lipids	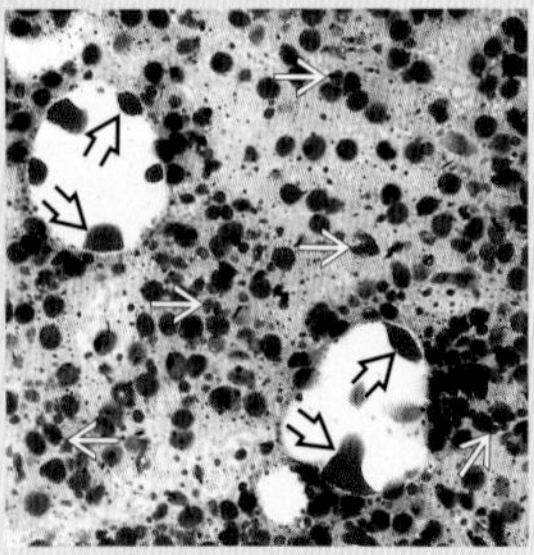 From *Diagnostic Pathology*. Copyright Elsevier.

TABLE 2 ■ **Special Histologic Stains—cont'd**

Special Stain	To Visualize	Example
Mucicarmine	Mucin	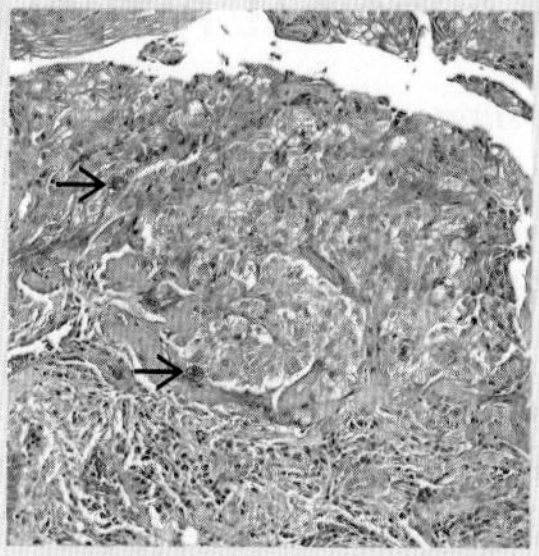 From *Diagnostic Pathology*. Copyright Elsevier.
Alcian blue	Mucin	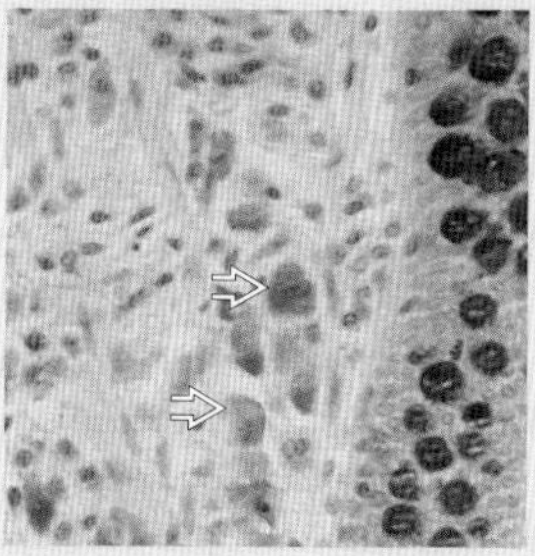 From *Diagnostic Pathology*. Copyright Elsevier.
Verhoeff-van Geison	Elastic	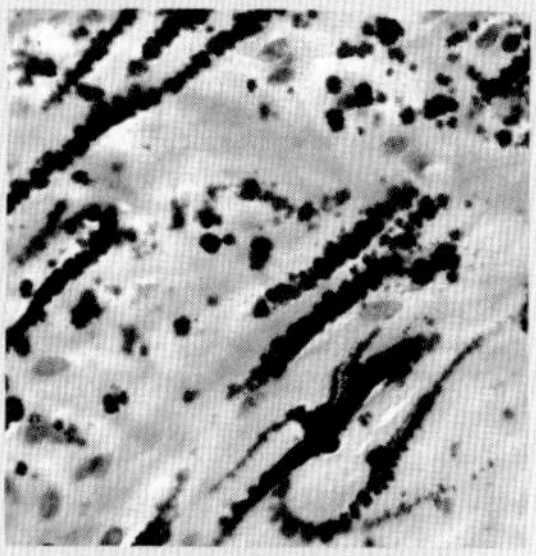 From *Diagnostic Pathology*. Copyright Elsevier.

- **Immunohistochemistry (IHC)** is a laboratory method that applies the principles and techniques of immunology to the study of cells and tissues. The method uses a monoclonal or polyclonal antibody labeled with an enzyme or a dye to check for the presence of an antigen in a sample of tissue. The technique has been revolutionary and is a powerful tool that is used to determine the presence and tissue distribution of antigens in health and disease. IHC has many applications in surgical pathology, such as aiding in the diagnosis of cancers, predicting the prognosis of tumors by identifying prognostic markers, and determining the site of origin for an unknown primary.
- **Molecular techniques** have a major impact, since they can be performed utilizing formalin-fixed paraffin embedded tissue routinely handled in clinical practice. These include in situ

hybridization, cytogenetics, polymerase chain reaction, array-based comparative genomic hybridization, and microdissection.

THE SURGICAL PATHOLOGY REPORT

"The surgical pathology report is an important medical document that should describe, as thoroughly and concisely as possible, not only all the relevant gross and microscopic features of a case but should also interpret their significance for the clinician. It should be prompt, accurate, and brief. The pathologist should avoid unnecessary histologic jargon that is of no significance to the case and concentrate on the aspects that bear a relation to therapy and prognosis." - Juan Rosai, in *Rosai and Ackerman's Surgical Pathology*, 9th ed, 2004; St Louis, MO: Mosby, p 5

The main purpose of the surgical pathology report is to communicate the histopathologic findings to the submitting physician while at the same time expect that the report will be read by many other members of clinical care team and even by patients. Since the report contains critical information required to direct patient care, it is imperative to understand the major components of the report and know where to find important information.

The typical surgical pathology report is composed of seven sections:

1. The **demographics section** includes information about the patient, submitting doctor, hospital, and laboratory.
2. The **clinical history section** is populated by information provided by the submitting doctor. The information should be accurate, brief, and include pertinent information about the nature of the problem that led to that particular procedure.
3. The **gross description section** is where the findings of the gross examination are recorded along with a key describing what sections were submitted for microscopic examination.
4. The **microscopic description section** is optional and is where details of histopathologic findings or laboratory techniques are described. Usually, this type of information is of lesser importance to the submitting physician and should be kept brief.
5. The **final diagnosis section** contains the most important information. This is where the pathologist communicates the diagnoses for the specimens submitted. Each specimen is listed separately titled by the "site, subsite, procedure." Beneath the title, diagnoses are listed for that specimen in outline format with the most important diagnosis first. Diagnoses are reported in a standardized format in accordance with guidelines published by the College of American pathologists (CAP) and the American Joint Commission on Cancer (AJCC).
6. The **comment (or note) section**. This section is also optional, but when used, it is a very important means of clinic-pathologic correlation. The pathologist may use this section to convey prognostic or therapeutic information, provide a differential diagnosis, enumerate reasons for arriving at a particular diagnosis, clarify important aspects of the case, or include pertinent references.
7. The **intraoperative consultation section** is included when a rapid diagnostic consultation is requested by the submitting physician while the patient is still on the operating room table. A key feature of this consultation is that the submitting physician is waiting for the diagnosis to direct his/her intraoperative management of the patient. Indications for intraoperative consultation can be placed into two general categories:
   a) **frozen section**—a microscopic review of the specimen or part of the specimen to establish a diagnosis, evaluate margins, determine extent of disease, determine adequacy for diagnosis and/or ancillary studies, or triage for ancillary studies. A frozen section is performed in a cryostat—an enclosed microtome kept at -20C.
   b) **intraoperative consultation**—a gross (non-microscopic) review of the specimen to establish a gross diagnosis, evaluate margins, confirm the presence of a lesion, triage tissue for ancillary studies or research, or preserve orientation.

TURNAROUND TIME (TAT): HOW LONG DOES IT TAKE TO GET A REPORT?

The **time from submitting a specimen to receiving a Surgical Pathology Report (TAT)** on an intraoperative consultation or **frozen sections** is rapid, usually 20 minutes or less, in comparison to diagnoses on routine histologic processed "**permanent**" sections. The TAT of specimens with routine histologic sections is usually 1 day or more depending on the specimen and diagnosis. In general, routine small biopsies are "signed out" within 24–48 hours while large complex resection specimens usually take 48–72 hours but may take up to a week. "**Sign out**" refers to the process in which the pathologist reviews, analyzes, and interprets the gross, microscopic, and ancillary studies, then renders a diagnosis, and finalizes the surgical pathology report with their electronic signature. When **ancillary studies** are performed, the TAT can be delayed from a day (for immunohistochemistry) to possibly weeks (for multigene expression panels). Occasionally, a preliminary diagnosis will be reported while the pathologist awaits the ancillary test results.

Neoplasia: Understanding Benign and Malignant

Neoplasia means "new growth." A new growth, or tumor, is called a **neoplasm**. Neoplasms can be benign, malignant, or intermediate. **Benign** tumors, designated by the suffix -oma, are relatively indolent, do not spread to other sites, and are amenable to surgical removal. Usually patients with benign diseases survive. **Malignant** tumors, more commonly known as **cancer**, can invade local structures and have the ability to spread to distant sites (**metastasize**). Malignant tumors can cause death, but if discovered early enough, they may be successfully be treated with surgery, chemotherapy, or radiation.

Carcinogenesis, the initiation of cancer formation, is a multistep process that involves accumulating genetic damage (tumor progression) that leads to excessive growth, invasion of local structures, and potentially distant spread. Genetic damage, or **mutations**, that leads to cancer can be initiated by environmental agents such as chemicals, radiation, physical injury, or viruses, or may be inherited through the germ line. Common genes that are mutated in cancer include (Table 3) the growth-promoting proto-oncogenes, growth-inhibiting tumor suppressor genes, regulators of programmed cell death (apoptosis), and genes involved in DNA repair. Although a tumor is initially formed by the clonal expansion of a single precursor cell, at the molecular level when a tumor progresses, it becomes more heterogeneous as mutations accumulate independently in different cells. This creates sub-clones within the tumor with varying abilities to grow and respond to therapy.

To determine the diagnosis and whether a tumor is benign or malignant, patients can undergo a variety of medical procedures and laboratory analysis to sample and/or therapeutically remove a tumor. These include biopsy (incisional or excisional), fine-needle aspiration (FNA), cytologic smear, and resection (excision). Once the tumor is biopsied or removed, the pathologist examines the specimen to determine the diagnosis.

Pathologic features of benign and malignant tumors. In most cases the pathologist has no trouble determining whether a tumor is benign or malignant based on morphologic gross and microscopic features. In general, benign and malignant tumors can be separated on the basis of their differentiation, rate of growth, local invasion, anaplasia, and metastasis. **Benign tumors** are usually well differentiated. This means that the neoplastic cells greatly resemble normal parenchymal cells. Benign tumors also have a slower rate of growth than malignant tumors and grow as cohesive units that remain localized to their site of origin. They do not invade or metastasize to distant sites. **Malignant tumors** can show a wide range of differentiation. Well differentiated malignant tumors closely resemble their normal counterparts and may be difficult to recognize.

TABLE 3 ■ **Common Genes That Are Mutated in Cancer**

Common Genes Mutated in Cancer	Mode of Action/Function and Associated Tumor
Growth Promoting Proto-Oncogenes	
INT2	Growth factor, overexpressed in bladder, breast, and skin cancer
RET	Growth factor receptor, point mutation in leukemia and MEN2A and B
KRAS	Signal transduction, point mutation in colon, lung, and pancreas cancer
C-MYC	Nuclear regulatory protein, translocation in Burkitt lymphoma
Cyclin D	Cell cycle regulator, amplified in breast and esophageal cancer
Growth Inhibiting Tumor Suppressor Genes	
e-cadherin	Cell surface adhesion, somatic mutation in stomach cancer
NF1	Inhibition of RAS signal transduction, inherited mutation in sarcomas
PTEN	PI3 kinase signal transduction, inherited mutation in Cowden syndrome
Genes Regulating Apoptosis	
P53	Cell cycle arrest in response to DNA damage, inherited mutation in Li-Fraumeni syndrome, many carcinomas and sarcomas
DNA Repair Genes	
BRCA1 and BRCA2	DNA repair, inherited in breast and ovarian cancer

Poorly differentiated tumors are easily recognized, since the tumor cells have a lack of differentiation (anaplasia). Anaplastic tumors contain cells with marked variation in size and shape (pleomorphism), dark staining hyperchromatic nuclei, irregularly shaped nuclei, abundant atypical or bizarre mitoses, and have disorganized architecture (i.e., tumor cells form sheets or masses). Some tumors fall into a gray zone in between benign and malignant and may need ancillary testing, expert consensus, or be classified as being of **intermediate or uncertain** malignant potential.

BASIC MECHANISMS OF INFLAMMATION

Inflammation is a nonspecific defensive host response that brings important cells and molecules from the circulation to sites where and when they are needed. The cardinal signs of inflammation are Rubor (redness), Tumor (swelling), Dolor (pain), and Functio laesa (loss of function).

Acute inflammation refers to the host's initial response to infection and tissue damage. It is rapid, develops within minutes to hours, lasts only for a few hours or days, leads to typical vascular and cellular events, and is composed primarily of neutrophils.

Inflammation usually progresses through a series of sequential vascular and cellular steps:

1) The infectious agent/tissue damage is recognized by host.
2) Cells and plasma proteins are recruited to the site of infection/injury.
3) The inflammatory response is activated by mediators of inflammation.

4) Once the offending agent is eliminated, the response is terminated.
5) Tissue damage is repaired.

The typical sequence of vascular reactions in acute inflammation includes reflex arteriolar vasoconstriction followed by vasodilation (mediated by histamine and vasodilators), increased permeability of venules, edema, and reduced blood flow. The typical sequence of cellular leukocyte reactions at the site of injury include margination, activation, adhesion, transmigration, chemotaxis, phagocytosis, and destruction of phagocytosed material. The principle chemical mediators of inflammation are summarized in Table 4.

TABLE 4 ■ **The Actions of the Principal Mediators of Inflammation**

Mediator	Principal Sources	Actions
Cell-Derived		
Histamine	Mast cells, basophils, platelets	Vasodilation, increased vascular permeability, endothelial activation
Serotonin	Platelets	Vasodilation, increased vascular permeability
Prostaglandins	Mast cells, leukocytes	Vasodilation, pain, fever
Leukotrienes	Mast cells, leukocytes	Increased vascular permeability, chemotaxis, leukocyte adhesion and activation
Platelet-activating factor	Leukocytes, mast cells	Vasodilation, increased vascular permeability, leukocyte adhesion, chemotaxis, degranulation, oxidative burst
Reactive oxygen species	Leukocytes	Killing of microbes, tissue damage
Nitric oxide	Endothelium, macrophages	Vascular smooth muscle relaxation, killing of microbes
Cytokines (TNF, IL-1)	Macrophages, endothelial cells, mast cells	Local endothelial activation (expression of adhesion molecules), fever/pain/anorexia/hypotension, decreased vascular resistance (shock)
Chemokines	Leukocytes, activated macrophages	Chemotaxis, leukocyte activation
Plasma Protein–Derived		
Complement products (C5a, C3a, C4a)	Plasma (produced in liver)	Leukocyte chemotaxis and activation, vasodilation (mast cell stimulation)
Kinins	Plasma (produced in liver)	Increased vascular permeability, smooth muscle concentration, vasodilation, pain
Proteases activated during coagulation	Plasma (produced in liver)	Endothelial activation, leukocyte recruitment

IL-1, interleukin-1; MAC, membrane attack complex; TNF, tumor necrosis factor.
(From Kumar V, Abbas A, Fausto N, Aster J. Chapter 2, "Acute and Chronic Inflammation" and "Neoplasia". In: *Robbins and Cotran Pathologic Basis of Disease*, p. 57, Table 2-4)

Morphologically, acute inflammation is manifested by dilation of blood vessels with accumulation of leukocytes and fluid in the extravascular space. Acute inflammation can be serous (thick and watery), fibrinous (deposits of fibrin), or purulent (pus-neutrophils with necrosis and edema).

If the acute response fails to clear the infection or repair tissue damage, the response can progress to **chronic inflammation**. Chronic inflammation has a slow onset, is composed primarily of monocytes, macrophages, and lymphocytes, and often results in further injury to tissues and progressive fibrosis. Chronic inflammation is the insidious, smoldering host response that is the cause of tissue damage in the most common and disabling human diseases such as rheumatoid arthritis, tuberculous, and pulmonary fibrosis and cancer progression. The causes of chronic inflammation are persistent infections, immune-mediated inflammatory diseases, and prolonged exposure to potentially toxic agents. The primary morphologic features of chronic inflammation are infiltration of tissues by mononuclear cells (macrophages, lymphocytes, plasma cells, eosinophils, and mast cells), tissue destruction, and healing by fibrosis and angiogenesis. Macrophages are the dominant cell type. Once activated, they serve to eliminate injurious agents and initiate the repair process. If microbes persist, some neutrophils may be present. For certain agents, in an attempt to contain them (leprosy, cat-scratch, syphilis, TB, berylliosis), granulomas may form. Granulomas can be caseating (with central necrosis), non-caseating (without central necrosis), or foreign body type.

Systemic effects of inflammation include fever, acute phase reaction, leukocytosis, increased pulse and blood pressure, decreased sweating, rigors, chills, anorexia, somnolence, and malaise. Sepsis may result if organisms and lipopolysaccharides in blood stimulate the production of high levels of tumor necrosis factor and IL-1 leading to disseminated intravascular coagulation, cardiovascular failure, and metabolic disturbance.

References

AJCC Cancer Staging Manual. 8th ed. Chicago: Springer; 2019.

CAP guidelines, 2020. *Cancer Protocol Templates.* Available at: https://www.cap.org/protocols-and-guidelines/cancer-reporting-tools/cancer-protocol-templates.

Intersociety Council for Pathology Information. *Pathology: A Career in Medicine. (ICPI).* Rockville MD: 2018.

Rosai J, editor. Rosai and Ackerman's Surgical Pathology. In: *Special Techniques in Surgical Pathology.* 9th ed. St. Louis, MO: Mosby; 2004:37-41.

Kumar V, Abbas A, Fausto N, Aster J. Chapter 2, "Acute and Chronic Inflammation" and "Neoplasia". In: *Robbins and Cotran Pathologic Basis of Disease*, 43-77 and Chapter 7, 259-330.

Gastrointesintal System, Liver, Pancreas

CASE 1

A 60-Year-Old Male with a Solid Pancreatic Mass

Maria Cecilia D. Reyes

A 60-year-old male visits an outpatient gastroenterology clinic for abdominal pain and jaundice. The abdominal pain is most pronounced in the epigastric region. The pain is localized and non-radiating. It is exacerbated after eating a fatty meal. He has also noted a 20-pound unintentional weight loss. He has a past medical history significant for high blood pressure and high cholesterol, for which he is maintained on medications. His social history is significant for working as a truck driver, eating on the road and drinking a six-pack of beer daily as well as approximately 1 pint of stronger alcohol on the weekends. He has also smoked one pack of cigarettes a day for 20 years. On physical examination, his blood pressure is 125/80 mmHg and pulse rate is 85 beats/min. There is diffuse tenderness on palpation in the mid left upper outer quadrant on examination. The remainder of the exam is normal.

What organs can be affected with a chief complaint of epigastric pain?

CLINICAL PEARL

The organs affected with epigastric pain include the pancreas, stomach, duodenum, gallbladder, liver, and bile ducts. Examples of other differential diagnoses in this category include peptic duodenal ulcer, peptic gastric ulcer, cholecystitis, hepatitis, and pancreatitis.

Case Point 1.1

The results of his laboratory testing demonstrate an elevated lipase level of 540 U/L and amylase of 210 U/L. The remainder of his blood work, including basic metabolic panel and blood cell counts with differential, are within normal limits. He is then referred to the local hospital due to the elevated lipase and amylase levels for which he undergoes a computed tomography (CT) scan with contrast. The CT scan demonstrated a solid 3.4 × 3.2-cm pancreatic head mass that abuts but does not invade the superior mesenteric vein. He is admitted to the hospital and is scheduled to undergo an endoscopic ultrasound-guided fine needle aspiration (EUS-FNA) in the morning.

What is the normal anatomy of the pancreas?

The pancreas is approximately 12–15 cm long and is divided into the head, neck, body, and tail (Fig. 1.1). The main pancreatic duct runs from the tail to the head of the pancreas. It receives small ducts and eventually joins with the common bile duct to form the ampulla of Vater, which enters the duodenum.

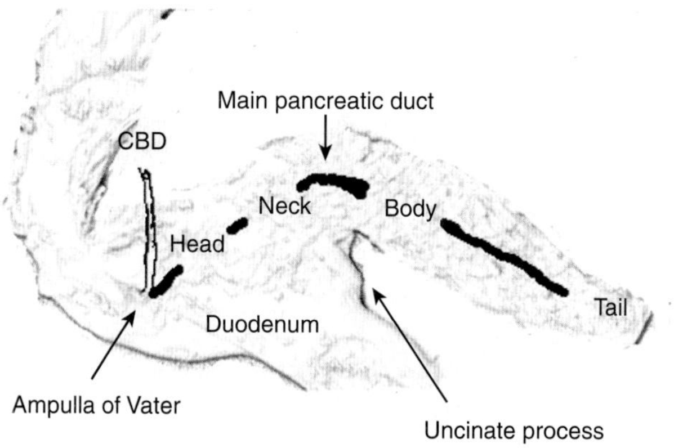

Fig. 1.1 Pancreatic anatomy showing the pancreatic head, neck, uncinate process, body, and tail. *CBD,* common bile duct.

What is the differential diagnosis of a solid pancreatic mass?

CLINICAL PEARL

The differential diagnosis for a solid pancreatic mass includes a pancreatic ductal adenocarcinoma, pancreatic neuroendocrine tumor, acinar cell carcinoma, solid pseudopapillary neoplasm, pancreatoblastoma, and metastasis.

What does normal pancreatic cytology show?

Normal pancreatic cytology will have benign pancreatic ductal and acinar cells (Figs. 1.2A–B). Ductal cells occur in flat, cohesive sheets with a uniform honeycomb appearance. Acinar cells occur in grape-like clusters with granular cytoplasm. Gastrointestinal tract mucosal contaminant may also be seen.

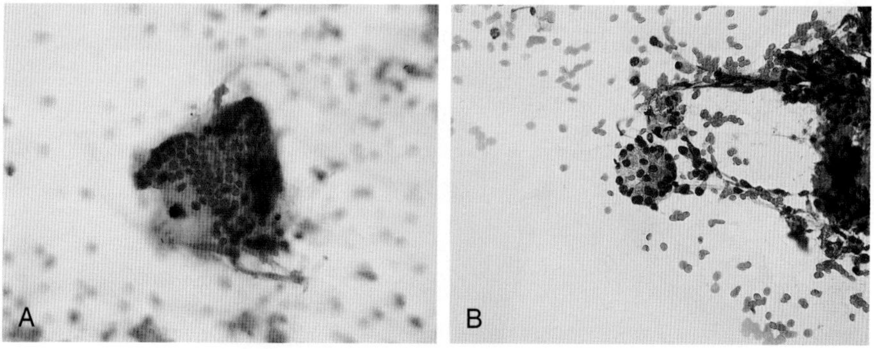

Fig. 1.2 (A) Normal pancreatic cytology showing normal pancreatic ductal cells with preserved honeycomb architecture (Pap 400x) and (B) normal acinar cells in grape-like architecture with granular cytoplasm (Pap 400x).

Case Point 1.2

The patient undergoes endoscopic US-FNA, and the cytology reveals clusters of malignant cells with the loss of honeycomb architecture, anisonucleosis, and single atypical cells (Fig. 1.3). A diagnosis of adenocarcinoma is made.

What are the risk factors for pancreatic ductal adenocarcinoma?

CLINICAL PEARL

The risk factors for pancreatic ductal adenocarcinoma include smoking, excessive alcohol consumption, obesity, diabetes, and family history of pancreatic cancer.

What are the criteria for pancreatic ductal adenocarcinoma on cytology?

CLINICAL PEARL

The criteria for the diagnosis of pancreatic ductal adenocarcinomas include the loss of honeycomb architecture, presence of atypical single cells, anisonucleosis of 4:1, nuclear contour irregularity, nuclear enlargement of 2–3x the size of a neutrophil or double the size of a red blood cell, chromatin clearing, and prominent nucleoli. A necrotic background is helpful but not necessary.

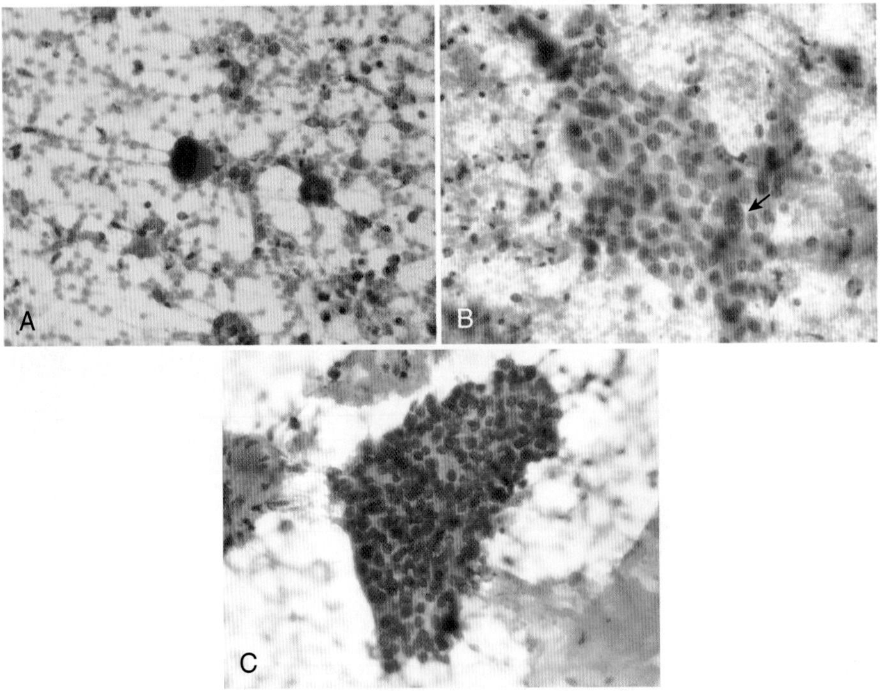

Fig. 1.3 (A) Pancreatic fine-needle aspiration showing an atypical single cell (Pap stain, 400x), (B) anisonucleosis of > 4:1 (arrow, Pap stain, 400x), and (C) loss of honeycomb architecture (Pap stain, 400x).

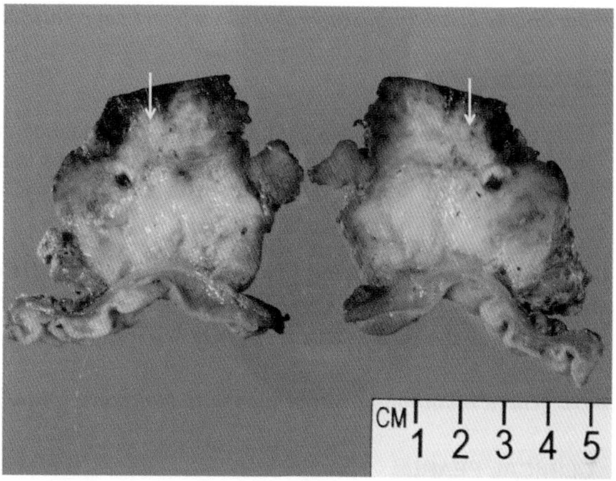

Fig. 1.4 Gross photograph of the pancreas with duodenum showing a white infiltrative tumor (arrows).

Case Point 1.3

He is referred to surgical oncology and undergoes a pancreaticoduodenectomy (Whipple procedure). The gross specimen shows a white infiltrative tumor (Fig. 1.4). Microscopic examination shows a haphazard arrangement of glands (Fig. 1.5).

What are the indications for a pancreaticoduodenectomy (Whipple procedure)?

CLINICAL PEARL

The indications for a pancreaticoduodenectomy (Whipple procedure) include malignancies of the pancreatic head, ampulla of Vater, duodenum, and distal end of the common bile duct, without evidence of arterial involvement or metastasis, as well as refractory pain from chronic pancreatitis.

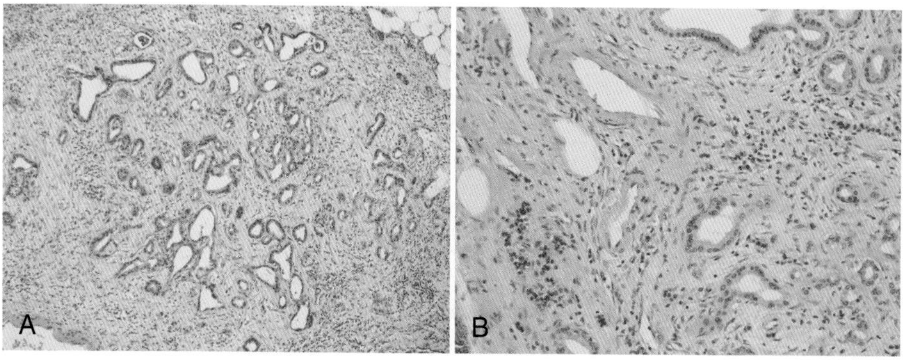

Fig. 1.5 (A) Section of the pancreas showing a haphazard arrangement of glands (H&E 200x) and (B) glands next to muscular vessels (H&E 200x).

What are the histologic features that can support pancreatic adenocarcinoma?

CLINICAL PEARL

Histologic features supporting a pancreatic ductal adenocarcinoma include a haphazard growth arrangement of glands, anisonucleosis of 4:1, glands next to muscular vessels, perineural invasion, vascular invasion, necrotic glandular debris, and incomplete lumina.

What is the American Joint Committee on Cancer (AJCC) pathologic staging of pancreatic carcinomas?

As per AJCC, the current staging of pancreatic carcinomas is shown in (Table 1.1).

What genetic mutations are associated with pancreatic ductal adenocarcinoma?

CLINICAL PEARL

Pancreatic ductal adenocarcinomas show mutations in KRAS, CDKN2A, TP53, and SMAD4.

What is the 5-year survival rate of pancreatic cancers?

The 5-year survival rate is 8.5%.

What are the other differential diagnoses for solid pancreatic neoplasms?

The differential diagnosis for solid pancreatic neoplasms includes pancreatic ductal adenocarcinoma, neuroendocrine neoplasm, solid pseudopapillary neoplasm, acinar cell carcinoma (ACC), pancreatoblastoma, and metastatic neoplasms. Pancreatic ductal adenocarcinoma comprise 85% of these pancreatic tumors. The other solid tumors are discussed below.

TABLE 1.1 ■ **Pathologic Staging of Pancreatic Carcinomas**

Primary Tumor (pT)	
pTx	Tumor cannot be assessed
p0	No evidence of primary tumor
pTis	Carcinoma in situ
pT1	Tumor limited to pancreas, ≤2 cm
pT1a	Tumor ≤0.5 cm
pT1b	Tumor >0.5 cm and <1 cm
pT1c	Tumor 1-2 cm
pT2	Tumor limited to panceas, >2 cm but ≤4 cm
pT3	Tumor limited to pancreas, >4 cm
pT4	Tumor involves the celiac axis, superior mesenteric, and/or common hepatic artery
Regional Lymph Nodes (pN)	
pNX	Regional lymph nodes cannot be assessed
pN0	No regional lymph node metastasis
pN1	Metastasis in 1-3 regional lymph nodes
pN2	Metastasis in 4 or more regional lymph nodes
Distant Metastasis (pM), if present pathologically	
pM1	Distant metastasis

Data from Burgart, with original data from Amin, M., Edge, SB, Greene FL, et al, eds., AJCC Cancer Staging Manual, 8th Edition. 2017, New York, NY: Springer.

TABLE 1.2 ■ **Grading of Pancreatic Neuroendocrine Tumors**

Neoplasm				Proliferation	
Type	**Differentiation**	**Definition**	**Grade**	**Ki-67 (% of ≥ 500 cells)**	**Mitotic count (per 2 mm²)**
Pancreatic neuroendocrine neoplasm	Well differentiated	Pancreatic neuroendocrine tumor	G1 G2 G3	<3 3–20 >20	<2 2–20 >20
	Poorly differentiated	Pancreatic neuroendocrine carcinoma Small cell type Large cell type	G3 by default	>20	>20

Data from Inzani, with original data from Klöppel G, Couvelard A, Hruban RH, et al. Neoplasms of the neuroendocrine pancreas. Introduction. In: Klöppel G, Osamura RY, Lloyd RV, et al, editors. WHO classification of tumours of the endocrine organs. Lyon (France): IARC; 2017. p. 211–4.

Pancreatic neuroendocrine neoplasms account for 4% of pancreatic tumors. It usually occurs in the pancreatic body/tail with a slight male predilection and mean age of 58. Pancreatic neuroendocrine neoplasms are now divided into well-differentiated pancreatic neuroendocrine tumors, graded from G1 to G3, and poorly differentiated pancreatic neuroendocrine carcinomas, which are automatically graded G3 (Table 1.2). Well-differentiated pancreatic neuroendocrine tumors are singly dispersed, plasmacytoid, with uniform round to oval nuclei and salt-and-pepper chromatin. Histologically, they have trabeculae, gyri, and rosettes of round uniform cells with salt-and-pepper chromatin (Figs. 1.6A–C). Poorly differentiated neuroendocrine carcinomas can have abundant cytoplasm and pleomorphic nuclei, like large cell neuroendocrine carcinoma, or minimal cytoplasm and nuclear molding, like small cell carcinoma. There is usually an infiltrative growth pattern, numerous mitotic figures, and necrosis. The diagnosis is made by pan-cytokeratin and neuroendocrine markers (synaptophysin, chromogranin, and CD56). Well-differentiated neuroendocrine tumors have mutations in MEN1, DAXX, and ATRX, whereas neuroendocrine carcinomas have mutations in Rb and TP53.

Solid pseudopapillary neoplasm represents 1-2% of pancreatic exocrine neoplasms and is a low-grade malignant neoplasm that occurs in the tail of the pancreas of young women. It is usually asymptomatic and found incidentally. Solid pseudopapillary neoplasms are large, encapsulated, and can have areas of hemorrhage, necrosis or cystic change. Histologically, they contain solid areas composed of sheets and cords of bland cells alternating with a pseudopapillary pattern and pseudorosettes (Figs. 1.7A–B). On cytology, they have fibrovascular cores and coffee bean nuclei with longitudinal grooves (Figs. 1.7C–D). They can stain for neuroendocrine markers Synaptophysin and CD56, and show nuclear staining for beta-catenin. They are positive for CD10, PR, and Vimentin and are associated with a mutation in the beta-catenin (CTNNB1) gene.

Acinar cell carcinoma (ACC) represents <2% of neoplasms of the exocrine pancreas and is an aggressive tumor that presents in the fifth to seventh decades of life, usually in males, with most common location in the pancreatic head. It is a solid neoplasm that is well circumscribed. It shows nodules of tumor cells with little or no stroma and can sometimes have a trabecular pattern. They are monotonous in appearance. Cytologic preparations will show sheets, clusters, and singly dispersed cells with granular cytoplasm (see Fig. 1.8). The nuclei in these cells have prominent nucleoli. ACCs show periodic acid–Schiff with diastase (PASD) staining and stain positive for trypsin, lipase, chymotrypsin, and bcl-10 immunohistochemical stains. ACCs can have an allelic loss of chromosome 11p or mutations in APC/beta-catenin.

Pancreatoblastomas occur in the pediatric population, most commonly in the first decade. The usual differentiation is acinar, but they can also have neuroendocrine and ductal differentiation. The architecture for acinar differentiation is lobular with intervening hypercellular stroma, and

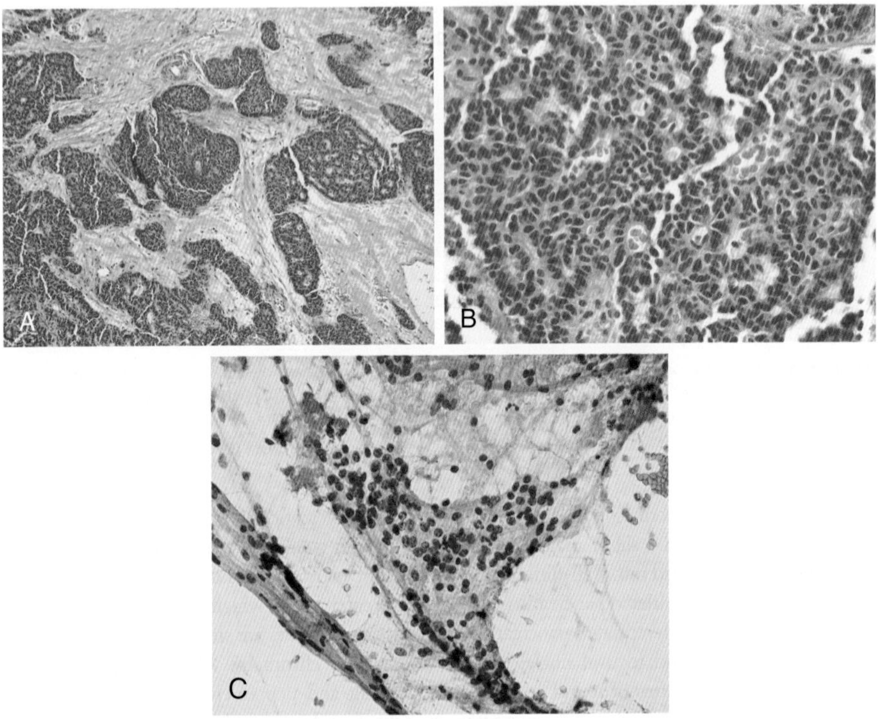

Fig. 1.6 (A and B) Pancreatic neuroendocrine tumor with rosettes of round uniform cells (H&E 100x, H&E 400x). (C) Cytology shows uniform singly dispersed cells (Pap 400x).

squamoid nests are a hallmark. Acinar differentiation can be confirmed by trypsin and chymotrypsin immunohistochemical stains, and it can exhibit nuclear and cytoplasmic staining staining with beta-catenin in squamoid morules. Pancreatoblastomas are associated with Beckwith–Wiedemann syndrome and can have genetic alterations in APC/beta-catenin.

The most common malignancy that metastasizes to the pancreas is renal cell carcinoma, specifically clear cell type. Other tumors that can metastasize include lung, colon, breast, liver, ovarian, melanoma, lymphoma, sarcoma, thyroid, and neuroendocrine tumor. The most common location for metastasis is the pancreatic head. Checking the patient's prior history of malignancy and recognizing uncommon cytologic morphologies are the keys to the diagnosis.

BEYOND THE PEARLS

- A combination of P53 positivity and SMAD4 loss on immunohistochemical stains may aid in the diagnosis of pancreatic adenocarcinoma.
- KRAS and CDKN2A mutations occur early in carcinogenesis for pancreatic ductal adenocarcinoma, whereas SMAD4 and TP53 occur late.
- A combination of Ki-67 and immunohistochemical stains for DAXX and ATRX will help grade a pancreatic neuroendocrine tumor.
- The differential diagnosis for tumors with vacuolated cytoplasm includes clear cell renal cell carcinoma, lipid-rich pancreatic neuroendocrine tumor, and pancreatic ductal adenocarcinoma with foamy gland pattern.
- The second most common malignancy to metastasize to the pancreas is lung.

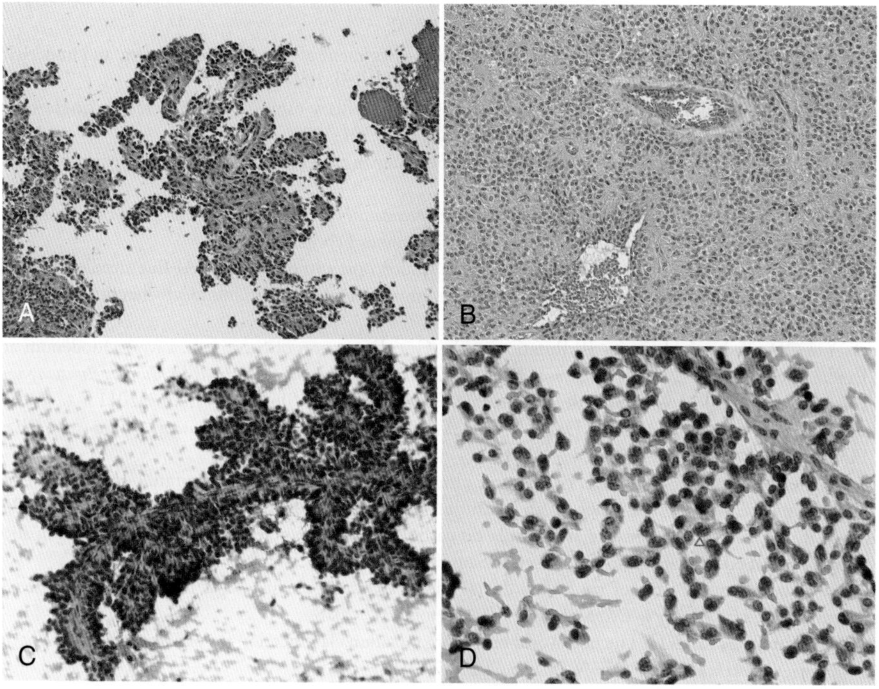

Fig. 1.7 (A) Solid pseudopapillary neoplasm showing pseudopapillary architecture and (B) an area with pseudorosettes (H&E 200x, H&E 200x). (C) Cytology shows a thin fibrovascular core and (D) coffee bean nuclei (arrowhead) (Pap 200x, Pap 400x).

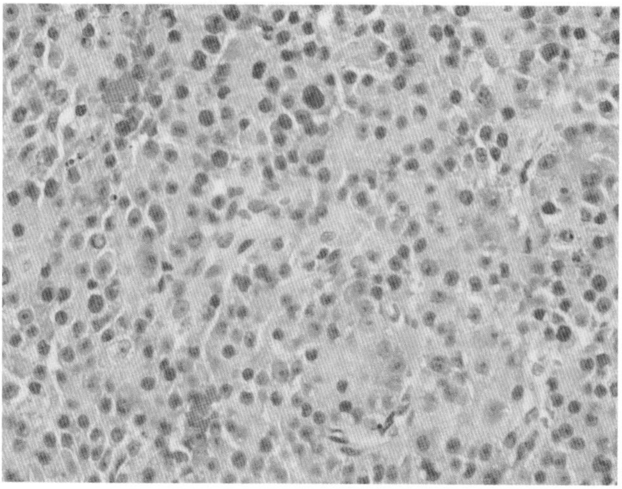

Fig. 1.8 Cytology of an acinar cell carcinoma showing solid or vague acinar architecture, granular cytoplasm, monotonous nuclei, and prominent nucleoli (H&E 400x).

References

Aier I, Semwal R, Sharma A, Varadwaj PK. A systematic assessment of statistics, risk factors, and underlying features involved in pancreatic cancer. *Cancer Epidemiol.* 2019;58:104-110.

Antoniou EA, Damaskos C, Garmpis N, et al. Solid pseudopapillary tumor of the pancreas: a single-center experience and review of the literature. *In Vivo.* 2017;31(4):501-510.

Brooks JC, Shavelle RM, Vavra-Musser KN, Life expectancy in pancreatic neuroendocrine cancer. *Clin Res Hepatol Gastroenterol.* 2019;43(1):88-97.

Burgart, L., Shi, C. et al. *Protocol for the Examination of Specimens From Patients With Carcinoma of the Pancreas.* College of American Pathologists Cancer Protocol Templates February 2020.

Chang F, Vu C, Chandra A, Meenan J, Herbert A. Endoscopic ultrasound-guided fine needle aspiration cytology of pancreatic neuroendocrine tumours: cytomorphological and immunocytochemical evaluation. *Cytopathology.* 2006;17(1):10-17.

Clemente CD. Abdominal Cavity II: Rotation of the Gut; Dissection of Stromach; Liver; Duodenum and Pancreas; Spleen. In: *Clemente's Anatomy Dissector Guides to Individual Dissections in Human Anatomy with Brief Relevant Clinical Notes.* 3rd ed. Philadelphia, PA: Lippincott William & Wilkins; 2011.

Drake, RL, Vogl AW. Abdomen. In: Drage R, Vogl AW, Mitchell A, eds. *Gray's Anatomy for Students.* 4th ed. Philadelphia, PA: Elsevier; 2020:249-412.

Hou Y, Shen R, Tonkovich D, Li Z. Endoscopic ultrasound-guided fine needle aspiration diagnosis of secondary tumors involving the pancreas: an institution's experience. *J Am Soc Cytopathol.* 2018:7(5):261-267.

Hruban R, Ali, SZ. Non-neoplastic and neoplastic pathology of the pancreas. In: *Gastrointestinal and Liver Pathology.* 2nd ed. Philadelphia, PA: Elsevier Saunders; 2012:514-556.

Hruban RH. The many faces of pancreatic ductal adenocarcinoma on histology. In: *66th Annual Scientific Meeting, American Society of Cytopathology.* Washington, DC: 2018.

Inzani F, Petrone G, Rindi G. The new world health organization classification for pancreatic neuroendocrine neoplasia. *Endocrinol Metab Clin North Am.* 2018;47(3):463-470.

Jahan, A., M.A. Yusuf, and A. Loya, *Fine-Needle Aspiration Cytology in the Diagnosis of Pancreatic Neuroendocrine Tumors: A Single-Center Experience of 25 Cases.* Acta Cytol, 2015. 59(2): p. 163-8.

Klimstra DS, Adsay V. Tumors of the pancreas. In: Odze RD, Goldblum JR, eds. *Surgical Pathology of the GI Tract, Liver, Biliary Tract, and Pancreas.* Philadelphia, PA: Elsevier Saunders; 2015:1081-1119.

Lin F, Staerkel G. Cytologic criteria for well differentiated adenocarcinoma of the pancreas in fine-needle aspiration biopsy specimens. *Cancer.* 2003;99(1):44-50.

Luo Y, Hu G, Ma Y, Guo N, Li F. Acinar cell carcinoma of the pancreas presenting as diffuse pancreatic enlargement: two case reports and literature review. *Medicine (Baltimore).* 2017;96(38):e7904.

Osbourne, NH, Colletti LM. Pancreaticoduodenectomy. In: Minter RM, Doherty GM, eds. *Current Procedures: Surgery.* The McGraw-Hill Companies; 2010.

Pitman MB. Pancreas and Biliary Tree. In: Cibas E, Ducatman BS, eds. *Cytology: Diagnostic Principles and Clinical Correlates.* 5th ed. Philadelphia, PA: Elsevier; 2021:451-478.

Reid MD, Centeno BA. Ancillary studies, including immunohistochemistry and molecular studies, in pancreatic cytology. *Surg Pathol Clin.* 2014;7(1):1-34.

Shattuck, T.M. and M.S. Waugh, *Lipid-rich variant of a pancreatic endocrine neoplasm in an endoscopic ultrasound-guided fine needle aspiration biopsy.* Diagn Cytopathol, 2013. 41(8): p. 703-4.

Smith AL, Odronic SI, Springer BS, Reynolds JP. Solid tumor metastases to the pancreas diagnosed by FNA: a single-institution experience and review of the literature. *Cancer Cytopathol.* 2015;123(6):347-355.

Swartz MH. The Abdomen. In: Swartz MH, ed. *Textbook of Physical Diagnosis.* 7th ed. Philadelphia, PA: Elsevier Saunders; 2014:429-467.

Ylagan LR, Edmundowicz S, Kasal K, Walsh D, Lu DW. Endoscopic ultrasound guided fine-needle aspiration cytology of pancreatic carcinoma: a 3-year experience and review of the literature. *Cancer.* 2002; 96(6):362-369.

A 54-Year-Old Female with Back Pain and an Incidental Pancreatic Cystic Mass Found on CT-Scan

Hasan Khatib

A 54-year-old female with history of non-insulin-dependent diabetes, obesity, obstructive sleep apnea, anxiety, and depression presented to the emergency department for back pain. The physical examination revealed abdominal sharp tenderness that radiated to the back. The vital signs are: temperature of 37.2°C (99°F), blood pressure 130/85 mm Hg, respiratory rate 20 breaths per minute. Initial laboratories studies were unremarkable, aside from a mild increase in serum amylase level. The patient underwent an abdominal magnetic resonance imaging (MRI), which revealed a cystic mass (2.1 × 1.5 cm) involving the tail of the pancreas (Fig. 2.1). Patient denies history of pancreatitis and drinks alcohol socially. Patient also mentioned 50 pounds of weight loss over the last 8 months.

What is the medical definition of the pancreatic cyst?

A pancreatic cyst is a cavity containing liquid and/or cellular debris. The pancreatic cyst may be lined with epithelium or may lack that epithelial lining (pancreatic pseudocyst). Most of pancreatic epithelial cysts are lined with serous, mucinous, or acinar epithelium.

What are the symptoms of pancreatic cysts?

The most common pancreatic cysts symptoms include abdominal pain (most common), weight loss, pancreatitis, jaundice, and back pain. Symptomatic pancreatic cysts are more likely to carry a potential malignant behavior.

What imaging techniques should be used to characterize a pancreatic cyst?

Magnetic resonance imaging (MRI) and magnetic resonance cholangiopancreatography (MRCP) are the tests of choice. These tests are noninvasive with low radiation dose and high accuracy in assessing pancreatic parenchyma and ductal system. Computed tomography (CT) and endoscopic ultrasound (EUS) are excellent alternatives in patients who are unable to undergo MRI.

What are the pathological classifications of pancreatic cysts?

Pancreatic tumors are categorized into two main subtypes—solid and cystic tumors. Pancreatic cystic neoplasms have a large differential diagnosis that can be broadly categorized as neoplastic versus non-neoplastic cysts and epithelial versus non-epithelial cysts.

CLINICAL PEARL

The diagnosis of pancreatic cyst type relies on clinical presentation, imaging studies, pathological characteristics, and for some cysts, on the cyst fluid analysis.

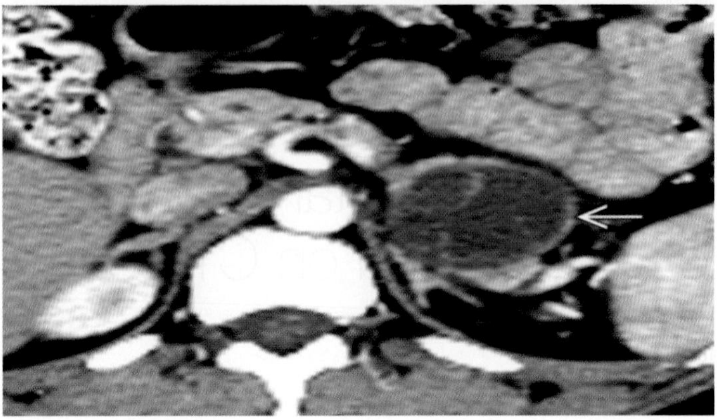

Fig. 2.1 Abdominal magnetic resonance imaging shows a well-defined cystic mass (arrow) in the pancreatic tail with enhancing wall and intracystic septa.

BOX 2.1 ■ Classifications of Pancreatic Cysts

Epithelial Neoplasms

Cysts with **mucinous** epithelium (exocrine neoplasm)

- Intraductal papillary mucinous neoplasms
- Mucinous cystic neoplasms

Mucinous non-neoplastic cysts: Mucocele and retention cysts

Cysts with **serous** epithelium (exocrine neoplasm)

- Serous cystadenoma SCA (microcystic, macrocystic, solid SCA)
- Von Hippel-Landau-associated pancreatic cysts
- Serous cystadenocarcinoma

Cysts lined by **acinar** cells (exocrine neoplasm)

- Acinar cell cystadenoma
- Acinar cell cystadenocarcinoma

Endocrine neoplasm with cystic component/degeneration

- Pancreatic neuroendocrine tumors

Epithelial neoplasms with multiple lines of differentiations

- Pancreatoblastoma (most common malignant pancreatic neoplasm of childhood)

Epithelial neoplasms of uncertain differentiations

- Solid pseudopapillary neoplasm
- Cysts with squamous epithelium: lymphoepithelial cysts; epidermoid cysts; dermoid cysts; squamoid cyst of pancreatic ducts
- Miscellaneous epithelial neoplasms: teratoma; heterotopic spleen

Non-Epithelial Neoplasms with Cystic Component/Degeneration

- Granular cell tumor; lymphangioma; cavernous hemangioma; sarcoma; leiomyoma; fibromatosis (desmoid tumor)

Non-Neoplastic Pancreatic Cysts

- **Congenital cyst:** foregut cyst; duodenal diverticulum; periampullary duodenal wall cyst (cystic dystrophy); cystic hamartoma; endometriotic cyst
- Pseudocyst (no lining), infection-related pseudocyst.

Secondary Neoplasms (Metastases to the Pancreas)

What is the clinical approach to evaluating pancreatic cysts?

When a pancreatic cyst is found on imaging, there is a clinical approach to further evaluation that considers the size of the cyst, location, and presence of a mural nodule (Fig. 2.2).

The patient underwent endoscopic ultrasound-guided fine-needle aspiration (EUS-FNA); what is the role of EUS-FNA?

In order to sample pancreatic cystic lesions, EUS-FNA of the pancreatic cyst is the procedure of choice with minimal invasion and cost-effectiveness. The rapid onsite evaluation of pancreatic

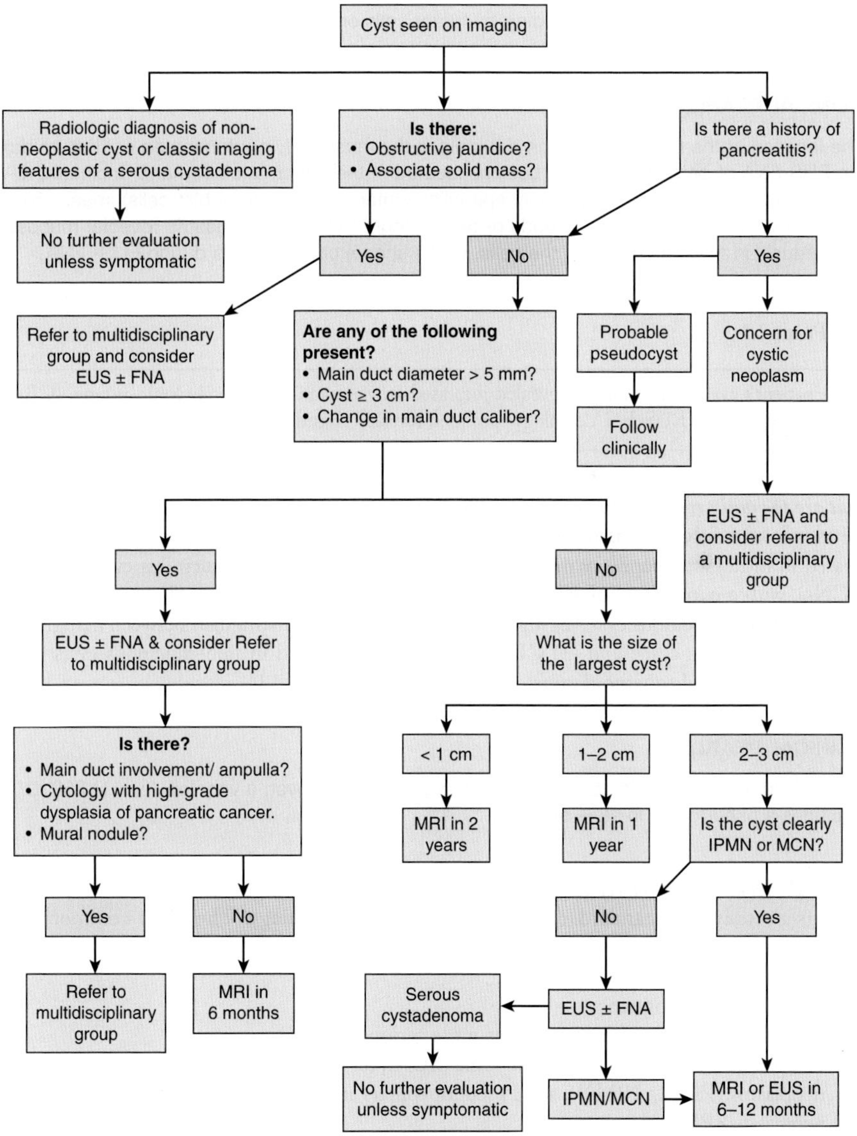

Fig. 2.2 The chart illustrates an approach to a patient with a pancreatic cyst according to American College of Gastroenterology guidelines.

EUS-FNA passes aid in obtaining adequate sample and lessening the nondiagnostic sample rates, and improve diagnostic yield. EUS-FNA has two potential roles: to obtain the cystic fluid for biochemistry and molecular studies, and to obtain cytology specimen (targeting cyst wall).

CLINICAL PEARLS

The most common complications of EUS-FNA pancreatic cyst are:

- Acute pancreatitis (up to 3%)
- Pancreatic duck leaks
- Hemorrhage
- Post-aspiration needle tract seeding by tumor cells or mucin is exceedingly (rare).

CLINICAL PEARLS

The location of the pancreatic lesion determines the most likely contaminated epithelium during EUS-FNA of pancreatic lesion. Lesions located in the pancreatic head and uncinate process are more likely to have duodenal epithelial contaminants (with goblet cells); meanwhile, lesions located in the pancreatic body or tail are more likely to have gastric foveolar mucosal cells (mucin in the upper third of the cells, U-like shape) contaminants during EUS- FNA.

Case Point 2.1

The patient's cystic fluid analysis revealed increased amylase and carcinoembryonic antigen (CEA) levels. The patient's EUS-FNA cytology specimen revealed abundant mucin with rare epithelial cells.

What are the main roles of pancreatic cystic fluid biochemical markers?

The most commonly used pancreatic cystic fluid markers are CEA and amylase. CEA levels are elevated in intraductal papillary mucinous neoplasms (IPMNs), and mucinous cystic neoplasms (MCNs), with a cutoff level of **192 ng/mL**. The limitations of CEA are: (1) low levels of CEA do not exclude a mucinous cyst; (2) high levels of CEA do not distinguish between benign versus malignant mucinous cysts; and (3) CEA levels may be elevated in non-mucinous cysts such as lymphoepithelial and squamoid cysts of pancreatic duct (Table 2.1).

CLINICAL PEARLS

Cystic fluid amylase levels can be useful to exclude pseudocyst; a very low level (<250 IU/L) excludes a pseudocyst in 98% of cases.

What is the terminology for reporting pancreatic cytology?

There is no universal standard reporting for pancreatic cytology. The most commonly used framework categories are:

- Nondiagnostic
- Negative (for malignancy)
- Atypical cell present (reactive versus more serious process)
- Neoplastic: benign [serous cystadenoma (SCA), teratoma] and others [pancreatic mucinous neoplasms (PMN), IPMNs, solid pseudopapillary neoplasms (SPNs), pancreatic endocrine neoplasms (PENs)]
- Suspicious for malignancy
- Positive/malignant

TABLE 2.1 ■ Features of the Pancreatic Cystic Lesions

Cyst Type	Clinical Association	Imaging & Fluid Analysis
Pseudocyst	Acute and/or chronic pancreatitis 50% cases resolve spontaneously	Imaging: cyst with fluid & debris fluid analysis: - High amylase/lipase (>250 IU/mL) - Low CEA (<200 ng/mL)
Serous cystadenoma	75% in women 6th decade	Imaging: well-defined microcystic / honeycomb. Fluid analysis: - Low CEA - Low amylase/lipase
Intraductal papillary mucinous neoplasm	Equal in men & women 7th–8th decade	Imaging: dilated ducts, mural nodules. Fluid analysis: - High CEA - High amylase
Mucinous cystic neoplasm	Almost exclusively in women 5th–7th decade	Imaging: body or tail, thick-walled, multilocular cyst with septations, wall calcification. **No main duct communication** Fluid analysis: - High CEA - Variable amylase
Solid pseudopapillary neoplasm	10:1 woman: men ratio Most commonly present in 20s.	Imaging: well-circumscribed neoplasm with solid & cystic components. Calcifications in 30%
Cystic pancreatic neuroendocrine neoplasm	Usually non-functioning Equal incidence in men & women 5th–6th decade May be associated with multiple endocrine neoplasia type 1 syndrome	Imaging: solid or solid/cystic, well-circumscribed, enhancing lesion Fluid analysis: - Low CEA - Low amylase/lipase

CEA, carcinoembryonic antigen.

What is the differential diagnosis of pancreatic mucinous cysts?

Cytology specimens of pancreatic cysts are usually very low cellular samples. Targeting the cyst wall by experienced gastroenterologists with standard needle gauge is the main factor in obtaining adequate cytology specimen. IPMNs and MCNs are the main pancreatic cysts with mucinous epithelium. Each of these two tumors has characteristic features (Table 2.2).

Case Point 2.2

The patient underwent Whipple procedure, and the surgery went smoothly without adverse side effects. The pancreatic gross examination revealed a well-demarcated, thick-walled, unilocular cystic pancreatic head mass with no grossly visible ductal communication (Fig. 2.3). The microscopic examination showed cyst lined by tall, columnar mucinous cells (Fig. 2.4) with underlying ovarian-type stroma. The cyst is entirely submitted for microscopic examination, and no dysplasia or stromal invasion identified. The diagnosis of MCN is rendered.

TABLE 2.2 ■ **Characteristic Features of Intraductal Papillary Mucinous Neoplasms (IPMNs) and Mucinous Cystic Neoplasms (MCNs)**

Features	MCNs	IPMNs
Age, y	50	60–70
Sex	Female (>95%)	Males ~ Females
Specific endoscopic findings	None	Mucin extrusion from ampulla
Specific radiologic findings	Multilocular thick-walled cyst	Cystic dilated ducts
Location	Tail (>90%)	Head (>80%)
Gross ductal communication	No	Yes
Specific **histologic** findings	Ovarian stroma	Dilated native duct with villous nodule

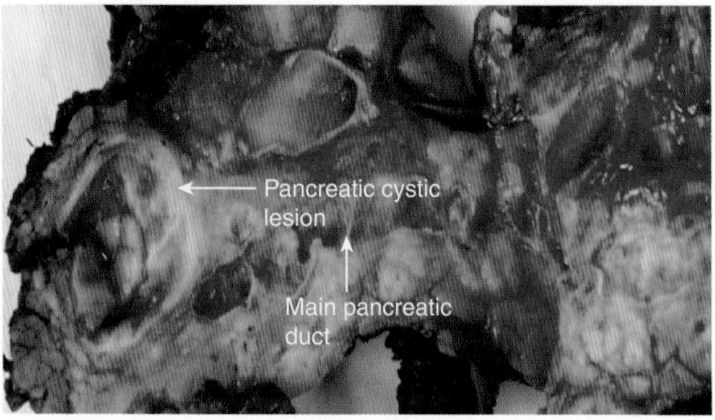

Fig. 2.3 Pancreatic head mass with well-demarcated, thick wall and with no communication to pancreatic ductal system (gross photograph).

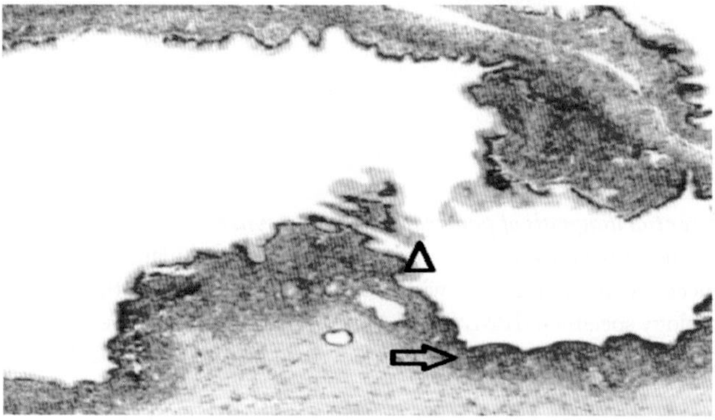

Fig. 2.4 Cyst wall lined by tall, columnar mucinous cells (arrow head) with underlying ovarian-type stroma (arrow) (H&E, 10x).

MCN is a mucin-producing lesion of the pancreas; it comprises 10% of pancreatic cystic lesions. Histologically, the lining epithelium shows crowding mucinous cells with underlying ovarian-type stroma, which is required for diagnosis of MCN. The lining epithelium may display low- or high-grade cytologic dysplasia. There is no communication with the pancreatic ductal system. MCNs occur predominately in females (male to female ratio ~20:1). MCNs with no dysplasia or invasion have a good prognosis.

What are the subtypes of IPMNs and what should a pathologist be aware of to document in the final report?

IPMNs are classified as main duct, branch duct type (most common type), or combined IPMN. Main duct IPMNs are much less common and appear to possess a higher risk of harboring high-grade dysplasia or pancreatic cancer. Microscopically, IPMNs have four epithelial subtypes (Fig. 2.5).

IPMNS have two dysplasia grading system (Fig. 2.6): (1) low-grade dysplasia—the tumor cells display mild atypia without complex architecture; and (2) high-grade dysplasia—the tumor cells display marked nuclear atypia, increased mitotic activity, and loss of polarity along with complex architectures.

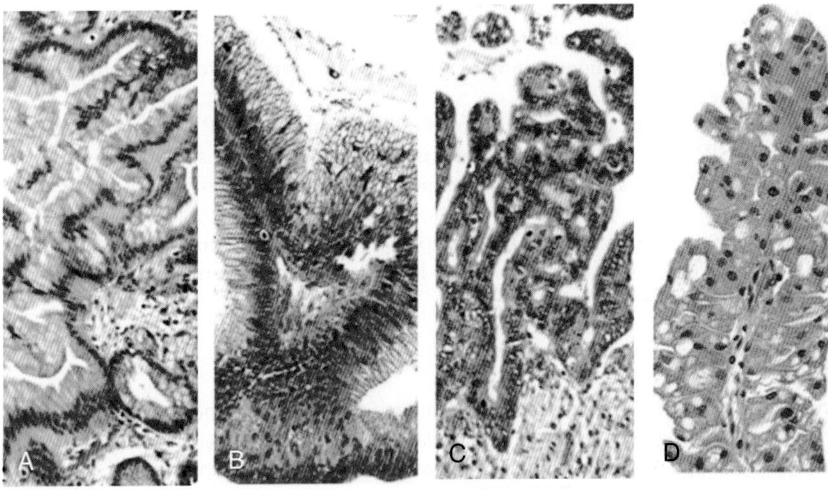

Fig. 2.5 IPMNs have four epithelial subtypes. (A) Gastric: Histologically low grade, apical cytoplasmic mucin. Diffuse MUC5 and MUC6 (basal glands). (B) Intestinal: Diffuse MUC2, common KRAS and GNAS mutations. (C) Pancreatobiliary: Thin, branching complex papillae. Focal MUC6 & MUC1 is positive. (D) Oncocytic: MUC 6 positive. MUC1/2 –/+. (H&E, 20x).

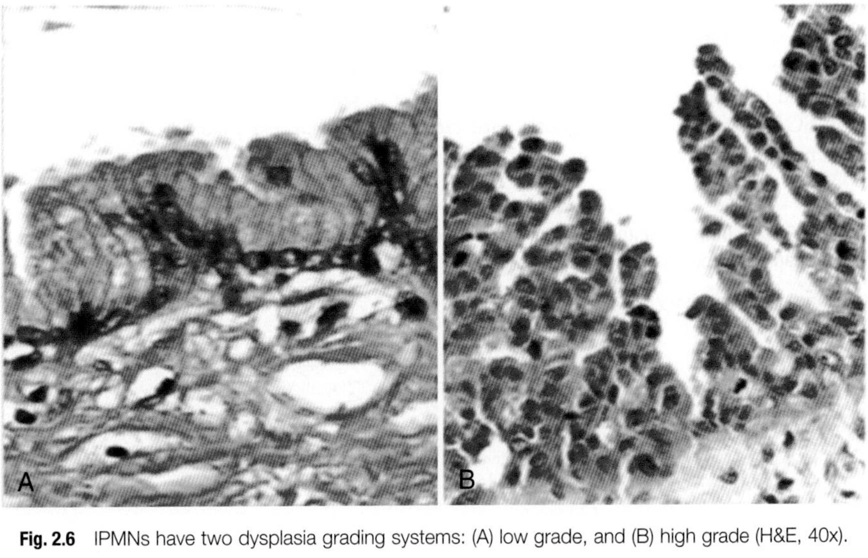

Fig. 2.6 IPMNs have two dysplasia grading systems: (A) low grade, and (B) high grade (H&E, 40x).

CLINICAL PEARLS

IPMNs may associate with focal foci of invasive adenocarcinoma; therefore, submission of the entire lesion for microscope examination is necessary. The intestinal-type IPMNs are associated with colloid carcinoma, while pancreatobiliary-type IPMNs are associated with tubular adenocarcinoma.

Solid Pseudopapillary Neoplasms (SPN) and Pancreatic Endocrine Neoplasms (PEN)

SPN is a low-grade malignant neoplasm of uncertain cellular differentiation. Clinically, SPNs present as indolent, slow-growing body/tail pancreatic tumors in young females (female-to-male incident ratio is 9:1).

PENs occur in the body or tail of the pancreas in adult patients with no sex predilection. PENs are considered to be malignant tumors, with 30% of metastatic disease at diagnosis, despite the tumor's slow-growing rate.

The cytologic characteristics of SPNs show similar morphology to PENs; cytoplasmic vacuoles are seen in SPNs, while nuclear chromatin is typically coarse with salt-and-pepper appearance characteristic of PENs. Immunohistochemistry may also aid in distinguishing SPNs from PENs (Table 2.3).

Well-differentiated PENs are subdivided into low grade (G1) and intermediate grade (G2). Low grade G1: <2 mitoses per 10 HPF or <3% Ki-67 index, while intermediate grade G2: 2–20 mitoses per 10 HPF or 3%–20% Ki-67 index.

CLINICAL PEARLS

Approximately 10% of PENs are associated with one of these syndromes:

- Multiple endocrine neoplasia type 1(MEN1): MEN1 gene on 11q13, younger age.
- Von Hippel-Lindau (VHL): VHL tumor suppressor gene on 3p25, younger age.
- Tuberous sclerosis complex (TSC): TSC1 tumor suppressor gene on 9q34 or TSC2 tumor suppressor gene on 16p13.3).
- Neurofibromatosis 1 (NF1): Microdeletion in neurofibromin gene on 17q11.2

The prognostic factors of PENs include mitotic count, Ki-67 proliferative index level, tumor size, extent of local invasion and/or metastases, and functional status.

Serous Cystadenoma

SCA is a benign, cystic epithelial neoplasm composed of numerous thin-walled cysts filled with serous fluid (microcystic) and lined by a single layer of cuboidal–flat cells with clear–pale cytoplasm. SCAs have excellent prognosis with recurrence rate of less than 2%. The symptomatic lesions required surgical resection.

TABLE 2.3 ■ **Immunohistochemistry of Pancreatic Endocrine Neoplasms (PENs) and Solid Pseudopapillary Neoplasms (SPNs)**

Immunohistochemistry	PENs	SPNs
E-cadherin	Positive	Negative
β-Catenin	Negative	Positive (nuclear)
CD56	Positive	Negative
CD10	Negative	Positive (cytoplasmic)
Progesterone receptor	Negative	Positive (nuclear)
Chromogranin	Positive	Negative
Synaptophysin	Positive	Negative

The main differential diagnosis of SCA is Von Hippel-Lindau-associated pancreatic cyst, which is an autosomal dominant disorder characterized by clear cell neoplasms with identical histology to SCA.

In contrast to SCA, Von Hippel-Lindau–associated pancreatic cysts do not form distinct lesions and present as irregular, multifocal scattered cysts in the pancreas.

CLINICAL PEARLS

The key question from a clinical perspective is whether a cyst is benign, has malignant potential, or harbors high-grade dysplasia or invasive carcinoma. This will guide patient case triage (discharged, undergo surveillance, or require surgical intervention).

Molecular Marker of Pancreatic Cyst Fluid

One of the problems with identifying mutations in pancreatic cysts is that the number of mutant alleles present is extremely low when compared with solid lesions.

Pancreatic cysts contain far fewer somatic mutations than pancreatic ductal adenocarcinoma, and each cyst type has a distinct mutational profile (Table 2.4).

Commercially, molecular tests for pancreatic cyst fluid are available with three components:

- KRAS mutation
- Loss of heterozygosity analysis: 15 preselected loci associated with tumor suppressor genes
- DNA quantity

TABLE 2.4 ■ **Molecular Markers of Pancreatic Cyst**

		Molecular Markers		
Type of Cyst	**Any of These present**	**Any of These Absent**	**Sensitivity (95% CI)**	**Specificity (95% CI)**
SCA	VHL chr3 LOH	KRAS GNAS RNF43 chr5p aneu chr8p aneu	100 (74–100)	91 (84–95)
SPN	CTNNB1	KRAS GNAS RNF43 Chr18 LOH	100 (69–100)	100 (97–100)
MCN	None	CTNNB1 GNAS chr3 LOH chr1q aneu chr22q aneu	100 (74–100)	75 (66–82)
IPMN	GNAS RNF43 chr9 LOH chr1q aneu chr8p aneu	None	76 (66–84)	97 (85–99.9)

aneu, aneuploidy; *chr,* chromosome; *CI,* confidence interval; *IPMN,* intraductal papillary mucinous neoplasm; *MCN,* mucinous cystic neoplasm; *SCA,* serous cystadenoma; *SPN,* solid pseudopapillary neoplasm.

What is the prognosis of the patient?

Dysplasia and stromal invasion are the histological features that possess predictive value of MCN. MCN without dysplasia or stromal invasion is with an excellent prognosis. Size of tumor, extent of tumor invasion (confined to tumor versus beyond tumor capsule), and patient age (>50 years) are also correlated to survival rate.

Case Point 2.3

Patient is reassured, and a follow-up routine checkup visit is scheduled within 6 months.

BEYOND THE PEARLS

Generally, pancreatic cysts with the following features harbor a high risk of malignancy:

- Jaundice secondary to the cyst
- Acute pancreatitis secondary to the cyst
- Elevated serum CA 19-9
- Mural nodule or solid component within the cyst on gross examination
- Main pancreatic duct diameter of >5 mm
- Cyst size >3 cm
- Cytology of high-grade dysplasia or invasion

References

Basturk O, Coban I, Adsay NV. Pancreatic cysts: pathologic classification, differential diagnosis, and clinical implications. *Arch Pathol Lab Med.* 2009;133(3):423-438.

Compagno J, Oertel JE. Mucinous cystic neoplasms of the pancreas with overt and latent malignancy (cystadenocarcinoma and cystadenoma). A clinicopathologic study of 41 cases. *Am J Clin Pathol.* 1978; 69(6):573-582.

Elta GH, Enestvedt BK, Sauer BG, Lennon AM. ACG clinical guideline: diagnosis and management of pancreatic cysts. *Am J Gastroenterol.* 2018;113(4):464-479.

Hruban RH, Verbeke CS. Pathology and classification of cystic tumors of the pancreas. In: Del Chiaro M, Haas S, Schulick R, eds. *Cystic Tumors of the Pancreas.* Cham, Switzerland: Springer; 2016:1-21.

Pitman MB, Centeno BA, Ali SZ, et al. Standardized terminology and nomenclature for pancreatobiliary cytology: the Papanicolaou Society of Cytopathology Guidelines. *Diagn Cytopathol.* 2014;42(4):338-350.

Volkan Adsay N. Cystic lesions of the pancreas. *Mod Pathol.* 2007;20(suppl 1):S71-S93.

Winner M, Sethi A, Poneros JM, et al. The role of molecular analysis in the diagnosis and surveillance of pancreatic cystic neoplasms. *JOP.* 2015;16(2):143-149.

Yeh MM. *Pancreas and Ampulla: Tumors, Mucinous Cystic Neoplasm.* Elsevier Expertpath, pathprimer.

CASE 3

A 41-Year-Old Man with a Liver Mass

Phoenix D. Bell ■ Aaron R. Huber

A 41-year-old man presents for evaluation of an incidentally discovered liver mass during cholecystectomy. A follow-up computed tomography scan is performed, which demonstrates a suspicious lesion measuring 3 cm in the right lobe of the liver. Laboratory examinations results reveal a serum α-fetoprotein level of 580 ng/mL. Subsequently, the patient undergoes wedge resection of the mass. His medical history is significant for obesity and prior gastric bypass surgery, perforated gastric ulcer, and ventral herniorrhaphy. The patient denies any history of liver disease.

What are the most common liver masses?

Worldwide, hepatocellular carcinoma (HCC) is the most common primary malignant tumor of the liver. The majority of HCC (80%) arise in a background of chronic liver disease or cirrhosis, primarily due to alcohol abuse and hepatitis B (HBV) or C (HCV) infection. HBV is the most common risk factor for HCC and has a direct oncogenic effect, regardless of the degree of background fibrosis. Other risk factors for HCC include nonalcoholic fatty liver disease and hereditary hemochromatosis. A minority of HCC occurs in patients without cirrhosis. Cirrhosis is defined, pathologically, as diffuse remodeling of the liver by fibrous septa that separate the hepatic parenchyma into nodules. Patients with HCC may present with weight loss, fatigue, abdominal pain, or jaundice, and most (70%–90%) have elevated serum α-fetoprotein levels (≥20 ng/mL). Treatment may include tumor resection, liver transplant, sorafenib (a tyrosine kinase inhibitor that has proven to be somewhat effective in advanced cases), ablation (radiofrequency or microwave ablation, options for small tumors), or transarterial chemoembolization (may prolong survival).

CLINICAL PEARL

Hemochromatosis is due to mutations in the HFE gene (most commonly C282Y), which impedes hepcidin function and results in increased iron absorption by enterocytes and thus iron overload. Patients are classically defined by the triad: cirrhosis, diabetes, and bronzing of the skin.

CLINICAL PEARL

The treatment for HCV has been rapidly expanding, and the particular agents chosen vary from patient to patient based upon certain variables including whether a patient has had treatment before or if they have cirrhosis. Most patients are treated with a combination of direct-acting antiviral agents, such as ledipasvir-sofosbuvir or sofosbuvir-velpatasvir, which inhibit various steps of the viral replication cycle.

Intrahepatic cholangiocarcinoma is the second most common primary liver tumor. It may develop from liver fluke infestation (*Opisthorchis viverrini or Clonorchis sinensis*), primary biliary (sclerosing) cholangitis, congenital anomalies of the biliary tree (Caroli disease, congenital hepatic fibrosis, choledochal cyst, and pancreaticobiliary maljunction), hepatolithiasis, or in association with cirrhosis, HCV, or HBV. Intrahepatic cholangiocarcinoma prevalence depends upon geographic distribution, and is most common in Asian countries. This tumor usually occurs in adult patients with a peak in the seventh decade of life. Similar to HCC, patients may present with weight loss, fatigue, abdominal pain, or jaundice and often have elevated serum CA19-9 levels. Notably, individuals with intrahepatic cholangiocarcinoma who lack the Lewis antigen will have undetectable CA19-9 in the serum and will therefore have a false-negative test. Patients with intrahepatic cholangiocarcinoma may be treated via surgical resection; however, the prognosis remains dismal.

CLINICAL PEARL

Clonorchis sinensis is a liver trematode that is found in raw or undercooked fish, specifically in Asia. Following consumption, the trematode lives within the bile ducts. In severe disease, they may cause blockage of the bile ducts, which can lead to cirrhosis or cholangiocarcinoma. The most effective treatment is Praziquantel.

CLINICAL PEARL

Primary sclerosing cholangitis is a disease of unknown etiology, most commonly affecting young to middle-aged men with a history of ulcerative colitis. Patients develop concentric fibrosis around intra- and extra-hepatic bile ducts, which causes a “beaded” appearance of the biliary tree on magnetic resonance cholangiopancreatography, as well as an “onion skin” appearance on histology.

Fibrolamellar carcinoma is a rare variant of HCC, accounting for less than 1% of these tumors. Classically, this malignancy is seen in teenagers and young adults, with 80% occurring in patients between 10 and 35 years of age, yet HCC remains the most common primary liver tumor in children and young adults. Fibrolamellar carcinoma is associated with a *DNAJB1-PRKACA* fusion transcript from an intra-chromosomal 19 deletion that leads to activation of protein kinase A.

Liver metastases are more common than primary liver malignancies. The most common carcinomas metastasizing to the liver include colon, breast, lung, pancreas, stomach, and uterine cervix. Melanoma and neuroendocrine tumors are also known for metastasis to the liver.

The most common benign tumor of the liver is a cavernous hemangioma. Cavernous hemangioma occurs more commonly in young women. Patients are usually asymptomatic; however, larger tumors may cause symptoms leading to surgical resection. Rare complications of cavernous hemangioma include rupture, acute thrombosis, or Kasabach–Merritt syndrome. Kasabach–Merritt syndrome refers to a rare consumptive coagulopathy associated with some vascular tumors, characterized by low platelets, hypofibrinogenemia, and elevated fibrin split products, which may be life-threatening.

Other benign hepatocellular lesions include hepatocellular adenoma (HCA) and focal nodular hyperplasia (FNH). HCA is a benign tumor of hepatocytes that is most common in young women taking oral contraceptives and young adults taking anabolic steroids. HCAs are also seen in patients with glycogen storage disease (types I and III) maturity onset diabetes of the young type 3. Patients most commonly present with abdominal pain; however, HCA can also be asymptomatic. Complications including rupture, hemorrhage, and malignant transformation are associated with HCA, depending on the subtype (Table 3.1).

CLINICAL PEARL

Glycogen storage diseases prevent the breakdown of glycogen to glucose, thus causing an accumulation of glycogen within cells. Glycogen storage disease type 1, also known as von Gierke disease, presents in infancy and is most commonly due to mutations in the G6PC gene, which is responsible for making glucose-6-phosphatase. These patients often have severe fasting hypoglycemia and lactic acidosis. Glycogen storage disease type 3, also known as Cori disease, also presents in infancy, due to mutations in the AGL gene, which is responsible for making the glycogen debranching enzyme. These patients often have hypoglycemia and hyperlipidemia.

FNH is the second most common benign hepatic lesion after cavernous hemangioma. This is not a hepatocellular neoplasm, but is thought to be a localized reaction to a vascular anomaly. FNH most commonly occurs in women aged between 30 and 40 years and is usually asymptomatic, with most lesions incidentally identified on imaging studies conducted for other medical reasons. Most cases of FNH are unifocal, but multiple lesions are not uncommon. Treatment is not required unless the patient is symptomatic.

What is the liver imaging reporting and data system?

The liver imaging reporting and data system (LI-RADS) is a system that standardizes interpretation and reporting nomenclature when evaluating computed tomography or magnetic resonance imaging scans of the liver in patients with cirrhosis who are at increased risk of HCC. LI-RADS

TABLE 3.1 ■ **Subtypes of Hepatocellular Adenoma**

Subtype	Clinical Features	Histologic Features	Immunohistochemical Features	Malignant transformation?
Hepatocyte nuclear factor-1 α inactivated	30% of tumors Associated with MODY-3	Steatosis	Loss of liver fatty acid-binding protein expression	Very rare
β-catenin mutated	10%–15% of tumors May occur in men Associated with anabolic steroids and glycogen storage disease	May have mild cytologic and architectural atypia	β-catenin nuclear positivity Glutamine synthetase positivity	50%
Inflammatory	IL6ST, STAT3, or GNAS mutations Most common subtype 35%–50% Associated with obesity and alcohol	Ductular reaction Inflammatory infiltrates Sinusoidal dilatation	Serum amyloid A positivity C-reactive protein positivity	May occur
Unclassifiable	10% of tumors No known mutation	No characteristic features	No characteristic features	Unknown

MODY-3, maturity onset diabetes of the young type 3.

combines arterial enhancement (HCC enhances more intensely than surrounding liver during arterial phase) with lesional size, venous washout, evidence of a capsule, and growth characteristics when compared with prior imaging studies. The categories are described as follows: category 1, definitely benign; category 2, probably benign; category 3, utilized for masses that do not meet criteria for the other categories and there is a moderate probability of being either benign or HCC; category 4, probably HCC; and category 5, diagnostic of HCC.

Case Point 3.1

The pathology from his original resection specimen reveals HCC. After 2 years, two new liver masses are identified on surveillance imaging, compatible with recurrent HCC.

What is the prognosis for patients with a diagnosis of HCC?

The prognosis is dependent on the stage at presentation with a 5-year survival of 30% for localized disease, 10% for regional disease, and less than 5% for patients with metastatic dissemination. For patients with localized disease who undergo liver transplantation, the 5-year survival rate is up to 60%–70%. Other clinicopathologic factors associated with a more favorable prognosis include age less than 50, female sex, a non-cirrhotic liver, well to moderate differentiation, and absence of vascular invasion

What are the gross and histologic findings of HCC?

Grossly, HCC shows green (due to bile staining) or tan to tan-brown cut surfaces, which are often bulging and distinct from the surrounding parenchyma (Fig. 3.1). Areas of hemorrhage and necrosis are common. There are four distinctive macroscopic growth patterns that may be seen: a single nodule, a dominant nodule with satellite nodules, multiple discrete nodules, or a diffuse pattern composed of abundant small tumor nodules. Histologically, HCC has both cytological and architectural features that help to distinguish malignant from benign lesions. The salient architectural features include a lack of portal triads within the tumor, abnormal (unpaired) arterioles or arteries within the tumor, trabecular growth pattern with thickening of the hepatocyte plates (versus the normal 1–2 cell thickness) separated by sinusoids, and pseudoacinar structures. The four major growth patterns in decreasing order of frequency include trabecular (Fig. 3.2),

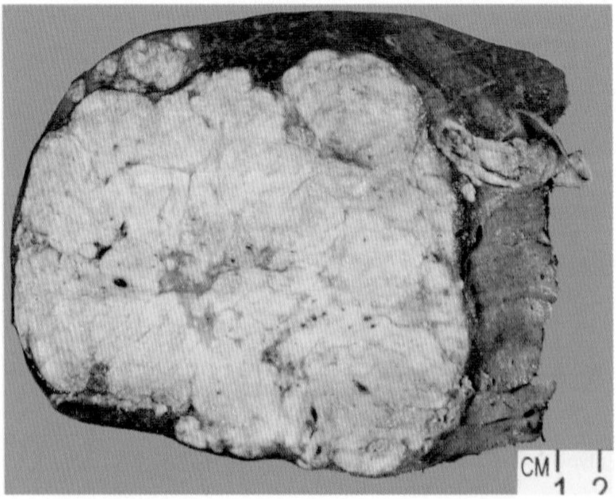

Fig. 3.1 Gross photograph of hepatocellular carcinoma showing a fairly well-circumscribed mass with lobulated, tan–white to yellow cut surfaces.

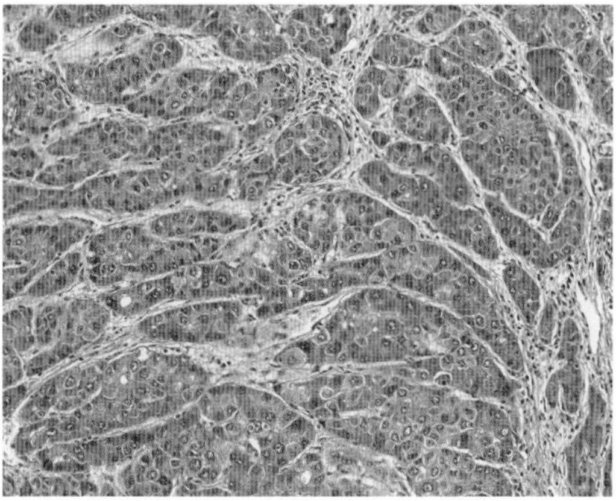

Fig. 3.2 Hepatocellular carcinoma, trabecular pattern (original magnification, 100x).

solid (compact), pseudoacinar (pseudoglandular) (Fig. 3.3), and macrotrabecular (defined as trabeculae that are ≥10 cells thick). Cytologically, the cells of HCC resemble hepatocyte, but show nuclear atypia including hyperchromasia and irregular nuclei with multinucleation, prominent nucleoli, and anisonucleosis. Cytoplasmic alterations include an increased nuclear–cytoplasm ratio, or the presence of glycogen, steatosis, Mallory–Denk bodies, hyaline bodies, or pale bodies. Additionally, HCC may show clear cell features (Fig. 3.4). HCC is typically graded on a three-tiered system as well differentiated, moderately differentiated, and poorly differentiated. The well-differentiated tumors (Figs. 3.5A–B) are difficult to distinguish from benign hepatocellular neoplasms, such as HCA. Moderately and poorly differentiated tumors are easily identified as malignant; however, poorly differentiated tumors may require stains to confirm hepatocellular differentiation, as they may appear like any poorly differentiated neoplasm (Fig. 3.6). If patients have been treated with transarterial chemoembolization, pathologic examination of tumor necrosis should be evaluated.

Special and immunohistochemical stains may be required to differentiate between benign neoplasms and HCC or to confirm that the tumor has hepatocellular differentiation in a poorly differentiated tumor. Use of the reticulin stain is very helpful in determining whether a well-differentiated hepatocellular lesion is benign or malignant. HCC will demonstrate loss of the

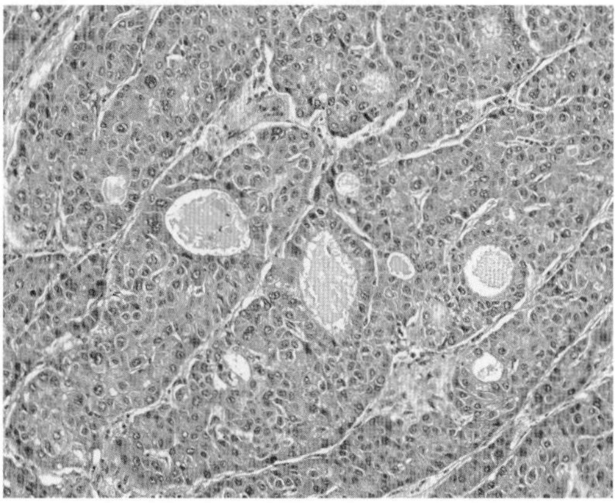

Fig. 3.3 Hepatocellular carcinoma, pseudoglandular pattern (original magnification, 100x).

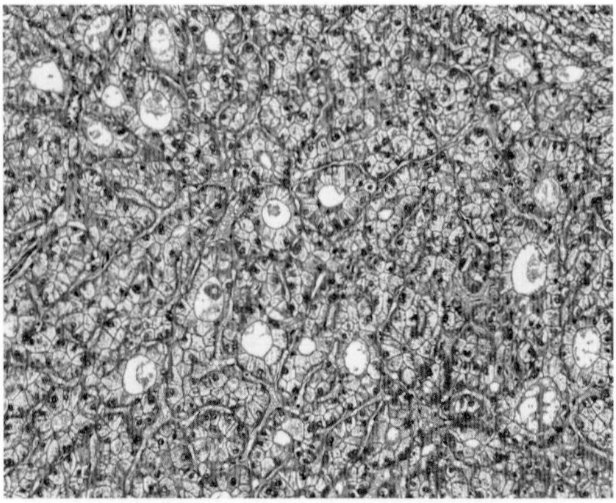

Fig. 3.4 Hepatocellular carcinoma with clear cell features (original magnification, 100x).

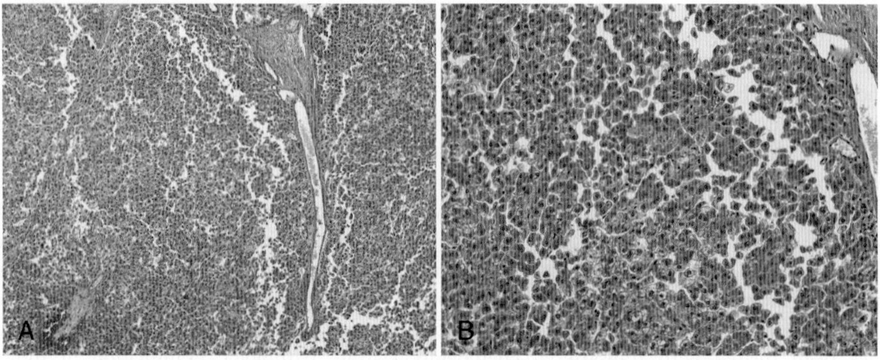

Fig. 3.5 (A) Well-differentiated hepatocellular carcinoma (HCC; original magnification, 40x). (B) Well-differentiated HCC (original magnification, 100x).

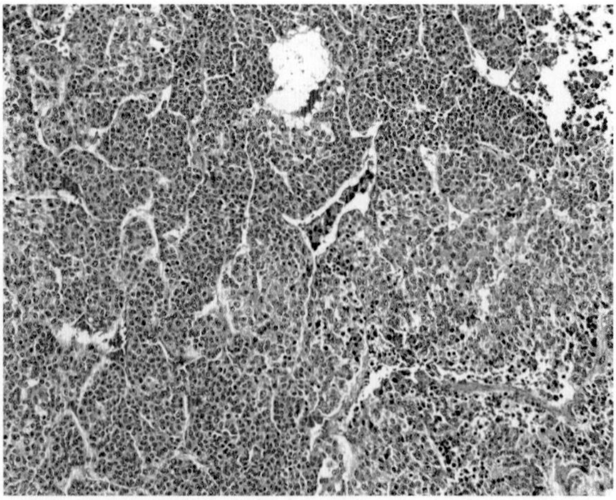

Fig. 3.6 Poorly differentiated hepatocellular carcinoma (original magnification, 100x).

reticulin framework and highlight the thickened or widened cell plates, while benign hepatocellular proliferations will demonstrate a retained reticulin framework and cell plates that are the normal 1–2 cells thick. Immunohistochemical stains confirming hepatocellular differentiation, helpful in poorly differentiated tumors, are HepPar1, arginase 1, and glypican 3. Older markers that have been used include CD10 and polyclonal carcinoembryonic antigen, which demonstrate a canalicular pattern of staining within HCC. Additionally, CD34 staining of the sinusoids is seen in HCC and is termed "capillarization," since normal hepatic sinusoidal endothelial cells do not express this marker (Fig. 3.7).

HepPar1 is an antibody directed against carbomyl phosphate synthetase 1, an enzyme in the urea cycle. A majority of HCCs (85%–95%) express cytoplasmic HepPar1 (Fig. 3.8); however, poorly differentiated tumors may lose this expression in around 50% cases. Benign hepatic parenchyma is also strongly positive, as well as other malignant tumors including hepatoid carcinoma from any site, gastric adenocarcinoma, ovarian clear cell and mucinous carcinomas, adrenal cortical carcinoma, lung adenocarcinoma, cholangiocarcinoma, and neuroendocrine carcinoma.

Arginase 1 is another antibody directed against a urea cycle enzyme, which is useful in confirming hepatocellular differentiation. Arginase 1 demonstrates cytoplasmic and/or nuclear

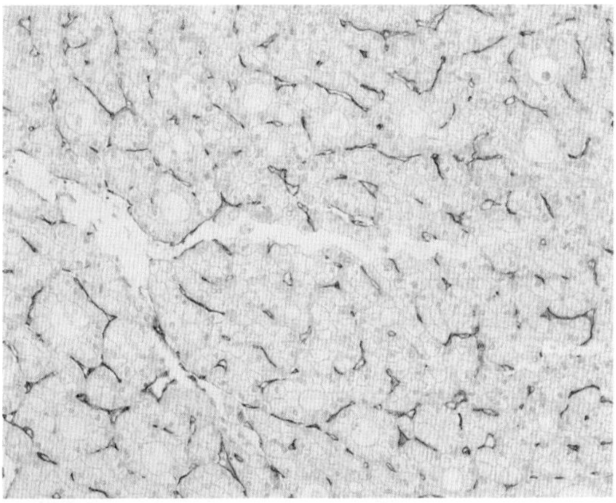

Fig. 3.7 Hepatocellular carcinoma with canalicular CD34 positivity (original magnification, 100x).

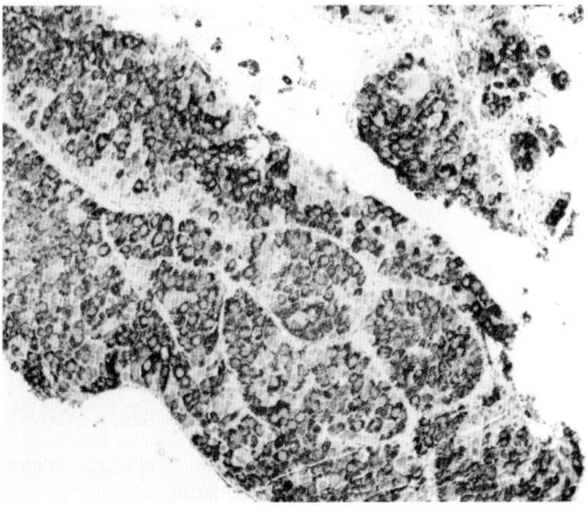

Fig. 3.8 Hepatocellular carcinoma biopsy with HepPar-1 positivity (original magnification, 100x).

expression in HCC and is more sensitive than HepPar1 for poorly differentiated tumors. Arginase 1, similar to HepPar1, is expressed in benign hepatocytes and other carcinomas including hepatoid carcinoma from any site, cholangiocarcinoma, breast carcinoma, pancreatic carcinoma, and colon carcinoma.

Glypican 3, a cytoplasmic stain, also supports hepatocellular differentiation. Most HCCs (80%–90%) express glypican 3; however, the positive staining may be focal and only 50% of HCC may show staining in cytologic or biopsy material. Additionally, glypican 3 may be negative in well-differentiated HCC, yet is expressed in poorly differentiated tumors. Notably, glypican 3 may be expressed in many other malignancies including yolk sac tumors, squamous cell carcinoma of the lung, chromophobe renal cell carcinoma, and cholangiocarcinoma. Glypican-3 should be negative in benign liver lesions such as HCA.

What are the gross and microscopic findings of other hepatocellular tumors listed in the pathologic differential diagnosis of HCC?

Intrahepatic cholangiocarcinoma can demonstrate three different patterns of growth, which are grossly classified as mass-forming (the most common) (see Fig. 3.9), periductal-infiltrating, or intraductal. Mass-forming intrahepatic cholangiocarcinoma appears as a distinct mass lesion within the hepatic parenchyma with firm, gray–white cut surfaces. The periductal-infiltrating type has either localized or diffuse bile duct obstruction. The cut surfaces are firm, and the lesion extends along the periductal connective tissue. The intraductal-growth type, as the name implies, shows tumor within a dilated bile duct, with a nodular or papillary appearance. Histologically, intrahepatic cholangiocarcinoma is a gland-forming neoplasm that may display one of several growth patterns, including glandular or tubular, solid, or papillary. There is a characteristic dense desmoplastic stroma that is absent in HCC, with the exception of the scirrhous variant. Intrahepatic cholangiocarcinoma is also graded as well, moderately, and poorly differentiated. Immunohistochemically, intrahepatic cholangiocarcinomas express numerous cytokeratins, but the most helpful to confirm a diagnosis are cytokeratins 7 and 19. Mucin core protein 1 (MUC1) is another useful marker as it is positive in 80% of tumors. Intrahepatic cholangiocarcinomas that

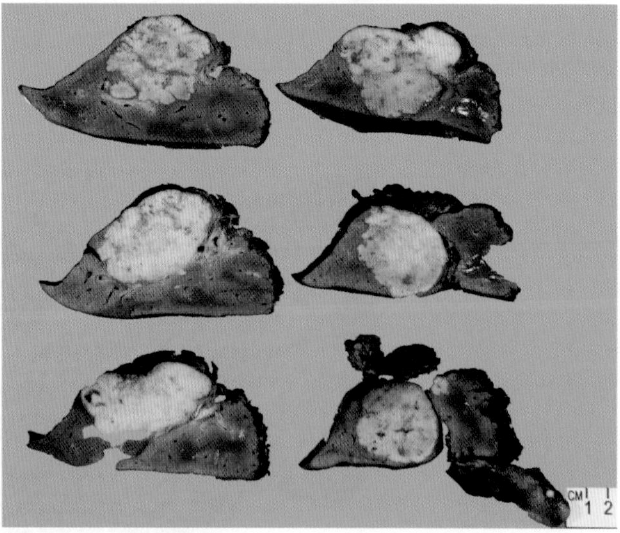

Fig. 3.9 Gross photograph of intrahepatic cholangiocarcinoma, revealing a well-circumscribed mass with tan–white to focally hemorrhagic cut surfaces.

express MUC1 are associated with a poor prognosis. Further, CA19-9 is expressed in approximately 60% of intrahepatic cholangiocarcinomas and is an important serum tumor marker utilized in the clinical setting to monitor for disease recurrence. Particularly important when differentiating this lesion from HCC, intrahepatic cholangiocarcinoma is negative for the markers of hepatocellular differentiation, specifically arginase 1, HepPar1, and glypican 3.

Combined HCC–cholangiocarcinoma, as defined by the World Health Organization (WHO) classification, is a tumor with intimately mixed unequivocal HCC and cholangiocarcinoma in the same tumor. This does not apply to separate tumors in the same liver or tumors adjacent to one another. This combined carcinoma occurs in patients with chronic liver disease and/or cirrhosis and has a worse prognosis than HCC, but a better prognosis than pure intrahepatic cholangiocarcinoma.

Fibrolamellar carcinoma is typically a single, large, well-circumscribed mass in a non-cirrhotic liver (70% of patients have masses over 10 cm). Grossly, it has pale tan to yellow cut surfaces, and a majority of cases demonstrate a central scar and calcification. Histologically, the cells of fibrolamellar carcinoma are large and polygonal with voluminous granular eosinophilic cytoplasm, well-demarcated cell borders, and prominent nucleoli. The cells are arranged in nests, cords, and/or trabeculae with characteristic lamellar fibrosis, described as dense parallel bands of fibrosis. The cytoplasm may have round or oval amphophilic inclusions, "pale bodies," which are composed of fibrinogen. Other eosinophilic inclusions, "hyaline bodies," may also be seen in the cytoplasm. Fibrolamellar carcinoma expresses both markers of hepatocellular and biliary differentiation. The tumor cells are positive for HepPar1 and arginase 1, as well as cytokeratin 1 and CD68, which can distinguish this entity from intrahepatic cholangiocarcinoma and scirrhous HCC, both of which are CD68 negative.

CLINICAL PEARL

Hepatocytes are regenerative and require a lot of ATP, which is generated by metabolic processes within the mitochondria. The abundant mitochondria within hepatocytes impart the eosinophilic granular cytoplasm that is seen on histology.

HCA are grossly unifocal or multifocal, predominantly subcapsular, and typically measuring 5–15 cm. Their appearance varies as they may be well demarcated from the surrounding hepatic parenchyma, or they may blend into it; however, the background liver is typically non-cirrhotic. The cut surfaces are soft and may be brown–tan, yellow, or green. The presence of more than 10 adenomas is termed "adenomatosis," which is common in patients with glycogen storage diseases. Histologically, HCAs are composed of cords of benign hepatocytes with normal thickness (one to two hepatocytes thick) (Figs. 3.10A–B). Similar to HCC, the tumor lacks portal triads, and unpaired arteries are present; the accumulation of fat or glycogen may also be seen. Importantly, HCAs lack cytologic atypia in comparison to HCC and are negative for glypican-3.

FNH may develop as a single lesion or may be multifocal. The lesion is well demarcated from the uninvolved hepatic parenchyma but lacks a capsule. A central scar, when present, is a characteristic gross feature. Histologically, FNH has the typical histologic findings of a central scar with radiating fibrous septa, nodules of hepatocytes in trabecula of normal thickness, a bile ductular reaction, abnormal thick-walled arteries, and a mixed inflammatory infiltrate (Figs. 3.11A–B). Of note, these features may not always be present in small biopsy specimens. If necessary, the immunostain glutamine synthetase, a member of the Wnt/β-catenin pathway, is an immunostain used for confirmation of the diagnosis. In FNH, the Wnt/β-catenin is activated, resulting in a "map-like" positivity in lesional cells.

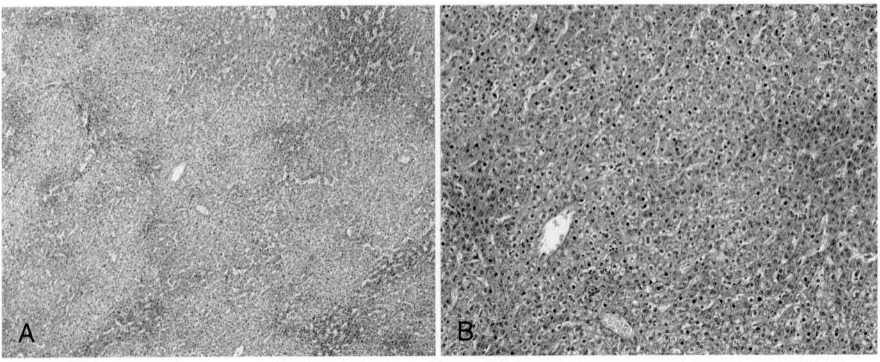

Fig. 3.10 (A) Hepatocellular adenoma (original magnification, 40x). (B) Hepatocellular adenoma (original magnification, 100x).

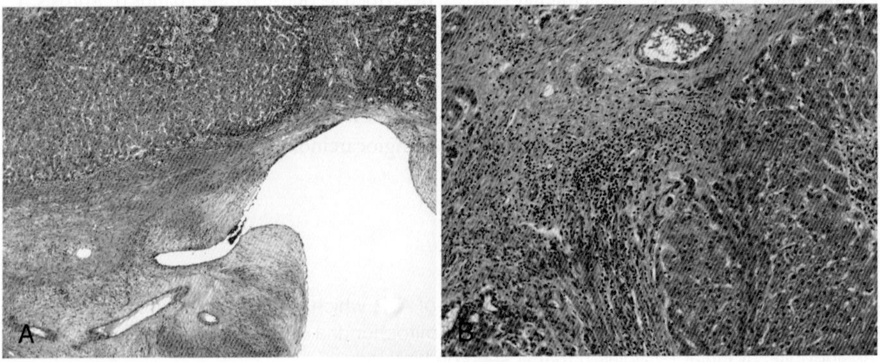

Fig. 3.11 (A) Focal nodular hyperplasia with central scar (original magnification, 40x). (B) Focal nodular hyperplasia with chronic inflammation (original magnification, 100x).

What are the subtypes of HCA and what is their molecular classification?

Relatively recently, the WHO has subclassified HCA into four groups: hepatocyte nuclear factor (HNF)-1 α inactivated, β-catenin mutated, inflammatory, and unclassified. As its name implies, the HNF-1 α inactivated group is defined by inactivation of the HNF-1 α gene and comprises 30% of HCA. This group is also characterized by macrovesicular steatosis histologically and a lack of liver fatty acid–binding protein (LFABP) immunohistochemically. They have the lowest risk of malignant transformation. The β-catenin mutated group is defined by mutations in β-catenin and comprise up to 15% of adenomas. Characteristic features are cytological and architectural atypia just short of a HCC diagnosis and β-catenin (nuclear) and glutamine synthetase expression. This group is also capable of malignant transformation. Inflammatory HCA is the most common subtype of HCA, comprising up to 50% of cases. The inflammatory group is defined by IL6ST, STAT3, or GNAS mutations and is associated with alcohol use and obesity. Histologically, the tumor demonstrates an inflammatory infiltrate with a ductular reaction at the tumor edges, as well as sinusoidal dilatation. Lesional cells expression serum amyloid A and C-reactive protein. Last, the unclassified HCA does not have histologic or immunohistochemical features of any of the other subtypes.

How should this patient be treated?

For patients with recurrent HCC (50% post-resection, 80% post-ablation), the treatment is not well defined. Patients may be referred for a partial hepatectomy or ablation of the lesion. In some cases, patients may undergo a salvage liver transplant, in which the initial tumor is surgically excised or ablated and then they are referred for a liver transplant if they have a recurrence. The course of management largely depends upon the patient's remaining liver function. This patient underwent a salvage liver transplant and is currently disease free.

BEYOND THE PEARLS

- The liver is functionally divided into three zones: Zone I (periportal), Zone II (intermediate), and Zone III (pericentral/centrilobular). Zone I is most affected by viral hepatitis, while Zone III is most affected by ischemia and alcohol.
- Cirrhosis is most commonly caused by alcohol abuse and HBV infection; however, other causes include nonalcoholic steatohepatitis and autoimmune hepatitis.
- Clinically, patients with cirrhosis may present with signs including jaundice, ascites, caput medusae, spider angiomas, gynecomastia, or palmar erythema.
- Aflatoxin, produced by Aspergillus, may cause HCC.
- The liver is one of the most common anatomic sites for metastasis.

References

Anatelli F, Chuang ST, Yang XJ, Wang HL. Value of glypican 3 immunostaining in the diagnosis of hepatocellular carcinoma on needle biopsy. *Am J Clin Pathol.* 2008;130:219-223.

Bioulac-Sage P, Sempoux C, Balabaud C. Hepatocellular adenomas: morphology and genomics. *Gastroenterol Clin North Am.* 2017;46:253-272.

Bosman FT, Carneiro F, Hruban RH, Theise ND. *WHO Classification of Tumours of the Digestive System.* 4th ed. France: IARC; 2010.

Bourlière M, Gordon SC, Flamm SL, et al. Sofosbuvir, velpatasvir, and voxilaprevir for previously treated HCV infection. *N Engl J Med.* 2017;376(22):2134-2146. doi:10.1056/NEJMoa1613512.

Brissot P, Pietrangelo A, Adams PC, et al. Haemochromatosis. *Nat Rev Dis Prim.* 2018;4:18016. doi:10.1038/nrdp.2018.16.

Butler SL, Dong H, Cardona D, et al. The antigen for Hep Par 1 antibody is the urea cycle enzyme carbamoyl phosphate synthetase 1. *Lab Invest.* 2008;88:78-88.

Dyson JK, Beuers U, Jones DEJ, Lohse AW, Hudson M. Primary sclerosing cholangitis. *Lancet.* 2018. doi:10.1016/S0140-6736(18)30300-3.

Jauze L, Monteillet L, Mithieux G, Rajas F, Ronzitti G. Challenges of gene therapy for the treatment of glycogen storage diseases type I and type III. *Hum Gene Ther.* 2019;30(10):1263-1273. doi:10.1089/hum.2019.102.

Jha RC, Mitchell DG, Weinreb JC, et al. LI-RADS categorization of benign and likely benign findings in patients at risk of hepatocellular carcinoma: a pictorial atlas. *Am J Roentgenol.* 2014;203:W48-W69.

Lin CC, Yang HM. Fibrolamellar carcinoma: a concise review. *Arch Pathol Lab Med.* 2018;142:1141-1145.

Mahajan P, Margolin J, Iacobas I. Kasabach-Merritt phenomenon: classic presentation and management options. *Clin Med Insights Blood Disord.* 2017;10:1-5.

Nakano M, Ariizumi SI, Yamamoto M. Intrahepatic cholangiocarcinoma. *Semin Diagn Pathol.* 2017;34:160-166.

Torbenson M, Zen Y, Yeh MM. *Tumors of the Liver.* Washington, DC: American Registry of Pathology; 2018.

Villanueva A. Hepatocellular carcinoma. *N Engl J Med.* 2019;15:1450-1462.

Yan BC, Gong C, Song J, et al. Arginase-1: a new immunohistochemical marker of hepatocytes and hepatocellular neoplasms. *Am J Surg Pathol.* 2010;34:1147-1154.

Zucman-Rossi J, Jeannot E, Nhieu JT, et al. Genotype-phenotype correlation in hepatocellular adenoma: new classification and relationship with HCC. *Hepatology.* 2006;43:515-524.

CASE 4

A 45-Year-Old Woman with Radiating Epigastric Pain

Jennifer J. Prutsman-Pfeiffer

A 45-year-old woman presents to the emergency department with a 6-hour history of severe epigastric and right upper quadrant abdomen pain radiating around to the upper back. The pain is worse lying down and is described as the worst pain she has ever had in her life. She has associated nausea and dry heaving, but is without symptoms of vomiting, diarrhea, fever, chills, chest pain, shortness of breath, dizziness, or palpitations. Tylenol has not alleviated her pain. She has not eaten since the night before. She has hypertension and takes enalapril; the only other medication is omeprazole. She has been eating healthier, resulting in an intentional weight loss of 36 pounds. She does not smoke, drink, or use illicit drugs. She does not have high cholesterol. She is 5'6" and weighs 260 pounds, with a body mass index of 42 kg/m^2, obesity class III (Table 4.1). She reports to have had similar symptoms on and off for 6 months which are worse with eating. Her primary care doctor diagnosed her with gallstones 2 months ago and referred her to a general surgeon for a cholecystectomy, scheduled in 2 weeks.

What are the differential diagnoses for this patient?
Differential diagnoses include biliary colic, cholecystitis, choledocholithiasis, pancreatitis, gastritis, peptic ulcer disease, gastroesophageal reflux disease, and less likely acute coronary syndrome, aortic dissection, renal colic, and pregnancy.

CLINICAL PEARL

Biliary colic is waxing and waning upper right quadrant pain due to the gallbladder contracting against a stone lodged in the cystic duct. Symptoms are relieved if the stone passes.

Renal colic is caused by a kidney stone lodging anywhere in the urinary tract (kidney, ureter, bladder, or urethra).

CLINICAL PEARL

Choledocholithiasis refers to the presence of one or more gallstones that are lodged in the common bile duct. Common bile duct obstruction may result in acute pancreatitis or obstructive jaundice.

Ascending cholangitis is a bacterial infection of the bile duct up to the liver, usually due to an ascending infection with enteric Gram-negative bacteria. Patients present with Charcot's triad: sepsis (high fever and chills), jaundice, and right upper abdominal pain. There is an increased incidence of ascending cholangitis with choledocholithiasis.

TABLE 4.1 ■ **Body Mass Index (BMI) and Obesity Class**

	BMI (kg/m^2)	Obesity Class
Underweight	<18.5	
Normal	18.5–24.9	
Overweight	25.0–29.9	
Obesity	30.0–34.9	I
	35.0–39.9	II
Extreme Obesity	40.0 +	III

CLINICAL PEARL

Acute cholecystitis is an acute inflammation of the gallbladder caused by an impacted gallstone in the cystic duct, resulting in dilation of the duct, pressure ischemia, and bacterial overgrowth, typically *E. coli*, with inflammation. Patients present with right upper quadrant pain often radiating to the right scapula, fever with increased WBC count, nausea, vomiting, and increased serum alkaline phosphatase. There is a risk of rupture if left untreated.

Chronic cholecystitis is chronic inflammation of the gallbladder due to chemical irritation from long-standing cholelithiasis, with or without bouts of acute cholecystitis, and is characterized histologically by herniation of the gallbladder mucosa into the muscular wall (Rokitansky–Aschoff sinus). Patients present with vague right upper quadrant pain after eating. A late complication of chronic cholecystitis is porcelain gallbladder, a shrunken, hard gallbladder due to chronic inflammation, fibrosis, and dystrophic calcification (Fig. 4.1).

Gallstone ileus results when a gallstone enters the small bowel and causes obstruction. The mode of entry for gallstone into bowel is due to cholecystitis with fistula formation between the small bowel and gallbladder.

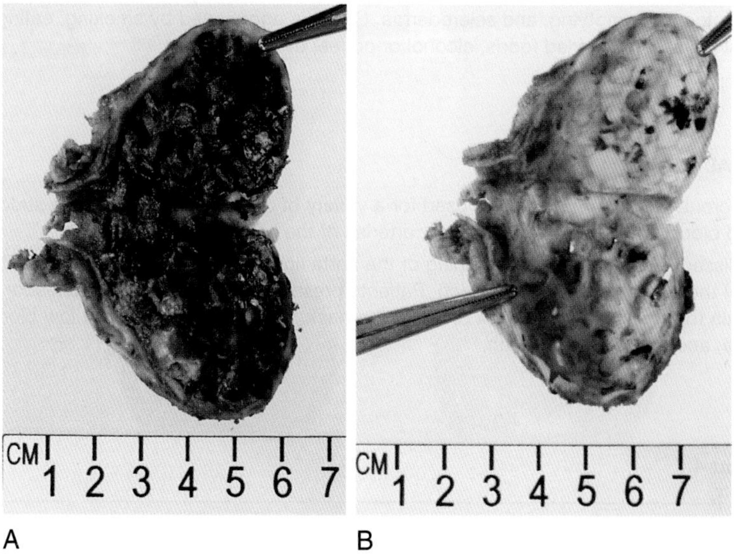

Fig. 4.1 (A) Bivalve gallbladder with numerous firmly packed gallstones. (B) Gallstones removed to show deep impressions in fibrotic mucosa; sectioning revealed focal areas of calcification. Diagnosis is chronic cholecystitis (porcelain gallbladder) with cholelithiasis.

CLINICAL PEARL

Pancreatitis is inflammation of the pancreas caused by the inability of pancreatic enzymes to be released into the small intestine, resulting in the digestive enzymes activating and attacking the pancreas. Patients with acute pancreatitis present with upper abdominal pain that radiates to the back (often aggravated by eating food high in fat), swollen and tender abdomen, nausea and vomiting, fever, and increased heart rate. Chronic pancreatitis has similar symptoms, with the exception of pain being constant. There may also be diarrhea and weight loss caused by malabsorption of food due to few digestive enzymes in the small bowel.
Both acute and chronic pancreatitis commonly present as a consequence of gallstones, heavy alcohol use, or medications.

CLINICAL PEARL

Gastritis is an irritation, inflammation, or ulceration (peptic ulcer disease) of the lining of the stomach caused by stress, chronic vomiting, excessive alcohol ingestion, or the use of aspirin or other antiinflammatory medications. Other causes include: *Helicobacter pylori*, a bacteria that lives in the mucous lining of the stomach; bile reflux, the backflow of bile into the stomach from the duodenum; and infections caused by bacteria and viruses.

CLINICAL PEARL

Gastroesophageal reflux disease (GERD) occurs when stomach acid refluxes across the lower esophageal sphincter and washes into the lower esophagus. Patients present with burning sensation in the chest (heartburn) usually after eating, chest pain, difficulty in swallowing, or regurgitation of food. Risk factors for GERD are obesity, hiatal hernia, pregnancy, delayed stomach emptying, and scleroderma. GERD is aggravated by smoking, eating large meals at night, fatty or fried foods, alcohol or coffee, or aspirin.

CLINICAL PEARL

Acute coronary syndrome is a term used for a variety of conditions that describe sudden and reduced blood flow through the coronary arteries of the heart.
Aortic dissection is when the inner lining of the aorta (intima) tears and blood causes the layers of the aorta to separate (dissect). Patients present with sudden severe chest or upper back pain that radiates to the neck or down the back, loss of consciousness, low blood pressure, and shortness of breath.

Case Point 4.1

Upon physical examination at triage, the patient demonstrates a blood pressure of 188/84 mm Hg (hypertensive), pulse rate of 72/min (normal range: 60–100 beats per minute), respiratory rate of 18/min (normal range: 12–20 breaths per minute), temperature of 36.5°C (97.7°F), and 100% oxygen saturation on room air.

TABLE 4.2 ■ **Liver Function Laboratory Test Results**

	Reference Range	Admission Day 1	Discharge Day 8	Follow-Up 4 Months
ALT	0–35 U/L	745 (H)	70 (H)	15
AST	0–35 U/L	632 (H)	18	12
Alkaline phosphatase	35–105 U/L	316 (H)	114 (H)	69
Amylase	28–100 U/L	1668 (H)		30
Direct bilirubin	0.0–0.3 mg/dL	3.7 (H)	0.3	
Total bilirubin	0.0–1.2 mg/dL	4.8 (H)	0.5	0.4
Lipase	13–60 U/L	>5000 (H)		25

(H) indicates elevated value.
ALT, aspartate transaminase; *AST,* aspartate transaminase.

Case Point 4.2

The patient is hemodynamically stable. A urine pregnancy test is negative. Her liver function tests are elevated and markedly deranged (Table 4.2) with total bilirubin of 4.8 mg/dL, direct bilirubin of 3.7 mg/dL, alkaline phosphatase of 316 U/L, aspartate transaminase of 632 units/L, alanine transaminase of 745 IU/L, and amylase 1668 U/L and lipase >5000 U/L. An abdominal ultrasound shows cholelithiasis and a mildly thickened gallbladder wall concerning for acute cholecystitis, and an 8-mm dilated common bile duct.

Case Point 4.3

The patient is diagnosed with gallstone pancreatitis given the ultrasound findings and the elevated liver enzymes (transaminitis) and elevated pancreatic enzymes (amylase and lipase) over three times beyond the upper limit. She is admitted to the hospital, is treated with ondansetron for nausea and vomiting and hydromorphone for pain, and has a general surgery consult. She is also treated with enoxaparin sodium for prophylactic deep vein thrombosis prevention.

What is the function of the gallbladder?

The function of the gallbladder, a pear-shaped luminal structure located on the inferior posterior surface of the liver, is to collect and store bile produced by the liver. Bile is released from the gallbladder to help in the digestion of lipids and to absorb fat molecules in the small intestine.

What is gallstone pancreatitis?

Gallstone pancreatitis is inflammation of the pancreas that results from a gallstone blocking the pancreatic duct. The gallstone must travel from the gallbladder through the cystic duct to the common bile duct (choledocholithiasis) and settles at the level of the sphincter of Oddi, a round muscle located at the opening of the bile duct into the small intestine at the ampulla of Vater. The stone prohibits outflow material from the upstream structures, the liver and pancreas, causing inflammation, which can be severe and potentially fatal.

What are the main types of gallbladder disease?

The main classifications of gallbladder disease are cholelithiasis (gallstones), inflammatory conditions (acute cholecystitis, chronic cholecystitis; Fig. 4.1), infections (ascending cholangitis),

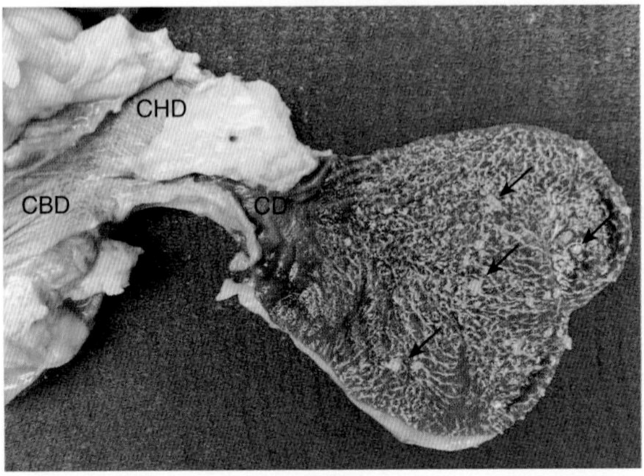

Fig. 4.2 Cholesterolosis of the gallbladder ("strawberry gallbladder"). Gallbladder and ducts opened. Yellow trabeculations of cholesterol and yellow cholesterol polyps (arrows) on mucosal surface of gallbladder. *CBD,* common bile duct; *CD,* cystic duct; *CHD,* common hepatic duct.

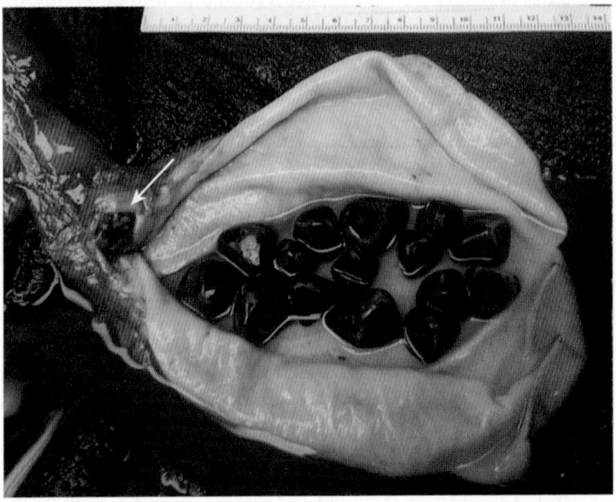

Fig. 4.3 Hydrops of gallbladder. Asymptomatic and unknown cholelithiasis in a 63-year-old male discovered at autopsy. Note multifaceted calculus wedged in cystic duct (arrow), clear mucinous bile, and pale fibrotic mucosa.

miscellaneous conditions (cholesterolosis, Fig. 4.2; hydrops of the gallbladder, Figs. 4.3 and 4.4), and biliary tract cancer.

CLINICAL PEARL

Miscellaneous conditions

Cholesterolosis: Accumulation of cholesterol-laden macrophages within the mucosa. Gross examination shows yellow stippling of the mucosa ("strawberry gallbladder", Fig. 4.2). Microscopically, there are lipid-laden macrophages of the lamina propria.

Hydrops of the gallbladder: Occurs when chronic obstruction blocks the neck or cystic duct of the gallbladder with associated production of large amounts of clear fluid (hydrops) or mucous (mucocele) (Figs. 4.3 and 4.4).

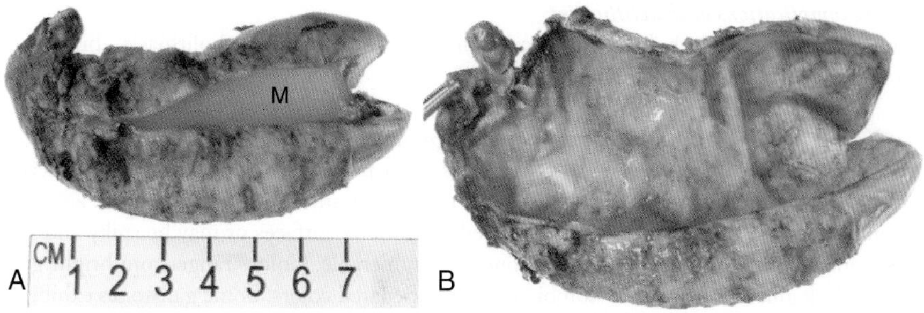

Fig. 4.4 (A) Gallbladder with mucocele, stones present, diagnosed as calculous cholecystitis. (B) Gallbladder with contents removed.

What is cholelithiasis?

Cholelithiasis is from the Greek root words chole—bile and lithos—stone. Gallstones are frequently asymptomatic (Fig. 4.5) but can cause biliary colic, right upper quadrant pain due to stone impaction in the gallbladder or bile ducts.

What are the symptoms of cholelithiasis?

Cholelithiasis is typically asymptomatic until there is an episode of biliary colic, when stones migrate into bile ducts. In this case, symptoms are sudden with rapid intensification of pain in the upper right portion or center of the abdomen (epigastric), with back pain between the scapulae or radiating to the right shoulder. There may be nausea or vomiting. The pain may last several minutes or persist for hours.

How is cholelithiasis diagnosed?

Gallstones are diagnosed by ultrasound as the majority of stones are not radiopaque. Unless calcium salts are present, gallstones are radiolucent and not easily seen on x-ray or computed tomography (CT) scan.

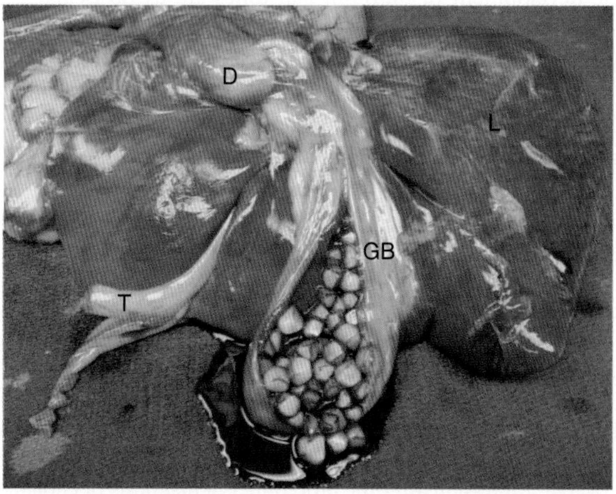

Fig. 4.5 Asymptomatic and unknown cholelithiasis in a 54-year-old female discovered at autopsy. Distended gallbladder with small amount of green–yellow viscous bile and numerous (>50) triangular yellow calculi with brown edges, up to 1 cm. *D,* duodenum; *GB,* gallbladder; *L,* liver; *T,* ligamentum teres.

What are complications of cholelithiasis?

Complications include cholecystitis (acute and chronic), choledocholithiasis, biliary tract obstruction, pancreatitis, and cholangitis.

What is the structural and chemical composition of gallstones?

Gallstones come in a variety of shapes and sizes from particulate, sand-like gritty material to ovoid, egg-shaped solid structures (Figs. 4.6A–F). Some are smooth and round, some are smooth and multifaceted, whereas others have lobulated or granular surfaces or may be spiky and spiculated. Numbers range from one solitary stone to innumerable. Colors range from bright golden yellow to dark green or black, or a combination of variegated colors. Some gallstones exhibit very interesting coloration and may include crystalline structures.

Chemically, gallstones are composed of cholesterol monohydrate or bilirubin; either type may have calcium salts. There have been recent attempts to further characterize gallstones by their chemical composition and expand the main chemical components to eight variants: cholesterol, pigment (bilirubin), calcium carbonate, phosphate, calcium stearate, protein, cysteine, and mixed. Cholesterol stones are the most common type and are typically yellow. Bilirubin stones are pigmented, usually radiopaque, and dark green to black. The formation of gallstones is due to the precipitation of these components in bile. Possible scenarios for formation include supersaturation of cholesterol or bilirubin, decreased phospholipids or bile acids that normally increase solubility, or stasis of bile.

What are the risk factors for cholelithiasis?

Risk factors for the development of cholesterol gallstones include a Western diet, age (over 40 years), estrogen (female sex, obesity, multiple pregnancies, oral contraceptives), clofibrate, Native American ethnicity, Crohn's disease, and cirrhosis.

CLINICAL PEARL

Clofibrate is used to treat hyperlipidemia (high cholesterol) and lower triglycerides and very-low-density lipoprotein (VLDL). It increases lipoprotein lipase activity to promote the conversion of VLDL to LDL. Long-term use of clofibrate is a risk factor for gallstone formation.

Risk factors for the development of bilirubin gallstones are extravascular hemolysis (increased bilirubin in bile), hemolytic anemia, cirrhosis, and biliary tract infection by bacteria or parasites. Infection of the biliary tract may be due to *Escherichia coli* (*E. coli*) bacteria. Parasitic infection may be due to *Ascaris lumbricoides* roundworm (found in areas with poor sanitation and fecal-oral transmission) or Clonorchis sinensis liver fluke (endemic in China, Korea, and Vietnam; a hazard as a food borne pathogen in fish-eating mammals including humans).

Case Point 4.4

The patient has continued elevated liver function tests and rising white blood cell count (WBC) 13.3 rising to 14.8 Th/mm^3 (reference range: 4.0–10.0 Th/mm^3). The patient has endoscopic retrograde cholangiopancreatography (ERCP). The procedure demonstrates an edematous major papilla of the duodenum and stone in the common bile duct (Fig. 4.7A). A biliary sphincterotomy is performed and the impacted stone is removed. Biliary sludge, dark bile, and pus flow from the major ampulla. The common bile duct is dilated up to 12 mm. A 10-cm-long straight plastic stent is placed in the common bile duct, with good flow of bile and contrast material from the stent (Fig. 4.7B). The overall impression after the procedure is a diagnosis of cholangitis and choledocholithiasis with an impacted stone and placement of internal common bile duct plastic stent. After 2 days, the patient has significantly improved pain and her liver function tests are trending down (Table 4.2). A laparoscopic cholecystectomy is performed the following day.

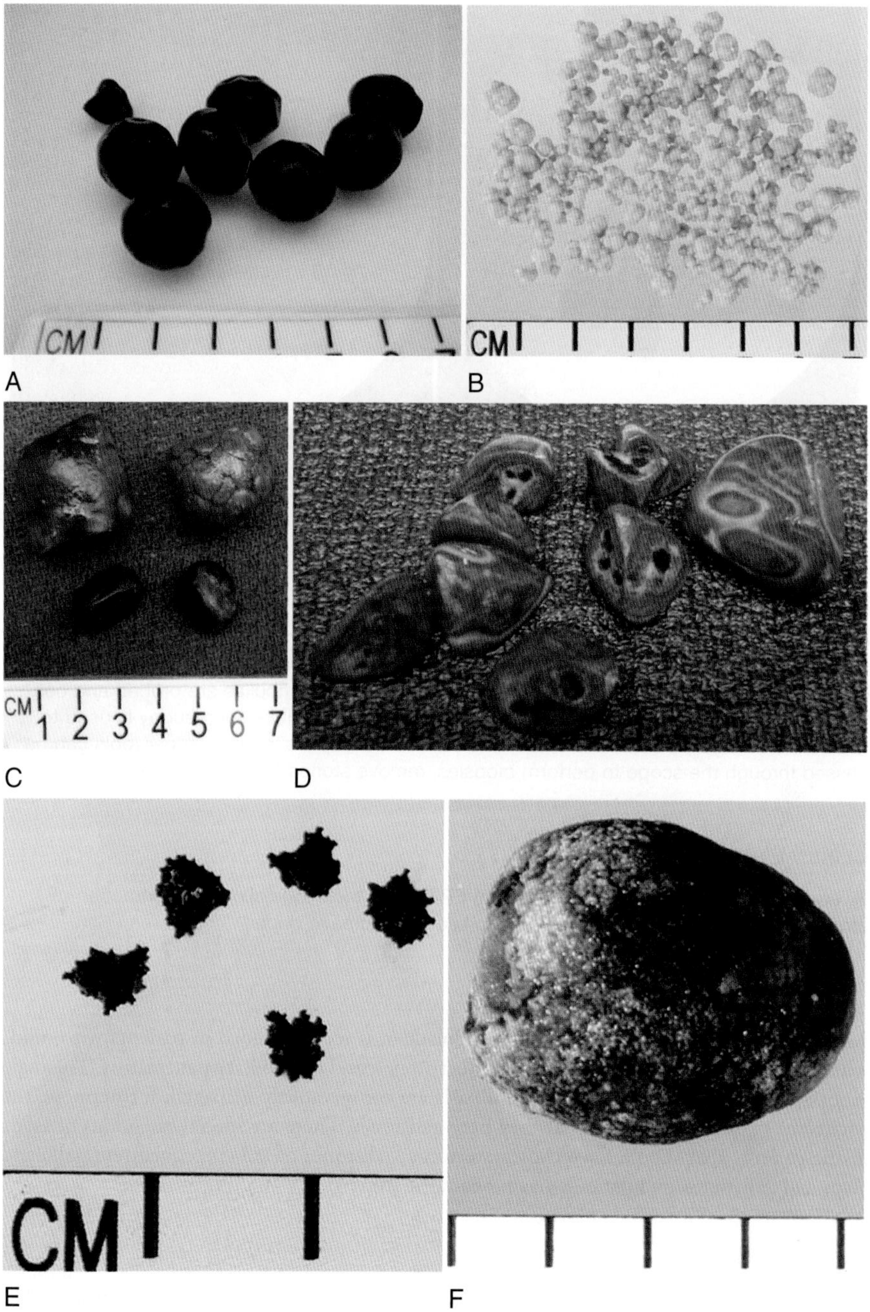

Fig. 4.6 Gallstones—shapes and composition: (A) round, bilirubin-phosphate; (B) lobulated, cholesterol; (C) multifaceted, mixed; (D) angular, calcium stearate-mixed; (E) spiculated, calcium carbonate; and (F) ovoid, mixed.

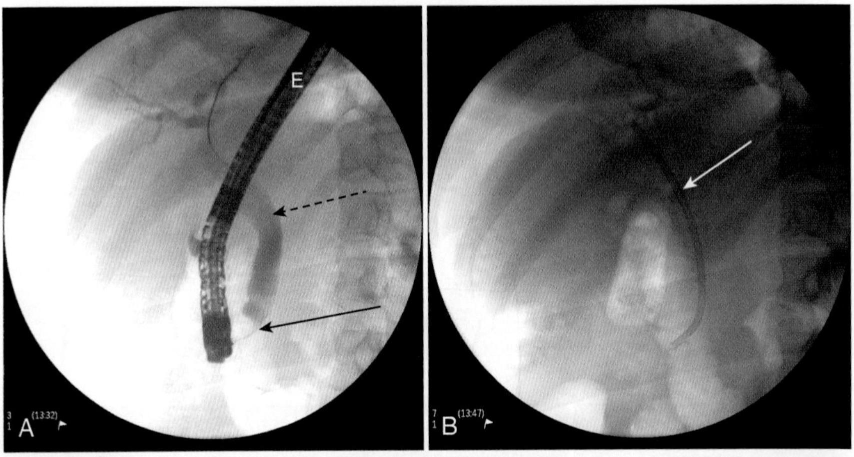

Fig. 4.7 Endoscopic retrograde cholangiopancreatography. (A) Dilated common bile duct with contrast media (dashed arrow), endoscope (E) and lucency (impacted calculus) at distal common duct (arrow). (B) Internal common bile duct stent in situ (arrow).

CLINICAL PEARL

ERCP is a diagnostic technique combining endoscopy and x-ray and is used to examine the bile and pancreatic ducts. A flexible, lighted endoscope is advanced from the mouth, down the esophagus, through the stomach to the duodenum. The ampullae are probed and contrast medium is injected into the ducts to make them more visible; fluoroscopy is used to evaluate blockages or narrowed areas. While the endoscope is in place, other tools can be passed through the scope to perform biopsies, remove stones, or insert stents.

CLINICAL PEARL

Biliary sphincterotomy is performed during ERCP. The technique allows for extraction of stones or for introduction of catheters into bile or pancreatic ducts.

What are the indications for cholecystectomy?

Cholecystectomy, surgical removal of the gallbladder, is recommended in patients with mild to moderate acute cholecystitis, common bile duct stones, and mild biliary pancreatitis. The majority of patients with asymptomatic cholelithiasis are conservatively managed; furthermore, these patients may not even be aware that they have gallstones. There are special categories of asymptomatic patients that should have cholecystectomy: gallstones of ≥3 cm, concurrent gallbladder polyps and gallstones, and patients having bariatric surgery.

CLINICAL PEARL

Gallbladder polyps are an incidental finding during pathologic examination of the surgically removed gallbladder. The majority of gallbladder polyps are benign. Patients with congenital polyposis syndromes (Peutz–Jeghers and Gardner syndromes) can develop gallbladder polyps. Risk factors for malignant gallbladder polyps include age over 60 years, presence of gallstones, and primary sclerosing cholangitis. Polyp characteristics for a higher risk of malignancy include solitary sessile polyps greater than 6 mm.

CLINICAL PEARL

Obesity and rapid weight loss are risk factors for gallstones. Bariatric patients should have prophylactic cholecystectomy during bariatric surgery, since future standard treatment with ERCP and extraction of gallstones may no longer be possible after anatomical rearrangements from surgery.

Case Point 4.5

The patient has laparoscopic cholecystectomy. The surgeon reports moderate pancreatitis and fluid surrounding the acutely inflamed and edematous gallbladder with adhesions. There is evidence of prior obstruction in the dilated neck and cystic duct of the gallbladder. During removal of the gallbladder, the wall ruptured in an area of inflammation. A percutaneous drain is placed in the subhepatic space near the gallbladder fossa and is secured with a suture. The gallbladder is sent to pathology.

CLINICAL PEARL

There is a five fold increase in biliary injury in laparoscopic cholecystectomy over open cholecystectomy. The critical view of safety (CVS) technique is a means of anatomical target identification of the cystic duct and artery during cholecystectomy. It was introduced in 1992 in an attempt to reduce biliary injuries. The three elements of CVS are to clear the hepatocystic triangle of fat and fibrous tissue, to take the lower part of the gallbladder off the cystic plate, and to see that two and only two structures are entering the gallbladder. CVS identification is effective in preventing biliary injury.

What are the macroscopic features of the gallbladder?

Case Point 4.6

The gallbladder measuring 10.5 × 3.6 × 1.5 cm is previously incised and disrupted. The serosa is tan-pink and smooth to slightly shaggy with focally adherent sparse yellow adipose tissue.

There is a 2.5 cm long staple line at the cystic duct resection margin. The gallbladder contains a 3 × 2.5 × 0.6 cm aggregate of green yellow multifaceted pearlescent calculi, ranging from 0.5 cm to 0.8 cm in greatest dimension (Fig. 4.8). The mucosa is maroon pink and trabeculated. The wall is up to 0.3 cm thick. An additional 7 × 5 × 2 cm aggregate of green–yellow pearlescent calculi, ranging from particulate to 1.1 cm in greatest dimension, are included in the specimen container with a 3 × 2.5 × 0.7 cm aggregate of tan fibromembranous bilious material.

What are the histopathologic features of the cholecystitis?

Case Point 4.7

The specimen is diagnosed as acute and chronic cholecystitis with cholelithiasis (Fig. 4.9). Microscopically, there is edema and fibrin deposition in and around the muscular layer with epithelial reactive changes and thrombi within small veins. There is mild chronic inflammation and mural necrosis with neutrophils and lymphoid aggregates, and Rokitansky–Aschoff sinuses.

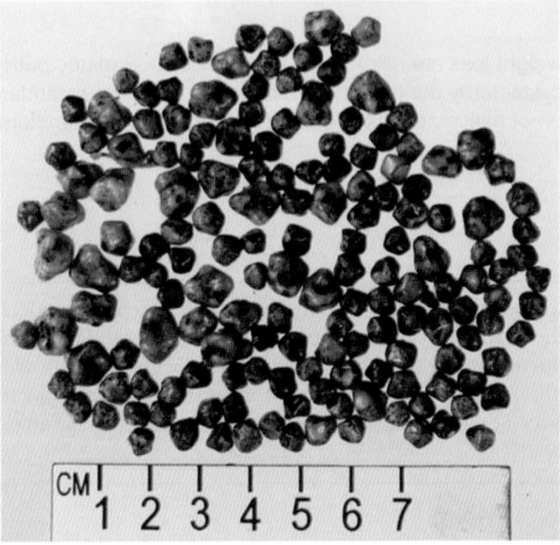

Fig. 4.8 Aggregate of green–yellow multifaceted pearlescent calculi, ranging from 0.5 to 0.8 cm in greatest dimension, mixed cholesterol-bilirubin.

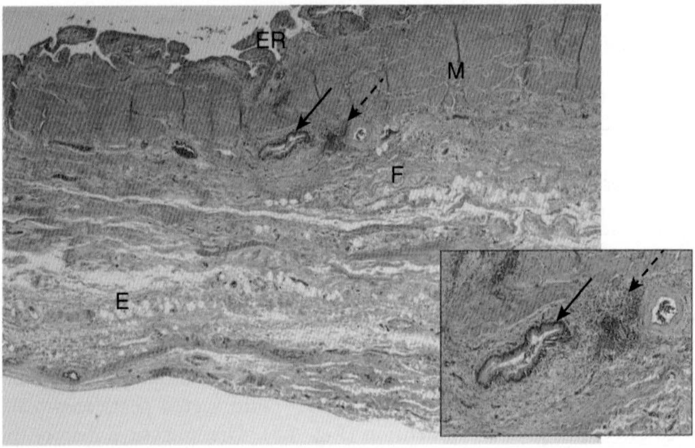

Fig. 4.9 Gallbladder fundus. Edema (E), muscular wall thickening (M), fibrosis (F), epithelial reactive change (ER), Rokitansky–Aschoff sinus (arrow), and lymphoid aggregate (dashed arrow). H&E stain 20x. Inset: H&E stain 40x.

CLINICAL PEARL

Microscopic features

Acute cholecystitis:

- Initial edema, congestion, hemorrhage, fibrin deposition in and around muscular layer
- Mucosal and mural necrosis with neutrophils (later stages)
- Variable reactive epithelial changes resembling dysplasia
- Myofibroblastic proliferation with chronic inflammatory infiltrate
- Fresh thrombi within small veins

Chronic cholecystitis:
- Mild chronic inflammation with Rokitansky–Aschoff sinuses, granulomas (from ruptured Rokitansky–Aschoff sinuses), smooth muscle hypertrophy
- Neuromatous hyperplasia, hyalinized collagen, dystrophic calcification, lymphoid aggregates (5%)
- Variable mucosal changes (normal, atrophic, ulcerated)
- Variable metaplastic change

Ascending cholangitis:
- Neutrophils within the lumina of interlobular bile ducts
- Large ducts may be destroyed and replaced by scar or atretic ducts

Case Point 4.8

The patient recovers over the next several days with improved liver function tests, and the percutaneous drain is removed. An abdominal CT scan with contrast reports acute pancreatitis. The patient is discharged on postoperative day 5. She returns 4 months later for ERCP removal of the internal common bile duct stent with no complications and normal liver function tests.

BEYOND THE PEARLS

Biliary atresia is typically diagnosed within the first 2 months postnatally, if not prenatally through early ultrasounds. Biliary atresia is the failure of formation or early destruction of the extrahepatic biliary tree. Biliary obstruction results in an infant presenting with jaundice, which may or may not progress to cirrhosis of the liver.

Biliary dyskinesia is a functional dysmotility of the gallbladder or the sphincter of Oddi at the duodenum. The diagnosis is based on biliary colic symptoms in the absence of cholelithaisis or cholicystitis.

A Phrygian cap deformity is an anatomic variant of the fundus of the gallbladder. A Phrygian cap is a slumped cloth hat with a pointed apex that falls over on itself. The distal gallbladder with a Phrygian cap deformity has a similar appearance (Fig. 4.10).

The laparoscopic approach is the gold standard for cholecystectomy, one of the most common procedures in gastrointestinal surgery. The advantages of laparoscopic surgery are faster recovery and better cosmetic results, yet the approach has a higher risk for iatrogenic bile duct injury and injury of the right hepatic artery. Iatrogenic bile duct injury is a complication associated with perioperative morbidity and mortality, reduced quality of life, and high rates of litigation should complications arise.

Gallbladder carcinoma is adenocarcinoma arising from the mucosal surface of the gallbladder. Adenocarcinomas account for 85% of gallbladder cancer and are diagnosed as one of three types: non-papillary adenocarcinomas (75% of adenocarcinomas), papillary adenocarcinomas, and mucinous adenocarcinomas. Squamous cell carcinoma is uncommon, as are sarcoma and lymphoma. Gallstones, especially those over 3 cm, are a major risk factor as is porcelain gallbladder. There is poor prognosis, and the classic patient presentation is an elderly woman with cholecystitis.

Cholangiocarcinoma (biliary tract cancer) can occur in any part of the biliary tree. Intrahepatic cancer begins in the hepatic (liver) bile ducts. Extrahepatic cancer begins in the bile ducts outside the liver (common hepatic, cystic, or common bile duct).

Gallbladder or cholangiocarcinoma is typically diagnosed at an advanced stage due to lack of symptoms with early disease. A blood test for the markers carcinoembryonic antigen and CA 19-9, if elevated, may indicate cancer. Imaging to include ultrasound, magnetic resonance imaging or CT scans, as well as interventional radiology tests of percutaneous transhepatic cholangiography or ERCP may be used to image bile flow and ductal anatomy with endoscopy and fluoroscopy.

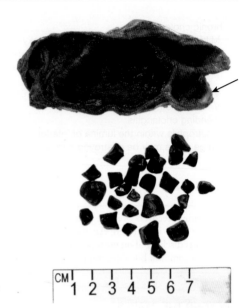

Fig. 4.10 Opened gallbladder with Phrygian cap deformity (arrow) and multifaceted calculi.

References

Andrén-Sandberg A. Diagnosis and management of gallbladder polyps. *N Am J Med Sci*. 2012;4(5):203-211.

Bakman Y, Freeman ML. Update on biliary and pancreatic sphincterotomy. *Curr Opin Gastroenterol*. 2012;28(5):420-426.

Lamberts MP. Indications of cholecystectomy in gallstone disease. *Curr Opin Gastroenterol*. 2018;34(2): 97-102.

Qiao T, Ma RH, Luo XB, Yang LQ, Luo ZL, Zheng PM. The systematic classification of gallbladder stones. *PLoS One*. 2013;8(10):e74887.

Renz BW, Bösch F, Angele MK. Bile duct injury after cholecystectomy: surgical therapy. *Visc Med*. 2017;33:184-190.

Sapmaz F, Başyiğit S, Başaran M, Demirci S. Non-surgical causes of acute abdominal pain. In: Garbuzenko D, ed. *Actual Problems of Emergency Abdominal Surgery*. 2016:95-107.

Strasberg SM. A perspective on the critical view of safety in laparoscopic cholecystectomy. *Ann Laparosc Endosc Surg*. 2017;2:91.

A 67-Year-Old Male with Dysphagia

Phoenix D. Bell ■ Aaron R. Huber

A 67-year-old male with past medical history of obesity, hypertension, hypercholesterolemia, and 10-year history of gastroesophageal reflux disease (GERD) presents with dysphagia and 15 lb weight loss over the past 6 months. He is also a current smoker with a 30 pack-year smoking history, but denies alcohol use. On physical examination, blood pressure is 142/90 mm Hg, pulse rate is 80 beats per minute, respiratory rate is 18 breaths per minute, and temperature is 37.2°C (99.0°F). Physical examination reveals a mildly distended abdomen, but is otherwise normal. Laboratory results show hemoglobin of 11 g/dL and hematocrit of 33%.

How do patients with GERD present clinically and what are the risk factors for the development of GERD?

Most patients with GERD typically complain of heartburn or regurgitation; however, some patients may present with dysphagia or chest pain. Risk factors for GERD include male sex, Caucasian race, age over 50 years, obesity, tobacco and alcohol use, and the presence of a diaphragmatic hernia.

CLINICAL PEARL

There are two main types of diaphragmatic hernia: sliding hiatal hernia (Type 1) and paraesophageal hiatal hernia (Type 2). Patients may present with heartburn or regurgitation symptoms, while others are asymptomatic and the hernia is an incidental finding. Most patients have a type 1 hernia, which is also the most common type seen in patients with GERD. In type 1, the stomach, including the GEJ, slides upward into the mediastinum. In contrast, type 2 hernias result in the proximal stomach displaced into the mediastinum, yet the GEJ remains below the diaphragm. Treatment includes lifestyle modifications, such as weight loss, and, in fewer cases, surgical intervention.

How is GERD treated?

For the modifiable risk factors, patients are counseled on lifestyle adjustments including weight loss, tobacco cessation, and decreased consumption of coffee, alcohol, carbonated beverages, chocolate, and spicy or acidic foods. Additionally, most patients are prescribed a proton pump inhibitor (PPI), such as omeprazole, to help alleviate their symptoms.

CLINICAL PEARL

PPIs impede the H^+/K^+ ATPase pump on the apical surface of the parietal cell membrane, which decreases H^+ production into to the stomach lumen, ultimately decreasing the formation of hydrochloric acid.

What are patients with GERD at risk of developing if not appropriately treated?

Patients with persistent symptoms of GERD are referred for upper endoscopy, as they are at a higher risk for the development of Barrett esophagus (BE). BE, also known as intestinal metaplasia, is a metaplastic change that occurs in the distal esophagus as a result of persistent acid reflux, which causes damage to the cells. Endoscopically, this is seen as salmon-colored "tongues" of mucosa (Fig. 5.1), extending at least 1 cm proximal to the gastroesophageal junction (GEJ). Histologically, the diagnosis is confirmed by identification of intestinal-type (columnar) mucosa with goblet cells (Fig. 5.2). It is important to identify the presence of intestinal metaplasia, since this can develop into low-grade dysplasia (LGD), high-grade dysplasia (HGD), and, ultimately, esophageal adenocarcinoma (EAC). On microscopic examination, dysplasia is defined by

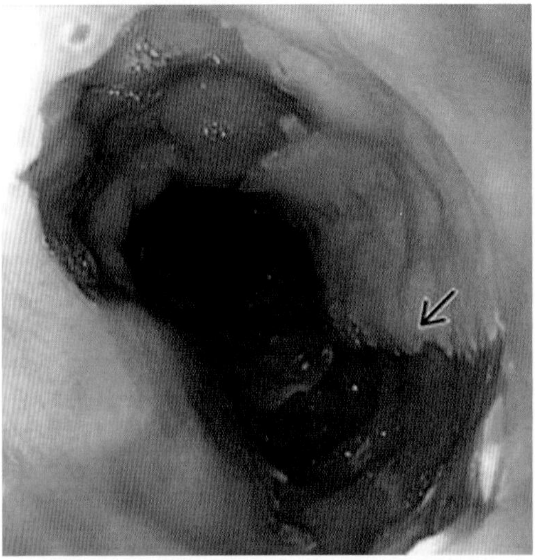

Fig. 5.1 Endoscopic appearance of Barrett mucosa, characteristically described as "salmon tongues" (arrow). (From *ExpertPath*. Copyright Elsevier)

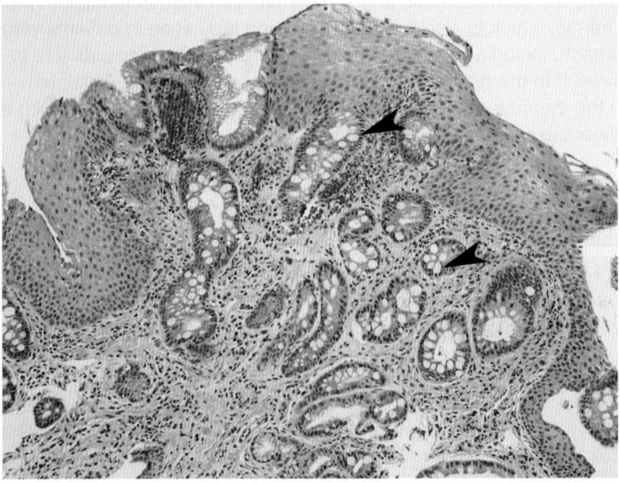

Fig. 5.2 Esophagusy biopsy with intestinal metaplasia (goblet cells at arrowheads) (H&E, 100x).

unequivocal neoplastic epithelium with both cytological and architectural atypia confined to the basement membrane. Architecturally, LGD displays minimal or absent architectural atypia. The cells of LGD maintain their polarity, yet the nuclei are hyperchromatic and do not show surface maturation (Fig. 5.3). In contrast, HGD demonstrates marked crowding of glands with loss of lamina propria and irregularly shaped glands. The cells of HGD have more rounded, hyperchromatic nuclei that lack surface maturation and that have lost their polarity (Fig. 5.4). Similar to biopsies with HGD, biopsies with invasive EAC show high-grade architectural and cytologic features; however, malignant cells invade beyond the basement membrane, for example, into the lamina propria, muscularis mucosae, submucosa, or beyond.

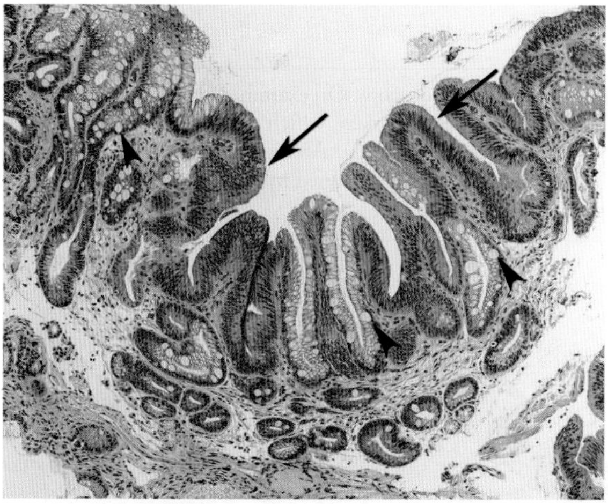

Fig. 5.3 Esophagus biopsy with areas of intestinal metaplasia (arrow heads) alternating with areas of low-grade dysplasia (arrows) (H&E, 100x).

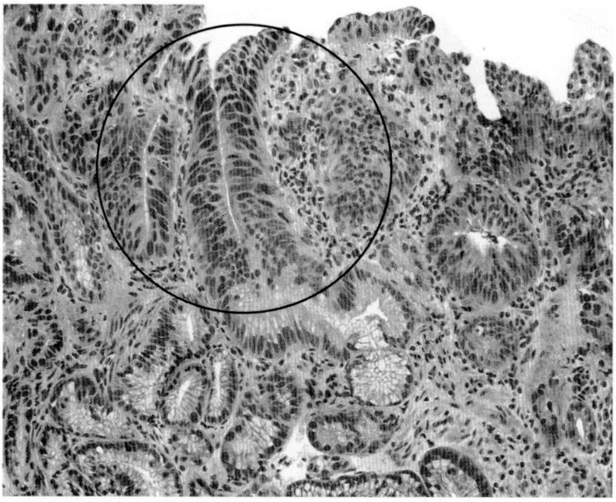

Fig. 5.4 Esophagus biopsy with high-grade dysplasia (circled) (H&E, 100x).

How are patients with intestinal metaplasia or dysplasia treated?

Determination of treatment relies upon several factors including the severity of their disease, age, and health status. Most patients with intestinal metaplasia usually prescribed a PPI and continued on regular endoscopic surveillance. Additionally, patients with low-grade or high-grade dysplasia may be treated with endoscopic techniques including ablation, endoscopic mucosal resection (EMR), or endoscopic submucosal dissection (ESD). Ablation is an endoscopic procedure that removes the superficial dysplastic cells using heat (radiofrequency) or cold (cryoablation). In contrast, EMR and ESD require resection of tissue. During EMR, saline is injected beneath the lesion to elevate it, so that it can be "snared" and removed (Fig. 5.5). ESD is similar to EMR, except it extends deeper into the esophageal wall. In superficial cases of EAC, such as tumor invading the lamina propria or muscularis mucosae, these procedures may also be considered.

Case Point 5.1

The patient is referred for upper endoscopy. On examination, there is a 2 × 2 cm area of nodularity at the GEJ (Fig. 5.6). Biopsies are taken, which demonstrate crowded irregular glands with areas of cribriform architecture (Fig. 5.7A). At higher power, the glands are surrounded by a desmoplasia and inflammation and they are lined by cells with pleomorphic nuclei that have lost their polarity (Fig. 5.7B).

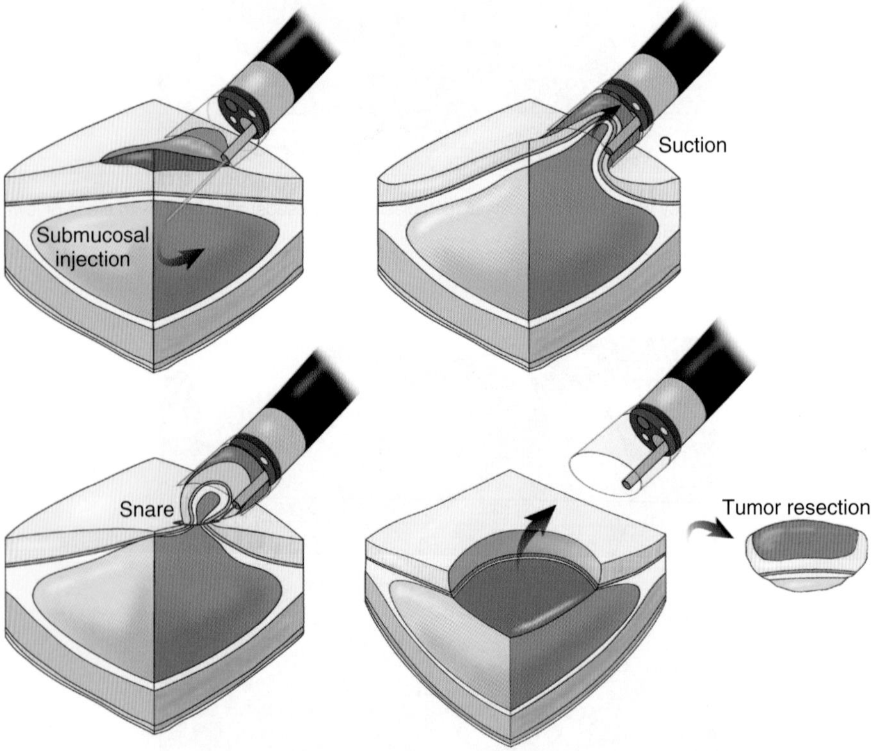

Fig. 5.5 Endoscopic mucosal resection technique. (From Chandrasekhara V, Ginsberg GG. Endoscopic Mucosal Resection: Not Your Father's Polypectomy Anymore, *Gastroenterology,* Volume 141, Issue 1, 2011, Pages 42-49, Figure 4.).

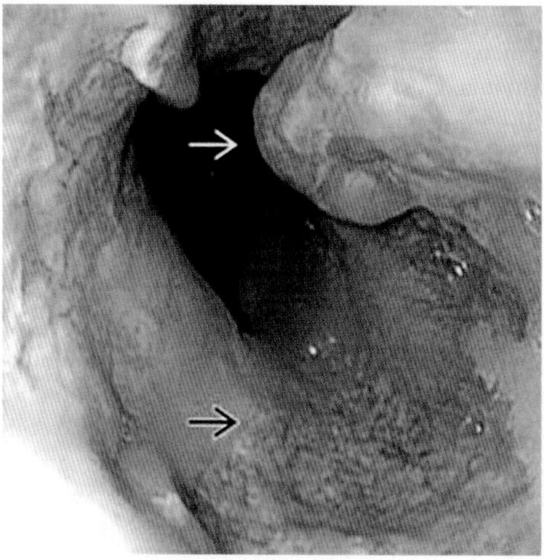

Fig. 5.6 Endoscopic appearance of an esophageal mass (white arrow) in the distal esophagus, adjacent to Barrett esophagus (black arrow). (From *ExpertPath*. Copyright Elsevier).

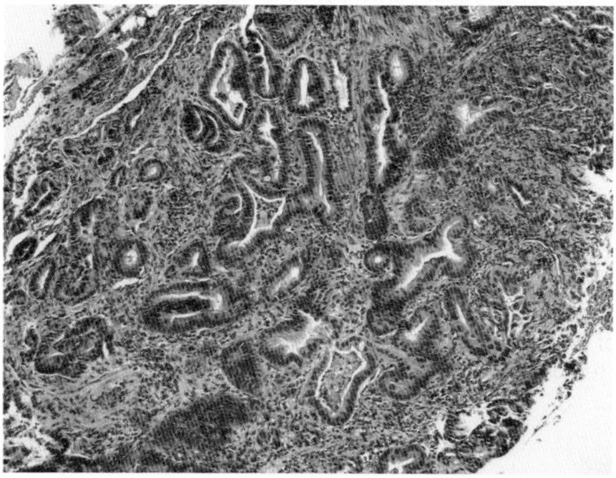

Fig. 5.7 Esophagus biopsy demonstrating crowded irregular glands with cytologic atypia and luminal necrosis (100x original magnification).

What is the differential diagnosis?

The cytologic and architectural features do not match those of normal esophageal mucosa. The glands are irregular and surrounded by desmoplasia. The cells are hyperchromatic, crowded, and show loss of polarity. These findings are suggestive of a high-grade lesion including HGD, esophageal adenocarcinoma, gastric adenocarcinoma, or metastatic adenocarcinoma. Differentiating HGD from EAC may be difficult as EAC can have background dysplasia and the muscularis mucosae can be duplicated. Histologic findings that help distinguish the two, as seen in this case, include the presence of desmoplasia and intraluminal necrosis. Additionally, single cells or glands may be seen invading beyond the basement membrane, which also supports a diagnosis of EAC.

Gastric adenocarcinoma may be considered in the histologic differential diagnosis, particularly the intestinal type; however, EAC can show signet-ring cell features which may mimic diffuse gastric adenocarcinoma. Gastric cancer is characterized by irregular glands with foveolar epithelium surrounded by desmoplastic stroma; however, moderately to poorly differentiated cancers can also mimic EAC. Gross examination of lesions near the GEJ is extremely important, as there are no good immunohistochemical markers to distinguish esophageal from gastric origin. Any lesions arising >2 cm distal to the GEJ should be considered gastric, while those arising <2 cm distal to the GEJ are esophageal.

It is also important to keep in mind, particularly in patients with a prior history, metastases from distant sites, which may include colon, breast, and lung primaries. Colon adenocarcinoma is composed of invasive glands with characteristic "dirty necrosis," and there may be tumor budding. Colon origin is supported by positive CK20 and CDX2 immunostains. Metastatic breast cancer may be seen as infiltrating tubules in a desmoplastic stroma, yet in comparison with EAC, there is less cytologic atypia. If the morphology is poorly differentiated, breast cancer tumor cells may be confirmed with GATA3 positivity, and some subtypes, with estrogen and progesterone receptor positivity. Lung adenocarcinoma that has metastasized may mimic EAC, again demonstrating atypical back-to-back glands with cytologic atypia. Diagnosis may be solidified with TTF-1 and Napsin A immunopositivity.

Lastly, an adenosquamous carcinoma should be considered in lesions characterized by the glandular features of EAC, as well as nests of atypical squamous cells with keratinization. The areas of squamous differentiation may be confirmed with cytokeratin 5/6 and p40, while the areas of glandular differentiation can be identified with a mucin stain, such as Kreyberg or mucicarmine.

Case Point 5.2

The patient is diagnosed with EAC.

CLINICAL PEARL

Tumor budding is a histologic feature seen in various gastrointestinal cancers, including colorectal, gastric, and esophageal carcinoma. Tumor budding is defined as single tumor cells or a group of up to four tumor cells present at the invasive front of the tumor. The presence of high tumor budding is associated with a worse prognosis.

CLINICAL PEARL

A duplicated muscularis mucosae is a microscopic feature of esophageal carcinoma, which results from continuous damage from reflux. This results in the normal muscularis mucosae, in addition to a second superficial smooth muscle layer. It is important for a pathologist to recognize a duplicated muscularis mucosae to avoid misdiagnosing submucosal invasion and upstaging the lesion.

What are the main clinicopathologic differences between EAC and esophageal squamous cell carcinoma (ESCC) (Table 5.1)?

The prevalence of EAC and ESCC varies by geographic location; EAC is more common in the United States, while ESCC is more prevalent worldwide, although the incidence of EAC is increasing. The main risk factor for EAC is GERD/BE, thus EAC is found in the distal

TABLE 5.1 ■ **Clinicopathologic Features of Esophageal Adenocarcinoma Versus Squamous Cell Carcinoma**

	Esophageal Adenocarcinoma	Esophageal Squamous Cell Carcinoma
Epidemiology	Most common esophageal cancer in the United States males > females, 60–70 years old	Most common esophageal cancer worldwide males > females, 60–70 years old
Risk Factors	Long-standing GERD/Barrett's esophagus	Tobacco and alcohol use
Anatomic Location	Lower one-third of the esophagus	Upper two-thirds of the esophagus
Histology	Irregular glands lined by hyperchromatic nuclei with loss of polarity; glands may be surrounded by a desmoplastic response	Squamous nests with abnormal keratinization; keratin pearls; intercellular bridges
Prognosis	Poor	Poor

one-third of the esophagus. The major risk factors for the development of ESCC are alcohol and tobacco use, and less commonly foods with nitrosamines, Plummer–Vinson Syndrome, achalasia, and consumption of hot beverages. ESCC is most common in the proximal two-thirds of the esophagus. EAC and ESCC are most commonly seen in males between 60 and 70 years, with dysphagia being the most common symptom for both. Grossly, EAC and ESCC may present as a mass lesion; however, their histologic characteristics are quite different. EAC forms irregular glands with cytologic atypia, whereas ESCC is characterized by nests of squamous cells with abnormal keratinization and characteristic squamous "pearls" or intercellular bridges (Fig. 5.8A–B).

CLINICAL PEARL

In South America, consumption of Mate tea, made from tree leaves, has been associated with ESCC. Often enjoyed by sipping the tea through a metal straw, the hot temperature of the tea is suspected to cause thermal injury, esophageal mucosal damage, and ESCC.

CLINICAL PEARL

Plummer–Vinson Syndrome is characterized by the triad of dysphagia, iron-deficiency anemia, and esophageal webs. Some patients may have atrophic glossitis. Patients are commonly middle-aged women who present with symptoms of iron-deficiency anemia, which may include fatigue, conjunctival pallor, koilonychia, or pica. The esophageal webs can be diagnosed on barium swallow. Patients are treated with oral iron supplementation and mechanical dilatation.

CLINICAL PEARL

Achalasia is caused by loss of the myenteric plexus in the esophageal wall resulting in the failure of the lower esophageal sphincter to relax. On barium swallow, achalasia is seen as a dilated esophagus ending in a narrowed distal esophagus giving the classic appearance of a "bird's beak."

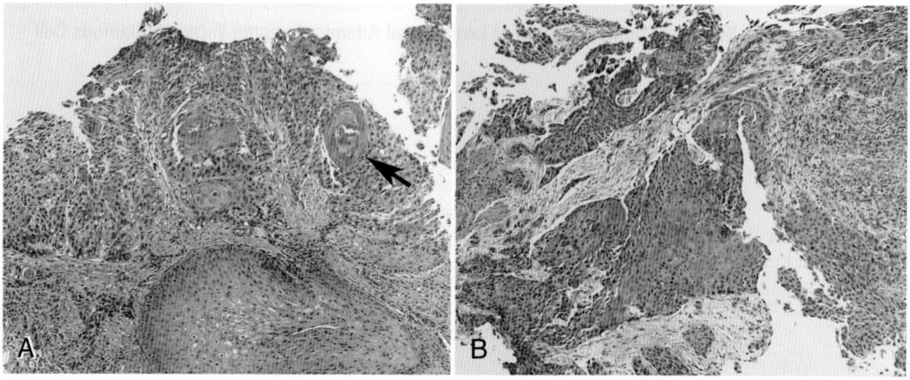

Fig. 5.8 (A) Esophagus biopsy showing squamous cell carcinoma with a characteristic keratin pearl (arrow), low power (H&E, 100x) (B) Irregular islands of squamous cell carcinoma invading the submucosa (H&E, 200x).

How should this patient be treated?

The histology demonstrates irregular glands and single cells extending into the submucosa; thus the patient has EAC. Patients diagnosed with EAC are first evaluated with an endoscopic ultrasound and positron emission tomography/computed tomography scan to assess for the presence or absence of locoregional and/or distant metastases. EAC most commonly metastasizes to the liver, lungs, bone, and adrenal glands. Although there is not one specific treatment for EAC, patients with surgically resectable disease are first given neoadjuvant chemoradiation, followed by esophagectomy (the distal esophagus is resected and the remaining esophagus is anastomosed to the proximal stomach). Chemotherapy agents that may be used include cisplatin, carboplatin, paclitaxel, or fluorouracil. Patients with tumors arising in the GEJ may be treated with a HER2 inhibitor if the tumor is inoperable, locally advanced, a recurrence, or metastatic. Additionally, patients who fail HER2 therapy or patients with disease progression who have failed two prior chemotherapy treatments may be treated with a PD-L1 inhibitor (pembrolizumab).

CLINICAL PEARL

Platinum-based chemotherapeutic agents, such as cisplatin and carboplatin, are alkylating agents that work by crosslinking purine bases on DNA. This prevents DNA repair, leading to DNA damage and cell death. The most common side effects of platinum-based agents include nephrotoxicity, ototoxicity, and neurotoxicity.

What is the prognosis for EAC?

The overall prognosis for EAC is poor and the 5-year relative survival rate for patients with EAC depends upon disease stage. Patients with localized disease have a 5-year relative survival rate of 45%, whereas those with regional and distant disease have 5-year relative survival rates of 24% and 5%, respectively.

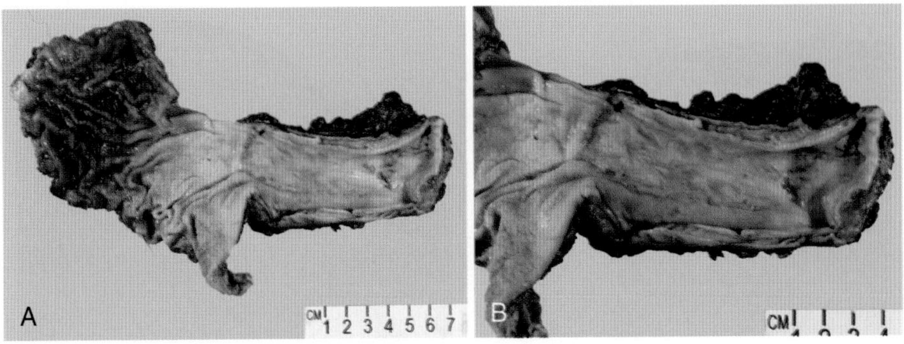

Fig. 5.9 (A and B) Gross examination of esophagectomy specimen post neoadjuvant treatment with no evidence of a mass lesion.

Case Point 5.3

The patient undergoes neoadjuvant chemoradiation followed by esophagectomy (Fig. 5.9A–B). Gross examination shows an irregularly defined area of mucosal flattening at the GEJ, with no discrete mass identified. Microscopic examination of this area of flattening reveals irregular glands extending into the submucosa surrounded by fibrosis and acute and chronic inflammation, with additional irregular glands and single cells present within the muscularis propria (Fig. 5.10).

How is the pathologic response to chemotherapy evaluated? What is the significance of the score?
The use of neoadjuvant chemoradiation causes changes in histomorphology, often resulting in extensive fibrosis. This treatment effect is evaluated by the pathologist and classified according to the Modified Ryan Scheme for Tumor Regression Score, under which the post-treatment specimen is given a score from 0 to 3: score 0, complete response; score 1, near complete response; score 2, partial response; or score 3, poor or no response. A complete response means that no tumor cells are identified. A near complete response reveals the presence of single cells or rare small groups of cancer cells, whereas a partial response suggests that there is residual cancer with evidence of regression, but it is greater than single cells or rare small groups of cells. Lastly, a poor or no response demonstrates extensive residual cancer and no evidence of tumor regression. The score is important, as it suggests that patients with a complete response have improved overall survival.

Case Point 5.4

The patient's treatment effect was graded as a near complete response. Four months later, he presented with dysphagia. A stricture at the esophagogastric anastomotic site was identified, and he was treated with balloon dilatation. There was no evidence of disease recurrence. Currently, he has no complaints.

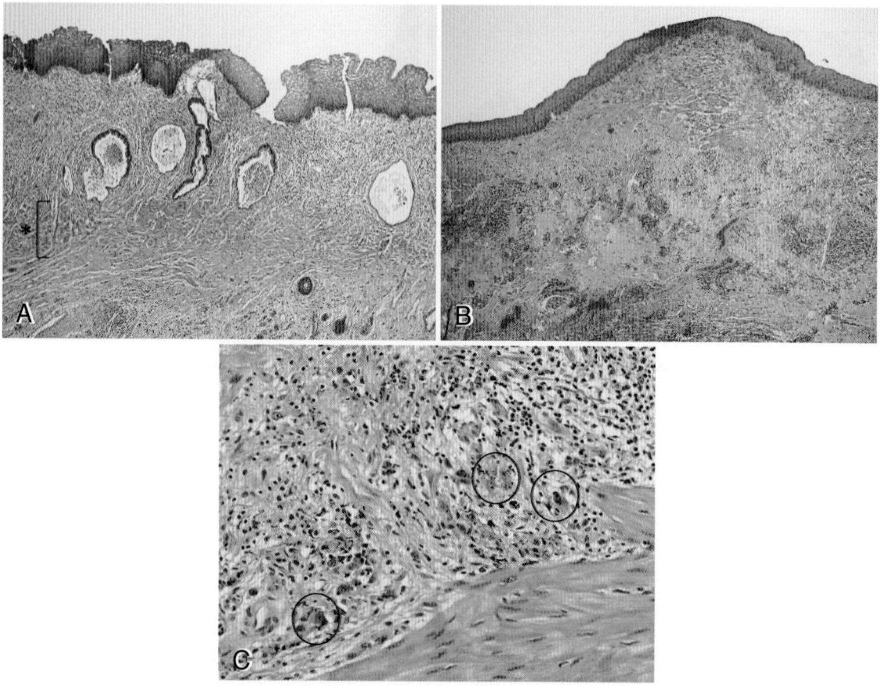

Fig. 5.10 (A) Atypical glands extending to the muscularis mucosae (*) (H&E, 40x). (B) Dense fibrosis with associated acute and chronic inflammation (H&E, 40x). (C) Residual tumor cells (circled) extending to, but not invading, the muscularis propria (H&E, 200x).

BEYOND THE PEARLS

- Patients with HER2-positive EAC have a better outcome if they are treated with Trastuzumab (HER2 monoclonal antibody).
- Histologically, cells containing neutral mucin may be mistaken for true goblet cells, thus they are called "pseudo-goblet cells." In contrast to true goblet cells, which are characterized by mucin distending the cytoplasm and imparting a pale blue color, pseudo-goblet cells are pale pink and more similar in size to the surrounding columnar cells. Additionally, true goblet cells will stain with Alcian blue, whereas pseudo-goblet cells will not.
- Mutations in the tumor suppressor gene, TP53, are seen in patients with dysplasia. The use of the p53 immunostain may identify patients at risk of developing HGD or EAC.

References

Chandrasekhara V, Ginsberg GG. Endoscopic mucosal resection: not your father's polypectomy anymore. *Gastroenterology*. 2011;141(1):42-49.

DeMeester SR. New options for the therapy of Barrett's high-grade dysplasia and intramucosal adenocarcinoma: endoscopic mucosal resection and ablation versus vagal-sparing esophagectomy. *Ann Thorac Surg*. 2008;85(2):S747–S750.

Hu Y, Bandla S, Godfrey TE, et al. HER2 amplification, overexpression and score criteria in esophageal adenocarcinoma. *Mod Pathol*. 2011;24(7):899-907.

Kahrilas PJ. Clinical practice. Gastroesophageal reflux disease. *N Engl J Med.* 2008;359(16):1700-1707.

Lewis JT, Wang KK, Abraham SC. Muscularis mucosae duplication and the musculo-fibrous anomaly in endoscopic mucosal resections for barrett esophagus: implications for staging of adenocarcinoma. *Am J Surg Pathol.* 2008;32(4):566-571.

Meltzer CC, Luketich JD, Friedman D, et al. Whole-body FDG positron emission tomographic imaging for staging esophageal cancer comparison with computed tomography. *Clin Nucl Med.* 2000;25(11):882-887.

Mizobuchi S, Tachimori Y, Kato H, Watanabe H, Nakanishi Y, Ochiai A. Metastatic esophageal tumors from distant primary lesions: report of three esophagectomies and study of 1835 autopsy cases. *Jpn J Clin Oncol.* 1997;27(6):410-414.

Odze RD. Update on the diagnosis and treatment of Barrett esophagus and related neoplastic precursor lesions. *Arch Pathol Lab Med.* 2008;132(10):1577-1585.

Pech O, May A, Manner H, et al. Long-term efficacy and safety of endoscopic resection for patients with mucosal adenocarcinoma of the esophagus. *Gastroenterology.* 2014;146(3):652-660.e1.

Rice TW, Chen LQ, Hofstetter WL, et al. Worldwide Esophageal Cancer Collaboration: pathologic staging data. *Dis Esophagus.* 2016;29(7):724-373.

Rice TW, Gress DM, Patil DT, Hofstetter WL, Kelsen DP, Blackstone EH. Cancer of the esophagus and esophagogastric junction—major changes in the American Joint Committee on Cancer eighth edition cancer staging manual. *CA Cancer J Clin.* 2017;67(4):304-317.

Rustgi AK, El-Serag HB. Esophageal carcinoma. *N Engl J Med.* 2014;371(26):2499-2509.

Salimian KJ, Waters KM, Eze O, et al. Definition of Barrett esophagus in the United States: support for retention of a requirement for goblet cells. *Am J Surg Pathol.* 2018;42(2):264-268.

Siegel RL, Miller KD, Jemal A. Cancer statistics, 2018. *CA Cancer J Clin.* 2018;68(1):7-30.

Simchuk EJ, Low DE. Direct esophageal metastasis from a distant primary tumor is a submucosal process: a review of six cases. *Dis Esophagus.* 2001;14(3-4):247-250.

CASE 6

A 45-Year-Old Female with Dyspepsia

Phoenix D. Bell ■ Aaron R. Huber

A 45-year-old Caucasian female presents to her primary care provider with a 6-month history of dyspepsia. She admits to intermittent episodes of nausea and bloating, but denies vomiting, diarrhea, abdominal pain, and weight loss. On physical examination, the abdomen is soft, non-tender, and non-distended. Her blood pressure is 130/70 mm Hg, heart rate is 80 beats per minute, and temperature is 37.1°C (98.8°F). A complete blood count (CBC) reveals hemoglobin of 7.5 g/dL and hematocrit of 30%. Other laboratory tests and physical examination findings are unremarkable.

What should be included in the differential diagnosis for patients with dyspepsia (Box 6.1)?
The differential diagnosis for dyspepsia should include gastroesophageal reflux disease (GERD), gastritis, peptic ulcer disease, and non-ulcer dyspepsia. There are many etiologic agents that contribute to the development of GERD, including structural abnormalities, such as decreased lower esophageal sphincter tone, impaired peristalsis, and delayed gastric emptying, as well as lifestyle factors, including obesity, diet (chocolate, caffeine, citrus fruits, and spicy foods), tobacco or alcohol use, and hot beverage consumption. Patients with GERD may present with heartburn, dysphagia, regurgitation, and nocturnal cough. In contrast, patients with gastritis, either acute or chronic, most often complain of epigastric pain. The most common causes of chronic gastritis are autoimmune gastritis and *Helicobacter pylori* infection, whereas acute gastritis is associated with frequent nonsteroidal antiinflammatory drug (NSAID) use, heavy alcohol consumption, and extended hospital stays (e.g. intensive care unit). Similarly, peptic ulcer disease is also seen in patients with long-term NSAID use, *H. pylori* infection, and extended hospital stays. Additionally, peptic ulcer disease is seen in patients with Zollinger–Ellison syndrome (ZES). Patients with peptic ulcer disease may be asymptomatic, with incidentally discovered anemia on a CBC, or they may be symptomatic, most commonly complaining of abdominal pain or hematemesis. Non-ulcer dyspepsia frequently causes indigestion; however, a particular etiology cannot be identified. Ultimately, non-ulcer dyspepsia is a diagnosis of exclusion.

CLINICAL PEARL

NSAIDs work by inhibiting cyclooxygenase (COX-1 and COX-2) as well as blocking prostaglandin E2 synthesis. Prostaglandins normally lead to decreased acid production; thus with NSAID inhibition, there is increased acid production and increased risk for mucosal damage, which can lead to gastritis.

CLINICAL PEARL

Patients with ZES have a gastrinoma (gastrin-secreting tumor), most often located in the small intestine, which leads to increased levels of gastrin and gastric acid output. Patients

BOX 6.1 ■ Differential Diagnosis for Dyspepsia

GERD

Acute vs. chronic gastritis

- Acute: frequent NSAID use, heavy alcohol consumption, extended hospital stays
- Chronic: autoimmune gastritis, *H. pylori*–associated gastritis

Peptic ulcer disease

- Long-term NSAID use
- *H. pylori* infection
- ZES
- Extended hospital (intensive care unit) stay (head trauma, intubation)

Non-ulcer dyspepsia

are diagnosed with the secretin suppression test. In this test, secretin administration in patients with ZES results in an increase in gastrin levels. In contrast, in normal patients, secretin administration results in a smaller increase or a decrease in gastrin levels.

What is the best next step in the management for this patient?

Patients presenting with symptoms of dyspepsia, particularly chronic, should be referred for an upper endoscopy to evaluate the esophagus, stomach, and duodenum. During this procedure, the gastroenterologist will evaluate the gastrointestinal tract mucosa and obtain tissue biopsies for histopathologic analysis. Endoscopically, mucosal findings in GERD are often normal, yet in some cases erythema or mucosal disruption may be seen. Similarly, in gastritis, endoscopy can range from unremarkable to erythematous, hemorrhagic, or erosive. Gastritis may also demonstrate a "varioliform" pattern, demonstrated by a nodular configuration with central erosions. Autoimmune gastritis is suspected on endoscopy when there is loss of the rugal folds in the antrum.

Case Point 6.1

During endoscopy, the gastroenterologist notes mild erythema in the stomach body and an atrophic-appearing antrum. Microscopically, the antral biopsy shows a superficial band of chronic lymphoplasmacytic inflammation within the lamina propria (Fig. 6.1). Upon further examination, slender curved rods are distributed throughout the epithelium and crypts (Fig. 6.2).

Based on the clinical history and microscopic findings, what is the most likely diagnosis?

The patient is presenting with dyspepsia, endoscopy shows mucosal flattening within the antrum, and rod-shaped bacteria are identified on histology. These findings support the diagnosis of *H. pylori*–associated chronic gastritis. *H. pylori* is a gram-negative bacterium that colonizes the gastric mucosa, particularly within the antrum. Microscopically, at low magnification, there is a dense lymphoplasmacytic infiltrate within the superficial lamina propria. At higher magnification, slender rods, sometimes referred to as "seagull-shaped," are seen within the mucin just above the epithelium or within the gastric crypts. Most of the time this diagnosis can be made on an H&E-stained slide, though there are *H. pylori* immunostains that can be used to highlight the presence of these organisms (Fig. 6.3). In addition to *H. pylori*, *H. heilmannii* may also result in identical clinical and histologic features; however, these bacteria are usually corkscrew-shaped and longer. If no microorganisms are identified, the main differential to consider is autoimmune atrophic gastritis. Autoimmune gastritis is due to antibodies against the H^+/K^+ ATPase on

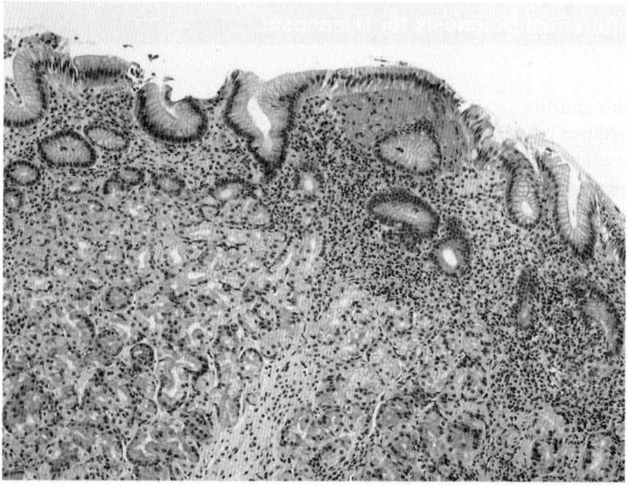

Fig. 6.1 Biopsy of the gastric antrum (H&E, original magnification 100x).

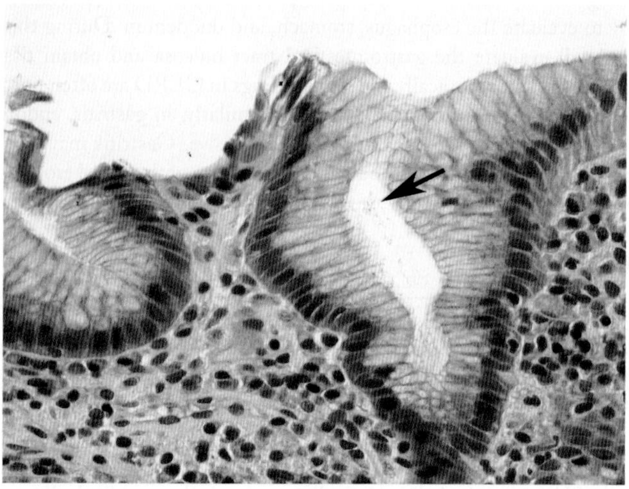

Fig. 6.2 Biopsy of the gastric antrum, arrow demonstrates *Helicobacter pylori* organisms (H&E, original magnification 400x).

parietal cells and antibodies against intrinsic factor, which leads to parietal cell loss and decreased hydrochloric acid production. This causes increased gastrin production by G cells in the antrum, resulting in enterochromaffin-like cell hyperplasia and neuroendocrine proliferation. Endoscopically, this is also seen as flattened mucosa within the antrum. Frequently, patients present with anemia, whereas some may present with vitamin B12 deficiency due to antibodies against intrinsic factor. Histologically, autoimmune gastritis is seen as lymphoplasmacytic infiltration in the lamina propria along with parietal cell loss within the fundus, G cell hyperplasia in the antrum, and possibly intestinal metaplasia.

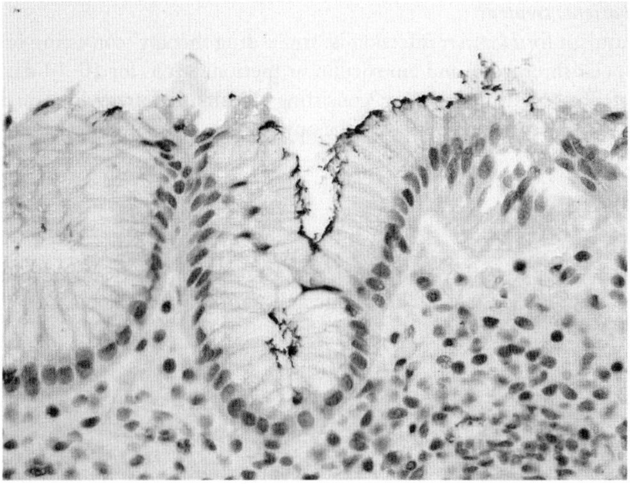

Fig. 6.3 Biopsy of the gastric antrum with *Helicobacter pylori* immunostain highlighting. *H. pylori* organisms in brown (H&E, original magnification 400x).

CLINICAL PEARL

H. pylori colonizes the gastric mucosa by hydrolyzing urea into ammonia, which neutralizes acid and allows the organism to thrive within the antrum.

CLINICAL PEARL

Intrinsic factor is produced by the parietal cells in the stomach and binds to B12 in the duodenum. This complex is absorbed in the terminal ileum. Antibodies against intrinsic factor cause decreased formation of the intrinsic factor-B12 complex, which leads to decreased B12 absorption and ultimately B12 deficiency.

What is the most common clinical manifestation of* H. pylori *infection?

H. pylori is present in greater than half of the world's population and is more common in developing and resource-poor countries than in developed countries. Despite its high prevalence, the majority of patients with *H. pylori* infection are asymptomatic. Of those with symptoms, presentation may include bloating, nausea, abdominal pain, or vomiting.

What are the possible consequences of an untreated* H. pylori *infection?

Following treatment, around 90% of patients with *H. pylori* achieve eradication of disease; however, 10%–20% of patients may develop peptic ulcer disease and 1%–2% may develop gastric adenocarcinoma. These patients are also at risk of developing mucosal-associated lymphoid tissue (MALT) lymphoma.

CLINICAL PEARL

Approximately 20%–50% of patients with a gastric MALT lymphoma will have the t(11;18)(q21;q21) / API2-MLT fusion, which is associated with persistent H. pylori gastritis or disease recurrence after eradication therapy.

How are these patients treated?

The current treatment for *H. pylori* infection is "triple-drug therapy" consisting of a proton pump inhibitor (PPI), clarithromycin, and amoxicillin or metronidazole for 10–14 days. Due to clarithromycin resistance, "quadruple therapy" consisting of bismuth, tetracycline, metronidazole, and a PPI for 10–14 days may be an alternative therapy.

CLINICAL PEARL

PPIs impede the H^+/K^+ ATPase pump on the apical surface of the parietal cell membrane, which decreases H^+ production into the stomach lumen, ultimately decreasing the formation of hydrochloric acid.

How is eradication of disease assessed?

Eradication of *H. pylori* is assessed using the stool antigen test or urea breath test. The stool antigen test assesses the presence of anti-*Helicobacter* antibodies and has a sensitivity and specificity of >92%. During the urea breath test, patients ingest ^{14}C-labeled or ^{13}C-labeled urea; if *H. pylori* is still present, the urease releases the label, which is compared with a baseline value. This test has a sensitivity and specificity of >95%.

Case Point 6.2

The patient is instructed to start triple-drug therapy and to follow up 1 month after finishing the regimen. Unfortunately, the patient is lost to follow-up. After 15 years, she presents to the emergency department with severe abdominal pain. A computed tomography scan of the abdomen is performed, which reveals a concerning lesion in the stomach. Per the patient, she never completed triple-drug therapy for her history of *H. pylori*. She is sent for endoscopy, which reveals a 2.5-cm mass in the gastric antrum. A biopsy of the mass is taken, which shows irregular glands within the submucosa that are lined by cells with a moderate amount of eosinophilic cytoplasm and pleomorphic nuclei. (Figs. 6.4A and 6.4B).

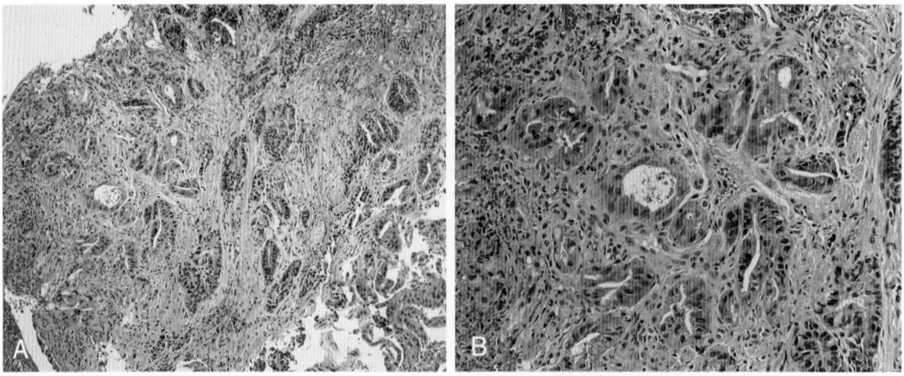

Fig. 6.4 Biopsy of the gastric antral mass (H&E, original magnification x40).

TABLE 6.1 ■ **Histologic Classification of Gastric Adenocarcinoma**

Lauren Classification	WHO Classification
Intestinal-type	Papillary, tubular, mucinous
Diffuse-type	Poorly cohesive carcinomas, including signet-ring cell carcinoma

What is the diagnosis?
Intestinal-type gastric adenocarcinoma.

What is the difference between intestinal- and diffuse-type gastric adenocarcinoma?
Histologically, gastric adenocarcinoma is most commonly classified using the Lauren or WHO classification schemes (Table 6.1). In terms of the Lauren classification, gastric cancer is usually categorized into intestinal or diffuse type. *H. pylori* is most commonly associated with intestinal-type gastric adenocarcinoma. On gross examination, these lesions may be crater-like with heaped-up edges or polypoid. Histologically, they are composed of variably sized glands with columnar and mucinous cells. In contrast, the diffuse-type gastric adenocarcinoma is grossly characterized by a diffusely thickened wall, particularly in the pre-pyloric region, deemed the "linitis plastica" appearance (Fig. 6.5). Histologically, single cells infiltrate the deeper layers of the stomach wall. This type is most commonly associated with "signet-ring cells," which show intracytoplasmic mucin and eccentrically placed nuclei (Fig. 6.6). In terms of prognosis, intestinal type is more favorable than diffuse type, since the diffuse type involves infiltration of single cells, which enables the cancer to escape early detection. With rapid advancements in molecular techniques, researchers have started classifying gastric cancer into molecular subtypes. For example, The Cancer Genome Atlas (TCGA) separates gastric cancer into the following molecular

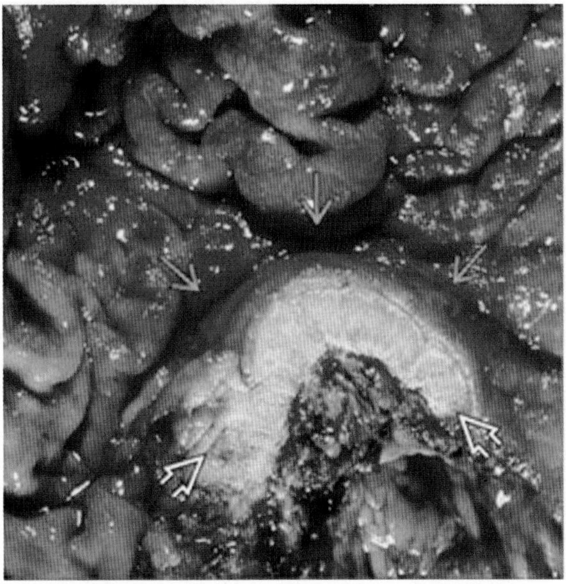

Fig. 6.5 Example of the linitis plastica appearance of diffuse-type gastric cancer. (From *ExpertPath*. Copyright Elsevier).

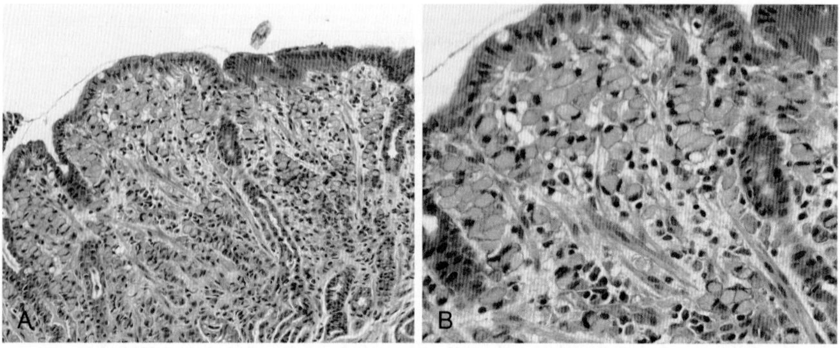

Fig. 6.6 Stomach biopsy. (A) Diffuse-type (signet-ring cell) gastric adenocarcinoma (original magnification 200x). (B) Diffuse-type (signet-ring cell) gastric adenocarcinoma (original magnification 400x).

subtypes: (1) Epstein–Barr virus (EBV)-associated, (2) microsatellite unstable, (3) genomically stable, and (4) chromosomal unstable. Currently, these genomic classifications are not incorporated into staging manuals; however, it is likely that they will be in the future.

CLINICAL PEARL

The diffuse-type gastric adenocarcinoma, particularly the signet-ring variant of diffuse type, may metastasize to the bilateral ovaries, which is known as "Krukenberg tumor." Patients with this type of metastasis have a poor prognosis.

CLINICAL PEARL

Approximately 9% of gastric cancers are related to EBV. EBV is a member of the herpes virus family and can be detected in tissue using EBV-encoded RNA. This subtype of gastric cancer is associated with PIK3CA mutations, as well as PD-L1 overexpression, and is associated with a better prognosis.

How should this patient be treated?

Treatment options for gastric cancer include surgical resection, chemoradiation, and superficial excision, depending upon the extent of disease. Unfortunately, many patients with gastric cancer present with advanced disease and are thus treated with gastrectomy. Tumors located in the upper two-thirds of the stomach often receive total gastrectomies, whereas tumors located in the distal one-third of the stomach undergo partial gastrectomies. Patients are not surgical candidates if there is proven metastatic disease, major vascular invasion, or the patient's medical history contradicts surgery. In patients with more superficial disease, newer treatment modalities include endoscopic mucosal resection and endoscopic submucosal dissection. These techniques are less invasive options to surgically excise the lesion. Additionally, some neoadjuvant, perioperative, and adjuvant chemoradiotherapy studies have showed an improved prognosis following their application; however, currently there are no strict guidelines for chemoradiotherapy administration in gastric cancer patients. More recently, trastuzumab and ramucirumab have been used in conjunction with chemotherapy in patients with advanced gastric cancer.

This patient underwent neoadjuvant chemotherapy followed by a subtotal gastrectomy. The resection specimen showed a fairly well-circumscribed polypoid lesion in the antrum (Fig. 6.7). Microscopically, the tumor was moderately differentiated and invaded the muscularis propria (Fig. 6.8). As there was extensive residual cancer, the treatment effect had a poor response.

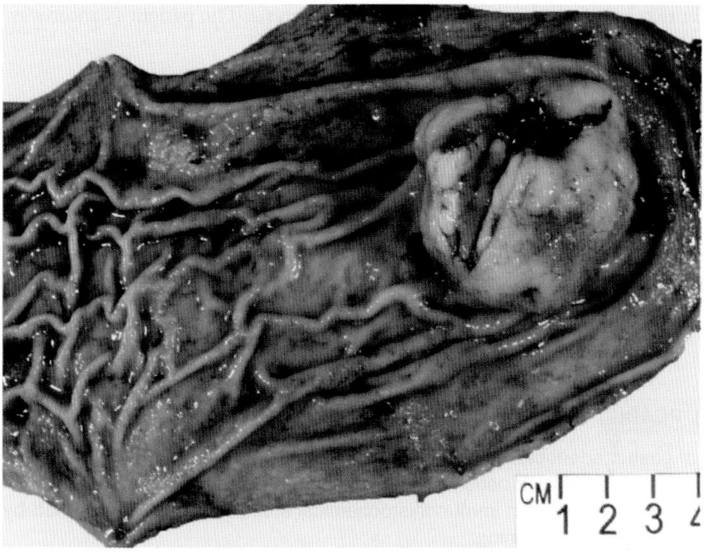

Fig. 6.7 Partial gastrectomy revealing a polypoid mass in the antrum.

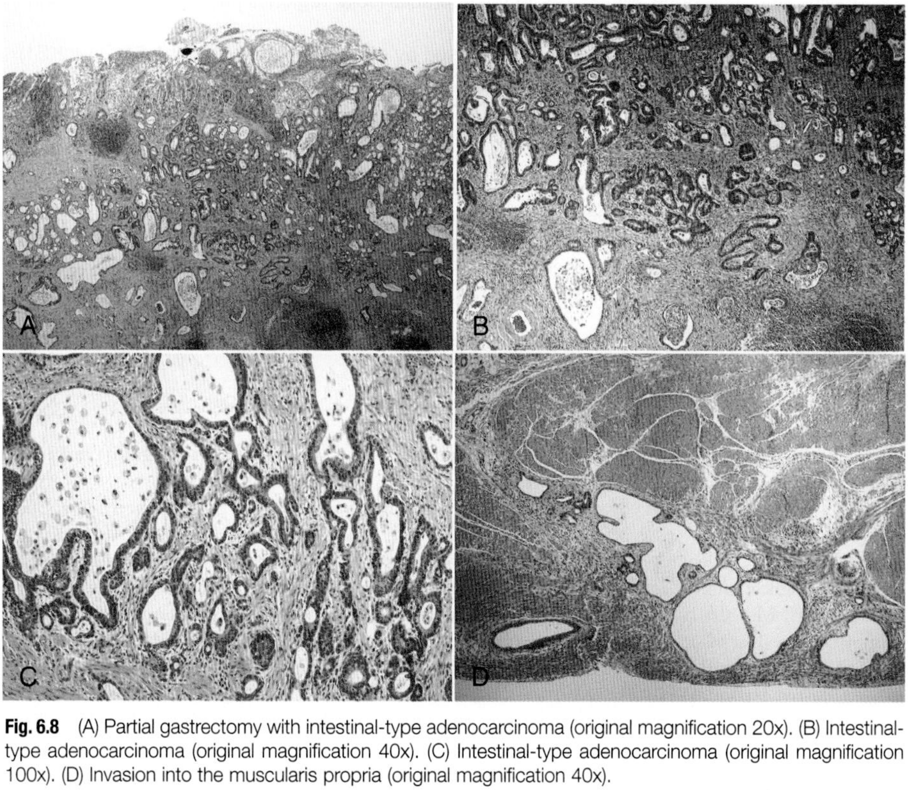

Fig. 6.8 (A) Partial gastrectomy with intestinal-type adenocarcinoma (original magnification 20x). (B) Intestinal-type adenocarcinoma (original magnification 40x). (C) Intestinal-type adenocarcinoma (original magnification 100x). (D) Invasion into the muscularis propria (original magnification 40x).

Additionally, two lymph nodes were positive for metastasis. The patient's cancer was thus staged as ypT2N1. Currently she is disease-free.

What is the prognosis?

Approximately 95% of gastric cancers are adenocarcinoma. The prognosis depends upon the extent of disease. Patients who present with early disease, limited to the mucosa and submucosa, are less likely to have lymph node involvement, and their 5-year survival rate is more favorable, around 80%–90%. As gastric adenocarcinoma progresses, involving the subserosal connective tissue, serosa, or adjacent organs, the 5-year survival rate progressively declines. The 5-year survival rate for patients with stage 4 (metastatic) disease is 15%–20%. For this patient, her cancer invaded the muscularis propria, but not into the serosa; thus she has an intermediate prognosis.

CLINICAL PEARL

A subset of gastric adenocarcinomas is HER2+. Trastuzumab is a HER2 inhibitor, which has shown to increase survival in patients with HER2+ gastric cancer (about 20%). HER2 expression is assessed using an immunohistochemical stain, with positivity defined by strong basolateral membranous staining.

BEYOND THE PEARLS

- The most common sites of metastasis from a primary gastric cancer are the liver, peritoneal cavity, lung, and bone. Metastasis to the supraclavicular region is known as "Troisier sign" or "Virchow node."
- Peutz–Jeghers syndrome is most often caused by germline mutations in the STK11 (LKB1) gene, which results in mucocutaneous pigmentation and hamartomatous polyps throughout the gastrointestinal tract. In addition to their increased risk of developing gastric adenocarcinoma, these patients are at higher risk of developing extra-gastrointestinal cancers; thus they must be followed closely.
- Hereditary diffuse gastric cancer is an autosomal dominant condition in which individuals are at an increased risk of developing diffuse-type gastric adenocarcinoma. Approximately 30%–40% of these patients have mutations in CDH1, which encodes for E-cadherin. These patients are also at increased risk of developing lobular breast carcinoma and signet-ring cell carcinoma of the colon.

References

Alfarouk KO, Bashir AHH, Aljarbou AN, et al. The possible role of *Helicobacter pylori* in gastric cancer and its management. *Front Oncol.* 2019;9:75.

Anderson ID, MacIntyre IM. Symptomatic outcome following resection of gastric cancer. *Surg Oncol.* 1995;4(1):35-40.

Arslan N, Yılmaz Ö, Demiray-Gürbüz E. Importance of antimicrobial susceptibility testing for the management of eradication in *Helicobacter pylori* infection. *World J Gastroenterol.* 2017;23(16):2854-2869.

Birkman EM, Mansuri N, Kurki S, et al. Gastric cancer: immunohistochemical classification of molecular subtypes and their association with clinicopathological characteristics. *Virchows Arch.* 2018;472(3):369-382.

Bosman FT, Carneiro F, Hruban RH, Theise ND, eds. *WHO Classification of Tumours of the Digestive System.* Geneva, Switzerland: WHO Press; 2010.

Ciesla MC. Atlas of gastrointestinal endoscopy and endoscopic biopsies. *Arch Pathol Lab Med.* 2000; 124(12):1857.

Crowe SE. *Helicobacter pylori* infection. *N Engl J Med.* 2019;380(12):1158-1165.
Cunningham D, Allum WH, Stenning SP, et al. Perioperative chemotherapy versus surgery alone for resectable gastroesophageal cancer. *N Engl J Med.* 2006;355(1):11-20.
Hawkey CJ. Nonsteroidal anti-inflammatory drug gastropathy. *Gastroenterology.* 2000;119(2):521-535.
Kamboj AK, Cotter TG, Oxentenko AS. *Helicobacter pylori*: the past, present, and future in management. *Mayo Clin Proc.* 2017;92(4):599-604.
Kim ST, Cristescu R, Bass AJ, et al. Comprehensive molecular characterization of clinical responses to PD-1 inhibition in metastatic gastric cancer. *Nat Med.* 2018;24(9):1449-1458.
Kwon CH, Kim YK, Lee S, et al. Gastric poorly cohesive carcinoma: a correlative study of mutational signatures and prognostic significance based on histopathological subtypes. *Histopathology.* 2018;72(4):556-568.
Lauren P. The two histological main types of gastric carcinoma: diffuse and so-called intestinal-type carcinoma. An attempt at a histo-clinical classification. *Acta Pathol Microbiol Scand.* 1965;64:31-49.
Liu H, Ye H, Ruskone-Fourmestraux A, et al. T(11;18) is a marker for all stage gastric MALT lymphomas that will not respond to *H. pylori* eradication. *Gastroenterology.* 2002;122(5):1286-1294.
Macdonald JS, Smalley SR, Benedetti J, et al. Chemoradiotherapy after surgery compared with surgery alone for adenocarcinoma of the stomach or gastroesophageal junction. *N Engl J Med.* 2001;345(10):725-730.
Mentis AA, Dardiotis E. *Helicobacter pylori* eradication for metachronous gastric cancer: an unsuitable methodology impeding broader clinical usage. *Front Oncol.* 2019;9:90.
Metz DC. Diagnosis of the Zollinger–Ellison syndrome. *Clin Gastroenterol Hepatol.* 2012;10(2):126-130.
Nakamura S, Matsumoto T, Nakamura S, et al. Chromosomal translocation t(11;18)(q21;q21) in gastrointestinal mucosa associated lymphoid tissue lymphoma. *J Clin Pathol.* 2003;56(1):36-42.
Nakamura T, Seto M, Tajika M, et al. Clinical features and prognosis of gastric MALT lymphoma with special reference to responsiveness to *H. pylori* eradication and API2-MALT1 status. *Am J Gastroenterol.* 2008;103(1):62-70.
Sinha M, Gautam L, Shukla PK, Kaur P, Sharma S, Singh TP. Current perspectives in NSAID-induced gastropathy. *Mediators Inflamm.* 2013;2013:258209.
Wanebo HJ, Kennedy BJ, Chmiel J, Steele Jr G, Winchester D, Osteen R. Cancer of the stomach. A patient care study by the American College of Surgeons. *Ann Surg.* 1993;218(5):583-592.
Wolfe MM, Jensen RT. Zollinger-Ellison syndrome. Current concepts in diagnosis and management. *N Engl J Med.* 1987;317(19):1200-1209.
Wu CW, Chiou JM, Ko FS, et al. Quality of life after curative gastrectomy for gastric cancer in a randomised controlled trial. *Br J Cancer.* 2008;98(1):54-59.
Yakirevich E, Resnick MB. Pathology of gastric cancer and its precursor lesions. *Gastroenterol Clin North Am.* 2013;42(2):261-284.

CASE 7

A 52-Year-Old Woman with an Incidental Terminal Ileum Mass

Phoenix D. Bell ■ Aaron R. Huber

A 52-year-old female with no significant past medical history is referred by her primary care provider for a screening colonoscopy. Physical examination reveals blood pressure of 140/74 mm Hg, heart rate of 62 beats per minute, temperature of 36.7°C (98.1°F), and respiratory rate of 16 breaths per minute. There are no signs of abdominal distension, tenderness to palpation, rebound, or guarding, and bowel sounds are normal. The patient reports intermittent diarrhea and hematochezia, but denies abdominal pain, constipation, nausea, vomiting, fever, and weight loss. Complete blood count and serum chemistries are within normal limits. Endoscopic evaluation reveals a 1-cm submucosal lesion within the terminal ileum. A biopsy of the lesion is taken.

What is the differential diagnosis for a submucosal mass in the small intestine?

The differential diagnosis for a submucosal mass in the small intestine includes leiomyoma, gastrointestinal stromal tumor (GIST), neuroendocrine tumor (NET), gangliocytic paraganglioma, adenocarcinoma, and lymphoma. A leiomyoma is a smooth muscle neoplasm arising from either the muscularis mucosae or muscularis propria. Histologically, it is characterized by a proliferation of spindle cells that have elongated nuclei with blunted ends, often termed "cigar-shaped," with abundant eosinophilic cytoplasm. These cells will stain positively for desmin and smooth muscle actin. A GIST is most commonly found in the stomach; however, it can also be seen throughout the gastrointestinal tract. Microscopically, it is described by a proliferation of bland spindle cells with eosinophilic cytoplasm, arranged in short fascicles. Often, cells will show paranuclear vacuoles. These cells will stain positively for discovered on GIST 1 (DOG1) and *c-Kit* (CD117). A NET arises from neuroendocrine cells and is most often seen as groups of cells arranged in nests or trabeculae, yet it may also form acini or glands. The cells are monotonous and have round to ovoid nuclei with moderate eosinophilic cytoplasm, as well as finely granular chromatin with a "salt-and-pepper" appearance. They stain positively for chromogranin and synaptophysin. Gangliocytic paraganlgiomas are submucosal tumors most commonly found in the second portion of the duodenum. They are composed of endocrine cells, Schwann cells, and ganglion cells in variable proportions, which is seen in their triphasic histologic appearance. Small intestine adenocarcinoma is uncommon, and arises from preexisting dysplasia. These tumors occur more commonly in certain settings, namely Crohn's disease, celiac disease, and polyposis syndromes including familial adenomatous polyposis (FAP), Lynch syndrome, Peutz–Jeghers syndrome, and neurofibromatosis type 1 (NF1). Microscopically, adenocarcinoma appears as irregular glands surrounded by a desmoplastic stroma. The glandular cells are pleomorphic and have lost their polarity, and there may be necrosis within the lumen. Lastly, lymphoma is characterized by the proliferation of malignant lymphocytes within the submucosa. The lymphocytes are discohesive and often infiltrate up into the epithelium.

CLINICAL PEARL

Lynch syndrome is the most common hereditary colorectal cancer syndrome, caused by germline mutations in DNA mismatch repair genes (MLH1, MSH2, PMS2, and MSH6). Lynch syndrome also has a risk of several other extra-colonic malignancies including the endometrium, ovaries, stomach, small intestine, hepatobiliary tract, urinary tract, and central nervous system.

FAP is the second most common hereditary colorectal cancer syndrome and is caused by a germline mutation in the APC gene, which is a tumor suppressor gene on chromosome 5q21-22 associated with the WNT signaling pathway. FAP patients have 100% lifetime risk of colon cancer without colectomy. Duodenal adenocarcinoma is the most common extra-colonic cancer in FAP patients and is a major cause of mortality.

Case Point 7.1

The biopsy reveals well-circumscribed nests of cells infiltrating the terminal ileum lamina propria (Fig. 7.1A). The nests are composed of a monotonous population of round cells with eosinophilic cytoplasm, evenly distributed chromatin, and inconspicuous nucleoli (Fig. 7.1B). No mitotic figures are identified. The neoplastic cells stain positively for chromogranin and synaptophysin (Fig. 7.2A–B).

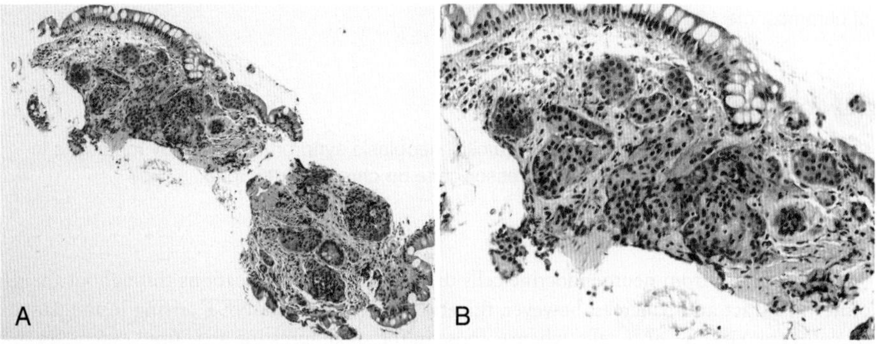

Fig. 7.1 (A) Terminal ileum biopsy low power (H&E, 100x). (B) Terminal ileum biopsy higher power (H&E, 200x).

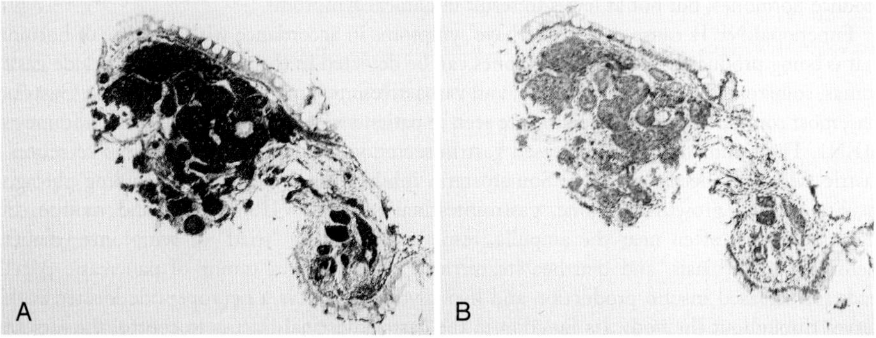

Fig. 7.2 (A) Terminal ileum biopsy with immunostain (chromogranin, 100x). (B) Terminal ileum biopsy with immunostain (synaptophysin, 100x).

What is the diagnosis?

The incidental finding of a small terminal ileal mass with the aforementioned microscopic findings is diagnostic of a small intestine NET. Most NETs are sporadic; however, some individuals are more prone to develop these tumors, including patients with multiple endocrine neoplasia type 1 (MEN1), NF1, von Hippel–Lindau syndrome, and tuberous sclerosis. The majority of gastrointestinal NETs are found in the small intestine, most commonly the terminal ileum, and approximately 30% of these are multifocal. NETs are discovered in older patients, around 60 years of age, as an incidental finding; however, patients with underlying obstruction or acute ischemia may present with abdominal pain. Around 50% of patients present with liver metastasis. Endoscopically, NETs are discreet submucosal nodules, occasionally with minimal overlying mucosal erosion. As mentioned, they are histologically characterized by nests of monotonous cells with eosinophilic cytoplasm and positive staining for synaptophysin, chromogranin, and CD56.

CLINICAL PEARL

NETs are also found in other locations throughout the body including the lungs (carcinoid, atypical carcinoid, small cell carcinoma, large cell carcinoma), thyroid (medullary carcinoma), adrenal gland (pheochromocytoma), and skin (Merkel cell carcinoma).

CLINICAL PEARL

The most common molecular alteration found in small intestine NETs is loss of heterozygosity of chromosome 18.

CLINICAL PEARL

Von Hippel–Lindau syndrome is a rare familial neoplasia syndrome caused by mutations in the VHL gene, which is a tumor suppressor gene on chromosome 3p25.

NET can arise from neuroendocrine cells distributed in many locations throughout the gastrointestinal tract and pancreas; however, the etiology is unknown. NET arising in the pancreas may come from α-, β-, or δ-cells, whereas those in the small intestine arise from enterochromaffin-like cells. These tumors can be classified as functional or nonfunctional based upon whether or not they are actively producing hormones. Of note, even those that are nonfunctional can still produce hormones, but not at levels to result in clinical symptoms.

Functional NETs cause patients to have symptoms in accordance with the type of hormone that is being produced, and these hormones can be detected in the serum. These include gastrinomas, somatostatinomas, insulinomas, and vasoactive intestinal peptide (VIPomas). Gastrinomas, most common in the duodenum, are seen in patients with Zollinger–Ellison Syndrome and MEN1. The tumor results in increased gastrin secretion, which leads to increased secretion of gastric acid, and ulcer formation. Somatostatin inhibits many hormones including glucagon, insulin, gastrin, growth hormone, gastrointestinal peptide, VIP, secretin, and motilin. Somatostatinomas, often near the ampulla, result in the classic "triad" of symptoms—diabetes mellitus, cholelithiasis, and diarrhea/steatorrhea. Insulinoma, a tumor of pancreatic β-cells, leads to increased insulin production and hypoglycemia. VIP is a neuropeptide located within nerves throughout the body. Its function in the gastrointestinal tract is to control the secretion of water and electrolytes into the gut lumen and to induce smooth muscle relaxation. Most VIPomas are located in the pancreas and lead to watery diarrhea, hypokalemia, and achlorhydria.

CLINICAL PEARL

MEN1 is an autosomal dominant condition characterized by pituitary gland tumors, pancreatic NET, and parathyroid tumors.

CLINICAL PEARL

The synthesis of insulin results in the production of C-peptide and insulin; thus patients with an insulinoma will have elevated levels of both C-peptide and insulin. In contrast, patients with exogenous insulin administration only have increased insulin.

Less than 10% of NETs of the small intestine result in carcinoid syndrome. Most often, carcinoid syndrome occurs when small intestine NETs metastasize to the liver. The tumors release biologically active amines and peptides that do not get broken down by the liver; instead, they enter systemic circulation. Specifically, the release of products of serotonin and kinins into the bloodstream causes patients to present with diarrhea, flushing, bronchospasms, and palpitations. In more severe cases, patients develop endocardial fibrosis of the right side of the heart, including the tricuspid valve, which can lead to heart failure.

What are the next steps in the management for this patient?

The patient should have radiologic imaging performed as NETs have the potential to metastasize. Imaging, including a computed tomography scan and an octreotide scan, assesses the extent of disease and the presence of metastasis.

CLINICAL PEARL

During an octreotide scan, a patient with a suspected NET is injected with octreotide. In the presence of a NET, the octreotide will bind to somatostatin receptors on the tumor and result in an area of enhancement on imaging.

How should this patient be treated?

Identification of a mass on radiology will most often lead to surgical resection of the portion of the small bowel containing the mass. In this patient's case, she should initially be sent for imaging and then a surgical consult. In symptomatic patients, symptomatic relief may be achieved with the use of somatostatin analogs, such as octreotide and lanreotide. Most patients with localized disease are treated with surgical resection followed by surveillance. Other treatment options, particularly for patients with metastasis, include everolimus (mTOR inhibitor) and sunitinib (tyrosine kinase inhibitor).

CLINICAL PEARL

In NET, the PI3K/Akt/mTOR pathway is activated by IGF-1. This leads to a signaling cascade that activates PI3K, AKT, and mTOR, which eventually results in neuroendocrine cell growth.

Case Point 7.2

A follow-up computed tomography scan of the abdomen is performed, which reveals mild wall thickening of the terminal ileum measuring up to 8 mm. An octreotide scan shows focal uptake in the terminal ileum with no evidence of metastatic spread of disease. The patient undergoes a right hemicolectomy.

Gross examination of the specimen shows a tan-brown polypoid lesion in the terminal ileum (circled) (Fig. 7.3). Microscopic assessment shows cells arranged in nests and trabeculae infiltrating the mucosa and submucosa (Fig. 7.4A). In some areas, they are arranged as pseudorosettes (Fig. 7.4B). The cells are monotonous with round nuclei, eosinophilic cytoplasm, and finely speckled chromatin (Fig. 7.4C). The mitotic rate is <2 mitoses/2 mm^2, the Ki-67 is <3%, and there is no lymph node metastasis. These findings are consistent with the previous biopsy findings of a NET.

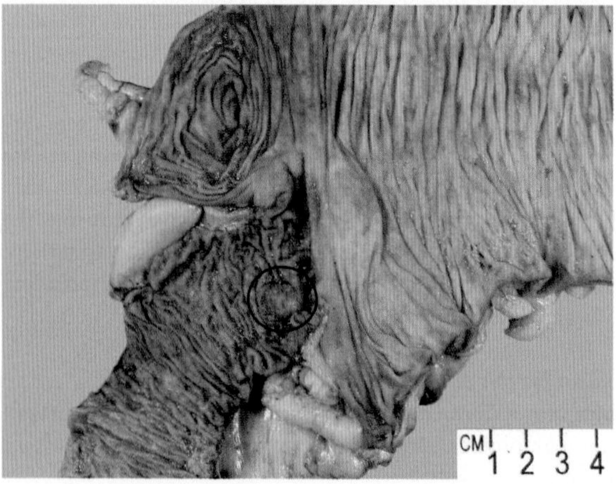

Fig. 7.3 Gross examination, right hemicolectomy specimen with a mass in the terminal ileum (circled).

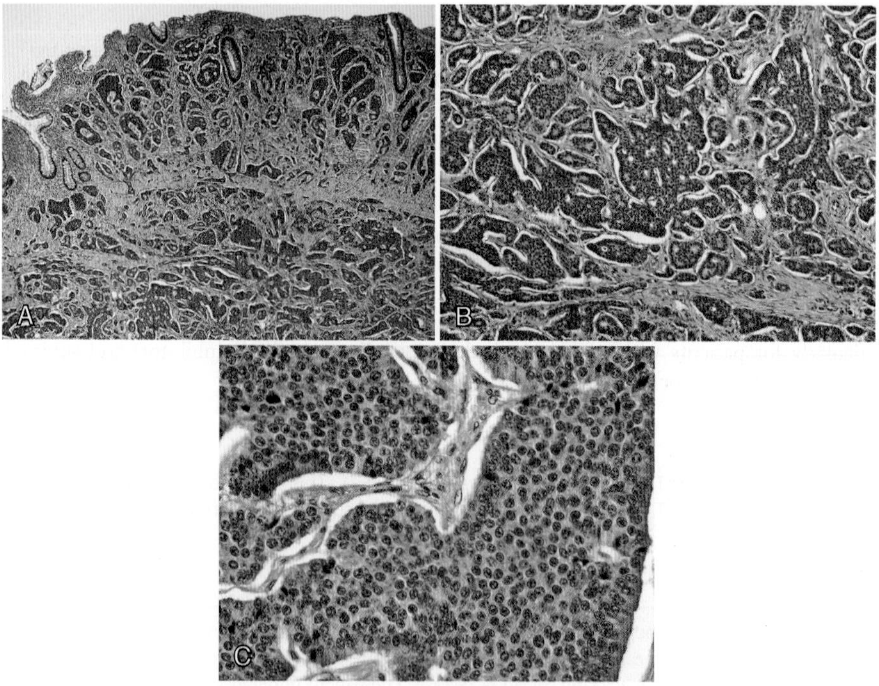

Fig. 7.4 (A) Neuroendocrine tumor (NET) terminal ileum low power (H&E, 40x). (B) NET terminal ileum higher power (H&E, 100x). (C) NET terminal ileum higher power (H&E, 400x).

TABLE 7.1 ■ **Grading of Gastrointestinal Neuroendocrine Tumors (WHO 2019)**

	Grade	Mitotic Rate (mitoses/2 mm^2)	Ki-67 index (%)
Well Differentiated			
G1	Low	<2	<3
G2	Intermediate	2–20	3–20
G3	High	>20	>20
Poorly Differentiated			
Small cell carcinoma Large cell carcinoma	High	>20	>20

How is a NET graded pathologically? (Table 7.1)

Recently, the World Health Organization (WHO) published new criteria for grading NETs of the small intestine, which is based on tumor differentiation, mitotic rate, and Ki-67 index. The well differentiated NET are graded as follows: G1 (low grade), G2 (intermediate grade), and G3 (high grade). G1 tumors have a mitotic rate <2 mitoses/2 mm^2 and a Ki-67 index of <3%. G2 tumors have a mitotic rate of 2–20 mitoses/2 mm^2 and a Ki-67 of index 3%–20%. G3 tumors have a mitotic rate of >20 mitoses/2 mm^2 and a Ki-67 index of >20%.

The poorly differentiated tumors are designated as neuroendocrine carcinomas, either small cell or large cell type. They are both high-grade tumors with a mitotic rate of >20 mitoses/2 mm^2 and a Ki-67 index of >20%. In addition to increased mitotic activity, neuroendocrine carcinomas are more likely to show necrosis and lymphovascular invasion. They are aggressive tumors with a poor prognosis.

What is this patient's prognosis?

The prognosis for NET is variable, currently best predicted by the grade and stage of the tumor. As mentioned previously, grade is dependent upon the mitotic activity and proliferation index. Well-differentiated tumors with lower mitotic counts and proliferation indices have a better prognosis than well-differentiated tumors with higher mitoses and Ki-67. With regard to stage, localized NETs have a better prognosis than NETs with lymph node or distant metastasis (5-year survival rate of 70%–100% and 35%–60%, respectively). The small cell– and large cell–type neuroendocrine carcinomas, with the poorly differentiated morphology, high mitotic rate, and elevated proliferation index, have a worse prognosis than well-differentiated tumors. Of note, nonfunctioning NETs tend to have a better prognosis than functioning NETs.

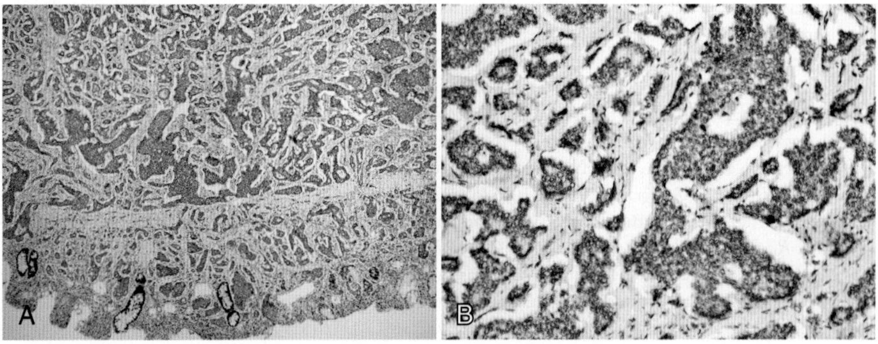

Fig. 7.5 (A) Neuroendocrine tumor (NET) terminal ileum immunostain for proliferation index, low power (Ki-67 100x). (B) NET terminal ileum immunostain for proliferation index, high power (Ki-67, 200x).

Case Point 7.3

This patient has a NET with a mitotic rate of <2 mitoses/2 mm^2 and a Ki-67 index of $<3\%$ (Fig. 7.5A–B); thus, it is graded as a well-differentiated (G1) NET and has a fairly good prognosis. The patient is currently being managed with surveillance. She reports occasional diarrhea/urgency, but is otherwise asymptomatic. She is instructed to report back yearly for surveillance scans and to report if she develops any symptoms.

BEYOND THE PEARLS

- The incidence of gastrointestinal NET is increasing, particularly those of the stomach and rectum, as detection methods have improved.
- In some patients, detection of chromogranin A or serotonin in the serum, as well as 5-hydroxyindole acetic acid (5-HIAA) (a metabolic of serotonin) in the urine, can aid in the diagnosis of gastrointestinal NET.
- A newer functional imaging technique for well-differentiated NETs is the ^{8}Ga tetraazacyclododecanetetraacetic acid–DPhe1-Tyr3-octreotate (DOTATATE) PET/CT that is preferred for initial diagnosis, selection of candidates for peptide receptor radionuclide therapy, and localization of tumors with an unknown primary site.
- (MiNENs) are rare gastrointestinal tumors that can be found throughout the gastrointestinal tract, most commonly in the pancreas. They are composed of two populations: one neuroendocrine population and one non-neuroendocrine population. In a resection specimen, each population must make up at least 30% of the neoplasm. In the small intestine, the most common type of MiNEN is a mixed adenocarcinoma-NEC.

References

Banck MS, Kanwar R, Kulkarni AA, et al. The genomic landscape of small intestine neuroendocrine tumors. *J Clin Invest.* 2013;123(6):2502-2508.

Caplin ME, Pavel M, Ćwikła JB, et al. Lanreotide in metastatic enteropancreatic neuroendocrine tumors. *N Engl J Med.* 2014;371(3):224-233.

Frilling A, Modlin IM, Kidd M, et al. Recommendations for management of patients with neuroendocrine liver metastasis. *Lancet Oncol.* 2014;15(1):e8-e21.

Glazer ES, Tseng JF, Al-Refaie W, et al. Long-term survival after surgical management of neuroendocrine hepatic metastasis. *HPB (Oxford).* 2010;12(6):427-433.

Grin A, Streutker CJ. Neuroendocrine tumors of the luminal gastrointestinal tract. *Arch Pathol Lab Med.* 2015;139(6):750-756.

Kanth P, Grimmett J, Champine M, Burt R, Samadder NJ. Hereditary colorectal polyposis and cancer syndromes: a primer on diagnosis and management. *Am J Gastroenterol.* 2017;112(10):1509-1525.

Kim JY, Hong SM. Recent updates on neuroendocrine tumors from the gastrointestinal and pancreatobiliary tracts. *Arch Pathol Lab Med.* 2016;140(5):437-448.

Nagtegaal ID, Odze RD, Klimstra D, et al. *WHO Classification of Tumours. Digestive System Tumours.* 5th ed. Vol. 1. Lyon, France: International Agency for Research on Cancer; 2019.

Sanli Y, Garg I, Kandathil A, et al. Neuroendocrine tumor diagnosis and management: ^{68}Ga-DOTATATE PET/CT. *AJR Am J Roentgenol.* 2018;211(2):267-277.

Shanbhogue KP, Hoch M, Fatterpaker G, Chandarana H. von Hippel-Lindau disease: review of genetics and imaging. *Radiol Clin North Am.* 2016;54(3):409-422.

Tang LH, Gonen M, Hedvat C, Modlin IM, Klimstra DS. Objective quantification of the Ki67 proliferative index in neuroendocrine tumors of the gastroenteropancreatic system: a comparison of digital image analysis with manual methods. *Am J Surg Pathol.* 2012;36(12):1761-1770.

von Wichert G, Jehle PM, Hoeflich A, et al. Insulin-like growth factor-I is an autocrine regulator of chromogranin A secretion and growth in human neuroendocrine tumor cells. *Cancer Res.* 2000;60(16):4573-4581.

Wang GG, Yao JC, Worah S, et al. Comparison of genetic alterations in neuroendocrine tumors: frequent loss of chromosome 18 in ileal carcinoid tumors. *Mod Pathol.* 2005;18(8):1079-1087.

Yao JC, Fazio N, Singh S, et al. Everolimus for the treatment of advanced, non-functional neuroendocrine tumours of the lung or gastrointestinal tract (RADIANT-4): a randomised, placebo-controlled, phase 3 study. *Lancet.* 2016;387(10022):968-977.

CASE 8

An 18-Year-Old Male with Right Upper Quadrant Abdominal Pain

Jennifer J. Prutsman-Pfeiffer

An 18-year-old male presents to the emergency department with a month-long progressive, constant pain of the right upper quadrant of the abdomen exacerbated with pressure, and a 12-pound weight loss. A computed tomography (CT) scan shows small bowel dilation, with an inflammatory complex in the right lower abdomen including small abscess pockets, a 2.5 × 1.5-cm phlegmon, fistula, and fecalization of the terminal ileum. The patient was diagnosed with Crohn's disease 4 years ago. He is on infliximab therapy every 6 weeks (last infusion 1 week ago). He takes mesalamine, vitamin D, and iron, and lives with his mother, father, and sister. A Crohn's flare is suspected, and he is transferred to a larger hospital for further monitoring and care. On physical examination, he is in no acute distress except for a tender right abdomen. His blood pressure is 104/71 mm Hg, heart rate is 76 beats per minute, temperature is 36.7°C (98.1°F), respiratory rate is 17 breaths per minute, and oxygen saturation is 100% on room air. Laboratory studies reveal a white blood cell (WBC) count of 11.8 × 1000/μL (high), platelet count of 510 × 1000/μL (high), erythrocyte sedimentation rate (ESR) of 53 mm/hour (high), and C-reactive protein (CRP) of 119 mg/L (high).

CLINICAL PEARL

Infliximab is a tumor necrosis factor blocker, initially designed as a chemotherapy drug that was found to be ineffective for the treatment of cancer. Infliximab is effective in reducing inflammation in IBD, rheumatoid arthritis, and psoriatic arthritis.

Mesalamine belongs to a class of drugs known as aminosalicylates, typically used to treat ulcerative colitis, in reducing the symptoms of diarrhea, rectal bleeding, and stomach pain. Its use has been efficacious in treating similar symptoms of Crohn's disease.

CLINICAL PEARL

Phlegmon is a term used to describe generalized inflammation of soft tissues. The phlegmon differs from abscess in that an abscess is self-contained and may have walled-off pus formation, whereas a phelgmon is a vascularized infection that has perfusion, typically without bacterial infection.

CLINICAL PEARL

CRP is a blood test marker for inflammation in the body. It is produced in the liver, and its level is measured by testing the blood. CRP is classified as an acute-phase reactant, which means that its levels will rise in response to inflammation.

ESR is a type of blood test that measures how quickly erythrocytes (RBCs) settle at the bottom of a test tube that contains a blood sample. Normally, RBCs settle relatively slowly. A faster-than-normal rate may indicate inflammation in the body.

A normal platelet count ranges from 150,000 to 450,000 platelets/μL of blood. Having more than 450,000 platelets is a condition called thrombocytosis; having less than 150,000 platelets is known as thrombocytopenia. Platelet numbers are reported in a routine blood test called a complete blood count (CBC).

The WBC count is another test reported in the CBC, and elevated levels of WBCs are an indication of infection.

What is Crohn's disease?

Crohn's disease is a chronic, relapsing, and remitting idiopathic immune-mediated disorder that can involve any part of the gastrointestinal (GI) tract from the mouth to the anus. This disorder is a subclassification of inflammatory bowel disease (IBD) that causes discontinuous granulomatous inflammation of the digestive tract, most commonly of the terminal ileum and colon. Crohn's disease is also known as regional enteritis, as it affects particular segments of the intestine, or granulomatous colitis due to the presence of granulomas. The inflammation affects the entire thickness of the bowel wall and can lead to associated fissures, fibrosis, neuromuscular hypertrophy, stricture, and fistulas, resulting in abdominal pain and cramping, severe diarrhea, rectal bleeding, weight loss, malnutrition, and fatigue. The etiology of Crohn's disease is unknown; a malfunctioning immune system, possibly due to an abnormal response to enteric flora, and heredity may play a role in the development of Crohn's disease. Smoking may double the risk of developing Crohn's disease; nonsteroidal antiinflammatory drugs (NSAIDs), antibiotics, and birth control pills may increase the risk of developing the disease. Diet and stress likely aggravate the symptoms. Western populations are most affected, and peak incidences occur during the adolescent years and again in the sixth and seventh decades of life. It is likely that a number of environmental triggers in a genetically predisposed individual can lead to the immune-mediated inflammatory injury to the GI tract seen in Crohn's disease.

What are the symptoms of Crohn's disease?

Abdominal pain, cramping, episodic mild bloody diarrhea, fatigue, fever, mouth sores, blood in stool, reduced appetite and weight loss, and anal fistula are symptoms of Crohn's disease. Anemia may be present if there is persistent loss of blood when the colon is affected. Symptoms are variable and may be progressive or of sudden onset, mimicking acute appendicitis or bowel perforation; after a flare, symptoms may go into remission. Extraintestinal symptoms include erythema nodosum, migratory polyarthritis, clubbing of the fingertips, sacroiliitis, ankylosing spondylitis, primary sclerosing cholangitis, pericholangitis, periureteral fibrosis, and occasional uveitis.

CLINICAL PEARL

Intestinal symptoms of Crohn's disease:	Extra intestinal symptoms:
Abdominal pain and cramping	Erythema nodosum
Episodic mild bloody diarrhea	Migratory polyarthritis
Fatigue	Clubbing of the fingertips
Fever	Sacroilitis
Mouth sores	Ankylosing spondylitis
Reduced appetite and weight loss	Primary sclerosing cholangitis
Anal fistulas	Pericholangitis
Anemia (blood in stool)	Periureteral fibrosis
	Occasional uveitis

What are complications of Crohn's disease?

Complications of Crohn's disease include fibrosing strictures of the terminal ileum and colon; fistulas to vagina, bladder, perianal skin, or other loops of bowel; generalized malabsorption and protein-losing enteropathy, vitamin B12 deficiency, bile salt malabsorption with steatorrhea; and toxic megacolon in a small percentage of patients (4%). Crohn's disease has been associated with tuberculosis (TB), sometimes acquired as a result of treatment of the bowel disease or conversely as a misdiagnosis of intestinal TB.

How is Crohn's disease diagnosed?

Crohn's disease is a diagnosis of exclusion, as symptoms mimic other causes of bowel inflammation. Low red blood cell (RBC) count may indicate anemia, and high WBC count may indicate inflammation. Fecal tests can be performed. Imaging studies, including CT scans and magnetic resonance imaging with contrast, may help diagnose abscess formation, fistulae, or small bowel obstruction. Endoscopic findings in the early stages of the disease include small aphthous lesions or erythematous ulcer, whereas later stages can include nodularity (cobblestone appearance), linear ulcers, stenosis, or strictures. Definitive diagnosis requires tissue biopsy that may require multiple serial biopsies with endoscopy. Terminal ileum involvement is a feature of the disease. Definitive diagnosis includes transmural lymphoid aggregates in areas not deeply ulcerated, and non-necrotizing granulomas. Suggestive features include skip lesions, linear ulcers, cobblestone mucosa, fat wrapping, and terminal ileum inflammation.

Case Point 8.1

The patient is treated with intravenous (IV) glucosteroids and IV antibiotics. Interventional radiology performs drainage of the abscess during CT imaging, and the culture grows yeast. A peripherally inserted central catheter (PICC) line is placed, and IV ertapenem antibiotics and glucosteroids are administered for 4 weeks, during which weekly laboratory draws and weekly abdominal ultrasounds will reassess the size of the abscess/phlegmon. Oral prednisone is continued at home (40 mg for 2 weeks and then taper to 5 mg per week). He continues omeprazole and iron supplementation. He is discharged with recommendation for follow-up with his primary care physician, pediatric gastroenterologist, and colorectal surgeon.

How is Crohn's disease treated?

The goals of treatment for Crohn's disease are management of symptoms and to decrease intestinal inflammation. Medicines that reduce symptoms include aminosalicylates (reduce inflammation in newly diagnosed patients), glucocorticoids (reduce the activity of the immune system and decrease inflammation in moderate-to-severe disease), immunomodulators (reduce immune system activity and decrease inflammation, prescribed if there is no response to other treatments or to promote remission), biologic therapies (target proteins made by the immune system, promote remission), acetaminophen (as NSAIDs can worsen the symptoms), antibiotics, and loperamide (antidiarrheal).

Bowel rest is important for severe symptoms. The most common indications for surgical approaches to Crohn's disease are after failure of medical treatment, and surgery may be indicated in severe disease complicated by fistulas, abscess formation, or intestinal obstruction. Most patients will need to undergo surgery at some point over the course of their disease. Crohn's will often recur in the pouch created after initial bowel resection; involvement of resection margins does not correlate with recurrence of the disease.

Case Point 8.2

The patient returns to the emergency department 3 weeks later with a Crohn's flare of 3 days with increased, sharp, constant abdominal pain radiating to the back, nausea, vomiting, and non-bloody

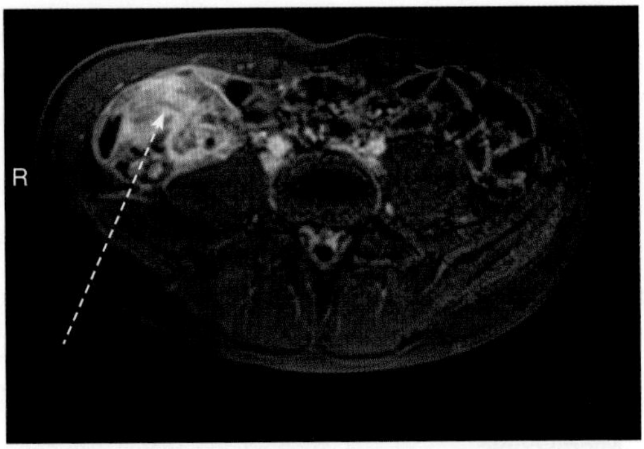

Fig. 8.1 Magnetic resonance enterography imaging showing fistula tract (arrow) between the terminal ileum and two adjacent right lower quadrant fluid collections.

diarrhea. Since previous discharge, laboratory and imaging findings have been worsening: laboratory studies reveal WBC count of 25.5 × 1000/μL (high), platelet count of 372 × 1000/μL (high), ESR of 44 mm/hour (high), CRP of 20 mg/L (high), and hemoglobin level of 11.8 g/dL (low). The right lower quadrant fluid collection is larger on ultrasound imaging, and magnetic resonance enterography demonstrates a fistula tract of the phlegmon (Fig. 8.1) and mild, partial small bowel obstruction of the terminal ileum. He is seen by colorectal surgery, and the narrowed segment is to be excised. TB antigen T-cell stimulation test is performed and found to be negative.

What is the relationship of Crohn's disease with granulomatous disease?

TB is caused by *Mycobacterium tuberculosis*, which favors the environment of the lungs. TB infection can be active or latent. Drugs used to treat IBD include immunosuppressing agents and antitumor necrosis factor therapies. The deactivation of the patient's immune system, therapeutic for the treatment of Crohn's disease, can leave patients more susceptible to acquiring TB or reactivating latent TB.

In countries where TB is endemic, intestinal TB can mimic Crohn's disease clinically, endoscopically, and histologically. Both intestinal TB and Crohn's disease are chronic granulomatous conditions.

What is the difference between Crohn's disease and ulcerative colitis?

Crohn's disease can occur anywhere from the mouth to the anus but typically occurs in the terminal ileum; ulcerative colitis begins in the rectum and may course proximally to the cecum. Crohn's disease has a discontinuous pattern with deep fissures, skip ulcerations, and may form fistulae and abscesses in the bowel wall that is typically thickened. Strictures and bowel obstruction may develop. Ulcerative colitis has a continuous pattern with pseudopolyps, and ulceration involves the mucosa and submucosa. Toxic megacolon may develop. See Table 8.1 for a detailed comparison of the two diseases.

Case Point 8.3

The patient returns in 1 month for surgery. The colorectal surgeon requests placement of a right ureteral stent as a temporary measure while operating in the right lower quadrant to help avoid injury to the right ureter. The open right hemicolectomy is performed, finding the distal small bowel, appendix, and cecum incased in an inflammatory phlegmon over the right pelvic sidewall with turbid fluid (without purulence or fecal material); there is no gross evidence of active Crohn's disease in the proximal bowel, and the transverse and left colon were normal. On postoperative day 5, the patient has the PICC line removed and is discharged home.

TABLE 8.1 ■ **Main Features of Crohn's Disease and Ulcerative Colitis**

	Crohn's Disease	Ulcerative Colitis
Location	Mouth to anus, most commonly terminal ileum	Begins in rectum, may extend proximally to cecum
Spread	Discontinuous/skip lesions	Continuous
Symptoms	Right lower quadrant pain with non-bloody diarrhea	Left lower quadrant pain with bloody diarrhea
Gross features	Cobblestone mucosa, linear fissures, focal aphthous ulcers with intervening normal mucosa, thickened bowel wall, strictures and fistulae, creeping fat	Pseudopolyps, extensive mucosal and submucosal ulceration, loss of haustra
Inflammation	Transmural	Limited to mucosa and submucosa
Microscopic features	Lymphoid aggregates with noncaseating granulomas (40% cases)	Crypt abscesses with neutrophils
Complications	Malabsorption with nutritional deficiency, calcium oxalate nephrolithiasis, fistula/sinus tract formation, strictures ("string sign" on barium imaging studies), abscesses, obstruction, carcinoma if colonic disease is present	Toxic megacolon, carcinoma risk based on extent of colonic involvement and duration of disease (>10 years)
Genetic association	Probable	Probable
Smoking	Increased risk for developing Crohn's disease	Protects against ulcerative colitis
Extraintestinal manifestations	Arthritis (peripheral joints, ankylosing spondylitis, sacroiliitis, migratory polyarthritis), primary sclerosing cholangitis, erythema nodosum, pyoderma gangrenosum, uveitis, perinuclear antineutrophil cytoplasmic antibodies	

What are the gross and microscopic features of Crohn's disease?

A segment of small bowel, typically ileum, is surgically removed in Crohn's disease and may or may not include cecum and appendix. Gross features include dull and granular serosa, creeping mesenteric fat wrapping around the serosal surface, thick and fibrotic bowel wall, strictures, and skip areas demarcating affected from normal areas. There may be fissures of the mucosal folds that lead to sinus tracts or fistulas, and linear serpentine ulcerations that result in a cobblestone appearance of the mucosa, and edematous mucosa and submucosa.

Histology may show superficial or deep ulcerations extending to the deep submucosa or below with granulation tissue; transmural inflammation with lymphoid aggregates throughout the bowel wall; sarcoid-like, noncaseating, poorly formed granulomas in all tissue layers adjacent to blood vessels or lymphatics; goblet cells; in early disease focal neutrophils in epithelium and overlying lymphoid aggregates and plasmacytosis, as disease progresses cryptitis, and crypt abscesses but no neutrophils in lamina propria; reduplication of muscularis mucosa in diseased segments, fibrosis and thickened bowel wall; may have neuronal hyperplasia; variable Paneth cells; and pyloric gland metaplasia.

CLINICAL PEARL

Gross features of Crohn's disease:

Dull and granular serosa
Creeping fat (mesenteric fat wraps around bowel surface)
Thickened and fibrotic bowel wall (due to edema, inflammation, fibrosis, and hypertrophy of muscularis propria)

Strictures (string sign on barium enema)
Sharp demarcation of affected segments from uninvolved bowel (skip areas)
Aphthous mucosal ulcers coalescing into long, serpentine linear ulcers along bowel axis to acquire cobblestone appearance
Fissures in mucosal folds leading to fistulas or sinus tracts
Rectal sparing and preferential right side colon involvement: disease less severe in distal than in proximal colon

CLINICAL PEARL

Microscopic features of Crohn's disease:

Superficial or deep ulceration with adjacent granulation tissue extending into deep submucosa or below
Transmural inflammation with lymphoid aggregates throughout the bowel wall
Sarcoid-like, noncaseating poorly formed granulomas in all tissue layers (50%–70% of cases, may need serial sections to detect) usually adjacent to blood vessels or lymphatics
Focal changes with intervening normal mucosa in bowel and throughout GI tract (mouth to anus)
Goblet cells present
Initially focal neutrophils in epithelium and overlying lymphoid aggregates and plasmacytosis, then cryptitis, crypt abscesses but usually no neutrophils in lamina propria
Edematous mucosa and submucosa
Reduplication of muscularis mucosa in diseased segments, fibrosis and thickened bowel wall; may have neuronal hyperplasia; variable Paneth cells; and pyloric gland metaplasia
Aphthous ulcer: lymphoid follicle with surface erosion

Note: Crohn's disease of colon resembles ulcerative colitis, but Crohn's colitis also has fistulas/sinus tracts, skip lesions, deep ulcerations, marked lymphocytic infiltration, serositis, granulomas, and fewer plasma cells.

Case Point 8.4

The patient undergoes open ileocecetomy and has surgical removal of a 20-cm-long segment of terminal ileum, 3 cm in diameter, attached to a 9-cm-long by 6.5-cm-diameter segment of cecum and an 8-cm-long tan-pink vermiform appendix, 0.6 cm in diameter. The terminal ileum serosa is tan-pink with adherent yellow mesentery; the serosa of the cecum is tan-pink to maroon and dull with a 7 × 6 × 5 cm firm and hemorrhagic area of serosa at the level of the ileocecal valve (ICV). The mucosa of the terminal ileum is tan and folded. There is a stricture, 0.5 cm in diameter, proximal to the ICV where the mucosa is yellow-tan and roughened with focally adherent yellow fibrinous exudate. A 4.5 × 4 cm extended area of mucosal ulceration surrounds the stricture. A probe patent defect within the ulcerated mucosa is identified that tracts to the firm hemorrhagic area of the serosa (Fig. 8.2). Sectioning reveals firm tan-white fibrous cut surfaces with irregular interspersed fistulae (Fig. 8.3). The cecal mucosa is tan, folded, and unremarkable. Histology shows viable resection margins and ulceration proximal and distal to ICV (Fig. 8.4) with stricture and underlying fistula, surrounding transmural chronic inflammation, fibrosis, and multifocal foreign body type giant cell reaction (Fig. 8.5A–B).

What are the differential diagnoses of Crohn's disease?

The differential diagnoses to consider in Crohn's disease are ischemic colitis, TB, and ulcerative colitis.

Ischemic colitis is a segmental disease arising in "watershed" areas of the vascular supply that can result in mucosal, mural, or transmural injury and can be caused by a long list of problems

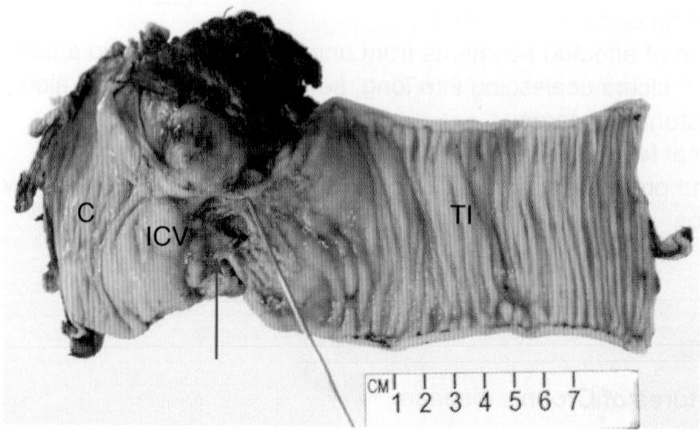

Fig. 8.2 Right hemicolectomy specimen, metal probe in fistula tract, arrow indicates stricture and ulceration. *C,* cecum; *ICV,* ileocecal valve; *TI,* terminal ileum.

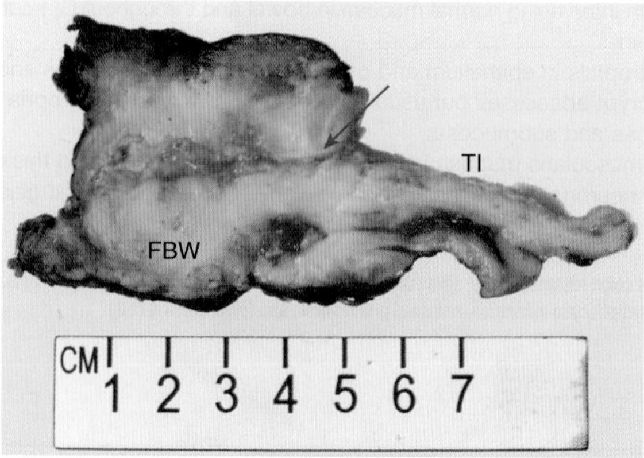

Fig. 8.3 Cut surface of terminal ileum (TI) at fistula tract (arrow) with thickened fibrotic bowel wall.

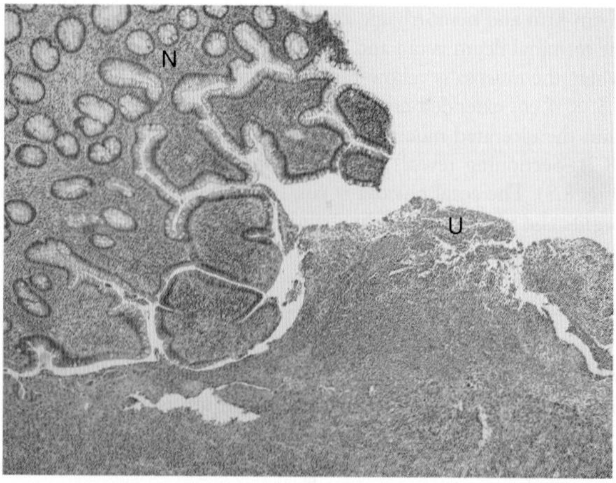

Fig. 8.4 Transition from normal terminal ileum mucosa (N) to ulcerated mucosa (U) (H&E stain 40x).

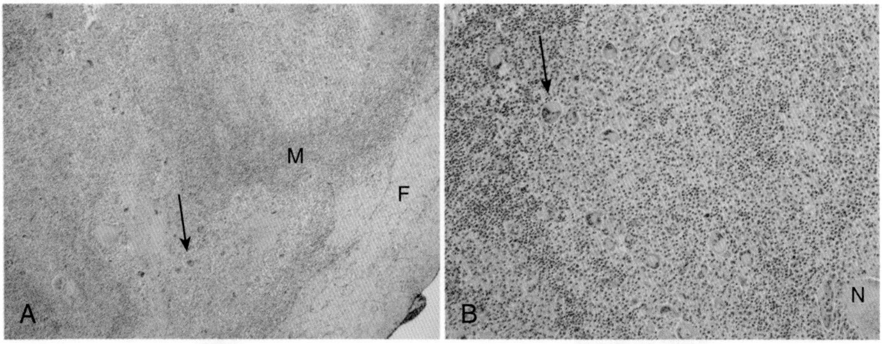

Fig. 8.5 Mixed inflammation (M), giant cells (arrow), fibrosis (F), and necrosis (N). (A) H&E stain 40x; (B) H&E stain 100x.

from bowel obstruction to vascular disease. The gross appearance can have serpiginous ulcerations with possible cobblestone pattern of the mucosa that resembles Crohn's disease.

Intestinal TB and Crohn's disease have granulomatous manifestations that overlap. In South African and Indian studies, features that distinguish patients with intestinal TB from those with Crohn's disease include confluent granulomas (>10 granulomas per biopsy site), caseous necrosis, acid-fast bacilli, granulomas exceeding 0.05 mm^2 in size, ulcers lined by bands of epithelioid histiocytes, disproportionate submucosal inflammation, and submucosal granulomas. The distribution of granulomas is submucosal in intestinal TB and mucosal in Crohn's disease.

Ulcerative colitis is an IBD that has a different distribution and pattern than that of Crohn's disease, as well as early and late stages of disease progression (Figs. 8.6 and 8.7). Ulcerative colitis is limited to the colon with a distal to proximal progression; no transmural involvement or bowel wall thickening; no strictures, fistulas, or fissures; and rare granulomas.

What is the prognosis for Crohn's disease?

Prognosis for people diagnosed with Crohn's disease is good. Education and management of symptoms are key factors in living with the disease. People with IBD have a higher risk for colon cancer; however, 90% of people with IBD will not develop colon cancer.

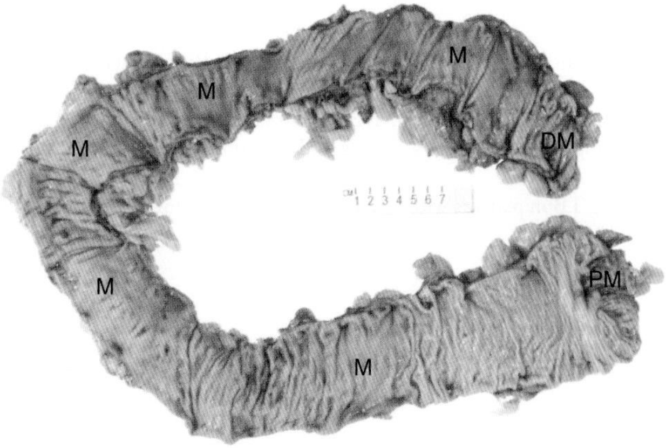

Fig. 8.6 Total colectomy specimen, early ulcerative colitis with diffuse granular friable mucosa (M). *DM,* distal margin; *PM,* proximal margin.

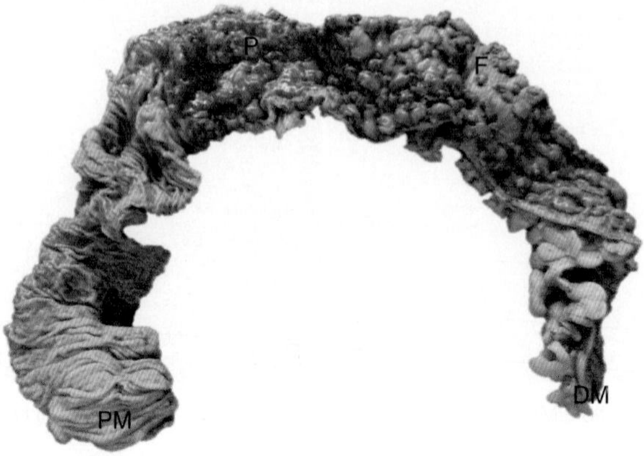

Fig. 8.7 Total colectomy specimen, late ulcerative colitis with extensive distal ulceration, flat mucosa (F) and pseudopolyps (P). *DM,* distal margin; *PM,* proximal margin. Photo credit: Kristen Weyhing, PA (ASCP)[CM]

BEYOND THE PEARLS

The distinction between Crohn's disease and ulcerative colitis cannot be made in approximately 10%–15% of patients. In these cases, the initial diagnosis is one entity and evolves into the opposite over time; the final diagnosis is then made as "indeterminate colitis."

Wireless video capsule endoscopy is a noninvasive technique used to visualize the small intestine. Magnification is greater than that of conventional endoscopy to the resolution of individual villi. Other advantages are examining the bowel in the natural physiological state, allowing passive movement of the capsule without inflation of the bowel. This technique is contraindicated in patients with strictures.

Perianal fistulae are caused by a penetrating, draining abscess that develops a fistula tract to the perianal skin. The fistulous openings are most common to the perianal skin but can extend to adjacent organs or sites, typically an adjacent bowel segment, vagina, bladder, or groin.

References

Aberra FN, Stettler N, Brensinger C, Lichtenstein GR, Lewis JD. Risk for active tuberculosis in inflammatory bowel disease patients. *Clin Gastroenterol Hepatol.* 2007;5:1070-1075.

Kirsch R, Pentecost M, Hall Pde M, Epstein DP, Watermeyer G, Friederich PW. Role of colonoscopic biopsy in distinguishing between Crohn's disease and intestinal tuberculosis. *J Clin Pathol.* 2006;59(8): 840-844.

Rampton DS. Preventing TB in patients with Crohn's disease needing infliximab or other anti-TNF therapy. *Gut.* 2005;54:1360-1362.

A 68-Year-Old Male with Hematochezia

Phoenix D. Bell ■ Aaron R. Huber

A 68-year-old man presents with a 15-pound weight loss and a 6-month history of intermittent hematochezia. Physical examination reveals blood pressure of 140/80 mm Hg, heart rate of 85 beats per minute, and respiratory rate of 14 breaths per minute. A complete blood count shows a hemoglobin level of 12 g/dL, hematocrit level of 36%, decreased serum iron and ferritin, and increased total iron-binding capacity. A fecal occult blood test is positive. The patient has no significant past medical or surgical history and is not on medications.

What conditions may contribute to the hematochezia seen in this patient?

Gastrointestinal tract (GIT) bleeding is commonly encountered in the clinical setting. Depending upon the source of bleeding, presenting signs and symptoms may differ. Lower GIT bleeding presents as hematochezia (bright red blood per rectum), whereas upper GIT bleeding presents as melena (black tarry stool). Most patients present with hematochezia, which is most commonly caused by diverticular disease, angiodysplasia, ischemic colitis, inflammatory bowel disease (IBD), infectious colitis, hemorrhoids, or colorectal carcinoma (CRC). This differential diagnosis can be narrowed depending on whether patients complain of associated abdominal pain. The conditions usually associated with abdominal pain include ischemic colitis, IBD, and infectious colitis.

CLINICAL PEARL

Common causes of upper GIT bleeding include peptic ulcer disease, esophageal varices, and Mallory–Weiss tear, whereas less common causes include esophagitis, Dieulafoy's lesion, and gastric antral vascular ectasia.

CLINICAL PEARL

Radiation proctitis may also cause lower GIT bleeding in patients who have received pelvic radiation in the past as a part of a prior cancer treatment. It is important to acknowledge this differential, as it histologically mimics ischemic colitis, thus emphasizing the importance of a clinical history.

Ischemic colitis is usually seen in patients > 60 years old and is caused by decreased perfusion to the watershed areas of the colon, which results in the sudden onset of abdominal pain followed by bloody diarrhea. Infectious colitis is usually caused by bacterial infections that result in acute-onset diarrhea with abdominal pain. The most common etiological agents for bloody diarrhea are *Shigella*, enterohemorrhagic *Escherichia coli*, and *Salmonella species*. Patients with IBD present in young adulthood (20s to 40s) with chronic relapsing and remitting abdominal pain and bloody diarrhea. They may also report mucus in their stool and symptoms of fecal urgency or weight loss.

CLINICAL PEARL

The arterial blood supply of the colon primarily comes from branches of the superior mesenteric and inferior mesenteric arteries. The most common watershed area—the area that receives minimal blood flow—is the splenic flexure. This is the most common site affected by ischemic colitis.

CLINICAL PEARL

IBD includes ulcerative colitis (UC) and Crohn's disease (CD). UC has a bimodal age distribution, occurring from 30–40 years or around 60 years, whereas CD is diagnosed in young adulthood at around 20–30 years. Both UC and CD can present with abdominal pain, diarrhea, and weight loss. UC can affect the entire GIT, whereas CD spares the rectum and often shows skip lesions (alternating areas of uninvolved and inflamed areas of mucosa). Patients with IBD have a higher risk for CRC, but it is more commonly seen in patients with UC than in those with CD.

Diverticular disease (diverticulosis) is most common in older adults (55–60 years old) and is usually asymptomatic; however, some patients may present with hematochezia. Diverticular disease is due to outpouchings in the colon wall that result from weakness in areas where small vessels penetrate. These vessels may rupture near the colon lumen, resulting in hematochezia. Fortunately, these cases are usually self-resolving. Angiodysplasia is seen in elderly patients and is caused by breakdown of capillaries and veins in the colon wall. The fragility of these vessels makes them more prone to rupture, which can cause intermittent hematochezia; however, in some cases, bleeding can be life-threatening. Patients with CRC present in middle age or older, either with an incidentally discovered lesion during routine colonoscopy surveillance, or with symptoms such as hematochezia and associated constipation/diarrhea, weight loss, and anemia. Lastly, internal hemorrhoids are seen in middle-aged adults and are painless, yet they can cause mild bleeding that is seen in stool or on toilet paper.

CLINICAL PEARL

Patients with aortic stenosis are more prone to have bleeding associated with angiodysplasia—this is known as Heyde's syndrome. The bleeding resolves following replacement of the aortic valve. The etiology is unknown but may be associated with von Willebrand factor.

Identifying the cause of hematochezia requires a thorough clinical workup including digital rectal examination, endoscopic evaluation with biopsies, stool cultures, and imaging studies.

What is the next best step in the management for this patient?

This patient is presenting with signs and symptoms of iron-deficiency anemia associated with hematochezia, which suggests the presence of a GIT bleed. Initially, some patients may undergo a digital rectal examination to inspect for hemorrhoids, fissures, or fistulae. Although most cases of lower GIT bleeding resolve spontaneously, most patients will be referred for endoscopy; immediately if the bleeding is severe or within the next few days or weeks if the bleeding is not

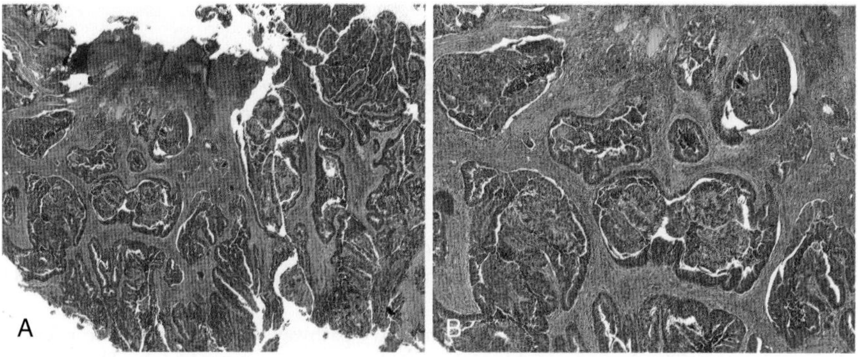

Fig. 9.1 (A) Biopsy of cecal mass (H&E, 40x). (B) Biopsy of cecal mass (H&E, 100x).

life-threatening. This patient should be sent for a colonoscopy, especially due to the evidence of iron-deficiency anemia.

Case Point 9.1

Endoscopic assessment shows a large nodular mass within the cecum. A biopsy of the mass is taken, which demonstrates haphazardly arranged, irregular glands with central necrosis, surrounded by a desmoplastic response (Fig. 9.1A–B). The patient is rendered a diagnosis of colon adenocarcinoma (arising within the cecum).

What are the risk factors associated with colon adenocarcinoma?

In the United States, CRC is the third most common cancer and the third leading cause of cancer-related death. When symptomatic, patients over 50 years old present with hematochezia, constipation or diarrhea, and weight loss. Further, there may be laboratory evidence of anemia or elevated levels of carcinoembryonic antigen (CEA) in their blood. There are several risk factors associated with the development of CRC. Environmental risk factors include a diet high in fat and low in fiber, sedentary lifestyle, obesity, and tobacco use. Patients with familial adenomatous polyposis (FAP), Lynch syndrome, juvenile polyposis syndrome, and Peutz–Jeghers syndrome are at a higher risk for CRC. Patients with IBD diagnosed for at least 8–10 years are also at a higher risk for CRC.

CLINICAL PEARL

The American Cancer Society recommends that patients at average risk begin screening colonoscopies at the age of 45 years, whereas the United States Preventive Services Task Force recommends surveillance starting at the age of 50 years.

CLINICAL PEARL

CEA is a protein that can be detected in the blood of patients with colon cancer. Clinically, it is used to monitor patients for disease progression, not for screening. Of note, CEA can also be elevated in other cancers such as those of ovarian and thyroid origin.

CLINICAL PEARL

Classic FAP is an inherited disorder caused by mutations in APC. Patients develop numerous (hundreds to thousands) gastrointestinal polyps, most commonly in the colon, but polyps can also be found in the small intestine and stomach. Polyps can be seen in the teenage years and often become cancerous around the age of 40 years. As a preventative measure, FAP patients will undergo prophylactic colectomy.

What is the molecular pathogenesis of colon adenocarcinoma?

CRC arises from one of two pathways: (1) the chromosomal instability (CIN) pathway or (2) the microsatellite instability (MSI) pathway.

The majority of CRC (85%) arises from the CIN pathway, also known as the adenoma–carcinoma sequence. The first step of this pathway is loss of APC gene, which leads to the development of a tubular adenoma (TA; a colon polyp with low-grade dysplasia). This is followed by alterations in KRAS, BRAF, and TP53, progressing from low-grade dysplasia to high-grade dysplasia and, ultimately, carcinoma. These are microsatellite-stable (MSS) and take approximately 10 years to develop.

Approximately 15% of CRC cases arise from the MSI pathway and are known as MSI-H. Microsatellites, also known as short tandem repeats, are small repeat DNA sequences made up of one to six base pairs. Normally, if there are errors in the microsatellite sequence during DNA replication, mismatch repair (MMR) enzymes (MLH1, PMS2, MSH2, and MSH6) will fix these errors; however, when these enzymes fail to properly repair a defect in the sequence, this results in MSI.

MSI cancers are due to either sporadic or germline mutations. Most cases of MSI are sporadic and are caused by hypermethylation of the MLH1 promoter. Approximately 50% of these cancers also have a BRAF V600E mutation. Sporadic MSI cancers frequently arise from sessile serrated polyps (SSPs). Conversely, less than 5% of MSI cancers are due to Lynch syndrome. Lynch syndrome is caused by a germline mutations in MMR genes, most commonly MLH1. These patients are at higher risk of developing other types of cancer including, but not limited to, endometrial, ovarian, stomach, and breast carcinomas. Identifying MSI CRC is important, as these tumors have a better prognosis and patients can be treated with PD-1/PD-L1 inhibitors (e.g., pembrolizumab).

CLINICAL PEARL

There are four molecular classifications for CRC that have been proposed by The Cancer Genome Atlas. These types are CMS1 (MSI immune), CMS2 (canonical), CMS3 (metabolic), and CMS4 (mesenchymal). BRAF mutations characterize the CMS1 type, which is associated with MSI, CIMP high cancers—these are associated with poorer prognosis. In contrast, KRAS mutations compose the CMS3 type, which is associated with CIMP low cancers, SCNA low, and mixed MSI status.

CLINICAL PEARL

PD-1 is a receptor found on the surface of T-cells, while PD-L1 is the respective ligand found on the surface of antigen presenting cells. Normally, PD-L1 binds to PD-1 and prevents cytotoxic T-cells from recognizing self antigens. Now, it is known that some tumor cells also express PD-L1, thus allowing them to evade the immune response and continue proliferating. PD-1/PD-L1 inhibitors prevent this interaction, enabling cytotoxic T-cells to fight off tumor cells.

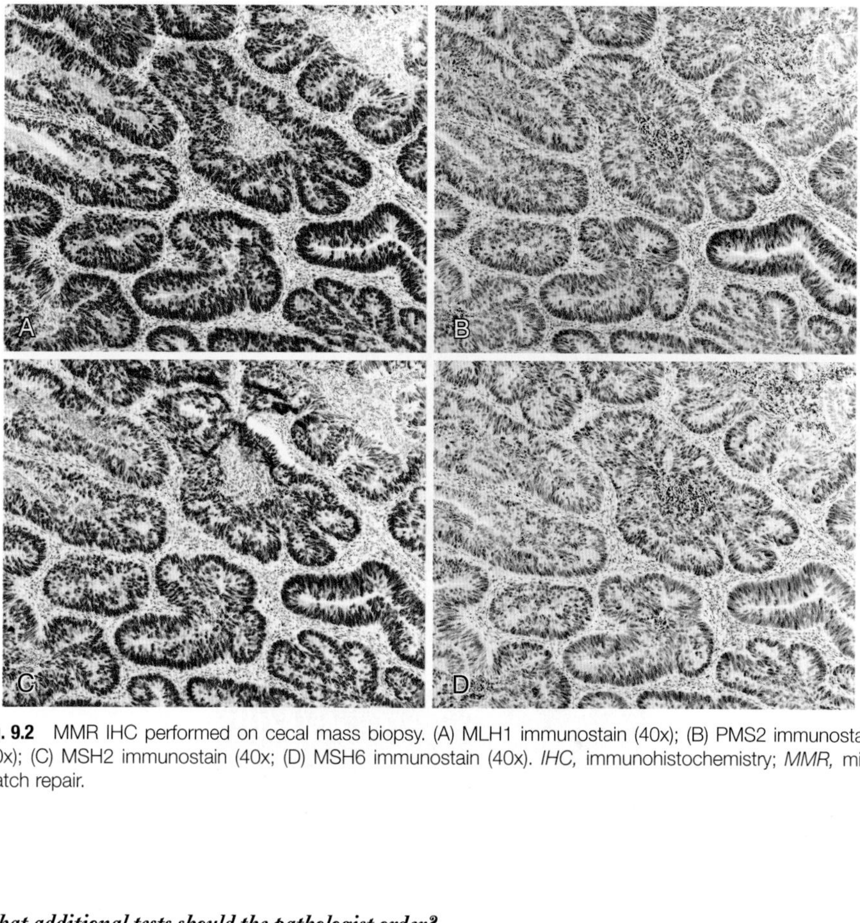

Fig. 9.2 MMR IHC performed on cecal mass biopsy. (A) MLH1 immunostain (40x); (B) PMS2 immunostain (40x); (C) MSH2 immunostain (40x; (D) MSH6 immunostain (40x). *IHC,* immunohistochemistry; *MMR,* mismatch repair.

What additional tests should the pathologist order?

Firstly, the pathologist should order MMR IHC on the biopsy material to determine whether the tumor is MSI. MSS tumors show intact MMR expression, i.e., there is positive nuclear staining for MLH1, PMS2, MSH2, and MSH6. Conversely, most MSI tumors show loss of MLH1 and PMS2. If the cancer is MSI by this immunoprofile, it must be sent for methylation or BRAF testing to determine whether the mutation is sporadic or germline. Sporadic tumors will show a mutation in BRAFV600E and/or promoter hypermethylation, while tumors caused by germline mutations will not.

MMR IHC performed on this patient's biopsy reveals intact MLH1, PMS2, MSH2, and MSH6 (Fig. 9.2 A–D); thus his cancer is MSS.

How should this patient be treated?

Most patients with CRC undergo surgical excision as the first line of treatment. Depending upon the location of the tumor, patients will undergo a subtotal colectomy or hemicolectomy. This patient has biopsy-proven adenocarcinoma of the cecum and therefore should be referred for a right hemicolectomy. In patients with advanced, unresectable disease, neoadjuvant chemoradiation is often offered prior to re-evaluation for surgical intervention.

Case Point 9.2

The patient undergoes a right hemicolectomy. The gross specimen shows a 5-cm exophytic, nodular, and focally ulcerated mass within the cecum (Fig. 9.3). Microscopic examination shows large irregular glands invading the submucosa and that are surrounded by a desmoplastic stroma (Fig. 9.4A and 9.4B). The glands are composed of cells with elongated and hyperchromatic nuclei surrounded intraluminal "dirty" necrosis (Fig. 9.4C).

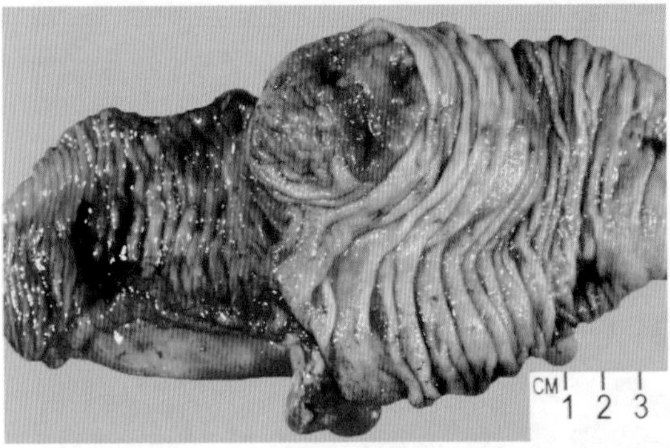

Fig. 9.3 Gross specimen showing a nodular, exophytic mass within the cecum.

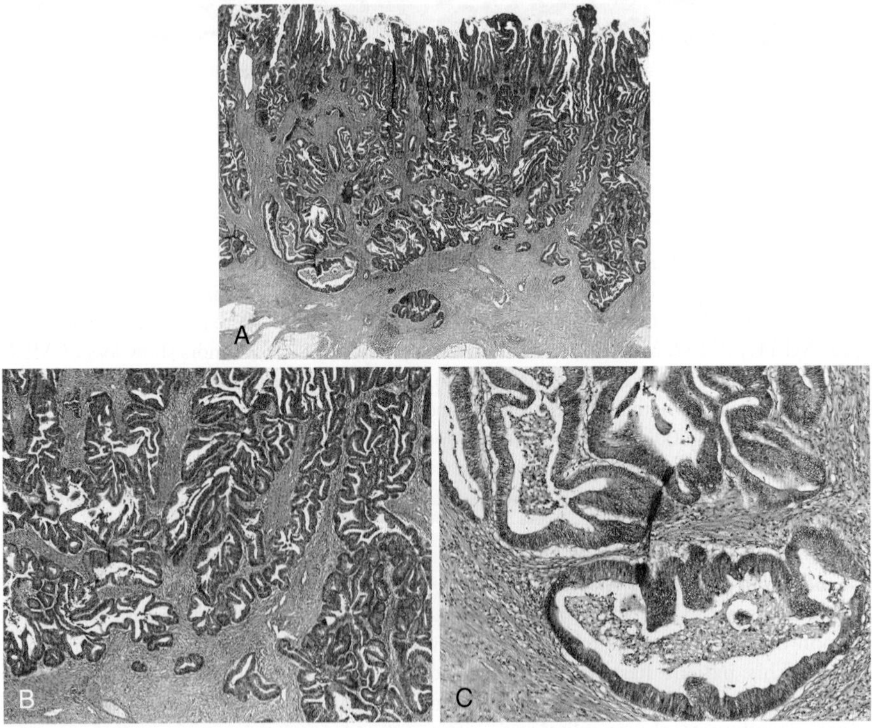

Fig. 9.4 Colon resection with adenocarcinoma (A and B) irregularly-defined glands invade the submucosa and are surrounded by desmoplasia (H&E, 20x and 40x) (C) the glands are composed of cells with elongated and hyperchromatic nuclei surrounding intraluminal "dirty" necrosis (H&E, 200x).

What are the gross and histologic findings of CRC?

Gross examination of CRC specimens usually shows ulcerated mucosal lesions with raised edges and an associated area of serosal puckering/retraction. Histologically, over 90% of CRC are adenocarcinomas characterized by irregular glands invading through at least the muscularis mucosae and surrounded by a desmoplastic stroma. The percentage of gland formation determines cancer grade. The percentages 95%, 50%–95%, and <50% correlate to grades 1, 2, and 3, respectively. Furthermore, colon cancers that are undifferentiated are termed as grade 4. Other distinguishing features of CRC include necrotic debris within the lumen of the glands ("dirty necrosis") and buds of single or small clusters of up to four cells at the tumor front ("tumor budding"). Immunohistochemical evaluation shows lesional cells are negative for cytokeratin (CK) 7 while positive for CK20 and CDX2. MSI tumors tend to show distinct histologic features. They are more likely to include more than one pattern (i.e., signet-ring or medullary), show a "Crohn-like pattern," and have associated intratumoral lymphocytes.

The World Health Organization outlines additional histologic patterns of CRC including mucinous, signet-ring cell, medullary, micropapillary, and adenosquamous. Rarely, squamous cell, spindle cell, neuroendocrine, and undifferentiated carcinomas may be seen. Mucinous carcinoma (10%–15% CRC) is characterized by malignant cells, singly or in groups, sitting within pools of mucin. More than 50% of the tumor must contain this mucinous component; otherwise the lesions should be designated as CRC with mucinous features. Signet-ring cell carcinoma is characterized by cells with abundant cytoplasmic mucin that displaces the nucleus to the periphery of the cell. Again, >50% of the cancer must be composed of these signet cells; otherwise the cancer is classified as CRC with signet-ring cell features. Medullary carcinoma is characterized by sheets of tumor cells with abundant eosinophilic cytoplasm, open chromatin, and prominent nucleoli, and is associated with increased intraepithelial lymphocytes. Micropapillary carcinoma is often seen with conventional CRC and is depicted by small clusters of pleomorphic tumor cells in open stromal spaces. Lastly, adenosquamous carcinoma shows features of both conventional CRC and squamous cell carcinoma.

The most common histologic differential for CRC, particularly on biopsies, is an adenoma with pseudoinvasion and, less commonly, metastasis. Pseudoinvasion shows dysplastic colonic epithelium with submucosal displacement. It is distinguished from invasive carcinoma by the lack of desmoplastic response, presence of stromal hemosiderin, and presence of adjacent normal epithelium. In cases of poorly differentiated adenocarcinomas, or in patients with a history of cancer, ruling out possible metastasis is necessary. This would include an immunohistochemical panel including stains for CRC and for the other cancers of interest.

What is the patient's prognosis?

CRC prognosis is associated with several histologic findings. Tumors with a greater depth of invasion have a worse prognosis, for example those with serosal involvement, colonic perforation, and invasion into nearby organs. Other adverse features include lymphovascular invasion, perineural invasion, high tumor budding, and no Crohn-like reaction. As mentioned earlier, patients with MSI-H tumors have a better prognosis. This particular patient's cancer extended through the muscularis propria and into the subserosa; however, there was no evidence of lymphovascular or perineural invasion, the budding score was low, and all lymph nodes were negative. The final pathologic stage was T3N0, which correlates to stage II clinical disease. Patients with stage II CRC have a 5-year survival rate of around 66%.

What is the next best step in management?

Patients with CRC cured by surgical resection (node negative disease) often do not require additional treatment. In patients with higher-stage lesions, chemotherapy may be considered particularly for patients with T3, T4, and lymph node–positive CRC. The use of adjuvant radiation in patients with

CRC is not routine, as no true benefit has been described; thus it is largely patient-dependent. Immunotherapy, by way of PD-1/PD-L1 inhibitors, can be used in patients with MSI-H cancers.

Case Point 9.3

This patient has stage II (node-negative) disease and has undergone surgical management. He should continue regular physical exams and colonoscopies as directed by his physician.

BEYOND THE PEARLS

- The sigmoid colon is the most common site for CRC.
- CRC most commonly metastasizes to the liver and lungs.
- The classic appearance of CRC on a barium x-ray is an "apple-core" lesion, which shows narrowing of the colonic lumen.
- *Streptococcus gallolyticus* infections have been associated with the development of CRC. This bacterium is a member of the group D streptococci (enterococci), which are catalase-negative and gram-positive organisms.
- Other syndromes associated with CRC include MYH polyposis, MSH3 polyposis, NTHL1 polyposis, polymerase proofreading-associated polyposis, PTEN hamartoma, and Li Fraumeni syndromes.
- The recommendations for colonoscopic surveillance following polyp detection vary depending upon the number and type of polyps found. If there are no polyps or hyperplastic polyps (<1 cm in the rectosigmoid), the patient can return in 10 years. In terms of TAs, if there are one to two TAs (<1 cm), the patient can return in 5–10 years. If there are 3–10 TAs, >10 TA, one or more TAs >1 cm, one or more villous adenomas, or an adenoma with high-grade dysplasia, recommended follow-up is 3 years. In regard to SSP, SSP <1 cm without dysplasia can follow up in 5 years, while those with SSP >1 cm or SSP with dysplasia or a traditional serrated adenoma should follow up in 3 years.
- Gardner syndrome is an autosomal dominant disease characterized by multiple adenomatous polyps, fibromatosis, osteomas, and epidermal inclusion cysts.
- Turcot syndrome is a rare variant of FAP associated with central nervous system gliomas.

References

Betge J, Pollheimer MJ, Lindtner RA, et al. Intramural and extramural vascular invasion in colorectal cancer: prognostic significance and quality of pathology reporting. *Cancer*. 2012;118(3):628-638.

Bosman FT, Carneiro F, Hruban RH, et al, eds. *WHO Classification of Tumours, Digestive System Tumours*. Lyon (France): International Agency for Research on Cancer; 2019. (WHO classification of tumours series, 5th ed.; vol. 1).

Cancer Genome Atlas Network. Comprehensive molecular characterization of human colon and rectal cancer. *Nature*. 2012;487(7407):330-337.

Cho YB, Chun HK, Yun HR, Kim HC, Yun SH, Lee WY. Histological grade predicts survival time associated with recurrence after resection for colorectal cancer. *Hepatogastroenterology*. 2009;56(94-95):1335-1340.

Dekker JP, Lau AF. An update on the streptococcus bovis group: Classification, identification, and disease associations. *J Clin Microbiol*. 2016;54(7):1694-1699. doi:10.1128/JCM.02977-15.

Dienstmann R, Salazar R, Tabernero J. Personalizing colon cancer adjuvant therapy: selecting optimal treatments for individual patients. *J Clin Oncol*. 2015;33(16):1787-1796.

Dinarvand P, Davaro EP, Doan JV, et al. Familial adenomatous polyposis syndrome an update and review of extraintestinal manifestations. *Arch Pathol Lab Med*. 2019;143(11):1382-1398. doi:10.5858/arpa.2018-0570-RA.

Eckmann JD, Chedid VG, Loftus CG. A rational approach to the patient with hematochezia. *Curr Opin Gastroenterol.* 2018;34(1):38-45.

Ghassemi KA, Jensen DM. Lower GI bleeding: epidemiology and management. *Curr Gastroenterol Rep.* 2013;15(7):333.

Greenson JK, Bonner JD, Ben-Yzhak O, et al. Phenotype of microsatellite unstable colorectal carcinomas: well-differentiated and focally mucinous tumors and the absence of dirty necrosis correlate with microsatellite instability. *Am J Surg Pathol.* 2003;27(5):563-570.

Grothey A, Sobrero AF, Shields AF, et al. Duration of adjuvant chemotherapy for stage III colon cancer. *N Engl J Med.* 2018;378(13):1177-1188.

Haupt B, Ro JY, Schwartz MR, Shen SS. Colorectal adenocarcinoma with micropapillary pattern and its association with lymph node metastasis. *Mod Pathol.* 2007;20(7):729-733.

Kang H, O'Connell JB, Maggard MA, Sack J, Ko CY. A 10-year outcomes evaluation of mucinous and signet-ring cell carcinoma of the colon and rectum. *Dis Colon Rectum.* 2005;48(6):1161-1168.

Kannarkatt J, Joseph J, Kurniali PC, Al-Janadi A, Hrinczenko B. Adjuvant chemotherapy for stage II colon cancer: a clinical dilemma. *J Oncol Pract.* 2017;13(4):233-241.

Knox RD, Luey N, Sioson L, et al. Medullary colorectal carcinoma revisited: a clinical and pathological study of 102 cases. *Ann Surg Oncol.* 2015;22(9):2988-2996.

Koelzer VH, Zlobec I, Lugli A. Tumor budding in colorectal cancer—ready for diagnostic practice? *Hum Pathol.* 2016;47(1):4-19.

Konishi T, Shimada Y, Hsu M, et al. Association of preoperative and postoperative serum carcinoembryonic antigen and colon cancer outcome. *JAMA Oncol.* 2018;4(3):309-315. doi:10.1001/jamaoncol.2017.4420.

Lee LH, Cavalcanti MS, Segal NH, et al. Patterns and prognostic relevance of PD-1 and PD-L1 expression in colorectal carcinoma. *Mod Pathol.* 2016;29(11):1433-1442.

Liebig C, Ayala G, Wilks J, et al. Perineural invasion is an independent predictor of outcome in colorectal cancer. *J Clin Oncol.* 2009;27(31):5131-5137.

Lugli A, Kirsch R, Ajioka Y, et al. Recommendations for reporting tumor budding in colorectal cancer based on the International Tumor Budding Consensus Conference (ITBCC) 2016. *Mod Pathol.* 2017;30(9):1299-1311.

Pyo JS, Sohn JH, Kang G. Medullary carcinoma in the colorectum: a systematic review and meta-analysis. *Hum Pathol.* 2016;53:91-96.

Sairenji T, Collins KL, Evans DV. An update on inflammatory bowel disease. *Prim Care.* 2017;44(4):673-692. doi:10.1016/j.pop.2017.07.010.

Santos C, López-Doriga A, Navarro M, et al. Clinicopathological risk factors of Stage II colon cancer: results of a prospective study. *Colorectal Dis.* 2013;15(4):414-422.

Smith RA, Andrews KS, Brooks D, et al. Cancer screening in the United States, 2018: a review of current American Cancer Society guidelines and current issues in cancer screening. *CA Cancer J Clin.* 2018;68(4):297-316.

Taliano RJ, LeGolvan M, Resnick MB. Immunohistochemistry of colorectal carcinoma: current practice and evolving applications. *Hum Pathol.* 2013;44(2):151-163.

Tjahjadi C, Wee Y, Hay K, et al. Heyde syndrome revisited: anaemia and aortic stenosis. *Intern Med J.* 2017;47(7):814-818.

Ueno H, Mochizuki H, Hashiguchi Y, et al. Risk factors for an adverse outcome in early invasive colorectal carcinoma. *Gastroenterology.* 2004;127(2):385-394.

Valle L, de Voer RM, Goldberg Y, et al. Update on genetic predisposition to colorectal cancer and polyposis. *Mol Aspects Med.* 2019;69:10-26. doi:10.1016/j.mam.2019.03.001.

Female Genital System

CASE 10

A 77-Year-Old Female Presenting with a Lesion in the Vaginal Area

Bradley M. Turner

A 77-year-old postmenopausal female presents to her primary care physician to discuss a lesion in her "vaginal area" that "just won't go away." She first noticed the lesion "several months ago." The lesion has started to hurt more over the last several weeks. She has no other complaints. The patient has a 120 pack-year smoking history. She does not report any medical problems and cannot remember any family history of medical problems. Her last Pap smear was over 10 years ago, and the patient reports it was "normal"; however, she does report a history of an abnormal Pap smear in the past, although it "was not cancer." Her temperature is 36.5°C (97.7°F), pulse rate is 95 beats per minute, respiration rate is 17 breaths per minute, and blood pressure is 147/92 mm Hg. Physical examination reveals a well-developed woman in no acute distress. Examination of the vaginal area reveals an ulcerating mass on the labia majora with whitish borders. The remainder of the physical examination is unremarkable.

What is the most common primary cancer of the vulva and vagina?

The most common primary cancer of the vulva and vagina is invasive squamous cell carcinoma (SCC; Figs. 10.1–10.3), accounting for 90% of vulvar and vaginal carcinomas.

CLINICAL PEARL

Invasive vulvar SCC accounts for approximately 5% of all gynecological cancers, whereas invasive vaginal SCC accounts for approximately 1% of all gynecological cancers.

What are other types of primary cancers of the vulva and vagina?

Other types of primary cancers of the vulva and vagina can be of epithelial origin, mesenchymal origin, and hematopoietic origin, among others (Table 10.1).

What are the precursor lesions associated with vulvar and vaginal SCC?

Two pathogenetic pathways are associated with vulvar invasive SCC of the usual type. The first pathway, more commonly associated with premenopausal women, is often associated with the precursor lesion usual vulvar intraepithelial neoplasia (uVIN, Fig. 10.4) and/or squamous neoplasia of the cervix or vagina. The second pathway, more commonly associated with postmenopausal women, is associated with lichen sclerosis (Fig. 10.5), squamous cell hyperplasia, and/or the precursor lesion differentiated VIN (dVIN, Figs. 10.6 and 10.7).

CLINICAL PEARL

Although two pathogenetic pathways have been associated with invasive vulvar SCC of usual type, the two pathways may act in synchrony. For example, lichen sclerosis associated with vulvar SCC may also be associated with uVIN.

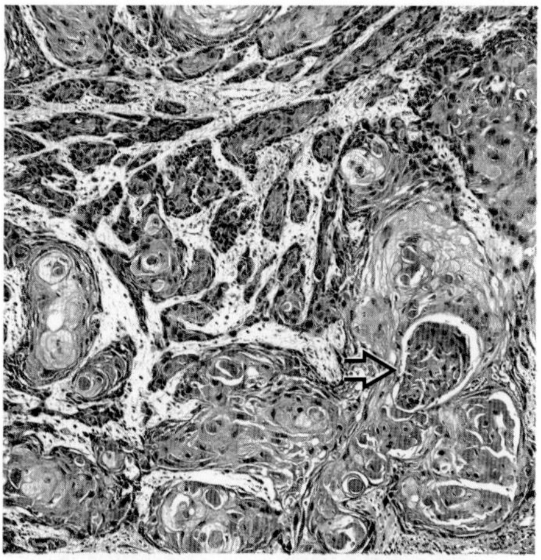

Fig. 10.1 Invasive squamous cell carcinoma (SCC) of the vulva (keratinizing subtype): Irregular, angulated nests infiltrate the dermis in a haphazard fashion in invasive SCC. Notice central keratinization (black open arrow). These tumors are sometimes erroneously designated as well differentiated, as they have abundant keratin, but cytologic atypia is often striking. From *Diagnostic Pathology*. Copyright Elsevier.

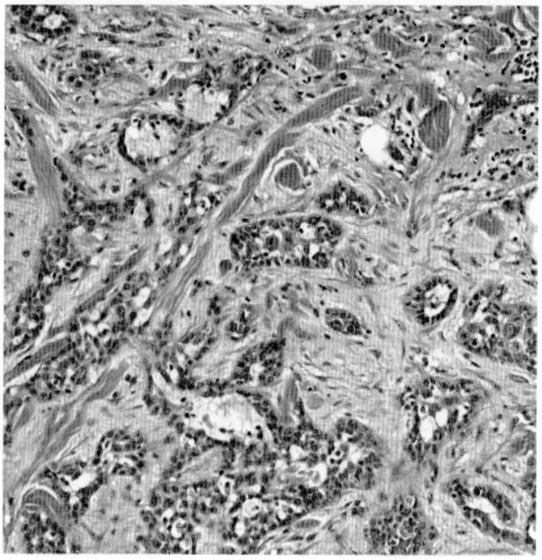

Fig. 10.2 Invasive squamous cell carcinoma (SCC) of the vulva: Invasive vulvar SCC may have an acantholytic morphology as seen at other locations. It may be confused with an adenocarcinoma, as it may contain luminal mucin, or as an angiosarcoma. p63 or p40 are helpful in establishing this diagnosis. From *Diagnostic Pathology*. Copyright Elsevier.

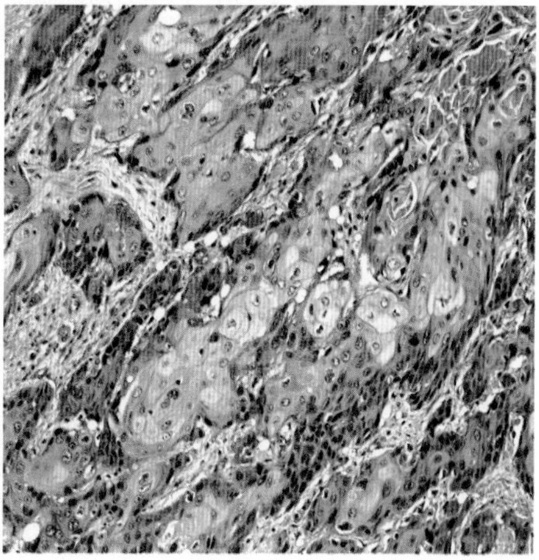

Fig. 10.3 Invasive squamous cell carcinoma (SCC) of the vagina (keratinizing subtype): Invasive vaginal SCC can show variable degrees of keratinization with formation of squamous pearls or individual cell keratinization (black solid arrow). Intercellular bridges may be seen. From *Diagnostic Pathology*. Copyright Elsevier.

TABLE 10.1 ■ **Primary Cancers of the Vulva and Vagina**

Vulva	Vagina
Squamous cell carcinoma	Squamous cell carcinoma
Basal cell carcinoma	Adenocarcinoma, non-clear cell type
Malignant melanoma	Clear cell adenocarcinoma
Bartholin gland carcinoma	Small cell carcinoma
Microcystic adnexal carcinoma	Malignant melanoma
Sebaceous carcinoma	Yolk sac tumor
Merkel cell tumor	Sarcoma
Sarcoma	Hematopoietic tumors
Hematopoietic tumors	

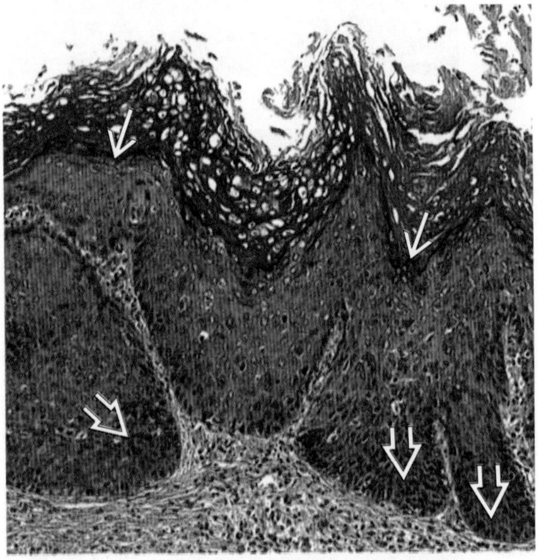

Fig. 10.4 Usual vulvar intraepithelial neoplasia (uVIN): Warty-type uVIN is characterized by hyperkeratosis, surface maturation, and koilocytotic change (white solid arrow) in addition to nuclear pleomorphism, hyperchromasia, and crowding in lower epithelial layers. Notice mitoses and apoptoses (white open arrow). From *Diagnostic Pathology*. Copyright Elsevier.

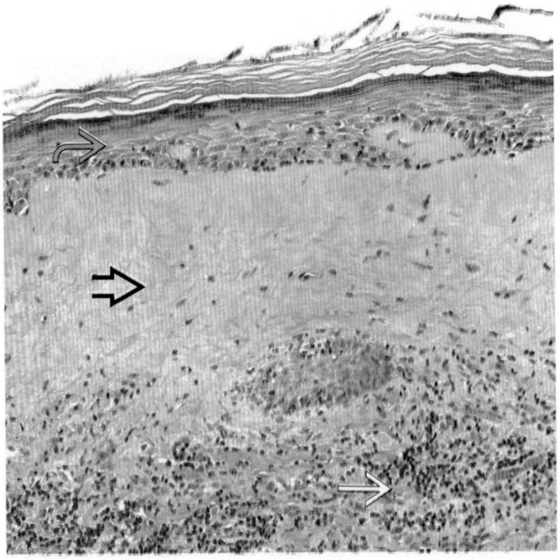

Fig. 10.5 Lichen sclerosus: Lichen sclerosus is characterized by a flattened epithelium (cyan curved arrow) and is often associated with basal cell damage, a band-like inflammatory infiltrate (white solid arrow), and homogenization of upper dermis (black open arrow). From *Diagnostic Pathology*. Copyright Elsevier.

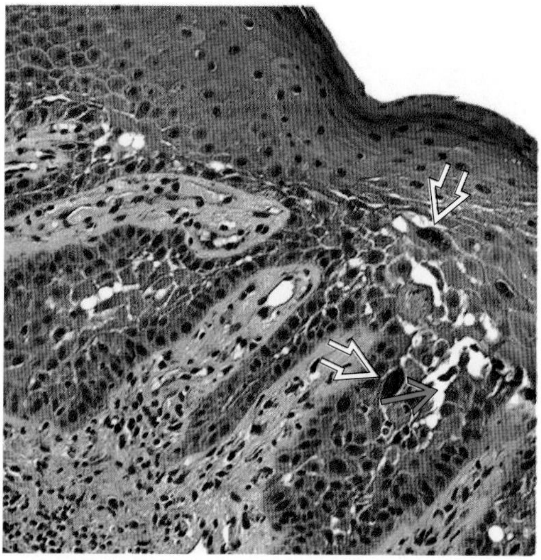

Fig. 10.6 Differentiated vulvar epithelial neoplasia (dVIN): Acantholysis (blue arrow) may be a prominent feature of dVIN and is secondary to loss of epithelial attachment rather than intercellular edema. Marked atypia of the basal epithelial layers is also apparent (white arrow). From *Diagnostic Pathology*. Copyright Elsevier.

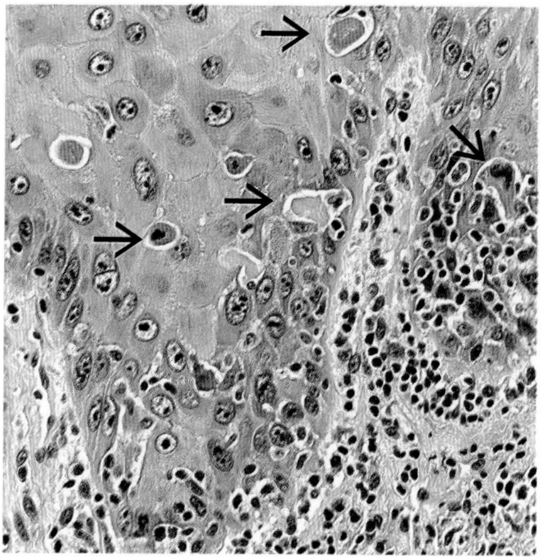

Fig. 10.7 Differentiated vulvar epithelial neoplasia (dVIN): In addition to basal epithelial atypia, dVIN also often shows abnormal keratinization, which may take the form of dyskeratotic cells (black arrows). Also notice "bright pink" cytoplasm of cells. From *Diagnostic Pathology*. Copyright Elsevier.

Vaginal intraepithelial neoplasia (VaIN) is the neoplastic counterpart of VIN and recognized as a precursor lesion for vaginal invasive SCC (Fig. 10.8). In most cases of vaginal invasive SCC, there is a previous or associated history of cervical or vulvar SCC.

What risk factors are associated with vulvar and vaginal SCC?

The precursor lesions, particularly VIN, VaIN, or any history of squamous neoplasia of the cervix, are the most important risk factors to consider for a synchronous or future invasive SCC of the vulva and vagina. The risk of vulvar cancer increases with age in women. Most cases of vulvar cancer occur in women aged over 70 years. Less than 20% of cases occur in women younger than 50 years. The human papillomavirus (HPV) has been linked with cancers of the vulva and vagina as well as cancers of the cervix, penis, anus, and throat (Table 10.2).

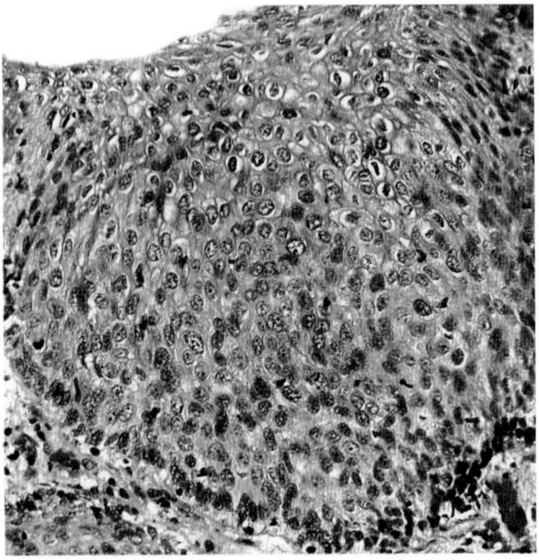

Fig. 10.8 Vaginal intraepithelial neoplasia (VaIN): High-grade squamous intraepithelial lesion (VaIN 2/3) shows increased cellularity, loss of maturation, and atypia throughout all epithelial layers. There is increased nuclear-to-cytoplasmic ratio, and nuclei show prominent nuclear membrane irregularities. From *Diagnostic Pathology*. Copyright Elsevier.

TABLE 10.2 ■ **Risk Factors Associated with Vulvar and Vaginal Squamous Cell Carcinoma**

Vulva	Vagina
Vulvar intraepithelial neoplasia	Vaginal intraepithelial neoplasia
Squamous neoplasia of the cervix or vagina	Squamous neoplasia of the cervix or vulva
Human papilloma virus	Human papilloma virus
Smoking	Smoking
Immune suppression	Immune suppression
Risk factors for cervical cancer	Risk factors for cervical cancer
Age	Pelvic radiation
	Vaginal adenosis

CLINICAL PEARL

Only high-risk HPVs (most commonly 16 and 18) are of concern with respect to increased risk of vulvar or vaginal carcinoma. Low-risk HPVs (6 and 11) are not implicated in an increased risk of vulvar or vaginal carcinoma.

Smoking also increases the risk of developing vulvar and vaginal cancer, particularly in women who are infected with a high-risk HPV. Immunocompromised women, particularly those infected with HIV, are at an increased risk for vulvar and vaginal cancer. All the risk factors associated with cervical squamous carcinoma are also the risk factors for vulvar and vaginal SCC. A history of prior pelvic radiation is also a risk factor for vaginal SCC.

CLINICAL PEARL

The pathogenetic pathway associated with uVIN is more commonly associated with high-risk HPV, p16 expression (Fig. 10.9), smoking, and cervical cancer risk factors. The pathogenetic pathway associated with dVIN may be associated with p53 mutations and p53 immunohistochemistry expression (Fig. 10.10).

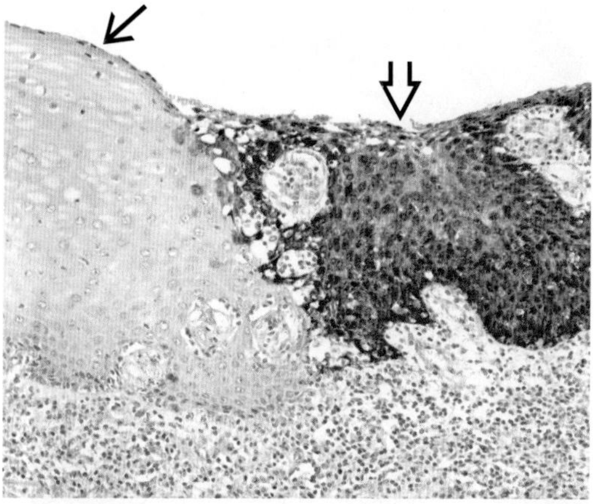

Fig. 10.9 p16 immunohistochemistry in usual vulvar intraepithelial neoplasia (uVIN): p16, a surrogate marker for high-risk human papillomavirus, shows block positivity in uVIN (black open arrow) and minimal positivity in nonneoplastic epidermis (black solid arrow). From *Diagnostic Pathology*. Copyright Elsevier. Courtesy E. Velazquez, MD.

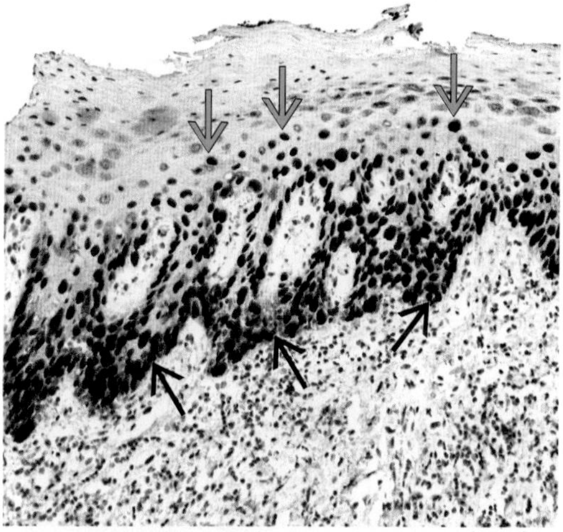

Fig. 10.10 p53 immunohistochemistry in differentiated vulvar intraepithelial neoplasia (dVIN): dVIN is strongly positive for p53 in the lower epithelial layers in a continuous pattern (black arrows) and shows increased positive cells in the upper levels of the epidermis (cyan arrows). From *Diagnostic Pathology*. Copyright Elsevier.

What findings might be present in a patient with vulvar and vaginal SCC?

Patients with vulvar or vaginal SCC will typically present with a mass, which may vary from being polypoid to ulcerating. Vaginal bleeding may be present, particularly with vaginal carcinomas. Occasionally patients with vulvar carcinoma will present with a groin mass. Presentation is often delayed, often resulting in tumors present at advanced stage. Clinical and gross examination of a suspected invasive vulvar SCC will often reveal a raised, white, occasional warty or ulcerated mass, most frequently present in the labia majora (Fig. 10.11). Clinical and gross examination of a suspected invasive vaginal SCC may show endophytic and/or exophytic growth grossly (Fig. 10.12).

Case Point 10.1

A biopsy is performed. The pathology reports a moderately differentiated SCC. The patient underwent a radical vulvectomy with groin lymph node dissection.

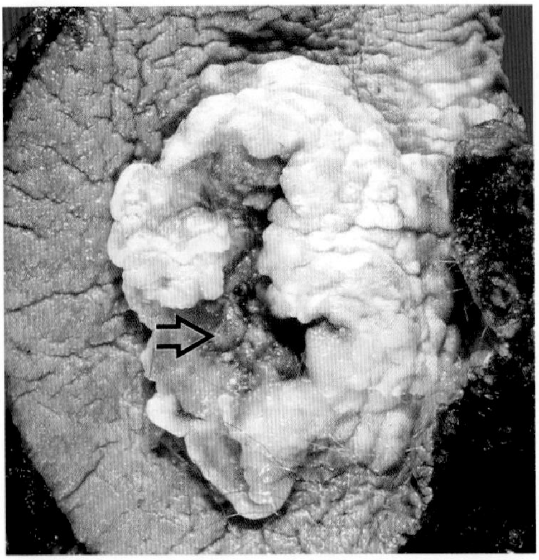

Fig. 10.11 Invasive squamous cell carcinoma (SCC) of the vulva (gross): Invasive vulvar SCC may present as a white (related to keratin), firm mass with raised borders. Central ulceration (black open arrow) may be seen. From *Diagnostic Pathology*. Copyright Elsevier.

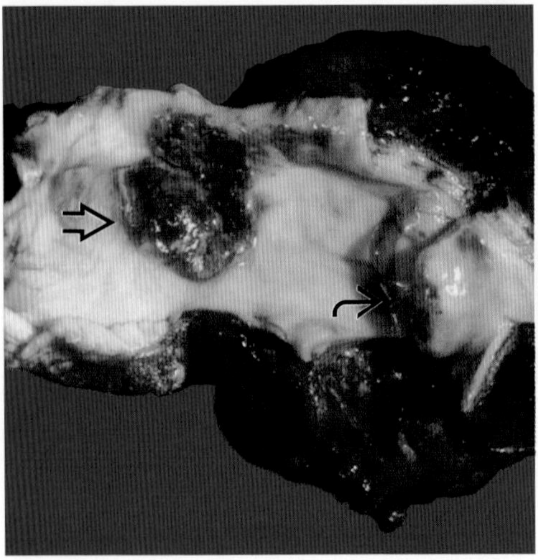

Fig. 10.12 Invasive squamous cell carcinoma (SCC) of the vagina (gross): Invasive vaginal SCC (black open arrow) may show endophytic and exophytic growths and has a hemorrhagic and friable appearance. It usually involves the upper half of the posterior vaginal wall. The uterine cervix (black curved arrow) is uninvolved. From *Diagnostic Pathology*. Copyright Elsevier.

What are the pathologic features of invasive SCC of the vulva and vagina?

The three main histologic subtypes of vulvar SCC include keratinizing (Fig. 10.1), basaloid (Fig. 10.13), and warty (Fig. 10.14). Occasionally, these subtypes coexist. A fourth type of SCC—verrucous carcinoma—must be considered in cases where there is mild but clear atypia with prominent hyperkeratosis, without frank invasion. Unlike the classic invasive SCCs, verrucous carcinoma rarely metastasizes.

CLINICAL PEARL

The keratinizing subtype of invasive vulvar SCC accounts for 65%–80% of invasive vulvar SCCs.

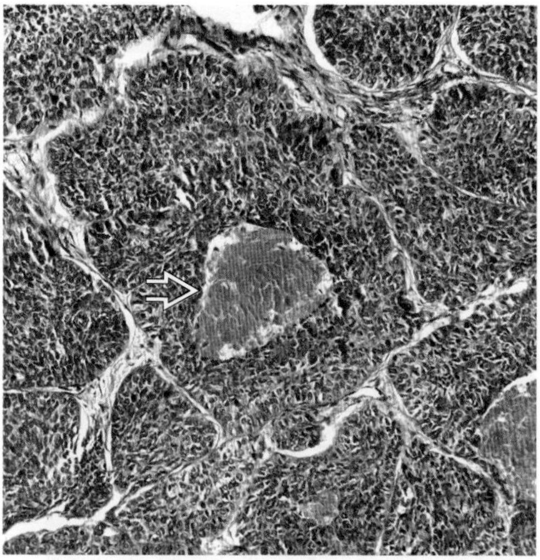

Fig. 10.13 Invasive squamous cell carcinoma (SCC) of the vulva (basaloid subtype): Basaloid SCC is composed of bulbous nests of cells with scant cytoplasm (white arrow), often showing peripheral palisading, and may be associated with central necrosis. From *Diagnostic Pathology*. Copyright Elsevier.

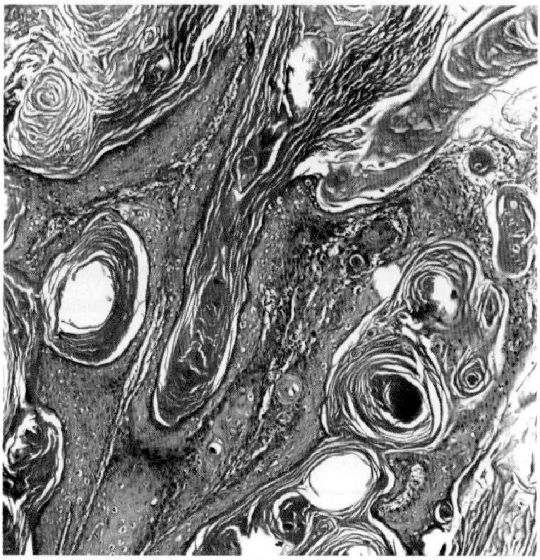

Fig. 10.14 Invasive squamous cell carcinoma (SCC) of the vulva (warty subtype): Warty SCC is characterized by a papillary growth that may closely simulate the appearance of a condyloma acuminatum, and thus may be confused with it in a superficial biopsy specimen. From *Diagnostic Pathology*. Copyright Elsevier.

The differential diagnosis of invasive vulvar SCC is detailed in Box 10.1.

Most invasive vaginal SCCs are typical keratinizing (Fig. 10.3) or nonkeratinizing (Fig. 10.15) types, with uncommon variants including verrucous, warty, papillary, sarcomatoid (spindled), lymphoepithelial-like carcinoma, and squamotransitional carcinoma. The differential diagnosis of invasive vaginal SCC is detailed in Box 10.2.

Case Point 10.2

The pathology report on the excision details a moderately differentiated SCC, keratinizing subtype, 3 cm in size, with a depth of invasion of 6 mm, without extension to any other submitted structures. Margins were all greater than 7 mm. All submitted lymph nodes were negative.

BOX 10.1 ■ Differential Diagnosis of Vulvar Squamous Cell Carcinoma

Amelanotic malignant melanoma
Epithelioid sarcoma
Basal cell carcinoma (versus basaloid vulvar subtype)
Metastatic small cell carcinoma
Merkel cell tumor
Verrucous carcinoma

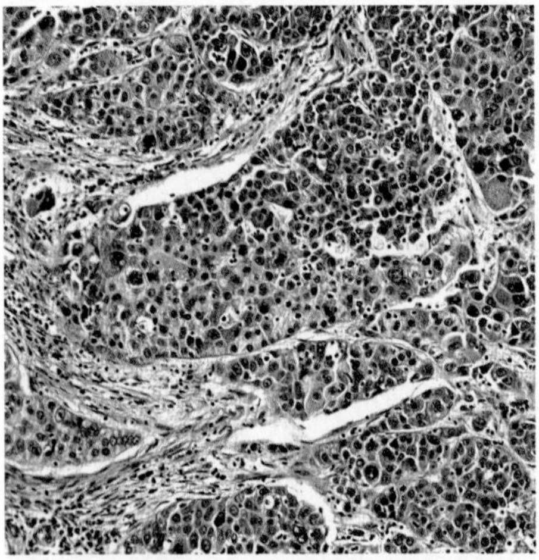

Fig. 10.15 Invasive squamous cell carcinoma (SCC) of the vagina (nonkeratinizing subtype): Nonkeratinizing SCC is more common than keratinizing SCC and is often associated with high-risk human papillomavirus. Tumor cells may be large with abundant cytoplasm, but there is no evidence of squamous pearls, individual cell keratinization, or intercellular bridges. From *Diagnostic Pathology*. Copyright Elsevier.

BOX 10.2 ■ Differential Diagnosis of Vaginal Squamous Cell Carcinoma

Cervical squamous cell carcinoma
Vulvar squamous cell carcinoma
Malignant melanoma
Sarcoma (versus spindle cell vaginal subtype)
Metastatic urothelial carcinoma

What are the prognostic factors in a patient with vulvar SCC?

The most important adverse prognostic factors of vulvar SCC are tumor size, depth of invasion, grade, lymphovascular invasion, and lymph node involvement.

CLINICAL PEARL

Vulvar SCCs invading 1 mm or less have <1% risk of nodal spread, whereas tumors invading more than 1 mm have a 10%–30% risk of nodal involvement.

Case Point 10.3

The patient received radiation therapy and continues to do well.

BEYOND THE PEARLS

- HPV infection tends to occur in premenopausal women and is more likely to be associated with uVIN.
- dVIN is not associated with HPV infection and is more likely to be found in postmenopausal women.
- Similar to uVIN, most vaginal SCCs are diffusely and strongly positive for p16 (Fig. 10.16), as they are related to high-risk HPV infection.
- As with dVIN, invasive vaginal SCCs may not be related to high-risk HPV and can overexpress p53 like dVIN (Fig. 10.17).

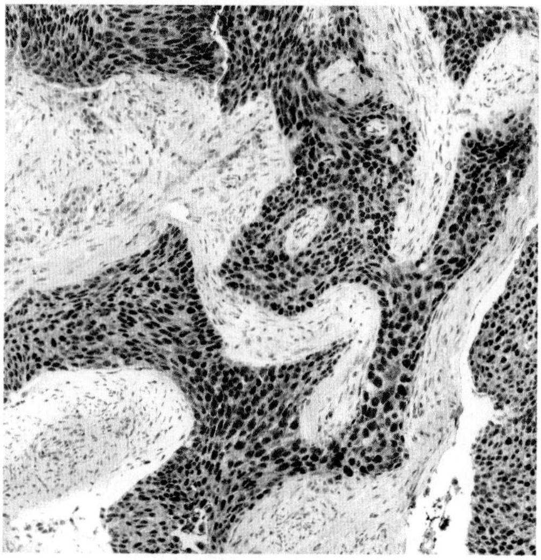

Fig. 10.16 p16 immunohistochemistry in vaginal cancer: Most vaginal SCCs are diffusely and strongly positive for p16, as they are related to high-risk human papillomavirus infection. From *Diagnostic Pathology*. Copyright Elsevier.

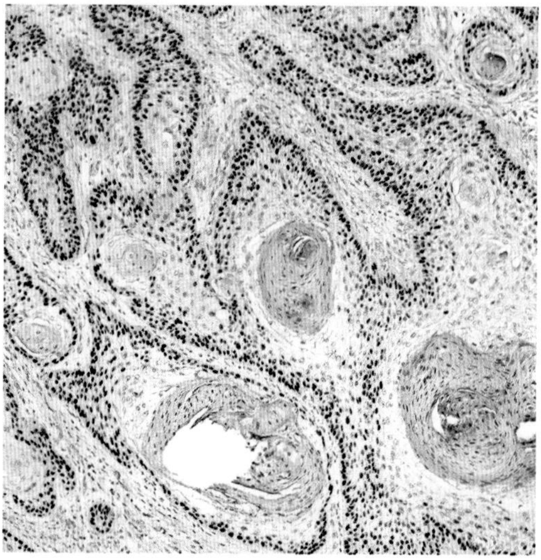

Fig. 10.17 p53 immunohistochemistry in differentiated vaginal cancer: Less frequently, invasive vaginal SCCs are negative for p16 but can overexpress p53 when not related to high-risk human papillomavirus infection. Positivity for p53 is typically seen in the lower layers of the neoplastic nests. Positivity should be strong and diffuse in these basal layers. From *Diagnostic Pathology*. Copyright Elsevier.

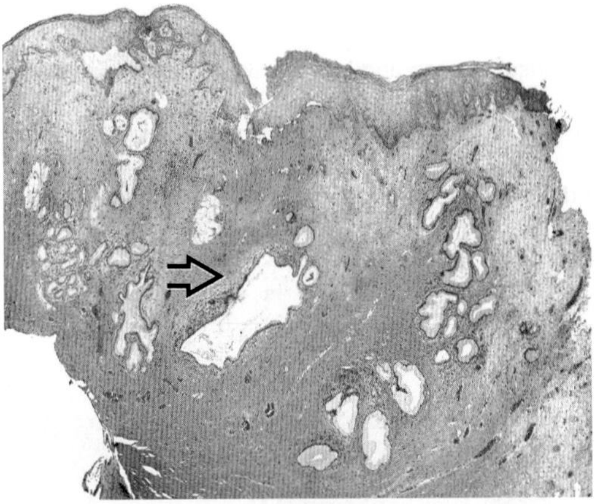

Fig. 10.18 Vaginal adenosis: Adenosis typically involves the surface epithelium or lamina propria as smoothly contoured glands that can be cystic (black open arrow) and may be focal or extensive (as seen here). From *Diagnostic Pathology*. Copyright Elsevier.

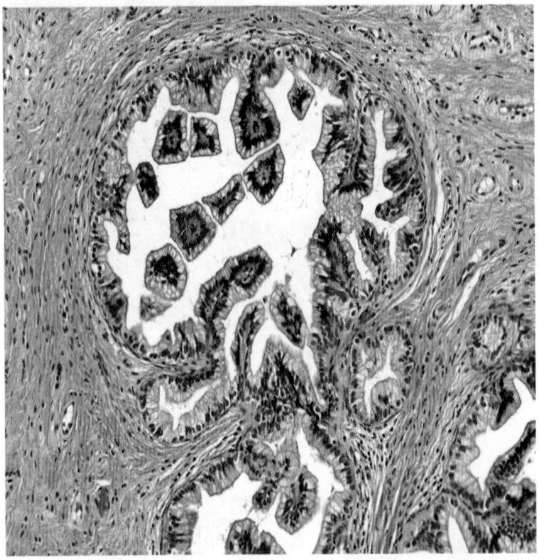

Fig. 10.19 Vaginal adenosis: Papillary growth may occur in florid vaginal adenosis and should not be misconstrued as malignant. From *Diagnostic Pathology*. Copyright Elsevier.

- Invasive vulvar SCCs involves, in descending order, labia majora, labia minora, perineal body, and clitoris. About 10% are multifocal.
- Basaloid subtype and p53 overexpression in vulvar carcinoma have been associated with worse prognosis.
- Most vaginal tumors arise in the upper third of the vagina.
- Vaginal adenosis (Figs. 10.18 and 10.19) is a risk factor for clear cell adenocarcinoma of the vagina.

References

Allbritton JI. Vulvar neoplasms, benign and malignant. *Obstet Gynecol Clin North Am*. 2017;44(3):339-352.

Bleeker MC, Visser PJ, Overbeek LI, van Beurden M, Berkhof J. Lichen sclerosus: incidence and risk of vulvar squamous cell carcinoma. *Cancer Epidemiol Biomarkers Prev*. 2016;25(8):1224-1230.

Clement PB, Young RH. *Atlas of Gynecologic Surgical Pathology*. 2nd ed. Philadelphia, PA: Elsevier; 2008.

Del Pino M, Rodriguez-Carunchio L, Ordi J. Pathways of vulvar intraepithelial neoplasia and squamous cell carcinoma. *Histopathology*. 2013;62(1):161-175.

Halonen P, Jakobsson M, Heikinheimo O, Riska A, Gissler M, Pukkala E. Lichen sclerosus and risk of cancer. *E Int J Cancer*. 2017;140(9):1998-2002.

Marfatia Y, Surani A, Baxi R. Genital lichen sclerosus et atrophicus in females: an update. *Indian J Sex Transm Dis AIDS*. 2019;40(1):6-12.

Nygård M, Hansen BT, Dillner J, et al. Targeting human papillomavirus to reduce the burden of cervical, vulvar and vaginal cancer and pre-invasive neoplasia: establishing the baseline for surveillance. *PLoS One*. 2014;9(2):e88323.

Pinto AP, Miron A, Yassin Y, et al. Differentiated vulvar intraepithelial neoplasia contains Tp53 mutations and is genetically linked to vulvar squamous cell carcinoma. *Mod Pathol*. 2010;23(3):404-412.

Reyes MC, Cooper K. An update on vulvar intraepithelial neoplasia: terminology and a practical approach to diagnosis. *J Clin Pathol*. 2014;67(4):290-294.

Satmary W, Holschneider CH, Brunette LL, Natarajan S. Vulvar intraepithelial neoplasia: risk factors for recurrence. *Gynecol Oncol*. 2018;148(1):126-131.

Serrano B, de Sanjosé S, Tous S, et al. Human papillomavirus genotype attribution for HPVs 6, 11, 16, 18, 31, 33, 45, 52 and 58 in female anogenital lesions. *Eur J Cancer*. 2015;51(13):1732-1741.

Shrivastava SB, Agrawal G, Mittal M, Mishra P. Management of vaginal cancer. *Rev Recent Clin Trials*. 2015;10(4):289-297.

Smith JS, Backes DM, Hoots BE, Kurman RJ, Pimenta JM. Human papillomavirus type-distribution in vulvar and vaginal cancers and their associated precursors. *Obstet Gynecol*. 2009;113(4):917-924.

Tan A, Bieber AK, Stein JA, Pomeranz MK. Diagnosis and management of vulvar cancer: a review. *J Am Acad Dermatol*. 2019;S0190-9622(19)32438–7. doi:10.1016/j.jaad.2019.07.055.

van de Nieuwenhof HP, Bulten J, Hollema H, et al. Differentiated vulvar intraepithelial neoplasia is often found in lesions, previously diagnosed as lichen sclerosus, which have progressed to vulvar squamous cell carcinoma. *Mod Pathol*. 2011;24(2):297-305.

van der Avoort IA, van de Nieuwenhof HP, Otte-Höller I, et al. High levels of p53 expression correlate with DNA aneuploidy in (pre)malignancies of the vulva. *Hum Pathol*. 2010;41(10):1475-1485.

Williams A, Syed S, Velangi S, Ganesan R. New directions in vulvar cancer pathology. *Curr Oncol Rep*. 2019;21(10):88.

CASE 11

A 26-Year-Old Female Patient Presents with Pap Smear of Atypical Squamous Cells of Undetermined Significance (ASCUS)

Hasan Khatib

A 26-year-old female patient presents to her physician for follow-up with regards to her Pap smear result. She was diagnosed with atypical squamous cells of undetermined significance (ASCUS), and her Pap smear 1 year ago showed a similar finding. Her past medical and surgical history is unremarkable, aside from a benign thyroid nodule with fine-needle aspiration results of multinodular goiter. The patient works as a laboratory technician in a community hospital, smokes five to six cigarettes a day for the last 7 years, and drinks socially. Medications include only multivitamins.

The patient has had three pregnancies and three vaginal deliveries. Her menstrual cycles are irregular with spotting between periods. She mentioned some vaginal spotting with intercourse, and she has had three sexual partners in the last year.

Upon physical examination, the patient's general appearance is normal; she is alert and cooperative with no obvious stress. The patient's vital signs include blood pressure of 118/82 mm Hg, pulse rate of 75 beats per minute, temperature of 36.3°C (97.3°F), and respiratory rate of 17 breaths per minute. The patient's height is 157.5 cm (5'2.01") and weight is 84.5 kg (186 lb 4.6 oz), with a body mass index of 34.06 kg/m^2. The patient denies chest pain, headache, and vision changes.

What are the risk factors for cervical cancer?

The last decades witnessed a remarkable decline in the mortality rate from cervical cancer; this accomplishment is significantly attributable to the implementation of the Papanicolaou test (Pap smear). The most common risk factors for developing cervical cancer are:

- Human papillomavirus (HPV) infection (the most important risk factor)
- Immune system deficiency (corticosteroid, organ transplantation, HIV infection, chemotherapy)
- Smoking
- Herpes infection
- Age: women younger than 20 years rarely develop cervical cancer. Most cervical cancer develops between early 20s to mid-30s
- Socioeconomic factors: cervical cancer is more common among women who are less likely to have access to screening for cervical cancer
- Multiple sexual partners

CLINICAL PEARL

Prevention of cervical cancer

- Delaying first sexual intercourse until the late teens or older
- Limiting the number of sex partners and practicing safe sex
- Quitting smoking

TABLE 11.1 ■ **Cancer Screening Guidelines**

Circumstances	Recommendation
Age to begin screening	Age 21, women younger than 21 years should not be screened, regardless of the age of sexual initiation
Women aged 21–29 years	Every 3 years with cytology alone
Women aged 30–65 years	Every 3 years with cytology alone, or every 5 years if contesting with cytology and human papillomavirus assay
Discontinuation of screening	Age 65 years if adequate prior screening and no history of cervical intraepithelial neoplasia (CIN-2 or CIN-3)
Screening after total hysterectomy	Not recommended if no history of CIN-2 or CIN-3

What are the current cervical cancer screening guidelines?

The purpose of cervical screening programs and systems is to rule out the presence of precancerous lesions or cervical cancer (Table 11.1). This is to reduce the mortality of cervical cancer and the rate of progressing precancerous lesion to cancer. Visual inspection with acetic acid, Pap smear test, and HPV test are the main screening tests for cervix. HPV test and Pap smear are performed on a sample of cervical cells.

CLINICAL PEARL

During visual inspection with acetic acid, a dilution of white vinegar is applied to the cervix. The physician then looks for cervical abnormalities on the cervix, which will turn white when exposed to vinegar, and the cervical sample should be taken from the changed area. This screening test is very useful in places where access to medical care is limited.

CLINICAL PEARL

Patient instructions to obtain an ideal pap specimen

- Avoid menstrual period time, at least 5 days after menstrual period stops
- No sexual intercourse for 2 days before the test
- Do not use tampons, birth control foams, jellies, or creams 2–3 days before the test

CLINICAL PEARL

- There are two types of Pap smears: conventional smear and liquid-based smear. There is no clinically important difference between them.
- A satisfactory squamous component must be present: 5000 squamous cells for liquid-based smears and 8000–12,000 squamous cells for conventional smears.

What is the etiology of developing cervical cancer?

The exocervix squamous epithelium growth is stimulated by estrogen. It is divided into three layers—basal, parabasal (intermediate), and superficial layer. The basal cells have scant cytoplasm and oval cuboidal nuclei. The parabasal cells are somewhat larger than the basal cells due to increased cytoplasm and larger nuclei. The superficial cells have small, rounded pyknotic nuclei with abundant cytoplasm. Glycogen accumulates in most intermediate cells and superficial cells.

The endocervix is lined by a single layer of mucin-secreting epithelium. Cervical transformation zone is the area between the endocervix and exocervix; the columnar cells of endocervix are constantly changing into squamous cells.

HPV infection is very well-known epidemiologic risk factor of cervical cancer. HPV is a DNA virus from the papillomavirus family, of which over 170 types are known. More than 40 types are transmitted through sexual contact. The genital HPVs are divided into low-risk and high-risk types. High-risk HPV strains include HPV 16 and 18, which cause about 70%–80% of cervical cancers. However, low-risk HPV strains, such as HPV 6 and 11, cause genital warts, which rarely develop into cancer.

CLINICAL PEARL

HPV infects the cervical transformation zone, which is an area of metaplastic tissue between the squamous epithelium of the vagina and the glandular tissue of the endocervical canal

The small HPV genome consists of about 8000 base pairs of circular double-stranded DNA. It codes for only eight genes, which are classified as early "E" or late "L" depending on the timing of their expression in the epithelium. HPV infection is established in the basal layers of the epithelium, where the HPV genome is maintained, with the expression of the E genes. As the epithelium matures toward the surface, gene amplification and viral assembly occur, with expression of L1 and L2, with eventual viral release.

CLINICAL PEARL

The E6 and E7 gene products play the most significant role in cervical oncogenesis. E6 inhibits apoptosis by binding to p53, and E7 binds to retinoblastoma tumor suppression protein pRB, which induces S-phase and leads to unscheduled cellular proliferation.

L1 is the major viral capsid protein and is the principal component of HPV vaccines.

The classic HPV infection cervical epithelial cell change is termed as koilocytosis. Koilocytosis is attributed to perinuclear halo appearance within the cell, along with enlarged irregular nuclei and increased nuclear-to-cytoplasmic ratio (Fig. 11.1).

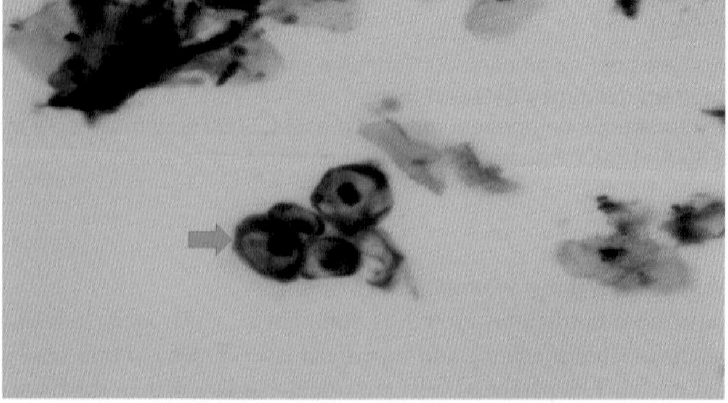

Fig. 11.1 Cervical Pap smear displays HPV-related cervical cell changes (arrow) referred as koilocytosis. (Liquid-based Pap smear, 200x).

What are the signs and symptoms of cervical cancer?

Unfortunately, lesions of cervix are asymptomatic until late advanced stages. Most of the cervical precancerous lesions are not visible to the naked eye. Some of these lesions present as exophytic polypoid or plaque-like mass.

The most worrisome signs or symptoms of cervical cancer:

- Blood spots or light bleeding between or following periods
- Longer and heavier than usual menstrual bleeding
- Painful intercourse, bleeding after intercourse or after a pelvic examination
- Increased vaginal discharge
- Menopausal bleeding
- Unexplained, persistent pelvic and/or back pain

Case Point 11.1

Patient's bimanual pelvic examination reveals no unusual changes in the external genital organs apart from mild pain upon moving the cervix. The external physical examination of the uterus and adnexa are unremarkable. The doctor repeats Pap smear and requests HPV typing test.

CLINICAL PEARL

The following tests may be used to diagnose cervical cancer:

- Bimanual pelvic examination
- Pap smear test
- HPV typing test: HPV testing alone is not enough for diagnosis of cervical cancer, it confirms the presence of HPV infection
- Colposcopy
- Biopsy: removal of a small amount of tissue for microscopic examination to render the definite diagnosis
- Imaging studies: Computed tomography (CT) scan, magnetic resonance imaging, positron emission tomography–CT scan
- Cystoscopy and sigmoidoscopy for advanced staged with suspicious cancer invading into adjacent visceral organs

What are the categories of the Bethesda system for reporting cervical cytology?

Bethesda system was developed in 1988 for reporting cervical/vaginal cytology. The system was modified several times subsequently. Box 11.1 illustrates the 2001 Bethesda system for reporting cervical cytology.

Case Point 11.2

The patient's Pap smear shows ASCUS, and HPV test reveals positive HPV 16.

CLINICAL PEARL

More than 40 HPV types infect the cervix, 13–15 high-risk and 4–6 low-risk HPV types account for majority of infections.

HPV test only tests for 13–14 high-risk HPV types

BOX 11.1 ■ The 2001 Bethesda System for Reporting Cervical Cytology

The 2001 Bethesda system for reporting cervical cytology

Specimen Adequacy

- A satisfactory squamous component must be present
- Note the presence/absence of endocervical/transformation zone component
- Obscuring elements (inflammation, blood, drying artifact) may be mentioned if 50%–75% of epithelial cells are obscured

General Categorization

- Negative for intraepithelial lesion or malignancy
- Epithelial cell abnormality
- Other

Interpretation/Results

Negative for intraepithelial lesion or malignancy

- Organism
  - *Trichomonas vaginalis*: Primitive, eukaryotic, parasitic protozoan. Sexually transmitted disease. Organism is pear-shaped (15–30 μm long), frequently staining blue–gray. Ill-defined, eccentrically located nucleus. Infrequently seen flagella (Fig. 11.2).
  - Fungal organisms (*Candida*): Bimorphic fungal organism, spearing of squamous cells, a feature that is readily appreciated at low power (shish-kebab-like morphology; Fig. 11.3)
  - Shift in flora suggestive of bacterial vaginosis: *Gardnerella vaginalis* or other short coccobacilli. Frequently associated with clue cells: squamous epithelial cells with coccobacilli on them, resulting in dark purple staining and cloudy, filmy appearance.
  - Bacteria morphologically consistent with *Actinomyces* species: Gram-positive anaerobic bacteria and typically related to intrauterine device (IUD) use (Fig. 11.4)
  - Cellular changes consistent with herpes simplex virus (HSV): Usually HSV type 2, sexually transmitted disease, present clinically with multiple vesiculopustular or small ulcerative lesions on external genitalia. Cytologically characterized by multinucleation, nuclear molding, and margination of chromatin (Fig. 11.5)
- Other non-neoplastic findings
  - Reactive cellular changes associated with inflammation radiation, IUD
- Glandular cells status post hysterectomy: benign-appearing endocervical type glandular cells that cannot be differentiated from those sampled from endocervix
- Atrophy

Epithelial Cell Abnormality

Squamous Cell

- Atypical squamous cell
  - Of undetermined significance
  - Cannot exclude high-grade squamous intraepithelial lesion
- Low-grade squamous intraepithelial lesion
- High-grade squamous intraepithelial lesion
- Squamous cell carcinoma

Glandular Cell

  - Atypical glandular cell (specify if endocervical, endometrial, or not otherwise specified)
  - Atypical glandular cells, favor neoplastic (specify if endocervical, endometrial, or not otherwise specified)

Endocervical adenocarcinoma in situ

Adenocarcinoma

Other

Endometrial cells in women older than 40 years.

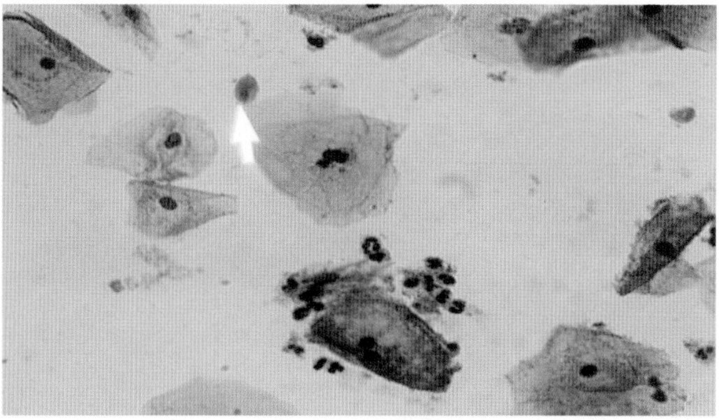

Fig. 11.2 Cervical Pap smear shows trichomonas vaginalis (arrow) (Liquid-based Pap smear, 200x).

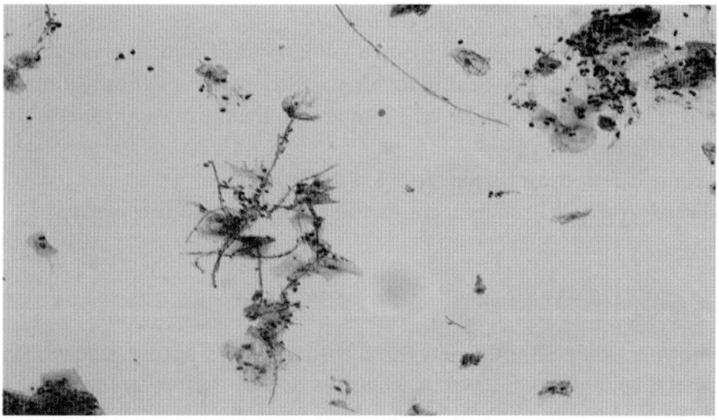

Fig. 11.3 Cervical Pap smear shows fungal organisms morphologically consistent with *Candida* species (Liquid-based Pap smear, 100x).

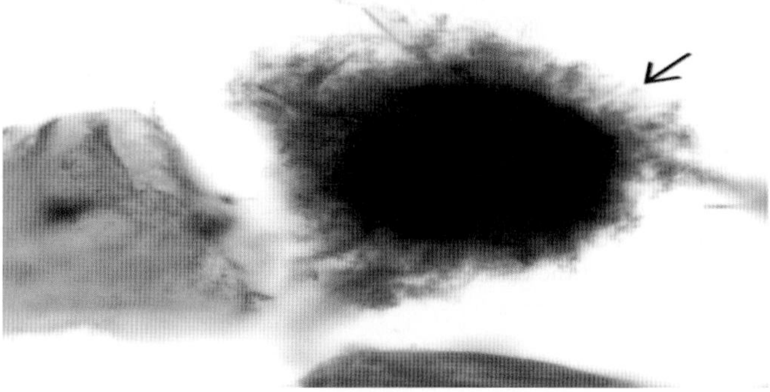

Fig. 11.4 Cervical Pap smear shows a fluffy ball-like structure from the periphery of which radiate fine filamentous bacteria (arrow) consistent with the *Actinomyces* species. (Surepath smear, 200x).

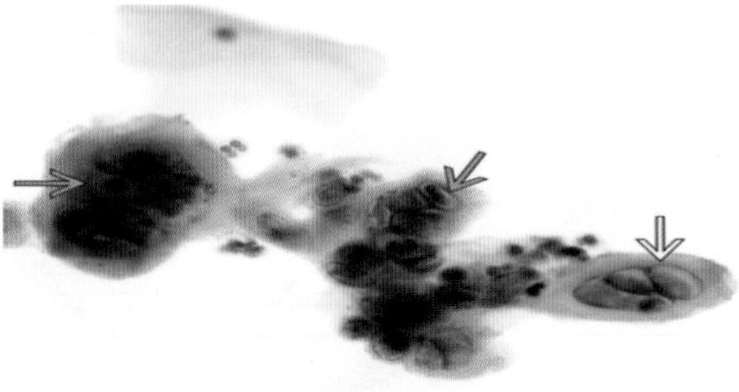

Fig. 11.5 Cervical Pap smear shows herpes viral cytopathic effect characterized by multinucleation, nuclear molding (white arrow), and chromatin clearing. Some cells have distinct eosinophilic intranuclear (Cowdry) inclusions (blue arrows) surrounded by clearing between the inclusion and nuclear membrane (Liquid-based Pap smear, 400x).

What is the definition of atypical squamous cell (ASC)?

ASC refers to cytological changes suggestive of low-grade squamous intraepithelial lesion (LSIL), which are qualitatively or quantitatively insufficient for a definitive interpretation. The interpretation of ASC requires that the cells in question demonstrate three essential features:

- Squamous differentiation
- Increased nuclear-to-cytoplasmic ratio
- Minimal nuclear hyperchromasia, chromatin clumping, and irregularity

CLINICAL PEARL

- ASCs cannot exclude HSIL (ASC-H). The high-grade cells appear singly or in small fragments of less than 10 cells. Ratio of nuclear-to-cytoplasmic may approximate that of high-grade lesions.
- LSIL criteria: Nuclear enlargement more than three times the normal intermediate nuclei. Binucleation and multinucleation. Nucleoli are absent usually. Irregular nuclear membrane with variable degree of nuclear hyperchromasia (Fig. 11.6)
- HSIL criteria: Cell size is variable, and ranges from cells similar in size to LSIL to quite small basal-type cells. Nuclear hyperchromasia with marked increase in nuclear-to-cytoplasmic ratio. Chromatin may be fine or coarsely granular, and nuclear membrane is quite irregular with frequent indentations or grooves (Fig. 11.7).

What is the follow-up for the patient?

A patient aged 26 years, who is not pregnant, with ASCUS on Pap smear, and positive for HPV should undergo colposcopy and biopsy (Fig. 11.8).

Colposcopy is used to help guide a cervical biopsy by magnifying the cells of the cervix and vagina to facilitate the view of the cervical lesion.

Case Point 11.3

The patient underwent colposcopy and biopsy. The microscopic evaluation of cervical biopsy reveals LSIL (Fig. 11.9).

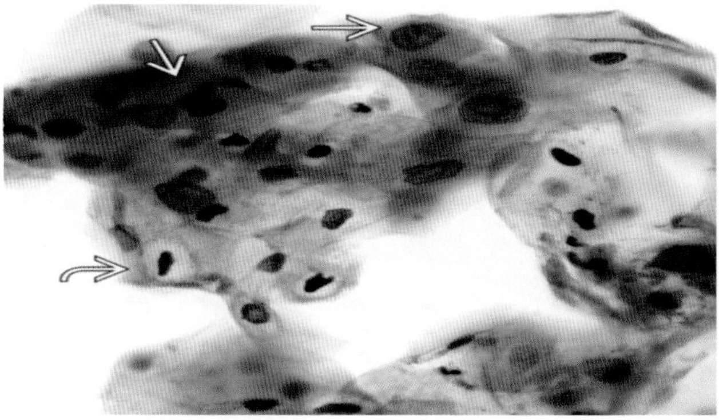

Fig. 11.6 ThinPrep smears show low-grade squamous intraepithelial lesion (LSIL), cells with nuclear enlargement and contour irregularities (arrows). Koilocytes are seen (curved arrow) (Liquid-base Pap smear, 200x).

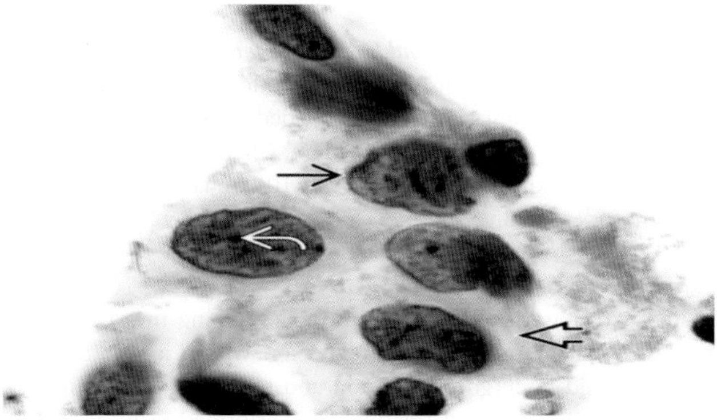

Fig. 11.7 ThinPrep smears shows high-grade squamous intraepithelial lesion (HSIL), cells with large nuclei and irregular nuclear membrane contours, and nuclear groove (black arrow). The cells display dispersed chromatin with chromocenters (curved white arrow), the cytoplasm is fragile (arrow head) (Liquid-base Pap smear, 400x).

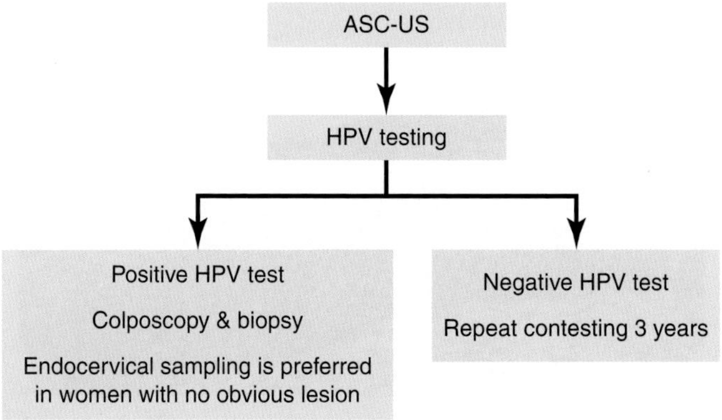

Fig. 11.8 Algorithm illustrates the management of women with atypical squamous cells of undetermined significance (ASCUS).

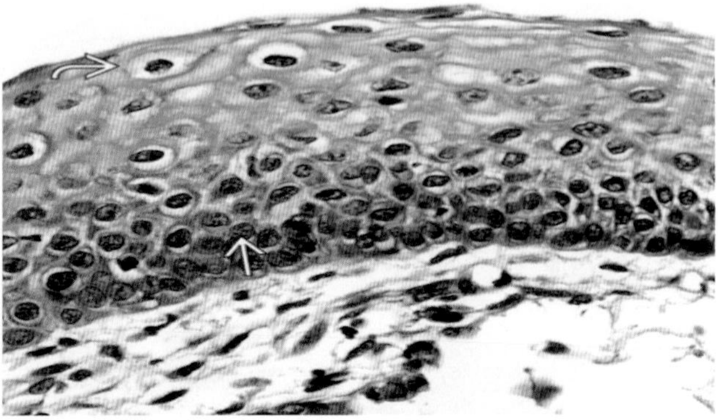

Fig. 11.9 Cervical biopsy shows low-grade cervical intraepithelial lesion (CIN-1), characterized by nuclear crowding and irregularity (straight arrow) limited to the lower one-third of the cervical epithelium. Koilocytes are seen in the upper half of the biopsy (curved arrow) (H&E, 400x).

What is the difference between high grade and low grade on cervical biopsy?

The proportion of cervical epithelium displaying dysplastic changes determine the grade of dysplasia. Cervical intraepithelial neoplasia (CIN) is divided into three grades: CIN-1 (low grade) involves the lower third part of the cervical epithelium, whereas CIN-2 and CIN-3 (high grade) involves two-thirds to full-thickness dysplasia (Fig. 11.10). Squamous cell carcinoma is diagnosed when stromal invasion is identified.

What are the treatment options for patient with CIN?

LSILs are associated with low risk of concurrent or developing invasive cancer. Most patients with CIN-1 have an excellent prognosis, as regression within a year is expected. Therefore, patients with CIN-1 should undergo observation and repeat co-testing in 1 year. If CIN-1 is persistent after 2 years, more advanced treatment is performed using lesion resection by loop electrosurgical excision procedure (LEEP) or cone biopsy with negative surgical margins.

High-grade squamous intraepithelial lesions (HSILs) CIN-2 or CIN-3 are associated with poor prognosis, and these patients should undergo further treatment. The treatment options include ablation or excision of abnormal cells. Excisional procedures for the treatment of CIN-2 and CIN-3 include LEEP, cold knife conization, and laser conization.

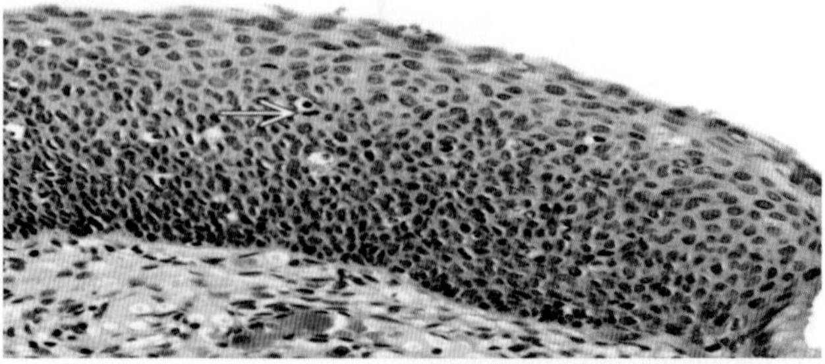

Fig. 11.10 Cervical biopsy shows high-grade cervical intraepithelial lesion (CIN-3), characterized by dysplastic changes involving full thickness of the epithelium (cells with mitotic activity pointed by arrow). (H&E, 200x).

CLINICAL PEARLS

There are several types of cervical excisional biopsies. LEEP and conization (a cone biopsy) are the most common types of cervical biopsies; they are used for diagnostic purpose and as treatment options. Negative surgical margin of dysplasia is very important in evaluating patient's cervical biopsy.

Excisional procedures may increase the risk for preterm labor due to cervical incompetence during pregnancy.

Bleeding, pain, infection, and, rarely, damaging surrounding tissues are the most common adverse effects.

Case Point 11.4

Healthcare providers and the patient discuss cervical cancer screening protocol and implement a reliable system for follow-up. The patient will undergo observation, and co-testing will be repeated in 1 year. The patient is advised to practice safe sex with consistent condom use to protect from HPV transmission. The patient is also advised to quit smoking with social work support offering smoking cessation aid with a support group system.

BEYOND THE PEARLS

- HPV infections are very common, affecting up to 80% of women in their early 20s.
- The factors that are associated with poorer prognosis and probably progress to high-grade lesion or cancer are HPV type 16, older age, immunosuppression, and smoking.
- American Society of Clinical Oncology recommends that all women receive at least one HPV test to screen for cervical cancer in their lifetime.
- Women aged 25–65 years should receive an HPV test once every 5 years. Women aged 65 years and older or who had a hysterectomy may stop screening if their HPV test results have been mostly negative over the previous 15 years.
- Most CIN-1 lesion will regress spontaneously within a year.
- Women treated for CIN-2 or CIN-3 should have a Pap smear and HPV testing 12 and 24 months after the procedure.

References

American Society for Colposcopy and Cervical Pathology. *Guidelines*. Updated February 12, 2019. Available at: www.asccp.org/Guidelines

Cervical Cancer Guide. *Cancer.Net Editorial Board*. American Society of Clinical Oncology; 2019.

Chantziantoniou N, Mody DR. *Elsevier Expertpath, Pathprimer. Infectious and Other Organisms in Pap Tests.*

Cibas ES, Ducatman BS. *Cytology: Diagnostic Principles and Clinical Correlates*. 4th ed.

Kurman RJ, Young RH. *WHO Classification of Tumours of Female Reproductive Organs*. 4th ed.

Mello V. *Cancer, Cervical Intraepithelial Neoplasia (CIN)*. State Pearls Knowledge Base. June 16, 2019.

Atkins KA, Hendrickson MR, Kempson RL. Normal histology of female genital organs. In: Mills SE, ed. *Histology for Pathologists*. 4th ed. 2012.

Solomon D, Nayar R. *The Bethesda System for Reporting Cervical Cytology*. 2nd ed.

CASE 12

A 61-Year-Old Woman with Postmenopausal Bleeding

Cynthia Reyes Barron

A 61-year-old female presents to her primary care physician complaining of vaginal bleeding. The bleeding has been ongoing for 3 months and varies from light to moderate, often soaking more than two feminine pads per day. She has passed several small clots and occasionally experiences cramp-like abdominal pain. She is nulliparous and experienced menopause at the age of 56. She was diagnosed with osteoporosis at the age of 58 and received estrogen hormone replacement therapy for 2 years. She is otherwise healthy with a body mass index of 20 kg/m^2 and works as an elementary school teacher. Her only medication is cetirizine for seasonal allergies.

What is the differential diagnosis of postmenopausal vaginal bleeding?
Postmenopausal vaginal bleeding may be due to various causes. First, the origin of abnormal bleeding should be confirmed. Bleeding from anatomic sites other than the uterus is considered. For example, pathologic conditions in the ureter, urethra, and bladder or anus and rectum may present with abnormal bleeding in the genital area. Malignancies in the fallopian tubes, ovaries, cervix, and vagina may also present with abnormal bleeding.

What is the most common clinical presentation in a patient with endometrial cancer?
Endometrial cancer may be asymptomatic, particularly in younger patients. However, postmenopausal vaginal bleeding is present in up to 90% cases.

What are the risk factors for endometrial cancer?
Unopposed estrogen has long been known to cause endometrial hyperplasia and increase the risk of endometrial carcinoma. The use of estrogen hormone therapy to treat menopausal symptoms and osteoporosis is linked to a significantly increased risk of developing endometrial carcinoma; the use of progesterone in combination with estrogen shows a protective effect.

CLINICAL PEARL

Tamoxifen, used to treat estrogen receptor- and progesterone receptor-positive breast cancer, has an anti-estrogen effect on the breast tissue and pro-estrogen effect on the endometrial tissue, leading to a slightly increased risk of endometrial carcinoma.

Obesity leads to increased circulating estrogen and thus an increased risk of endometrial carcinoma. Diabetes and polycystic ovary syndrome, both associated with obesity, are considered risk factors, while exercise decreases the risk.

BASIC SCIENCE PEARL

Aromatase is an enzyme critical for the conversion of androgens to estrogen, specifically androstenedione to estrone and testosterone to estradiol. Among other tissues, aromatase is found in adipose, resulting in increased levels of circulating estrogen in obese patients.

Reproductive factors play a role in endometrial cancer risk. Prolonged exposure to estrogen from early menarche, late menopause, low parity, or nulliparity is associated with an increased risk. In contrast, use of oral contraceptives with combined estrogen and progesterone and intrauterine devices have a protective effect and decreased risk as does increased parity and breastfeeding. Estrogen secreting tumors, such as thecomas and granulosa cell tumors of the ovary, are linked to an increased risk although they are rare.

Case Point 12.1

The patient has no family history of endometrial cancer. Her father had prostate cancer, and her sister was diagnosed with breast cancer.

What genetic syndromes are associated with an increased risk of endometrial cancer?

Cowden syndrome and mismatch repair deficiencies, including Lynch syndrome, are associated with an increased risk of endometrioid endometrial carcinoma. Cowden syndrome results from an autosomal dominant defect in the PTEN gene. Lynch syndrome (hereditary nonpolyposis colorectal cancer) results from an autosomal dominant genetic defect in the mismatch repair genes MSH2, MLH1, MSH6, and/or PMS2. Germline mutations in BRCA1/BRCA2 and Lynch syndrome also increase the risk for serous endometrial carcinoma.

BASIC SCIENCE PEARL

Lynch syndrome is a disease arising from mutations in the DNA proofreading genes MLH1, PMS2, MSH2, and MSH6 that function in MMR, and is associated with microsatellite instability. Microsatellites are short segments of DNA; microsatellite instability can be detected as repeats of these short segments. Patients with Lynch syndrome have an 80% lifetime risk of developing colorectal cancer and 40%–60% risk of developing endometrioid cancer. The risk is also increased for cancers of the ovaries (clear cell and endometrioid), adrenals, prostate, kidneys, ureters, bladder, skin, brain, and blood (leukemia). Diagnosis of Lynch syndrome and genetic counseling help patients and clinicians formulate a cancer surveillance plan.

Case Point 12.2

Physical examination shows a distended, non-tender abdomen in an otherwise thin woman. There are no genital lesions; however, there is a small amount of red–brown vaginal discharge.

Endometrial cancer is the most common gynecological malignancy in developed countries and is at the top of the differential diagnosis, particularly in postmenopausal women. However, there are many benign uterine entities that will also cause postmenopausal vaginal bleeding such as endometrial polyps, submucosal fibroids (leiomyomata), mucosal atrophy, and benign uterine hyperplasia.

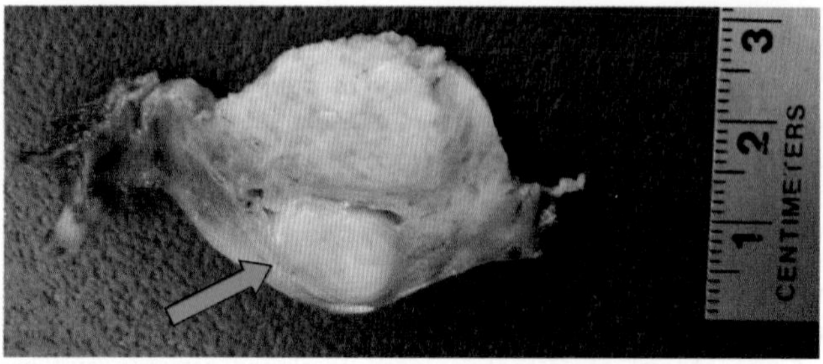

Fig. 12.1 Gross photograph of a well-circumscribed, white-whorled intramural mass, consistent with a leiomyoma designated by a green arrow.

Leiomyoma (fibroid) is a benign smooth muscle tumor that is very common and seen in approximately 70% of hysterectomy specimens, with a higher incidence in premenopausal women. They are often multiple and may have subserosal, intramural, or submucosal locations. They are typically well-circumscribed, firm, tan–white nodules with whorled, homogeneous cut surfaces. Their size can vary widely from microscopic foci to >30 cm; however, typically a decrease in size in postmenopausal women is noted (Fig. 12.1).

CLINICAL PEARL

Several variants of leiomyomata exist, including cellular, myxoid, epithelioid, lipomatous, mitotically active, and leiomyoma with bizarre nuclei. Although they may metastasize and be found years after a hysterectomy, they are benign and do not progress to leiomyosarcomas.

Endometrial polyps are also a common benign source of uterine bleeding. They consist of an abnormal proliferation of endometrial stroma with benign glands and thick-walled blood vessels forming a polypoid mass that is often exophytic. The glands may be cystically dilated and of various sizes and shapes. The stroma is more fibrous than in normal endometrium, and the cells are bland (Fig. 12.2).

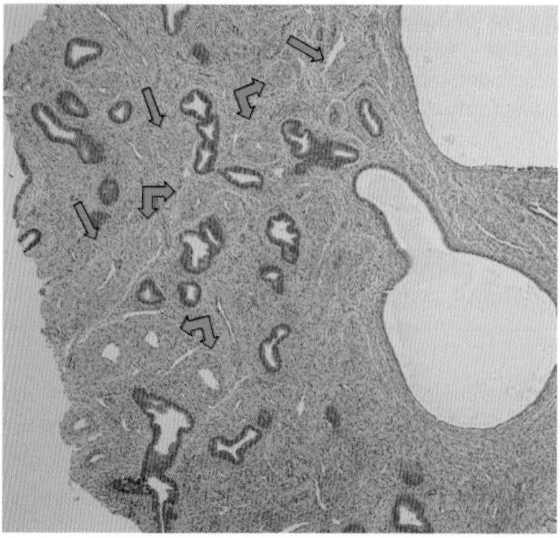

Fig. 12.2 Endometrial polyp histology showing cellular stroma, glands that are irregular and glands that are cystically dilated. Green arrows point to examples of thickened blood vessels. (H&E stain, 40x).

CLINICAL PEARL

Atypical endometrial hyperplasia and endometrial carcinoma may be present within an endometrial polyp. A careful search for atypia is important.

Postmenopausal hormone therapy, including therapy with combined estrogen and progesterone, may affect endometrial blood vessels and lead to vaginal bleeding, particularly during the first 6 months of treatment, independent of endometrial hyperplasia. Anticoagulant therapy presents a slight risk of abnormal uterine bleeding. Other factors such as trauma and infection should also be considered.

In general, endometrial hyperplasia is defined as a proliferation of endometrial glands so that the gland-to-stroma ratio exceeds 50%. The World Health Organization classifies endometrial hyperplasia into two categories: hyperplasia without atypia and atypical hyperplasia. The former is non-neoplastic and bears no increased risk of becoming malignant. Atypical endometrial hyperplasia, on the other hand, is a precancerous lesion. Not only is the gland-to-stroma ratio >50%, the epithelial cells may exhibit atypical features including enlarged size, nuclear hyperchromasia, prominent nucleoli, and clumped chromatin.

CLINICAL PEARL

Atypical endometrial hyperplasia is synonymous to endometrial intraepithelial neoplasm (EIN). EIN terminology is used in some classification systems. Women with either diagnosis should undergo further evaluation for concurrent endometrial carcinoma. Some studies have shown that over 30% of women with atypical hyperplasia will have endometrial carcinoma in the hysterectomy specimen.

Distinguishing atypical endometrial hyperplasia from endometrial carcinoma in a biopsy may be challenging. Both may exhibit metaplasia, frequently squamous metaplasia. However, only carcinoma will have confluent sheets of glands with no intervening stroma and invasion of the myometrium. Unlike serous endometrial carcinoma, p53 will be wild type. Mutations in PTEN and /or PAX2 may be present in either entity. In hysterectomy specimens with a history of atypical hyperplasia and no definite mass lesion, the entire endometrium is submitted for histologic evaluation.

Endometrial carcinoma has been divided into type I and type II. Type I carcinoma arises in a background of endometrial hyperplasia and is strongly associated with unopposed estrogen, typically endometrioid carcinoma. Type II carcinoma arises in atrophic endometrium and is typically the more aggressive serous carcinoma. Clear cell carcinoma is also classified as type II. The association of type II with unopposed estrogen and aforementioned risk factors has been debated; however, recent studies have shown that the risk factors are likely the same for both type I and type II carcinomas.

Case Point 12.3

Transvaginal ultrasound imaging shows a thickened, heterogeneous endometrium. A computerized tomography scan confirms the presence of an enlarged uterus that is thick walled and heterogeneous. The patient undergoes dilatation and curettage with endometrial biopsy. The biopsy is diagnostic for malignancy, and the patient proceeds to total laparoscopic hysterectomy with bilateral salpingo-oophorectomy and sentinel lymph node dissection.

What are the histologic types of endometrial (epithelial) tumors of the uterus?

Endometrioid endometrial carcinoma is the most common uterine carcinoma (approximately 80% of cases). Grossly, the tumor consists of a polypoid, exophytic mass commonly on the posterior wall, but may fill the uterine cavity and extend to the dome and anterior wall as well (Fig. 12.3). The tumor has back-to-back glands with varying degrees of nuclear atypia (Fig. 12.4). Higher-grade lesions have solid components and are classified by the International Federation of Gynecology and Obstetrics (FIGO) grade according to proportion of solid architecture, excluding squamous differentiation (Table 12.1). High-grade nuclear atypia in a tumor with low-grade architecture increases the FIGO grade by 1; therefore, a FIGO grade 2 tumor can become FIGO grade 3 based on nuclear atypia. Besides squamous, variants include mucinous (<50% mucinous differentiation), tubular, secretory, villoglandular, and others that are extremely rare (Table 12.2). Myometrial invasion is measured from

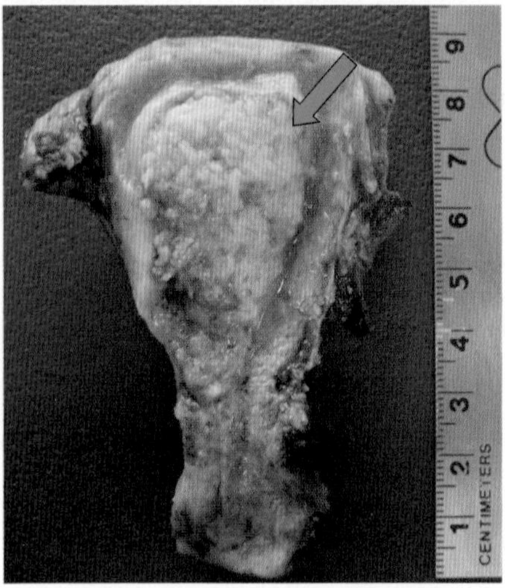

Fig. 12.3 Gross photograph of uterus with exophytic endometrioid endometrial carcinoma occupying the entire uterine cavity designated by a green arrow.

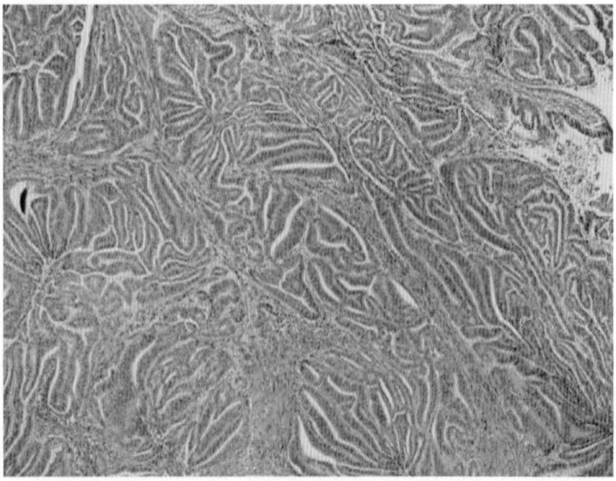

Fig. 12.4 Endometrioid endometrial carcinoma with back-to-back glands. (H&E stain, 40x).

TABLE 12.1 ■ **The International Federation of Gynecology and Obstetrics (FIGO) Grading Scheme**

FIGO Grade	Solid Growth Pattern (%)
1	≤5
2	6–50
3	>50

TABLE 12.2 ■ **Classification and Features of Endometrial Carcinomas**

Carcinoma Types	Microscopic Features	Ancillary Studies
Endometrioid	Glandular (usually proliferative-phase type) with acinar, papillary, or solid growth; nuclei may be uniform to pleomorphic	p53 usually wild type; p16 usually negative or patchy; ER/PR usually positive
Squamous differentiation	May have focal keratinization and/or necrosis, intercellular bridges or solid sheets of cells with abundant eosinophilic cytoplasm and distinct cell borders	
Villoglandular	Long and slender papillae with fibrovascular cores lined by low-grade cells	
Secretory	Glands are large and may have luminal scalloping; supranuclear vacuoles are present	
Other rare variants	Sertoliform, microglandular, tubular	
Mucinous	Abundant cytoplasmic mucin in >50% of cells; bland and basally located nuclei; glandular or papillary architecture; minimal mitotic activity	Vimentin, ER/PR usually positive Somatic KRAS mutations in most
Serous	Papillary, pseudoglandular, and solid architecture; irregular branching papillae with cellular budding; non-cohesive cells; high-grade nuclear atypia and brisk mitoses	p53 and p16 usually diffusely positive; pax-8 usually positive; ER/PR and WT1 often negative or weak
Clear cell	Mixed tubulocystic, papillary, and solid architecture; primarily clear cells with large, round hyperchromatic nuclei with prominent nucleoli and variable mitoses	C-erb-B2, HNF-1, Napsin-A and racemase positive; ER/PR usually negative; WT1, p16 and p53 variable
Neuroendocrine	Varies—low-grade carcinoid, high grade with small cell or large cell morphology	Synaptophysin, chromogranin, NSE, and CD56-positive
Mixed cell	Composed of at least two histologic types (one of which is type II); most commonly endometrioid and serous	Variable depending on components
Undifferentiated	Sheets of cells with no gland formation and no histologic features of other subtypes; mitoses are brisk	Pancytokeratin positive, CK18 and EMA positive; SMARCA4 loss
Dedifferentiated	Contains component of undifferentiated as well as other histologic subtype	Variable
Carcinosarcoma (malignant mixed Müllerian tumor)	Endometrial carcinoma with metaplastic sarcomatous component	Variable depending on components; p16 and p53 frequently positive in both

ER, estrogen receptor; PR, progesterone receptor.

the endomyometrial junction, excluding exophytic portions of the tumor, to the deepest point of invasion (Fig. 12.5).

Approximately 10% of endometrial carcinomas are serous carcinomas. Unlike endometrioid endometrial carcinomas, they occur in a background of atrophic endometrium instead of hyperplasia. Serous carcinoma is a high-grade aggressive malignancy that typically has a mutation in the p53 gene and a high mitotic rate. It is morphologically similar to its ovarian/fallopian tube counterpart. The most common architectural pattern is papillary with irregularly shaped papillae that may be closely packed, resulting in a slit-like appearance. Cellular budding from tips of papillae can be readily identified. Poorly formed glands and solid sheets of dyscohesive cells may also be present. The cells are high-grade and pleomorphic, with a high nuclear-to-cytoplasmic ratio, hyperchromatic nuclei, frequent prominent nucleoli, and eosinophilic cytoplasm (Fig. 12.6). Serous endometrial carcinomas are high-grade by convention, so the FIGO grading scheme is not used.

CLINICAL PEARL

Serum CA-125 is elevated in serous endometrial carcinoma as in advanced serous ovarian carcinoma. The endometrial and ovarian variants may be identical morphologically requiring careful consideration to determine a primary serous endometrial carcinoma from a metastatic ovarian carcinoma to the uterus.

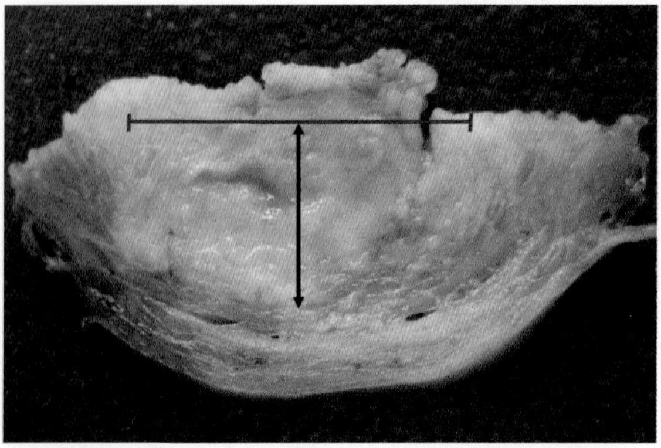

Fig. 12.5 Depth of invasion in myometrial invasive endometrioid endometrial carcinoma. The red bar is at the endomyometrial junction and the black arrows indicate the greatest depth of invasion.

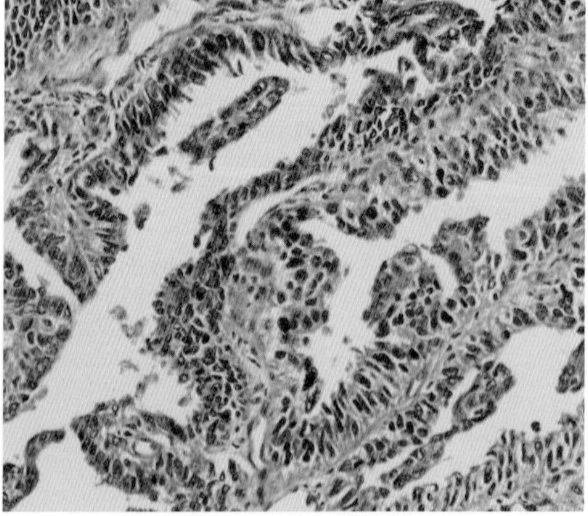

Fig. 12.6 Serous endometrial carcinoma with papillary architecture and high-grade nuclei (H&E stain, 200x).

Carcinosarcoma, formerly known as malignant mixed Müllerian tumor, is a biphasic tumor with a carcinomatous component and usually a minor sarcomatous component with an abrupt transition. The carcinomatous component is typically high grade and can be endometrioid, serous, clear cell, squamous, or mixed. The sarcomatous component may be homologous (leiomyosarcoma or fibrosarcoma) or heterologous (rhabdomyosarcoma or chondrosarcoma).

Other endometrial carcinomas include mucinous (>50% mucinous differentiation), clear cell, neuroendocrine, mixed cell adenocarcinoma, undifferentiated, and dedifferentiated carcinomas (Table 12.2). These entities are rare, occurring in <10% of cases in total.

CLINICAL PEARL

Although benign leiomyomata are very common, malignant smooth muscle tumors, leiomyosarcomas, are not. Mesenchymal tumors of the uterus are generally rare. Other mesenchymal tumors include benign and low-grade endometrial stromal tumors and high-grade sarcomas, undifferentiated sarcomas, inflammatory myofibroblastic tumors, perivascular epithelioid cell proliferations, and uterine tumors resembling ovarian sex cord tumors.

Case Point 12.4

The patient's hysterectomy specimen is opened to reveal an exophytic, papillary, tan-white friable tumor filling the majority of the uterine cavity and involving both the anterior and posterior walls. Sectioning reveals that the tumor invades >50% of the myometrial wall thickness. Multiple well-circumscribed subserosal and intramural leiomyomata with firm, tan-white cut surfaces and no hemorrhage or necrosis are identified.

Histologically, approximately 70% tumor consists of well-defined proliferative-type glands in a back-to-back arrangement, whereas 20% consists solid sheets of tumor cells displaying squamous differentiation (Fig. 12.7). The remaining tumor (10%) consists of solid sheets of tumor cells without gland formation (Fig. 12.8).

Case Point 12.5

A diagnosis of endometrioid endometrial carcinoma, FIGO 2, is rendered.

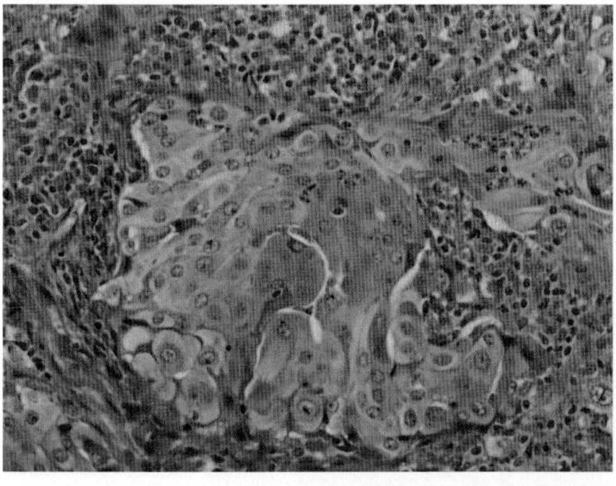

Fig. 12.7 Endometrioid endometrial carcinoma with squamous differentiation (H&E stain, 200x).

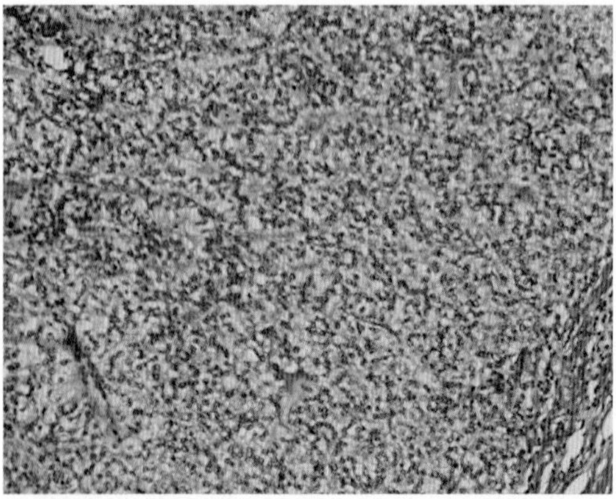

Fig. 12.8 Endometrioid endometrial carcinoma with solid growth pattern (H&E stain, 100x).

What are the factors to consider when staging endometrial carcinoma?

Myometrial invasion (whether greater or less than 50%), involvement of the cervix, serosa, adnexa, vagina, parametrium, bladder mucosa, and bowel mucosa are considered for staging. Regional lymph node metastasis to para-aortic and pelvic lymph nodes is reported as well.

Case Point 12.6

The extent of myometrial invasion, 84%, is calculated grossly and confirmed microscopically. The lower uterine segment is involved, but the cervical and soft tissue margins, adjacent structures, and regional lymph nodes are free of tumor. However, lymphovascular invasion is identified (Fig. 12.9).

The staging is pT1b N0.

What additional testing should be performed on endometrial carcinomas?

Case Point 12.7

Immunohistochemical testing for MMR proteins is performed.

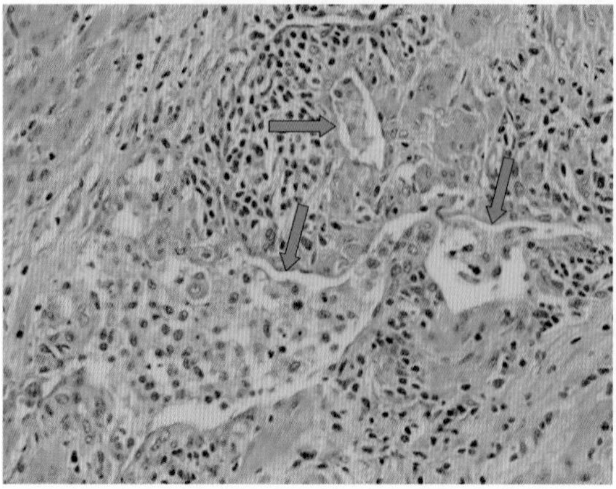

Fig. 12.9 Lymphovascular invasion in endometrioid endometrial carcinoma. The green arrows indicate invasive tumor cells within vessels (H&E stain, 200x).

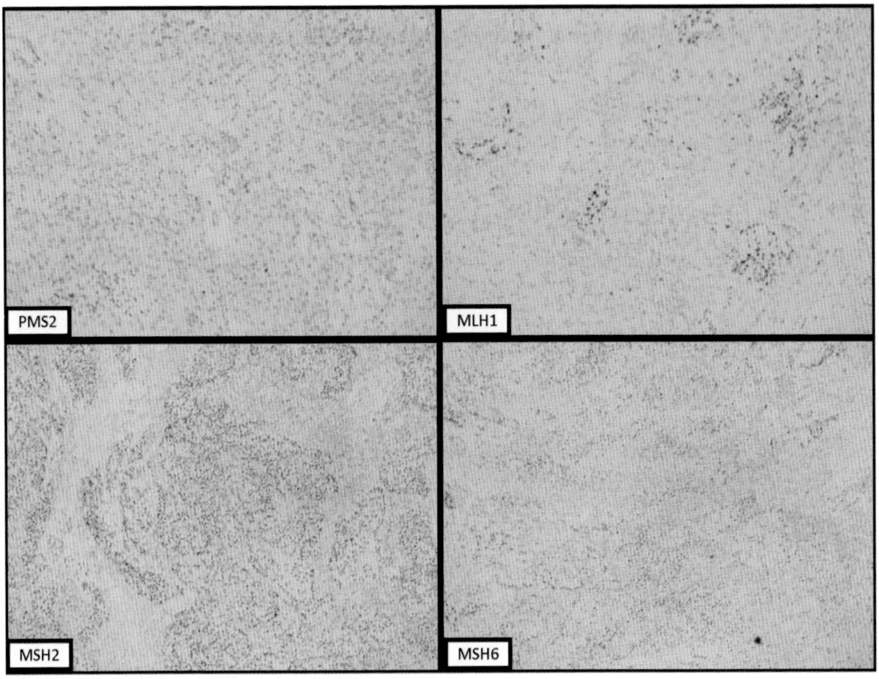

Fig. 12.10 Results of mismatch repair deficiency immunohistochemical studies showing retained expression of MSH2 and MSH6 and loss of PMS2 and MLH1.

The four MMR proteins evaluated are MLH1, PMS2, MSH2, and MSH6. Loss of MSH2/MSH6 indicates the presence of a germline mutation, and genetic counseling is recommended. If MLH1/PMS2 is lost, MLH1 promoter methylation testing is recommended. Hypermethylation indicates likely sporadic inactivation rather than germline.

Case Point 12.8

MSH2 and MSH6 have intact nuclear expression, whereas MLH1 and PMS2 show loss of nuclear expression (Fig. 12.10). MLH1 methylation promoter testing is ordered and is positive indicating that the patient is unlikely to have Lynch syndrome and the microsatellite instability is due to a sporadic MMR deficiency mutation.

How does stage determine treatment recommendations?

In young patients, with low-grade tumors, who wish to preserve fertility, progestin hormonal therapy and observation may be preferred. However, surgery with hysterectomy and salpingo-oophorectomy is standard for treatment and staging purposes.

CLINICAL PEARL

Prognosis of endometrioid endometrial carcinoma worsens with increasing FIGO stage, age, histologic grade, and depth of myometrial invasion. Presence of lymphovascular invasion is also associated with worse prognosis.

TABLE 12.3 ■ **General Overview of Treatment Approach for Endometrial Carcinomas**

Risk	Definition	Treatment Approach	5-Year Survival Rate (%)
Low	Grade 1 or 2 (endometrioid), confined to endometrium or invading <50% of myometrium; no lymphovascular invasion	Total hysterectomy and bilateral salpingo-oophorectomy	80–90
Intermediate	Confined to uterus with involvement of myometrium >50% or cervical stromal invasion	Total hysterectomy and bilateral salpingo-oophorectomy followed by observation or pelvic radiation therapy depending on additional factors including age, grade 2 or 3 histology, and presence of lymphovascular invasion	70–80
High	Serous or clear cell carcinoma, some grade 3 endometrioid carcinomas; tumors extending beyond uterus (including serosa, adnexa, vagina, parametrium, bladder, or bowel)	Total hysterectomy followed by chemotherapy and pelvic radiation therapy	20–60

Stage helps stratify risk of recurrence and metastasis. Pelvic radiation therapy and chemotherapy are considered for higher-stage tumors based on pathologic findings (Table 12.3).

BEYOND THE PEARLS

- Pap smears may detect abnormal glandular cells and raise suspicion for endometrial carcinoma. Glandular cells seen in cytologic preparations in women older than 45 years of age are routinely reported.
- p53 is a tumor suppressor gene that codes for a protein important for detection of DNA damage and halting cell cycle progression in response to stress signals. Mutations in p53 are the most common mutations in malignant neoplasms across tissue types. Serous endometrial carcinoma and high-grade endometrioid carcinomas often harbor an inactivating p53 mutation. Immunohistochemical stains for p53 will either be diffusely positive or completely negative if mutated.
- Germline mutations in BRCA1/BRCA2 result in deficient homologous recombination DNA double-strand break repair and are known to increase the risk of breast and ovarian cancer. Risk of serous endometrial cancer also increases.
- Smoking actually decreases the risk of endometrial carcinoma.
- Ki67immunohistochemical studies provide an indication of tumor mitotic activity and help differentiate between low-grade carcinoid tumors and high-grade neuroendocrine carcinomas.
- The uterus is not a common site for metastasis; however, metastatic gastrointestinal malignancies such as colon and stomach may be histologically similar to endometrioid or mucinous endometrial carcinomas.

References

Carcangiu ML, Herrington CS, Young RH. *Who Classification of Tumours of Female Reproductive Organs.* 2014.

Clarke MA, Long BJ, Del Mar Morillo A, Arbyn M, Bakkum-Gamez JN, Wentzensen N. Association of endometrial cancer risk with postmenopausal bleeding in women: a systematic review and meta-analysis. *JAMA Intern Med.* 2018;178(9):1210-1222. doi:10.1001/jamainternmed.2018.2820.

College of American Pathologists. *Protocol for the Examination of Specimens from Patients with Carcinoma and Carcinosarcoma of the Endometrium.* 2018.

Felix AS, Brinton LA. Cancer progress and priorities: uterine cancer. *Cancer Epidemiol Biomarkers Prev.* 2018;27(9):985-994. doi:10.1158/1055-9965.EPI-18-0264.

Goldblum JR, Lamps LW, McKenney JK, et al. *Rosai and Ackerman's Surgical Pathology.* Elsevier; 2018.

Setiawan VW, Yang HP, Pike MC, et al. Type I and II endometrial cancers: have they different risk factors? *J Clin Oncol.* 2013;31(20):2607-2618. doi:10.1200/JCO.2012.48.2596.

CASE 13

A 56-Year-Old Female with Pelvic Mass

Cynthia Reyes Barron

A 56-year-old woman presents to her physician after noticing a mass palpable above her pubic bone. She also complains of acute urinary retention. She denies nausea, vomiting, changes in bowel habits, abdominal pain, and tenderness. Her surgical history is significant for a supracervical hysterectomy and left oophorectomy, for symptomatic leiomyomas, over 20 years ago. Then 9 years ago, she underwent abdominal surgery for lysis of adhesions causing small bowel obstruction. She is otherwise healthy and her only medications are vitamin supplements. Upon physical examination, there is a palpable, non-tender, pelvic mass. There are no genital lesions or vaginal discharge. Her chemistry panel, cell count, and vitals are within normal limits.

What is the differential diagnosis of a pelvic mass in a woman?

Whether found incidentally or symptomatically (urinary retention, bowel obstruction, pain), most pelvic masses are benign. For premenopausal women, two etiologies that require urgent intervention and need to be ruled out are ectopic pregnancy and ovarian torsion. However, these typically present with severe pain. In a postmenopausal woman with a painless pelvic mass, both benign and malignant etiologies are in the differential (Table 13.1). Ovaries are one of the main organs to consider and are composed of four tissue types: epithelium, germ cells, sex cords, and stroma. Neoplasms of ovarian origin are classified into categories based on these four tissue types. Each category is further subdivided and has entities that are benign, borderline, or malignant (Table 13.2).

CLINICAL PEARL

Benign ovarian tumors are well differentiated and consist of cells that are histologically similar to normal cells.

Borderline ovarian tumors consist of cells with cytologic atypia, but lack invasion.

Malignant ovarian tumors are distinguished from others by the presence of invasion and often have high-grade histologic features including pleomorphism, increased nuclear size, prominent nucleoli, and a high mitotic rate.

What familial syndromes carry an increased risk of ovarian cancer?

Hereditary breast and ovarian cancer syndrome (HBOCS) and Lynch syndrome are associated with an increased risk of ovarian cancer. HBOCS results from germline mutations in BRCA1 or BRCA2 and causes an increased risk of high-grade serous carcinoma of the ovary. Lynch syndrome results from germline mutations in DNA mismatch repair (MMR) proteins. Patients with Lynch syndrome have an increased risk of developing clear cell carcinoma and endometrioid carcinoma.

TABLE 13.1 ■ **Differential Diagnoses of Pelvic Masses**

Origin	Benign	Malignant
Ovarian	Cysts (functional, corpus luteal, theca lutein, polycystic ovarian disease, cystadenoma) Pregnancy luteoma Endometrioma Germ cell tumor (benign type) Sex cord-stromal tumor (benign type)	Epithelial carcinoma or borderline tumor Germ cell tumor (malignant type) Sex cord-stromal tumor (malignant type)
Tubal	Ectopic pregnancy (urgent intervention required) Hydrosalpinx	Epithelial carcinoma Serous tubal intraepithelial neoplasia
Other	Uterine leiomyoma Abscess (appendiceal, diverticular, pelvic) Diverticula (bladder, ureteral, intestinal) Constipation Peritoneal cyst Nerve sheath tumor	Appendiceal adenocarcinoma Gastrointestinal malignancy Retroperitoneal sarcoma Lymphoma Metastatic endometrial carcinoma Other metastases (breast, gastric, colon)

TABLE 13.2 ■ **World Health Organization Classification of Ovarian Neoplasms**

Histologic Type	Subtype	Benign	Borderline	Malignant
Epithelial	Serous	Cystadenoma Adenofibroma Surface papilloma	Borderline (variants)	Low- or high-grade carcinoma
	Mucinous	Cystadenoma Adenofibroma	Borderline	Carcinoma
	Endometrioid	Cyst Cystadenoma Adenofibroma	Borderline	Carcinoma
	Clear cell	Cystadenoma Adenofibroma	Borderline	Carcinoma
	Brenner	Benign	Borderline	Malignant
	Seromucinous	Benign	Borderline	Malignant
	Undifferentiated			Carcinoma
Mesenchymal				Low- and high-grade endometrial stromal sarcoma
Mixed epithelial and mesenchymal				Adenosarcoma Carcinosarcoma
Sex cord-stromal tumors	Pure stromal tumors	Fibroma Thecoma Sclerosing stromal tumor Signet-ring stromal tumor Microcystic stromal tumor Leydig cell tumor Steroid cell tumor		Fibrosarcoma Steroid cell tumor—malignant

Continued on following page

TABLE 13.2 ■ **World Health Organization Classification of Ovarian Neoplasms** (Continued)

Histologic Type	Subtype	Benign	Borderline	Malignant
	Pure sex cord tumors	Sertoli cell tumor: benign Sex cord tumor with annular tubules: benign		Sertoli cell tumor: malignant (rare) Adult granulosa cell tumor Juvenile granulosa cell tumor Sex cord tumor with annular tubules: malignant (rare)
	Mixed sex cord-stromal tumors	Sertoli-leydig cell tumor (variants)		May be malignant
	Sex cord-stromal tumors, NOS	Usually benign		Malignant (rare)
Germ cell tumors		Mature teratoma		Dysgerminoma Yolk sac tumor Embryonal carcinoma Choriocarcinoma Immature teratoma Mixed germ cell tumor
Germ cell-sex cord-stromal tumors	Gonadoblastoma	Benign		With malignant germ cell tumor component

CLINICAL PEARL

Mutations in DNA MMR proteins MLH1, PMS2, MSH2, and/or MSH6 are associated with Lynch syndrome, the most common familial cause of cancer. The risk increases for several epithelial cancers, most notably colon cancer and endometrial cancer. The MMR deficiency results in microsatellite instability. Microsatellites are short DNA repeats produced by the replication errors from MMR deficiency.

CLINICAL PEARL

BRCA1 and BRCA2 genes encode proteins essential to DNA double-strand break repair. Patients diagnosed with ovarian high-grade serous carcinoma should undergo genetic testing because 15%–20% will have a germline mutation in BRCA1 or BRCA2. Patients with BRCA1/BRCA2 mutations should undergo increased monitoring for breast cancer as well.

Case Point 13.1

Although several first-degree relatives have been diagnosed with aortic aneurysms, the patient has no family history of cancer.

What patient characteristics are important for determining the risk of malignancy?

Low parity increases the risk for certain tumors including serous carcinoma. In addition, age and menopausal status help narrow the differential diagnosis of a pelvic mass. Ovarian cysts are physiologic lesions related to ovulation and more commonly seen in premenopausal women, although they may present in postmenopausal women, particularly within the first 5 years of

TABLE 13.3 ■ **Features of Common Ovarian Neoplasms**

Diagnosis	Average Size	Laterality	Mean Age at Diagnosis (Years)
High-grade serous carcinoma	Variable, often large	65% Bilateral	63
Mucinous carcinoma	Mean 19 cm	Usually unilateral	45
Endometrioid carcinoma	Mean 15 cm	40% Bilateral	58
Clear cell carcinoma	Mean 15 cm	40% Bilateral	55
Brenner tumor	Usually <2 cm	Usually unilateral	Variable (mostly 40–70)
Fibroma	Variable	Unilateral (unless syndromic)	48
Granulosa cell tumor	Variable, mean 10 cm	Unilateral	53
Dysgerminoma	>10 cm	Usually unilateral	Children and young women, mean 22
Yolk sac tumor	Variable, usually >10 cm	Usually unilateral	19
Embryonal carcinoma	Mean 15 cm	Usually unilateral	Average <15
Mature teratoma	5–10 cm	15% Bilateral	Variable (most during reproductive years)
Immature teratoma	Mean 17 cm	Unilateral	Usually <30

menopause. Germ cell tumors, such as teratomas and dysgerminomas, are more likely to occur in children and young adults. Both benign and malignant ovarian epithelial tumors are typically seen in adults (Table 13.3).

CLINICAL PEARL

Germ cell tumors are the most common ovarian tumors in females younger than 20 years, and approximately 95% are benign mature cystic teratomas. However, the younger the patient, the more likely the tumor is malignant. Approximately 8% are mixed germ cell tumors composed of two components, most frequently dysgerminoma and yolk sac.

What role does imaging play in evaluating pelvic masses?

Ultrasound is routinely performed to assess suspected pelvic masses and is usually the initial diagnostic test. To begin with, imaging may identify the origin of the mass whether it is arising from a gynecological structure such as ovary, uterus, or fallopian tube, or other structures such as bladder, bowel, or soft tissue. Ultrasound and/or magnetic resonance imaging (MRI) may provide a diagnosis with fair certainty in some cases of adnexal masses such as paratubal or paraovarian cysts and hemorrhagic cysts, which have characteristically cystic appearances with no solid components. Mature cystic teratomas have various echogenic and shadowing qualities that point to the diagnosis. The most important feature of a malignant mass is a solid component. This component may be papillary, nodular, or manifest as thickened septae within a cystic lesion. Another feature of malignancy is strong color Doppler flow measured by ultrasound. Benign cystic lesions typically have no visible blood flow. Size and laterality are also features that guide the differential (Table 13.3). Epithelial tumors, in particular, are frequently bilateral. Malignant serous tumors are bilateral approximately in 60% cases, whereas clear cell and endometrioid carcinomas are bilateral in 40% cases. Imaging may also identify evidence of metastasis and pelvic implants.

Case Point 13.2

Given the patient's previous surgical history, MRI studies are performed instead of ultrasound. MRI shows a cystic mass of 13 × 10.3 × 9.8 cm in the pelvis. There is a small amount of free fluid without any evidence of other masses or peritoneal nodules.

CLINICAL PEARL

Biopsy is generally not indicated for adnexal masses because disruption of a malignant tumor may adversely affect prognosis. Malignant cell spillage into the peritoneum increases stage.

What serum biomarkers are important for evaluation?

Because biopsy plays no role in the diagnosis of ovarian tumors, there is great interest in the use of serum biomarkers in the evaluation of pelvic masses. No single biomarker is sufficiently sensitive and specific to diagnose ovarian carcinomas, yet results of several biomarkers are diagnostically useful.

Cancer antigen 125 (CA125) is the most widely used biomarker for evaluation of adnexal masses. CA125 levels are elevated in epithelial ovarian cancers, with a general increase in value with increase in the disease stage; however, it is neither sensitive nor specific enough to be used for definitive diagnosis. CA125 is used to calculate the risk of malignancy in several risk score assessments. Levels of CA125 may also be followed to monitor treatment response.

Like CA125, the human epididymis protein 4 (HE4) level is elevated in epithelial ovarian cancers and is a factor in several risk assessment calculations. HE4 levels may also be followed to monitor treatment response.

Germ cell or sex cord-stromal tumors may secrete hormones that are detectable in serum. For example, patients with embryonal carcinoma or choriocarcinoma have elevated levels of human chorionic gonadotropin, whereas those with yolk sac tumors have elevated levels of alpha-fetoprotein. Inhibin levels are elevated in granulosa cell tumors, and sertoli-leydig tumors secrete androgens that typically cause virilization.

Case Point 13.3

The patient's CA125 level is 71 (normal range: 0–34) U/mL and HE4 level is 44 (normal range: 0–140) pmol/L.

How are biomarker panels and risk assessments utilized in patient evaluation?

Multiple algorithms, which take into account serum biomarker values and other factors, are available for clinicians to calculate the risk that a given adnexal mass is malignant. Many of these algorithms factor a patient's menopausal status as well as ultrasound findings (Table 13.4). The results help guide patient management. Patients with a low risk by calculation may be monitored if asymptomatic, while patients with a high risk are likely to undergo surgery.

Case Point 13.4

The risk of ovarian malignancy algorithm (ROMA) score is low risk.

TABLE 13.4 ■ **Algorithms for Risk Assessment**

Assessment	Serum Tests	Imaging Features	Other Factors
ADNEX	CA125	Size, solid tumor, cysts, papillary projections, acoustic shadows, ascites	Age, treatment center
Overa	Follicle-stimulating hormone, human epididymus protein 4 (HE4), apolipoprotein A-1, transferrin, cancer antigen (CA125)		
Risk of malignancy index I	CA125	Multilocular cysts, solid tumor, metastases, ascites, bilaterality	Menopausal status
ROMA	CA125 and HE4		Menopausal status
Simple rules		Cyst loculations, size, ascites, blood flow, papillary structures	

ROMA, risk of ovarian malignancy algorithm.

What specimens are analyzed for staging purposes of an ovarian malignancy?

To begin with, a sample is collected for peritoneal cytology once the cavity is incised to assess the presence of malignant cells. The sample may consist of ascites fluid or pelvic washings obtained by instilling saline into the peritoneal cavity and removing it by suction. It is important to determine the presence of peritoneal implants, particularly for staging of serous and seromucinous borderline tumors. The peritoneal surfaces, upper abdomen, and bowel mesentery are evaluated for involvement, and biopsies may be taken at the time of salpingo-oophorectomy. Diaphragmatic scrapings are also taken for cytology evaluation. An omentectomy is performed for full pathologic evaluation of omental implants. Surgeons make every effort to remove the ovary/ovarian tumor and fallopian tube intact. Seeding of the peritoneum by intraoperative rupture may have an impact on prognosis and is reported by the staging designation. Finally, bilateral lymph node dissection of periaortic and pelvic nodes is important for staging.

Case Point 13.5

The patient is scheduled for surgery. Cell block and cytospin preparations are examined for the patient's pelvic washings and diaphragmatic scrapings that are sent to cytopathology. No malignant tumor cells are identified.

CLINICAL PEARL

Cytology plays an important role in staging of ovarian carcinoma. Peritoneal washings are analyzed for the presence of malignant cells. High-grade serous carcinomas, tumors involving the ovarian surface, and tumors at advanced stage are more likely to have positive cytological findings.

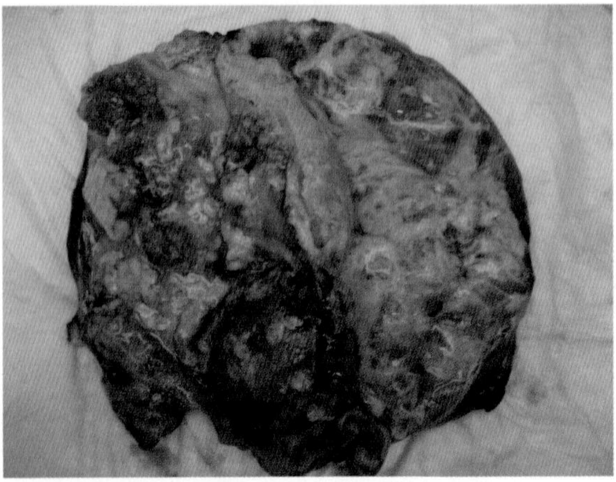

Fig. 13.1 Gross photograph of a transected ovarian tumor.

Case Point 13.6

The right fallopian tube, ovary, and cervix are resected and sent for pathological evaluation. The specimen is received intact and the tumor is identified arising from the right ovary. The fallopian tube and omentum are not involved by the tumor. Multiple biopsies of pelvic tissue including the round ligament, bladder, and anterior abdominal wall are submitted for evaluation, and results are negative for malignancy. Seven lymph nodes are examined, and are all negative for malignancy. Grossly, the ovary is 15 cm in greatest dimension and cystic (Fig. 13.1). Sectioning reveals a multiloculated cystic mass with tan-brown gritty fluid and cyst walls that are predominantly smooth. There are two solid components consisting of lobulated excrescences. A frozen section of a representative sample of a solid area of the tumor is performed. The section of tumor frozen for immediate assessment is diagnosed as carcinoma.

CLINICAL PEARL

Intraoperative frozen section diagnosis aids in tumor assessment and guides further surgical management. Tissue sent to surgical pathology is immediately frozen and a thin section cut and mounted onto a glass slide. The slide is processed and stained. Although it may not be possible for the evaluating pathologist to make a definitive diagnosis on the frozen section tissue, malignant features are often apparent. The surgeon typically receives an answer within 20 minutes.

Case Point 13.7

Histologically, the solid components of the tumor consist of tubulocystic, papillary, and solid sheets of malignant cells with a fibrous stroma (Fig. 13.2). There is focal necrosis. The papillae are short with hyalinized cores that lack hierarchical branching (Fig. 13.3). Some of the nuclei of the cells lining the papillae protrude into the lumina resulting in a "hobnail" appearance. The nuclear contours are irregular, and the cells have prominent nucleoli. The cytoplasm is eosinophilic or clear (Fig. 13.4). Immunohistochemistry shows strong staining for napsin-A, while p53 shows wild-type staining.

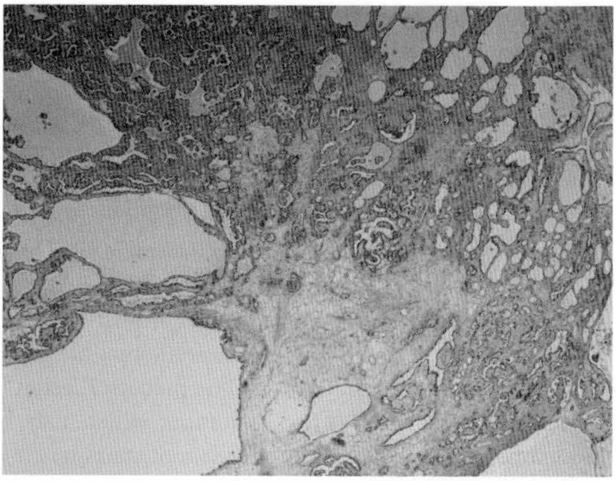

Fig. 13.2 Histologic section of the patient's tumor demonstrating tubulocystic, papillary, and solid architectural growth patterns (H&E, 20x).

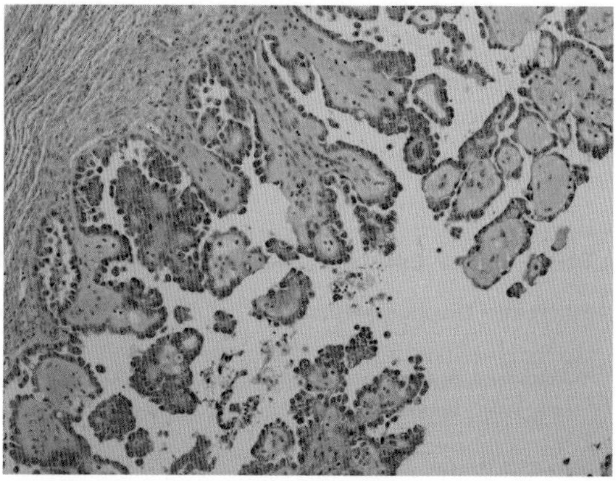

Fig. 13.3 Histologic section of the patient's tumor demonstrating papillae with hyalinized cores (H&E, 100x).

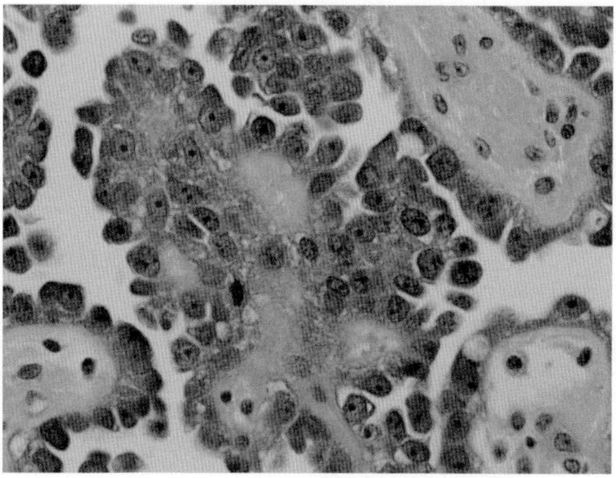

Fig. 13.4 Histologic section of the patient's tumor demonstrating nuclear atypia and prominent nucleoli (H&E, 400x).

What is the histological differential diagnosis?

Several primary ovarian neoplasms may display papillary and solid architecture. The features of the papillae including branching and hyalinization of the vascular cores help differentiate between entities. Although multiple lesions, including metastatic renal cell carcinoma, may have clear cell features, immunohistochemistry is a valuable tool for distinguishing malignancies (Table 13.5).

High-grade serous carcinomas may have papillary, glandular, or solid patterns of growth. When papillae are present, they typically vary in size; have hierarchical branching, cellular tufting, and budding. Necrosis and psammoma bodies may be readily identified in some cases. The nuclei are typically pleomorphic, large, hyperchromatic, and may have multinucleation. Mitoses are usually abundant (Fig. 13.5). Serous carcinomas are generally believed to arise from the fallopian tube, typically the fimbriated end. The precursor lesion is serous tubal intraepithelial carcinoma. These tumors harbor a TP53 mutation, which may be apparent by diffuse staining of p53 immunohistochemistry or complete loss of staining.

Endometrioid carcinoma usually has a glandular architecture, similar to its uterine counterpart, but may also have papillary and solid architecture (Fig. 13.6). Variants include tumors with squamous differentiation or clear cell change. Most tumors are low grade, and cytologic atypia is moderate. The cells are usually columnar with pseudostratified nuclei and may have nuclear grooves. The International Federation of Gynecology and Obstetrics or FIGO grading scheme, based on percentage of solid growth, used for endometrial endometrioid carcinoma is also used for the ovarian counterpart.

TABLE 13.5 ■ **Differential Diagnoses of Ovarian Tumors With Clear Cell Features**

Differential Diagnosis	Histology	Immunohistochemistry	Other
High-grade serous carcinoma with clear cell change	Stratified epithelium with tufting, very high mitotic rate, marked nuclear atypia	Positive: WT1, p53, ER Negative: Napsin-A	
Serous borderline tumor or low-grade carcinoma	Hierarchical branching of papillae, cellular stratification and budding	Positive: WT1, ER Negative: Napsin-A	
Endometrioid carcinoma with clear cell change	Low-grade nuclear atypia, columnar cells, glandular and solid growth	Positive: ER, PR Negative: Napsin-A	
Clear cell carcinoma	Tubulocystic, papillary, and solid growth; no hierarchical branching, small papillae with hyalinized cores; flat, cuboidal, or hobnail cells; low mitotic rate	Positive: CK7, EMA, Napsin-A, HNF1β Negative: WT1, p53 (wild-type)	
Yolk sac tumor	Reticular architecture with loose myxomatous stroma, Schiller–Duval bodies may be seen	Positive: SALL4 Negative: CK7 and EMA	Young age (20s—30s)
Metastatic renal cell carcinoma (RCC)	Cells in nests, cysts, or solid sheets; branching fibrovascular septations, high-grade nuclei	Positive: AE1/AE3, EMA, CD10, RCC, CA9	Renal mass or history of RCC
Dysgerminoma	Primitive cells in nests, lymphocytes in fibrous septae	Positive: SALL4, OCT4	Young age (average 19 years)

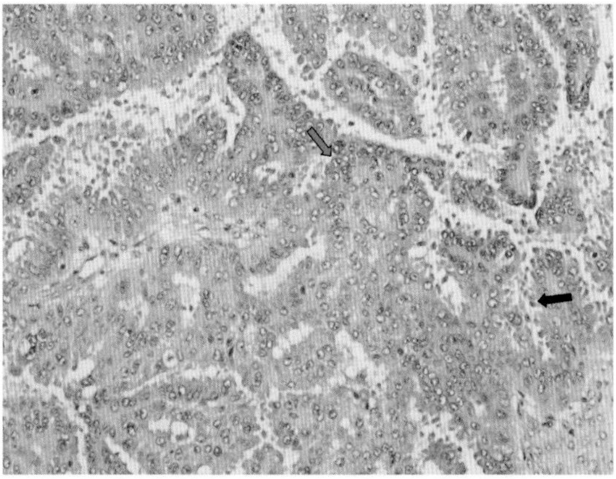

Fig. 13.5 Example of papillary high-grade serous carcinoma with high-grade nuclei, atypical mitoses (green arrow), and cellular tufting around papillae (black arrow) (H&E, 200x).

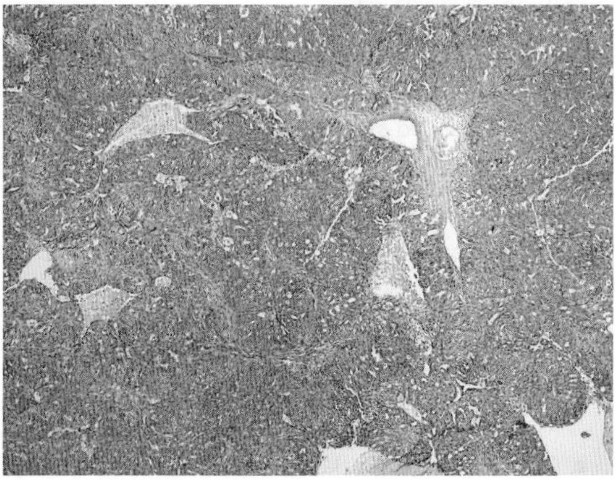

Fig. 13.6 Example of endometrioid ovarian carcinoma with glandular and solid growth (H&E, 40x).

Clear cell carcinoma characteristically consists of cells with clear or eosinophilic cytoplasm that is rich in glycogen. Tumors usually have variable papillary, solid, or tubulocystic growth patterns. The papillae are small with hyalinized, edematous, fibrovascular cores. Unlike serous carcinomas, there is no hierarchical branching or cell tufting. The mitotic activity is relatively low, but the cells may possess marked nuclear atypia. The cells are flattened, cuboidal, or hobnail.

CLINICAL PEARL

Clear cell and endometrioid carcinomas of the ovary are associated with endometriosis, while serous carcinoma is not.

CLINICAL PEARL

Clear cell carcinoma is associated with paraneoplastic syndromes including hypercalcemia, thromboembolism, subacute cerebellar degeneration, and bilateral diffuse uveal melanocytic proliferation.

What is the pathologic staging of ovarian carcinoma?

Staging is based on tumor involvement of peritoneal structures including ovaries, fallopian tubes, extension or implants to the uterus and other pelvic intraperitoneal tissues, spread to the peritoneum outside of the pelvis, involvement of retroperitoneal lymph nodes, and distant metastases or involvement of extra-abdominal organs including lymph nodes outside the abdominal cavity. As mentioned earlier, intraoperative surgical spill of malignant cells increases the stage as does the presence of malignant cells in ascites or peritoneal washings not caused by surgical intervention.

Case Point 13.8

A diagnosis of clear cell carcinoma is rendered, and the pathologic stage is pT1aN0. After surgical resection the patient receives chemotherapy with paclitaxel and carboplatin.

BEYOND THE PEARLS

- Combined chemotherapy regimens are very effective in treating germ cell tumors, with an overall survival greater than 95%.
- Overall, ovarian carcinoma has a poor prognosis because most carcinomas are diagnosed at an advanced stage and are high-grade serous carcinomas.
- Surgery is a mainstay of therapy with salpingo-oophorectomy and possible hysterectomy. Chemotherapy is used when indicated in the neoadjuvant or adjuvant setting.
- The integrity of the surgical specimen and involvement of the ovarian and/or fallopian tube surfaces are consistently noted in pathology reports to help assess the risk of peritoneal seeding and best treatment options.
- When salpingo-oophorectomies are performed for risk reduction in patients with BRCA1/BRCA2 mutations, the ovaries and fallopian tubes are serially sectioned and entirely submitted for histologic evaluation.
- Napsin-A is a helpful immunohistochemical stain that will be positive in ovarian clear cell carcinoma as well as pulmonary adenocarcinoma and most papillary renal cell carcinomas.
- Oral contraceptives, later age at menarche, earlier age at menopause, and increased parity decrease the risk of developing high-grade serous carcinoma.
- The ovarian ROMA incorporates CA125, HE4, and menopausal status to assign women that present with an adnexal mass into a high-risk or low-risk group for finding an ovarian malignancy.

References

Berek JS, Kehoe ST, Kumar L, Friedlander M. Cancer of the ovary, fallopian tube, and peritoneum. *Int J Gynaecol Obstet.* 2018;143(suppl 2):59-78.

Carcangiu ML, Herrington CS, Young RH. *Who Classification of Tumours of Female Reproductive Organs.* 2014.

College of American Pathologists. *Protocol for the Examination of Specimens From Patients With Primary Tumors of the Ovary, Fallopian Tube, or Peritoneum.* 2018.

Elattar A, Bryant A, Winter-Roach BA, Hatem M, Naik R. Optimal primary surgical treatment for advanced epithelial ovarian cancer. *Cochrane Database Syst Rev.* 2011;(8):CD007565. doi:10.1002/14651858.CD007565.pub2.

Goldblum JF, Lamps LW, McKenney JK, et al. *Rosai and Ackerman's Surgical Pathology.* Elsevier, 2018.

Kumar V, Abbas A, Fausto N, Aster J. *Robbins and Cotran Pathologic Basis of Disease.* 8th ed. Elsevier, 2010.

Timmerman D, Van Calster B, Testa A, et al. Predicting the risk of malignancy in adnexal masses based on the Simple Rules from the International Ovarian Tumor Analysis group. *Am J Obstet Gynecol.* 2016;214:424-437.

Male Genital System

CASE 14

A 37-Year-Old Man with a Left Testicular Swelling

Numbereye Numbere

A 37-year-old Caucasian man presents to his primary care physician with complaints of 4 weeks of progressive, painless swelling in his left testis. He is otherwise healthy and denies any history of testicular trauma, surgery, weight loss, and back pain. He participates in regular games of golf three times a week. He is not on any medications, he is a lifelong teetotaler, and he neither smokes nor uses illicit drugs. His family history is noncontributory. Physical examination is notable for a 3.5-cm, nontender, firm left testicular mass; his right testis is normal. A left testicular ultrasonogram and serum tumor markers are ordered, and a follow-up appointment is scheduled for 1 week.

How should a scrotal mass be evaluated clinically?
The clinical approach to the evaluation of a scrotal mass is illustrated in Fig. 14.1.

What are the differential diagnoses of a scrotal mass?
The causes of a scrotal mass run the gamut from congenital structural abnormalities to aggressive malignant neoplasms. Age, clinical history (e.g., the presence or absence of pain), and findings on physical examination (e.g., intratesticular vs. paratesticular location of the lesion) help pare the myriad possibilities. Hydroceles, spermatoceles, varicoceles, tumors, and uncomplicated inguinal hernias present as painless scrotal masses. Pain occurs with incarcerated inguinal hernias, torsion of the testicular appendix, torsion of the testis, infections, and trauma.

Hydroceles, Spermatoceles, and Hematoceles

Hydroceles, spermatoceles, and hematoceles are intrascrotal fluid collections. The classic case of hydrocele presents as a painless, cyst-like transilluminable paratesticular swelling in a neonate or infant. A hydrocele is an accumulations of fluid between congenitally nonfused layers of the tunica vaginalis. A hematocele is a collection of blood in the tunica vaginalis; it is most commonly caused by trauma. A spermatocele is an intraepididymal retention cyst that contains spermatozoa. Surgery is curative for all three lesions.

Testicular Torsion

Patients with acute testicular torsion present with sudden, severe testicular pain associated with an abnormally higher situation of the testis within the scrotum (high-riding testis), loss of the cremasteric reflex, and a negative Prehn sign (no relief of pain with testicular support). It occurs from the twisting of the vas deferens, which leads to impaired testicular vascular perfusion. The absence of blood flow on Doppler ultrasonography is confirmatory. Emergency surgery with untwisting of the vas deferens and prophylactic anchoring of the testis within the scrotum (orchiopexy) should be carried out within 6 hours to prevent infarction.

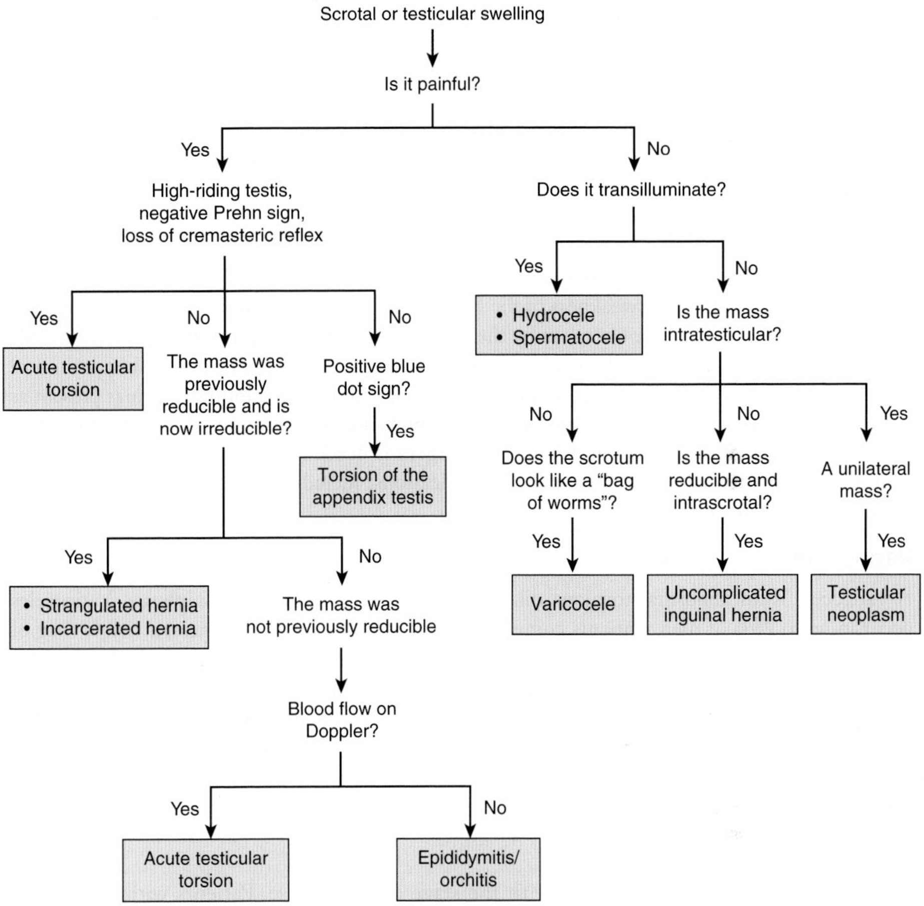

Fig. 14.1 A diagnostic algorithm for scrotal/testicular swellings.

Torsion of the Appendix Testis

The appendix testis is situated at the upper pole of the testis. Patients with torsion of the appendix testis present with acute onset of severe unilateral scrotal pain. In contradistinction to testicular torsion, a high-riding testis is not seen. When present, the blue dot sign (blue discoloration of the scrotum over the superior pole of the testis) is virtually diagnostic, but its absence does not exclude the diagnosis. An ultrasonogram is helpful for confirmation. Pain relief is paramount. The condition is self-limited, but scrotal exploration is indicated when testicular torsion cannot be excluded.

Epididymitis, Orchitis, and Epididymo-Orchitis

Patients with acute epididymitis, orchitis, or epididymo-orchitis complain of unilateral scrotal or testicular swelling and pain that may radiate to the flank along the spermatic cord. Patients may also have urethral discharge. A positive Prehn sign (relief of pain with testicular support) and an intact cremasteric reflex are seen. In young, sexually active men, the disease is usually sexually transmitted and caused by infection with *Chlamydia trachomatis* and/or *Neisseria gonorrhoea*. In older men and men who have sex with men, enteric organisms (e.g., *Escherichia coli* and *Pseudomonas aeruginosa*) are the usual cause. Orchitis may also be caused by infection with the mumps or HIV viruses. Treatment is with empiric ceftriaxone and doxycycline when the disease is sexually transmitted and ciprofloxacin when enteric organisms are the culprit.

Hernias

In the case of direct hernias, abdominal contents protrude "directly" through the anterior abdominal wall via a point of weakness in the Hesselbach triangle. Indirect hernias follow a more "indirect" path via the same route taken by the descending testis during intrauterine life. In children, the pathway of descent is the persistent processus vaginalis. In adults, protruding peritoneal contents forge a new route through the inguinal canal. Uncomplicated indirect hernias present as reducible, painless scrotal masses. Pain and irreducibility herald the onset of incarceration with the attendant risk of strangulation. Emergency surgery is needed in incarcerated hernias to prevent a host of potentially life-threatening complications, including sepsis, intestinal gangrene, small bowel obstruction, and intestinal perforation.

Varicocele

A varicocele is an abnormal tortuous dilation of the pampiniform venous plexus. Varicoceles occur in up to 20% of men. Patients complain of dull scrotal pain or heaviness, a visible "bag of worms" appearance of the scrotum, and/or infertility. The more frequent occurrence of varicoceles on the left (78%–93% of cases) is explained by chronically increased hydrostatic pressure resulting from the slower right-angled drainage of the longer left testicular vein into the left renal vein. Incompetent venous valves are also contributory. The rare occurrence of an isolated right-sided varicocele should raise suspicion for an intraabdominal tumor. Treatment is by excision (varicocelectomy) or embolization.

Tumors

Symptoms of testicular tumors vary with the stage of the disease. Patients with early-stage lesions present with a painless swelling of a unilateral testis, but may also complain of a sensation of scrotal heaviness. Symptoms concerning for metastasis include unintentional weight loss and pain due to bony metastasis. Rarely, patients may manifest symptoms brought on by the elaboration of biologically active substances by the tumor. Serum tumor markers and testicular ultrasonography (Fig. 14.2) are performed to clarify the clinical impression. Abdominopelvic computed tomography (CT) scans or magnetic resonance imaging (MRI) are used to search for metastases.

CLINICAL PEARL

A painless, unilateral testicular mass in an adult is considered cancerous until proved otherwise. Germ cell tumors (GCTs) are most common between the ages of 15 and 40 years. From the age of 60, lymphoma and spermatocytic tumor are of greater concern.

CLINICAL PEARL

The absence of a testicular mass by palpation is not sufficient to rule out a testicular tumor. An ultrasound scan must be performed.

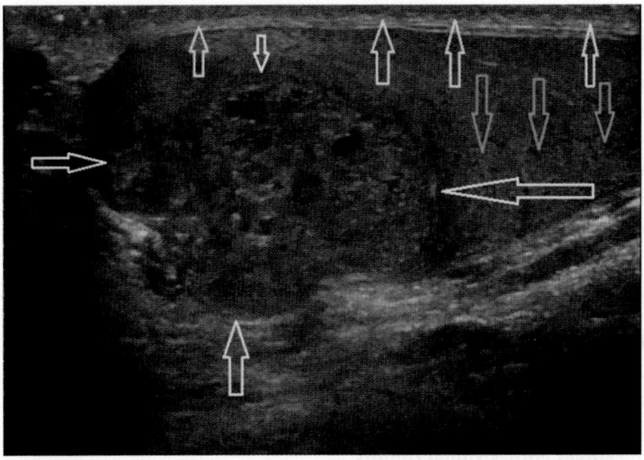

Fig. 14.2 An ultrasonographic image of a mixed germ cell tumor. A heterogeneous right testicular tumor (yellow arrows), adjacent uninvolved testicular parenchyma (green arrows), and the scrotum (blue arrows) are seen. (Image courtesy of Thomas Marini, MD, University of Rochester Medical Center).

Case Point 14.1

The patient returns for follow-up. The testicular ultrasonogram shows a 2.6 × 2 × 1.9-cm heterogeneous intratesticular mass with calcifications. Serum tumor markers show alpha-fetoprotein (AFP) of 149 ng/mL (reference range: 0–10 ng/mL), human chorionic gonadotropin (hCG) of 420 IU/L (reference range: 0–5 U/L), and lactate dehydrogenase (LDH) of 128 U/L (reference range: 338–610 U/L). A clinical impression of a testicular germ cell tumor (GCT) is made. Chest and abdominopelvic CT scans are ordered.

CLINICAL PEARL

Due to a significant risk of iatrogenic seeding of the tumor with resultant local cancer recurrence, biopsies are not performed if testicular cancer is suspected.

What are the types of testicular tumors? (Box 14.1)

CLINICAL PEARL

Spermatocytic tumor is unique for arising only in the testis. Histologically identical GCTs of all other types (except spermatocytic tumor) can also arise primarily in the ovary and midline sites like the pineal gland and soft tissues of the anterior mediastinum, retroperitoneum, and lower vertebra.

Although rare (1%–2% of all cancers in men), testicular tumors are the most common malignant neoplasms in men aged between 15 and 44 years and account for about 10% of cancer deaths in this cohort.

BOX 14.1 ■ Common Testicular Tumors

1. **Germ cell tumors**
   A. Seminoma
   B. Nonseminomatous germ cell tumors
      - Embryonal carcinoma
      - Yolk sac tumor
      - Choriocarcinoma
      - Teratoma
      - Spermatocytic tumor (formerly known as spermatocytic seminoma)
      - Mixed germ cell tumors
2. **Sex cord-stromal tumors**
   A. Leydig cell tumor
   B. Sertoli cell tumor
   C. Fibroma
3. **Mixed germ cell/sex cord-stromal tumors**
4. **Lymphomas**
5. **Secondary (metastatic) tumors**

Testicular tumors are classified according to their cell of origin. GCTs arise from their namesake germ cells that are the forebears of spermatozoa. GCTs account for 95% of testicular tumors. Sex cord-stromal tumors arise from somatic sex cord cells and stromal cells, which provide metabolic support for germ cells and constitute the supportive stroma of the testis, respectively. GCTs are, for the most part, malignant; sex cord-stromal tumors are most commonly benign.

What are the risk factors and etiology of testicular tumors?
Although much remains unknown, established risk factors for testicular GCTs include cryptorchidism and personal/family history of testicular cancer. Factors not associated with testicular cancers include physical activity, trauma, tight underwear, heat, and vasectomy.

What is the pathogenesis of GCTs?
GCTs arise from abnormal *in utero* development of testicular germ cells. Many associated genetic aberrations have been identified, but their exact roles in pathogenesis are not fully understood. Except for prepubertal yolk sac tumor, prepubertal teratoma, and spermatocytic tumor, the precursor lesion of GCTs is the germ cell neoplasia in situ (GCNIS). Akin to carcinoma in situ, the neoplastic cells of GCNIS are noninvasive and confined within the basement membrane of seminiferous tubules. GCNIS is seen in histological sections as large atypical cells with well-defined cell borders, abundant clear cytoplasm, and central nuclei with prominent nucleoli.

Case Point 14.2

The patient expresses sadness over his diagnosis and asks if something could have been done to prevent the tumor or detect it earlier.

Tumor markers are soluble substances produced by a tumor and detectable in body fluids or tissues. They are used for screening, diagnosis, prognostication, monitoring the response to treatment, and surveillance for recurrence after therapy. Examples of testicular serum tumor markers include LDH, AFP, and hCG (Table 14.1). Serum tumor markers are elevated in about 60% of testicular tumors.

TABLE 14.1 ■ **Testicular Serum Tumor Markers**

Tumor Marker	Tumor With Elevated Serum Levels
Alpha-fetoprotein	Yolk sac tumor; less often in embryonal carcinoma.
Human chorionic gonadotropin	Very high levels (>100,000 IU/L) occur in choriocarcinoma; also elevated in embryonal carcinoma; lesser degrees of elevation (<500 IU/L) are seen in 20% of seminomas.
Lactate dehydrogenase	All germ cell tumors.

Due to the rarity and high rate of cure of testicular tumors, routine screening of asymptomatic men without risk factors is not recommended. Screening with serum tumor markers or testicular palpation may be warranted in symptomatic men or men with risk factors like cryptorchidism. Testicular tumors are not preventable.

Case Point 14.3

The CT scans show no evidence of metastatic disease. The patient is offered sperm banking but declines. He is scheduled for surgery in 1 week.

What is the treatment of testicular GCTs?

GCTs are managed with radical inguinal orchiectomy followed by adjuvant chemotherapy with agents like bleomycin, etoposide, and cisplatin, or radiotherapy (for seminomas). Cryopreservation of sperm for maintenance of fertility is offered to all patients before the commencement of treatment.

Case Point 14.4

The patient undergoes a radical inguinal orchiectomy, and the specimen is submitted for histopathologic evaluation.

What are the clinical, gross, and histological features of testicular tumors?

Seminoma

Seminoma is the most common testicular tumor, accounting for 40%–50% of GCTs. Serum levels of LDH may be elevated. Grossly, the tumor consists of one or more nodules of soft, light tan/yellow tissue (Fig. 14.3A). On histology, the tumor is partitioned into lobules by lymphocyte-rich fibrous septa (Fig. 14.3B). Tumors cells have well-defined cell borders, ample clear cytoplasm due to intracellular accumulation of glycogen, and prominent central nuclei with conspicuous nucleoli. Granulomas occur in 50% of cases. Multinucleated trophoblastic giant cells are seen in up to 20% of cases, their presence correlating with mildly elevated serum hCG levels.

CLINICAL PEARL

The distinction of seminoma from other GCTs is clinically important because seminomas are uniquely exquisitely radiosensitive, and patients are more likely to present with earlier-stage disease than in other GCTs.

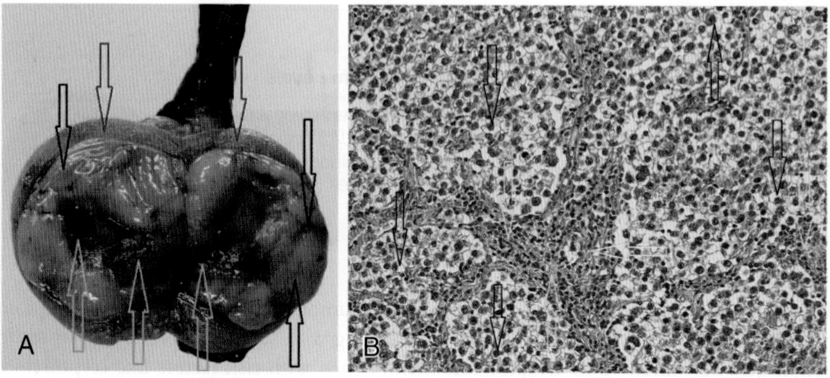

Fig. 14.3 (A) This gross photograph shows a bisected testis with a seminoma (black arrows) and a surrounding rim of uninvolved tissue (red arrows). The cut surface of the seminoma is nodular, bulging, light tan, and shiny with a central area of hemorrhage (green arrows). (B) On microscopy, tumor cells of seminoma (black arrows) have abundant clear cytoplasm and distinct cell borders. The tumor is partitioned by fibrovascular septa studded with lymphocytes (yellow arrows) (H&E 200x).

Spermatocytic Tumor

Spermatocytic tumor (formerly known as spermatocytic seminoma) is rare, accounting for 1% of all GCTs. Spermatocytic tumor has distinct clinical, epidemiologic, pathogenetic, and morphologic features that set it apart from other GCTs. Patients are older, presenting in their late 50s to 70s. It is not linked to cryptorchidism. Serum tumor markers are not elevated. It arises only from the testis and not from extragonadal sites or the ovary. It is not associated with GCNIS, and it occurs in pure form only, not associated with other GCTs.

On gross examination, the tumor is circumscribed, soft, and light tan and bulges on sectioning. On histology, the tumor is arranged in sheets of three cell types: large, small, and intermediate-sized cells (Fig. 14.4). Unlike seminomas, the stroma is scant, and septa are delicate and inconspicuous. It is an indolent tumor with an excellent prognosis.

Yolk Sac Tumor

Yolk sac tumor is the most common pediatric testicular tumor. It usually presents as a rapidly enlarging testicular mass in a child. Seventy-five percent of cases in children occur in pure form,

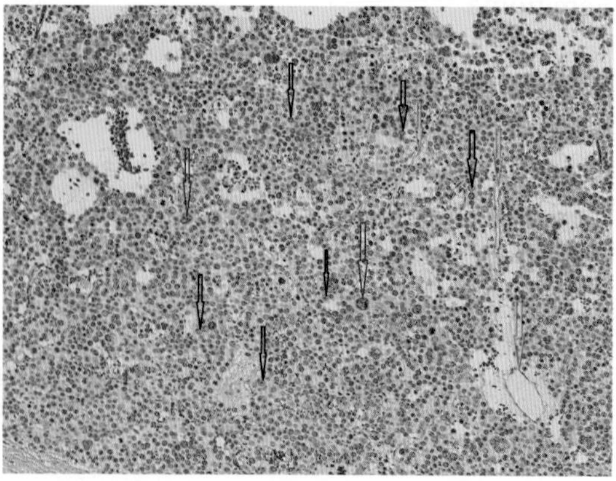

Fig. 14.4 Spermatocytic tumor. A solid growth of predominantly intermediate-sized cells (black arrows) is traversed by delicate fibrous stroma and blood vessels (green arrows). Few small cells and fewer large cells with spireme nuclei (red arrows) are seen (H&E 100x).

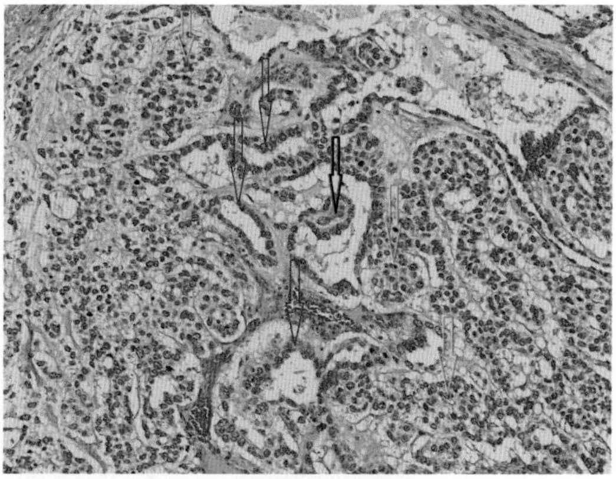

Fig. 14.5 Endodermal sinus pattern of yolk sac tumor with a pathognomonic Schiller–Duval body (black arrow). Schiller–Duval bodies have a central capillary lined by inner and outer layers of neoplastic cells that are separated by a clear space. It is believed to be an attempt to form yolk sacs. The remainder of the tumor consists of cuboidal tumor cells arranged in clusters (green arrows) and acinar structures (red arrows) (H&E 100x).

but 99% of tumors in adults occur as constituents of mixed GCTs. The gross tumor is a poorly circumscribed, soft, lobulated, and yellow-white mass with mucoid cut surfaces. Many histological growth patterns occur (reticular, endodermal sinus, tubular, etc.). Eosinophilic hyaline globules may be seen. The pathognomonic glomeruloid Schiller–Duval body is present in only 20%–50% of cases (Fig. 14.5).

Teratoma

Teratoma is the second most common pediatric testicular tumor. Teratoma is a common component of mixed GCTs. The gross tumor is firm and heterogeneous with solid and cystic areas (Fig. 14.6). Yellow sebaceous material, hair, cartilage, teeth, and bone occur frequently. On microscopy, mature (skin, gastrointestinal, and respiratory epithelia) and/or immature (neural, blastomatous) tissue elements derived from more than one embryonic germ cell layer are present (Fig. 14.6). Serum tumor marker levels are usually not elevated. Adult teratomas are frequently malignant; pediatric teratomas are most commonly benign.

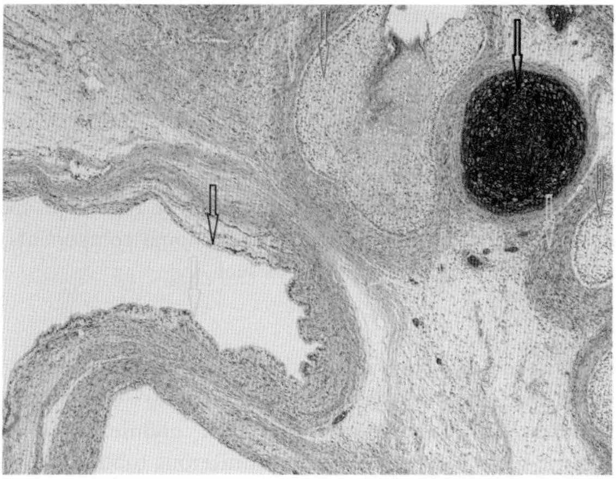

Fig. 14.6 Histologic section of a teratoma showing an island of cartilage (black arrow), islands of stratified epithelia (green arrows), and glandular epithelium (red arrows) within fibrous stroma (yellow arrows) (H&E 40x).

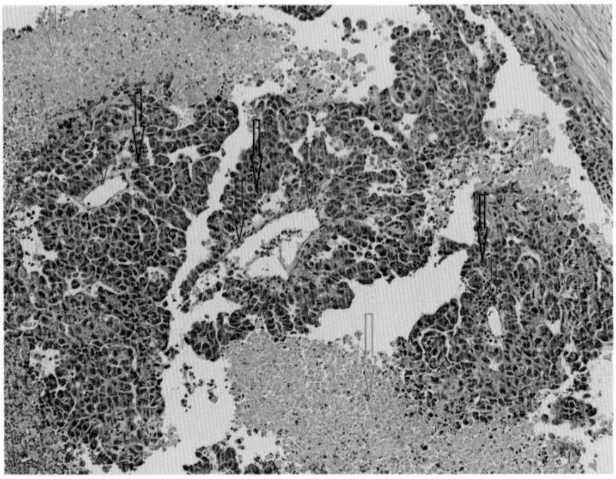

Fig. 14.7 Embryonal carcinoma. There is crowding of large high-grade malignant tumor cells (black arrows) around blood vessels (red arrows) with necrosis of cells farther afield (green arrows) (H&E, 100x).

Embryonal Carcinoma

Embryonal carcinoma is a frequent component of mixed GCTs—only 2% of cases occur in pure form. Patients usually present in their 20s and 30s with a painless enlarging testicular mass. An estimated 60% of patients have metastatic disease at presentation. It appears grossly as a soft, poorly demarcated mass with areas of hemorrhage and necrosis. On histology, poorly differentiated epithelioid cells are arranged in various architectural patterns, including solid, glandular, and papillary. Tumor necrosis is prominent (Fig. 14.7).

Choriocarcinoma

Choriocarcinoma occurs more frequently as a component of mixed GCTs and only rarely (0.5% of cases) in pure form. Patients often present with symptoms of metastasis like hemoptysis and gastrointestinal bleeding. Common sites of spread include the lung, liver, and bone. The gross tumor is a hemorrhagic tan nodule. On microscopy, mononucleated cytotrophoblasts and intermediate trophoblasts, and multinucleated syncytiotrophoblasts are identified (Fig. 14.8).

Mixed Germ Cell Tumor

Mixed GCT is the second most common testicular tumor, accounting for about 40% of GCTs. It occurs as a combination of any of the other types of GCTs, except spermatocytic tumor (Fig. 14.9). Tumors with mixed seminoma and nonseminoma components have the biologic behavior of nonseminomas and are thus managed as such.

Lymphoma

Testicular lymphoma is the most common testicular tumor in the elderly. It presents most commonly as bilateral testicular neoplasms in men 60 years of age and older. The gross tumor is a well-demarcated, firm, light tan "fish flesh" nodule. Microscopy reveals dense infiltration of neoplastic lymphocytes between seminiferous tubules with relative sparing of the tubules.

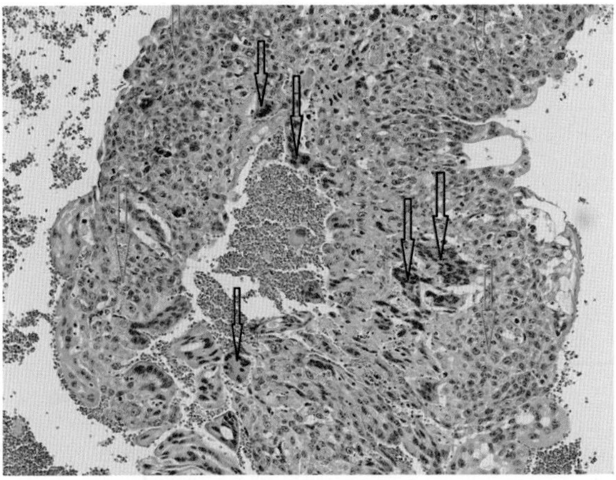

Fig. 14.8 Choriocarcinoma. There is an admixture of syncytiotrophoblasts (multinucleated cells with irregular, smudged, hyperchromatic nuclei; black arrows) and more numerous cytotrophoblasts (mononucleated cells with rounded nuclei and prominent nucleoli; green arrows). Note the areas of hemorrhage. In some cases, hemorrhage and tumor cell necrosis may be marked so as to obscure tumor cells (H&E 100x).

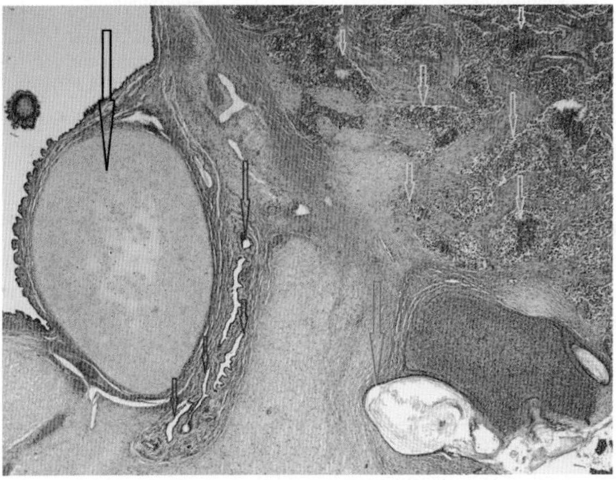

Fig. 14.9 Mixed germ cell tumor. Teratoma is identified by an island of cartilage (black arrow), keratinized stratified squamous epithelium (green arrow), and glandular epithelia (red arrows) in a bland fibrous stroma. Irregular, interconnected nests of distinctly basophilic embryonal carcinoma (yellow arrows) are seen in the upper right of the field (H&E 100x).

What are the immunohistochemical features of testicular tumors?

Fig. 14.10 presents a summary of important immunohistochemical profiles of select testicular tumors.

Case Point 14.5

Postoperatively, the patient feels well and is discharged from the hospital, and follow-up visits are scheduled.

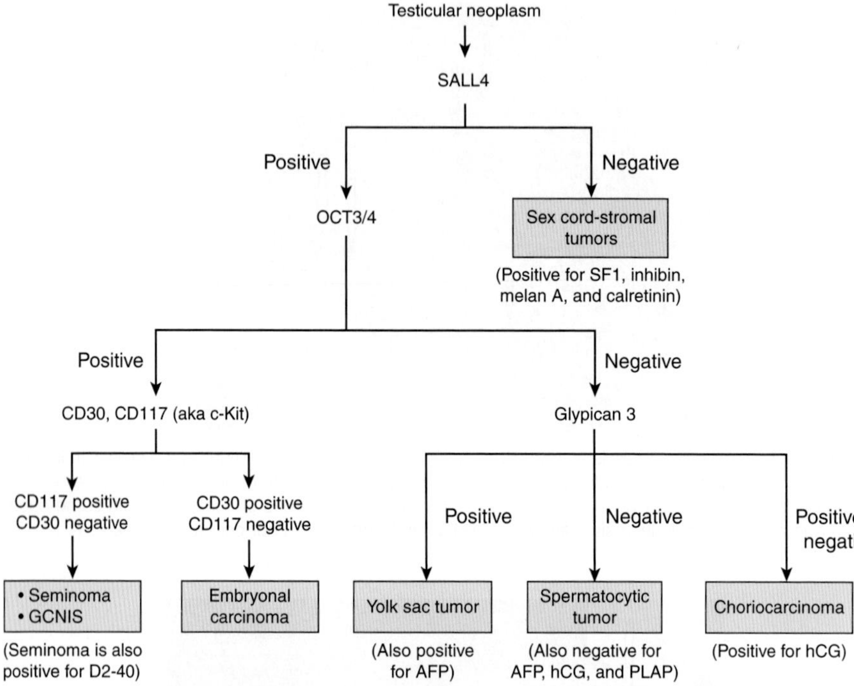

Fig. 14.10 Immnunohistochemical characterization of testicular tumors. *AFP,* alpha-fetoprotein; *hCG*, human chorionic gonadotropin; *PLAP,* placental alkaline phosphatase; GCNIS, germ cell neoplasia in situ.

How are patients with GCTs followed-up after surgery?

Surveillance for recurrence is performed with periodic history, physical examinations, and serum tumor markers (AFP, LDH, and hCG). Abdominopelvic CT and MRI as well as chest radiographs are also performed.

Case Point 14.6

The patient presents for his first follow-up 2 weeks after surgery. His surgical pathology report is ready, and he is informed of the diagnosis—mixed GCT.

What is the prognosis of GCTs?

Prognosis indicators for GCTs can be divided into factors that affect early-stage (stage I) disease and factors that impact metastatic disease. Stage I seminomas have excellent outcomes, but size greater than 4 cm and rete testis invasion are associated with increased rates of relapse. Lymphovascular invasion and a predominant component of embryonal carcinoma are predictors for recurrence in stage I nonseminomas.

The International Germ Cell Consensus Classification Group stratifies patients with metastatic disease into good, intermediate, and poor-risk groups based on the presence of nonpulmonary visceral metastasis and tumor marker studies (Table 14.2).

In the American Joint Committee on Cancer scheme, patients are stratified into five prognostic groups based on the size of the primary tumor, the presence or absence of nodal and extranodal metastasis, and the results of tumor marker studies (Table 14.3).

TABLE 14.2 ■ **Summary of the IGCCCG Risk Classification of Metastatic Germ Cell Cancer* and Corresponding Survival Statistics**

Risk Status	Nonseminoma	Seminoma	5-Year Overall Survival (%)
Good risk	• Absence of nonpulmonary visceral metastasis **AND** • Presence of post-orchiectomy tumor markers at ALL of the following levels: • AFP < 1,000 ng/mL, hCG < 5,000 IU/L, and LDH < 1.5x upper limit of normal	• Absence of nonpulmonary visceral metastasis. **AND** • Presence of normal levels of AFP • Any level of hCG and LDH	~ 90
Intermediate risk	• Absence of nonpulmonary visceral metastasis **AND** • Presence of postorchiectomy tumor markers at ANY of the following levels: • AFP 1,000 – 10,000 ng/mL, hCG 5,000 – 50,000 IU/L, and LDH 1.5 – 10x upper limit of normal	• Presence of nonpulmonary visceral metastasis **AND** • Presence of normal levels of AFP • Any level of hCG and LDH	~ 75
Poor risk	• Presence of nonpulmonary visceral metastasis **OR** • Presence of postorchiectomy tumor markers at ANY of the following levels: • AFP >10,000 ng/mL, hCG > 50,000 IU/L, and LDH > 10x upper limit of normal	A poor risk classification for seminoma does not exist	~ 45

*Applies to tumors of any primary site – both testicular and nontesticular

AFP α-fetoprotein; hCG - human chorionic gonadotropin; LDH - lactate dehydrogenase; IGCCCG - International Germ Cell Consensus Classification Group

TABLE 14.3 ■ **Summary of the American Joint Committee on Cancer Prognostic Stage Groups for Testicular Neoplasms**

Stage	Features
Stage 0	Intratubular germ cell neoplasia No spread to lymph nodes or distant sites
Stage I	Direct spread of tumor beyond the seminiferous tubules, including invasion of surrounding structures (e.g., epididymis, hilar soft tissue, tunica vaginalis, intratesticular blood vessels or lymphatics, spermatic cord, and scrotum) No spread to lymph nodes or distant sites Serum tumor marker levels are normal, have not been performed, or are not available
Stage IS*	Primary tumor of any stage without lymph node or distant metastasis Serum markers remain higher than normal after the tumor is removed
Stage II	Spread to regional (retroperitoneal) lymph nodes but not distant lymph nodes or organs Serum markers are unavailable, normal, or only slightly high
Stage III	Spread to distant lymph nodes or any organ

*Stage IS nonseminomas are treated the same as stage III tumors.

BEYOND THE PEARLS

- On occasion, patients with testicular tumors may present with endocrine abnormalities. This is more common with sex cord-stromal tumors than with GCTs.
  - Precocious pseudopuberty can be caused by androgenic steroids elaborated by Leydig cell tumors.
  - Gynecomastia may occur from by estrogenic steroids produced by Leydig cell and Sertoli cell tumors.
  - Rarely, hyperthyroidism or gynecomastia can occur in patients with choriocarcinoma. This is due to the stimulatory action of hCG on thyrocytes or mammary ductal epithelium, respectively.
- The oxymoron – monodermal teratoma – refers to a rare variant of teratoma that is derived from only one embryonic germ layer. Examples include epidermoid cyst (ectodermally derived squamous epithelium without skin adnexa) and carcinoid tumor (derived from ectodermal neural crest cells).
- Primary brain tumors histologically identical to testicular seminomas are known as germinomas. Morphologically identical tumors arising in the ovary are known as dysgerminomas.
- Syndromes associated with testicular masses/tumors:
  - PTEN hamartoma tumor syndrome (caused by germline mutations of *PTEN* on 10q23.3) is associated with lipomatous testicular hamartomas.
  - Peutz-Jeghers syndrome (caused by germline mutation of *LKB1/STK11* on 19p13.3) is associated with some rare variants of Sertoli cell tumors.
  - Testicular dysgenesis syndrome is associated with testicular GCTs. The other components of the syndrome are cryptorchidism, hypospadias, and poor sperm quality.
- On rare occasions, testicular GCTs undergo spontaneous partial or complete regression, while still maintaining viable metastatic lesions. The mechanisms governing this phenomenon still remain a subject of conjecture.
- Patients with pure seminomas and elevated serum levels of AFP are managed clinically as non-seminomatous germ cell tumors.
- Critical elements in a pathology report of a testicular GCT include (but are not limited to) the tumor size, regional lymph node status, rete testis stromal invasion, the state of the resection margin, and the stage.

References

Albers P, Albrecht W, Algaba F, et al. Guidelines on testicular cancer: 2015 update. *Eur Urol.* 2015;68;1054-1068.

Cook MB, Akre O, Forman D, Madigan MP, Richiardi L, McGlynn KA. A systematic review and meta-analysis of perinatal variables in relation to the risk of testicular cancer—experiences of the son. *Int J Epidemiol.* 2010;39;1605-1618.

Crawford P, Crop JA. Evaluation of scrotal masses. *Am Fam Physician*. 2013;89;723-728.

Leman ES, Gonzalgo ML. Prognostic features and markers for testicular cancer management. *Indian J Urol.* 2010;26;76-81.

Park JS, Kim J, Elghiaty A, Ham WS. Recent global trends in testicular cancer incidence and mortality. Medicine (*Baltimore*). 2018;97;e12390.

Skakkebæk NE, Meyts ER-D, Main KM. Testicular dysgenesis syndrome: An increasingly common developmental disorder with environmental aspects. *Hum Reprod.* 2001;16;972-978.

Ulbright TM, Berney BM. Testicular and paratesticular tumors. In: Mills SE, ed. *Sternberg's Diagnostic Surgical Pathology*. Philadelphia, PA: Wolters Kluwer Lippincott Williams & Wilkins, 2015.

Ulbright TM, Tickoo SK, Berney DM, Srigley JR, Members of the ISUP Immunohistochemistry in Diagnostic Urologic Pathology Group. Best practices recommendations in the application of immunohistochemistry in testicular tumors: Report from the international society of urological pathology consensus conference. *Am J Surg Pathol.* 2014;38;e50-e59.

Oral Cavity/ENT

CASE 15

A 72-Year-Old Female with a White Plaque on Her Left Lateral Tongue

Anna-Karoline Israel

A 72-year-old woman with a complex medical history including hypertension, hyperlipidemia, hypothyroidism, essential tremor, and breast cancer presents to the clinic with a white lesion on her left lateral tongue. She drinks alcohol socially but has never smoked. Her vitals are within normal limits, and her other medical problems are maintained with medications. On physical exam, she has a white plaque measuring 2 × 1 cm on the lateral tongue. The decision is made to take a biopsy of the lesion.

What is leukoplakia?

Leukoplakia refers to a white patch in the oral cavity, which cannot be rubbed off. Histologically, it is characterized by hyperkeratosis and parakeratosis, which leads to the typical gross appearance. The prevalence of leukoplakia is approximately 2% in the Western world; in less than 25% of these cases, dysplasia is found on biopsy.

Hairy leukoplakia is a distinct entity that shows white patches with corrugated surfaces, which also cannot be rubbed off. Histologically, it demonstrated epithelial hyperplasia, hyperkeratosis, acanthosis, and balloon cells. It is related to Epstein–Barr virus infections and nearly always occurs in immunocompromised patients.

In contrast, oral candidiasis, which is the most common fungal infection in the oral cavity, can manifest with white patches that tend to bleed if scraped off.

Case Point 15.1

The patient's biopsy demonstrates skin with orthokeratosis and parakeratosis. There is a band-like lymphocytic infiltrate and focal vacuolar change of the basal keratinocyte layer. Infectious organisms, dysplasia, or invasive carcinoma are not identified (Fig. 15.1). The diagnosis is consistent with oral lichen planus.

CLINICAL PEARL

Lichenoid reaction pattern

- Synonym: Interface dermatitis
- Variety of inflammatory skin conditions that all show keratinocyte apoptosis and either a dense lymphocytic infiltrate or a vacuolar pattern at the dermal–epidermal junction
- The lymphocytic infiltrate may further extend into the deep dermis in some entities.

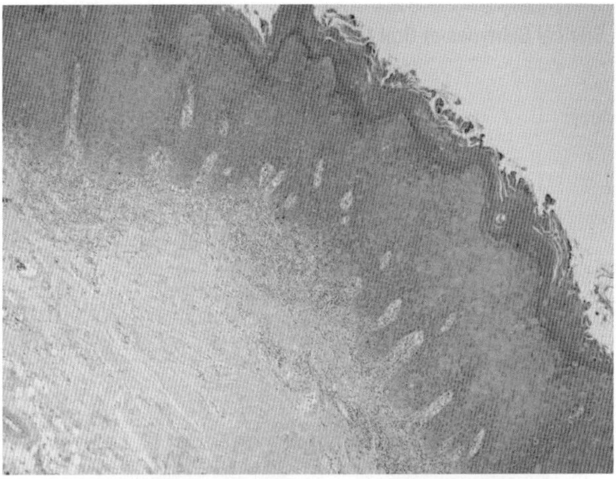

Fig. 15.1 Band-like lymphocytic infiltrate at dermal-epidermal junction (H&E, 40x).

CLINICAL PEARL

Lichen is formed by algae, cyanobacteria, and fungi that live in a mutualistic relationship.

- Lichens can present with many shapes and forms.
- The medical terminology refers to the morphology of lichen that appears in nature.

Where does lichen planus usually occur and who is affected by the disease?

Lichen planus may affect the skin, scalp, nails, and mucous membranes. It can occur virtually anywhere in the body and can affect the genital area, esophagus, and oral cavity. The terminology may alter depending on the affected site, such as cutaneous lichen planus, vulvar lichen planus, oral lichen planus, and lichen planopilaris. Oral lichen planus occurs multifocal and most commonly involves the buccal mucosa. Gingiva, dorsal tongue, and lower lip can also be affected. Oral lichen planus affects more commonly middle-aged adults and shows a predilection to females.

What is the etiology and pathogenesis of lichen planus?

The precise cause of lichen planus is unknown. It is thought that activated CD8+ T cells induce apoptosis in basal keratinocytes. Several drugs have been associated with the onset of lichen planus. However, lesions do not always resolve when the offending drug is discontinued.

CLINICAL PEARL

Lichenoid drug eruption

- In addition to the classic lichenoid reaction pattern, focal parakeratosis and eosinophils may be present.
- A variety of different drugs have been associated with a lichenoid drug eruption; the most common are gold, thiazide, beta blockers, angiotensin-converting enzyme inhibitors, antimalarials, and griseofulvin.
- Lichenoid reaction to dental amalgam develops in areas of direct mucosal contact to amalgam.

TABLE 15.1 ■ **Clinical Subtypes of Oral Lichen Planus**

Subtype	Presentation
Reticular lichen planus	Fine white lace-like striae (Wickham striae) Usually asymptomatic Multifocal Fig. 15.2
Erythematous lichen planus	Atrophic, red discolored mucosa Ulcerations may be present
Erosive lichen planus	Pain while eating May be confined to the gingiva
Bullous lichen planus	Unusual variant with bullae formation

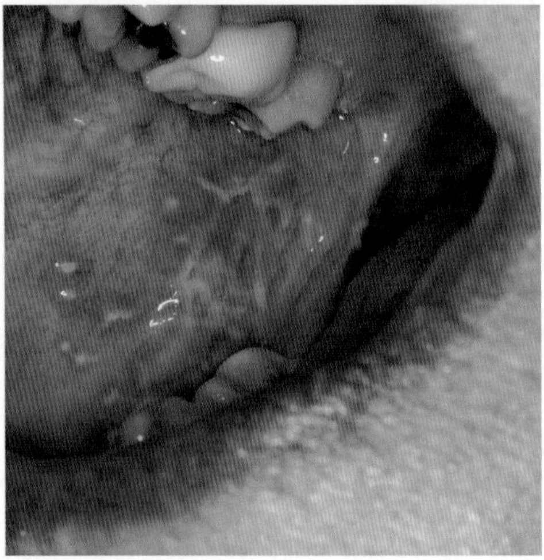

Fig. 15.2 Reticular lichen planus (From *ExpertPath*. Copyright Elsevier).

What are the subtypes of oral lichen planus?

Oral lichen planus may present with reticular, erythematous, erosive, and bullous patterns. Multiple simultaneous morphologies may be identified (Table 15.1).

What are the classic histologic features of lichen planus?

Lichen planus classically demonstrates a band-like lymphocytic infiltrate at the dermal–epidermal junction that consists primarily of T cells with destruction of the epithelial basal cell layer. The basal cell layer shows vacuolar change and degenerating keratinocytes, which are also called civatte bodies (Fig. 15.3). The overlying epidermis shows varying degrees of orthokeratosis and parakeratosis. Atrophy, acanthosis, and acantholysis of the epidermis may be present. Erosive lichen planus demonstrates ulceration and sub-basal separation.

What features can be seen on immunofluorescence?

Immunofluorescence may show unspecific deposition of fibrin and fibrinogen at the basement membrane zone. Bullous forms may rarely show nonspecific IgG and C3 in the basement membrane area.

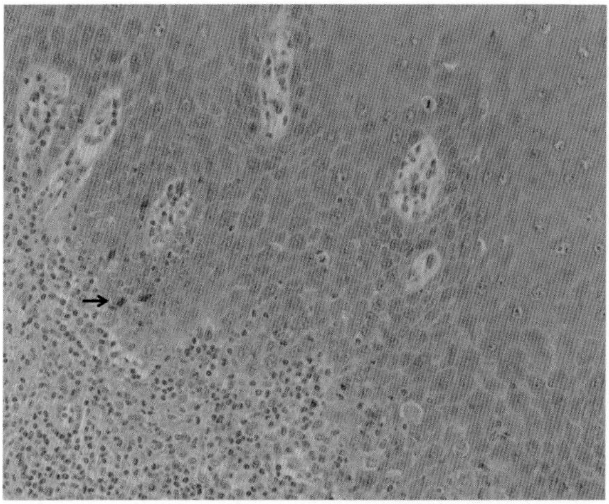

Fig. 15.3 Vacuolar change and degenerating keratinocytes (civatte bodies, arrow) at dermal-epidermal junction (H&E, 200x).

What are the differential diagnoses of oral lichen planus?

The leading differential diagnoses are mucous membrane pemphigoid, lupus erythematosus, pemphigus vulgaris, chronic graft-versus-host disease, linear immunoglobulin A disease, lichenoid drug reaction, and chronic ulcerative stomatitis (Table 15.2).

In addition to routine histologic exam, direct immunofluorescence may be helpful in distinguishing those entities. Lichen planus is usually not solitary. Thus, solitary lesions should undergo biopsy to assess for dysplasia.

TABLE 15.2 ■ **Differential Diagnosis of Oral Lichen Planus**

Entity	Key Differentiating Features
Mucous membrane pemphigoid	Subepithelial clefting DIF shows linear band of IgG or C3, and less commonly IgM or IgA at basement membrane zone
Lupus erythematosus	Superficial and deep perivascular lymphocytic infiltrate Dermal mucin Fibrin deposition around vessels and thickening of the basement membrane
Pemphigus vulgaris	Suprabasilar split of squamous epithelium IgG in intercellular desmosomal areas on DIF
Chronic graft-versus-host disease	Superficial lymphocytic infiltrate Prominent vacuolar change at basement membrane zone
Linear IgA disease	Tense vesicles and bullae Subepidermal blisters with neutrophils and eosinophils By definition, DIF shows linear IgA at dermal–epidermal junction
Lichenoid drug reaction	Eosinophils Melanin incontinence Offending medication
Chronic ulcerative stomatitis	Granular perinuclear IgG in lower one-third of epithelium on DIF

DIF, direct immunofluorescence; *Ig,* immunoglobulin.

CLINICAL PEARL

Risk factors for oral dysplasia and squamous cell carcinoma of the oral cavity

- Chronic abuse of tobacco (increases risk 5–17 times)
- Chronic abuse of alcohol
- Betel quid chewing
- Sun exposure for squamous cell carcinoma of the vermillion border
- Human papillomavirus, particularly type 16 and 18

What is the prognosis of oral lichen planus?

Oral lichen planus is a chronic condition with waxing and waning symptoms. However, rarely it can undergo spontaneous remission.

How is lichen planus treated?

Reticular lichen planus does not need to be treated, particularly if asymptomatic. Topical and systemic steroids are used for erosive lesions. Tacrolimus can be used for steroid-resistant oral lichen planus.

Case Point 15.2

The patient is treated with clobetasol and monitored for several years. At a follow-up appointment, extension of the white plaque with multiple speckled reddish foci is noted.

Another biopsy is taken. The diagnosis of invasive squamous cell carcinoma is made (Figs. 15.4 and 15.5 A, B). The patient is treated with a partial glossectomy. A complete excision with negative margins is achieved, and the neck dissection does not reveal any lymph node metastasis. Thus, further treatment is not required.

CLINICAL PEARL

Erythroplakia/Erythroplasia

- Red patch in oral cavity
- Less common than leukoplakia

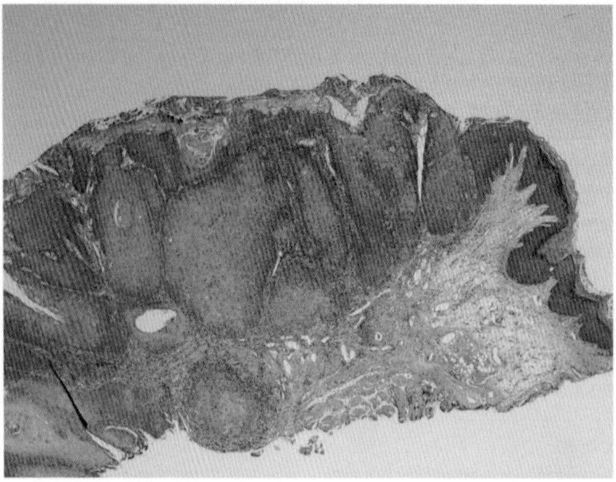

Fig. 15.4 Squamous cell carcinoma arising in the background of lichen planus (H&E, 20x).

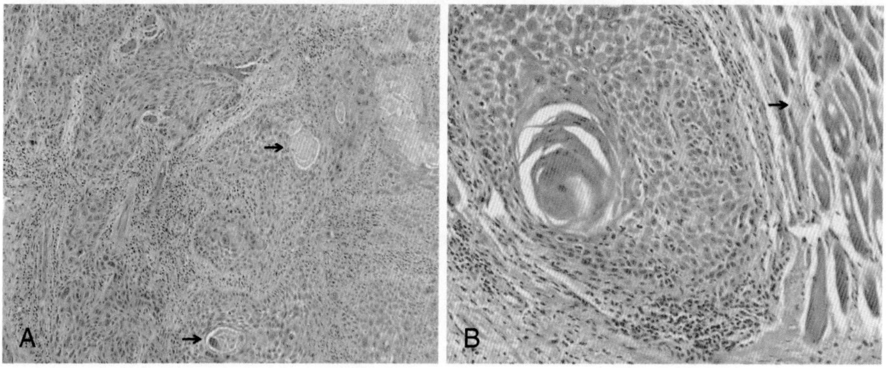

Fig. 15.5 (A) Islands and cords of invasive squamous cell carcinoma with central keratin pearls (arrow) (H&E 100x) (B) Island of squamous cell carcinoma with central keratin pearl invading into muscle (arrow) (H&E 200x).

- May exist in combination with leukoplakia (erythroleukoplakia)
- Most erythroplakia/erythroplasia will undergo malignant transformation, if not completely excised (90%).

BEYOND THE PEARLS

- 40% patients with oral lichen planus will develop cutaneous lichen planus.
- Scalp and nail involvement is rare in patients with oral lichen planus.
- Oral lichen planus has been associated with hepatitis C.
- Lichen planus in general has also been associated with human herpesvirus 6, dental amalgam, immunodeficiency, and malignancy.
- Malignant transformation of oral lichen planus is controversial, but may occur in chronic ulcerated areas.
- Single lesions and lesions that undergo morphologic change should undergo biopsy to evaluate for dysplasia.

References

Johnston R. *Weedon's Skin Pathology Essentials*. 2nd ed. Philadelphia, PA: Elsevier, 2017.
Patterson J, Hosler GA. *Weedon's Skin Pathology*. 4th ed. Edinburgh: Churchill Livingstone Elsevier; 2016.
Thompson L, Bishop J. *Head and Neck Pathology*. 3rd ed. Philadelphia, PA: Elsevier; 2019.
Wenig B. *Atlas of Head and Neck Pathology*. 3rd ed. Philadelphia, PA: Elsevier; 2016.

CASE 16

A 49-Year-Old Man with a Neck Mass

Phillip Huyett ■ Daniel Faden

A 49-year-old man presents to his primary care physician with 2 months of a right-sided neck mass. He first noticed the mass while shaving. When the mass did not resolve spontaneously, he was started on a 5-day course of azithromycin by his primary care physician. He thinks that it is slowly enlarging, but it is not painful. He has not experienced hoarseness, dysphagia, or dyspnea. He does endorse a mild throat discomfort that partially responds to omeprazole. He also notes intermittent right ear pain. He denies fevers, chills, night sweats, and unintentional weight loss. He has diet-controlled hyperlipidemia but is otherwise healthy and on no medications. He smoked cigarettes briefly in college on weekends but quit over 30 years ago. He estimates he smoked a half-pack per day for 2 years. He consumes four glasses of wine per week, but was never a heavy drinker. Vital signs are within normal limits. His physical exam is normal except for a right-sided, firm, nontender, partially mobile mass measuring 2–3 cm in the right neck level 2. The thyroid gland is smooth, and there are no palpable nodules. Oral cavity exam does not reveal any concerning mucosal lesions. His cranial nerves II-XI are intact.

What is the differential diagnosis of a neck mass in adults?
A new neck mass in an adult represents a malignancy until proven otherwise. Approximately 80%–90% of neck masses in adults are malignant in nature. This contrasts starkly with the pediatric population where ~90% of neck masses are benign, with benign reactive lymphadenopathy representing the most common etiology. History and physical exam are instrumental in narrowing a differential diagnosis list. The mnemonic "KITTENS" can be very helpful to systematically categorize differential diagnoses (Table 16.1).

What is the most appropriate next step in the management for an adult with a head and neck mass?
Imaging would be an appropriate first step. Ultrasound, CT with contrast, or MRI with contrast would be the most appropriate first imaging step, with CT being the most commonly performed. If thyroid carcinoma is suspected, a thyroid and lateral neck ultrasound is preferred. A patient such as the one presented here also requires a tissue diagnosis of the neck mass and a search for the primary tumor location if the biopsy reveals metastatic malignancy. The vast majority of neck masses can be adequately biopsied with a fine-needle aspiration (FNA) biopsy with or without ultrasound guidance. An open surgical (incisional/excisional) or core biopsy may also be used in certain scenarios, such as when lymphoma is high on the differential diagnosis. The identification of primary tumor site begins with the physical exam: examination of the scalp, face, and neck for cutaneous lesions, oral cavity and oropharynx for mucosal irregularities, and the thyroid gland for nodules.

Ultimately, this patient requires a referral to an otolaryngologist who specializes in head and neck surgical oncology for a more detailed physical exam including bedside endoscopy (flexible fiberoptic laryngoscopy) to examine the nasal cavity, nasopharynx, oropharynx, hypopharynx, and larynx in detail. Referral of an adult with a persistent neck mass to an otolaryngologist prior to

TABLE 16.1 ■ **Differential Diagnosis of Neck Masses**

Kongenital	Thyroglossal duct cyst, branchial cleft cyst, dermoid cyst, lymphatic or venous malformation, teratoma
Infectious/inflammatory	Deep neck space infection (abscess), benign reactive lymphadenopathy, tuberculosis (scrofula), atypical tuberculosis infection
Trauma	Neck hematoma, traumatic fibroma/neuroma
Toxins	
Endocrine	Thyroid nodule (benign or malignant), parathyroid malignancy, or adenoma
Neoplasms	Metastatic head and neck squamous cell carcinoma, paraganglioma/schwannoma/nerve sheath tumor, lymphoma, lipoma, salivary gland tumors, metastases from other body sites
Systemic	Granulomatous disease
Other	Laryngocele, skin-based cysts, submandibular gland, sialodenitis/sialolithiasis, plunging ranula

imaging and biopsy is also an option and may be preferred in situations where the optimal imaging studies or biopsy techniques are not obvious.

Case Point 16.1

The patient undergoes a CT scan with contrast that reveals a partially cystic conglomerate of lymph nodes (Fig. 16.1A). Additionally, there is a 2-cm mass of the right palatine tonsil with possible extension onto the base of the tongue (Fig. 16.1B). An FNA biopsy of the right neck mass is performed and returns as positive for squamous cell carcinoma (SCC).

CLINICAL PEARL

The most common causes of cystic or partially cystic neck masses in an adult are regional metastases from papillary thyroid carcinoma, cutaneous SCC (nonmelanoma skin cancer), and HPV-associated oropharyngeal SCC. Common benign cystic lesions include congenital cysts such as thyroglossal duct cysts and branchial cleft cysts.

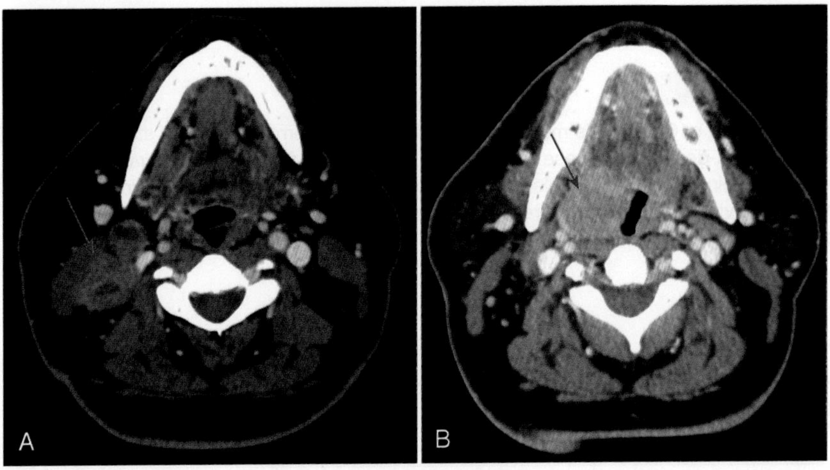

Fig. 16.1 (A) Axial computed tomography scan of the neck with contrast demonstrating conglomerate of partially cystic right neck masses and (B) enlarged right tonsil.

What is head and neck cancer?

Head and neck cancer represents the sixth most common cancer in adults in the United States, with an estimated 65,000 new cases per year. The term *head and neck cancer* typically refers to cancers of the nasopharynx, paranasal sinuses, oropharynx, hypopharynx, larynx, and oral cavity. Over 90% of head and neck cancers are SCCs (HNSCCs) arising from the mucosal lining of these anatomic regions. Cancers of the salivary glands, thyroid and parathyroid glands, advanced melanoma and nonmelanoma skin cancer, and skull base tumors are also types of head and neck cancer and arise from a diverse array of other histologic categories. There is significant morbidity associated with HNSCCs given the critical functions of the upper aerodigestive tract and the fact that disruption of these structures by a cancer or treatment for a cancer can result in impairments in speaking, swallowing, breathing, and/or cosmesis. The traditional risk factor for HNSCC is carcinogen exposure (tobacco smoking and heavy alcohol consumption). Heavy smoking increases one's risk by 5.8x and heavy drinking by 7.4x; when both exposures are present, the risk is increased by 38x in males and 100x in females.

Since this patient does not have a significant smoking or alcohol history, how does human papilloma virus (HPV) play into his diagnosis and what other diseases does it cause?

HPV is the most prevalent sexually transmitted virus in the world. Exposure and infection are nearly universal through oral, vaginal, and anal secretions. Most acute infections are cleared within several months to years, but a small subset of patients has persistent infection. Traditionally, HPV was most notable as the causative agent in cervical SCC, which led to the development of the first Food and Drug Administration (FDA)-approved vaccine against a cancer-causing virus (HPV quadrivalent vaccine). HPV is also the causative agent in most SCCs of the oropharynx, anus, penis, vagina, and vulva as well as papillomas (warts) of the skin, airway, genitals, and anus.

CLINICAL PEARL

The process by which HPV causes cancer is complex, but it is important to know that two of the proteins expressed by HPV, E6 and E7, inhibit the tumor suppressor genes p53 and Rb, respectively. Thus, E6 and E7 are oncoproteins that lead to cellular immortalization.

CLINICAL PEARL

Staining for the p16 protein is most commonly used to determine the HPV status of HNSCC. p16 is a cyclin-dependent kinase that acts on Rb. With the functional inactivation of Rb by the viral protein E7, p16 accumulates in HPV-positive HNSCC and thus is a good surrogate for HPV activity. One can also directly test for the presence of HPV, although this is less frequently done due to the cost involved.

Case Point 16.2

Immunostaining for p16, which is a surrogate marker for HPV, is performed on the patient's FNA biopsy and the cells are p16-positive (Fig. 16.2).

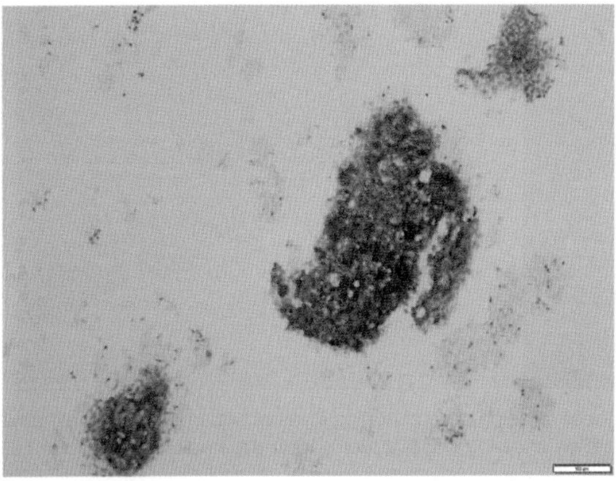

Fig. 16.2 Immunostain for p16 highlighted in brown of right neck mass fine-needle aspiration.

What is HPV-positive HNSCC?

HPV-positive HNSCC most often refers to SCC of the oropharynx that is caused by HPV infection. The oropharynx is the area bounded by the soft palate superiorly, vallecula inferiorly, and the circumvallate papillae of the tongue and hard–soft palate junction anteriorly. The lymphoid tissues of the oropharynx (palatine tonsils and lingual tonsils/base of tongue) are the most commonly affected sites by HPV-positive HNSCC. In contrast to most other types of HNSCC, which are on the decline due to decreasing smoking rates in the US, HPV-positive HNSCC has shown a dramatic rise in prevalence rates over the past 15 years. Approximately 70% of oropharyngeal carcinomas in the US are related to HPV. In fact, the incidence rate of HPV-positive HNSCC has now surpassed HPV-mediated cervical cancer, making it the most common HPV-mediated malignancy in the US.

Which HPV subtypes are most commonly implicated in HPV-positive HNSCC?

HPV 16 is the most common genotype in HNSCC, causing ~87% of all infections. Types 18, 33, and 35 make up the remainder. HPV 6 and 11 are considered low-risk genotypes and are associated with genital warts and respiratory papillomas. HPV 6, 11, 16, and 18 were the genotypes covered by the original quadravalent vaccine.

What is the prognostic significance of HPV positivity in HNSCC?

Survival rates for HPV-positive HNSCC are superior to those for equivalently staged HPV-negative HNSCC. HPV-positive HNSCC tends to present in younger patients, males more frequently than females, and with bulky lymph node metastases. The primary tumor site is often surprisingly small and can be challenging to identify even with PET/CT and operative endoscopy. These findings are reflected in the most recent staging guidelines for head and neck cancer, which effectively down-stages HPV-positive HNSCC with new HPV-specific T and N staging. This is also reflected in ongoing clinical trials to examine whether de-intensification of therapy (i.e., decreased radiation dose) yields similar survival rates and decreased rates of treatment-related side effects. The younger median age of diagnosis for HPV-positive HNSCC and better survival equates to a longer life expectancy with radiation-related toxicities (neck fibrosis, trisumus, xerostomia, dental caries, osteoradionecrosis of the mandible, and dysphagia) that occur at higher, traditional radiation doses.

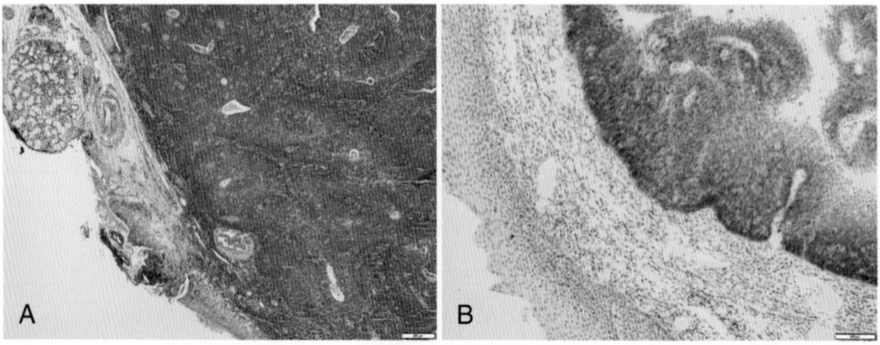

Fig. 16.3 (A) Right transoral robotic surgery tonsil excision demonstrating invasive squamous cell carcinoma (H&E, 40x). (B) Immunostain highlighted in brown showing positivity for p16 in the invasive squamous cell carcinoma (p16, 40x).

Case Point 16.3

The patient elects to undergo transoral robotic surgery (TORS) to remove the primary tumor and a neck dissection to remove the lymph nodes in the right side of the neck. The right tonsil is removed and submitted for frozen section diagnosis. The frozen section confirms that the tonsil is indeed the site of the primary cancer. This returns as SCC, and again the p16 staining is strongly positive (Figs. 16.3A–B).

What is the appearance of HNSCC on histopathology?
SCCs are composed of nests of squamous epithelial cell, often with abundant eosinophilic cytoplasm and large vesicular nuclei. Variable amounts of keratinization can be seen. They are also characterized by nuclear atypia, mitotic figures, and basement membrane invasion.

CLINICAL PEARL

Nonkeratinizing SCC is more typical of HPV-positive HNSCC, whereas keratinizing SCC is more often HPV-negative HNSCC.

What are the treatment options for HPV-positive HNSCC?
Treatment of early-stage HPV-positive HNSCC most commonly involves TORS and a neck dissection or radiation therapy with concurrent chemotherapy. Advanced-stage HPV-positive HNSCC is most commonly treated by radiation with concurrent chemotherapy.

What is the effect of smoking in an HPV-positive HNSCC?
A patient with HPV-positive HNSCC who also smokes progressively returns to a worse expected survival with increasing cigarette exposure. In general, a smoking history of less than 10 pack-years does not seem to alter the outcomes of HPV-positive HNSCC. Smoking during treatment (both surgical and chemoradiation) leads to worse outcomes, highlighting the importance of smoking cessation.

What are critical aspects to consider in a patient with HNSCC undergoing treatment?

The safety of the airway must be established for all patients with HNSCC both during diagnosis and throughout treatment. For some patients, a tracheostomy is necessary regardless of whether surgical or nonsurgical treatment is pursued. Swallowing function also needs to be evaluated by history and sometimes with imaging (chest x-ray, CT) or swallowing studies (modified barium swallow, function endoscopic examination of swallowing) if there is concern for aspiration. Swallowing function universally declines with radiation and/or surgery, and sometimes a gastrostomy is needed. Swallowing therapy, delivered by a head and neck cancer-focused speech and language pathologist is frequently utilized. Cancer patients have heightened nutritional requirements, especially during treatment, so ensuring adequate caloric intake and quality is critical.

Are HPV vaccines effective at preventing HPV-positive HNSCC?

It is currently unknown whether HPV vaccination will reduce HPV-positive HNSCC. Given the HPV genotype coverage of the HPV 9-valent vaccine, it stands to reason that the vaccine should prevent against infection and therefore malignant transformation in the oropharynx as well as the cervix. The risk-potential benefit of the vaccine for this indication is one of several motivations for expanding the vaccine series to adolescent males in addition to females, especially considering the higher incidence of HPV-positive HNSCC in men.

CLINICAL PEARL

The quadrivalent and 9-valent HPV vaccines are noninfectious recombinant vaccines prepared from the purified virus-like particles of the major capsid protein L1 from each of the genotypes covered.

BEYOND THE PEARLS

- HNSCC is traditionally associated with heavy cigarette and/or alcohol use.
- HPV-associated oropharyngeal SCC is markedly on the rise. HPV 16 and 18 are the most commonly implicated HPV subtypes associated with this malignancy.
- The prognosis for HPV-associated HNSCC is better than that for a comparably staged non-HPV-associated HNSCC.
- Treatment options include surgery (often TORS), radiation, and chemotherapy.
- Treatment-related toxicities include xerostomia and dysphagia. Given the inherently better prognosis, de-escalation of therapy (e.g., reducing radiation dose) is one strategy to minimize treatment-related side-effects.

References

Bonner JA, Harari PM, Giralt J, et al. Radiotherapy plus cetuximab for squamous-cell carcinoma of the head and neck. *N Engl J Med.* 2006;354:567-578.

Centers for Disease Control and Prevention. *Human Papillomavirus (HPV).* September 30, 2015. Available at: https://www.cdc.gov/hpv/index.html.

Chaturvedi AK, Engels EA, Pfeiffer RM, et al. Human papillomavirus and rising oropharyngeal cancer incidence in the United States. *J Clin Oncol.* 2011;29:4294-4301.

Gillison ML, Lowy DR. A causal role for human papillomavirus in head and neck cancer. *Lancet.* 2004;363(9420):1488-1489.

Gillison ML, Broutian T, Pickard RK, et al. Prevalence of oral HPV infection in the United States, 2009-2010. *JAMA.* 2012;307:693-703.

Gillison ML, Koch WM, Capone RB, et al. Evidence for a causal association between human papillomavirus and a subset of head and neck cancers. *J Natl Cancer Inst.* 2000;92:709-720.

Gillison ML, Zhang Q, Jordan R, et al. Tobacco smoking and increased risk of death and progression for patients with p16-positive and p16-negative oropharyngeal cancer. *J Clin Oncol.* 2012;30:2102-2111.

Jemal A, Simard EP, Dorell C, et al. Annual Report to the Nation on the Status of Cancer, 1975-2009, featuring the burden and trends in human papillomavirus (HPV)-associated cancers and HPV vaccination coverage levels. *J Natl Cancer Inst.* 2013;105:175-201.

Kreimer AR, Pierce Campbell CM, Lin HY, et al. Incidence and clearance of oral human papillomavirus infection in men: the HIM cohort study. *Lancet.* 2013;382:877-887.

Langendijk JA, Doornaert P, Verdonck-de Leeuw IM, Leemans CR, Aaronson NK, Slotman BJ. Impact of late treatment-related toxicity on quality of life among patients with head and neck cancer treated with radiotherapy. *J Clin Oncol.* 2008;26:3770-3776.

Mehanna H, Beech T, Nicholson T, et al. Prevalence of human papillomavirus in oropharyngeal and nonoropharyngeal head and neck cancer—systematic review and meta-analysis of trends by time and region. *Head Neck.* 2013;35:747-755.

National Cancer Institute. Surveillance, Epidemiology and End Results Program. *Cancer Statistics.* Available at: www.seer.cancer.gov.

Vent J, Haidle B, Wedemeyer I, et al. p16 expression in carcinoma of unknown primary: diagnostic indicator and prognostic marker. *Head Neck.* 2013;35:1521-1526.

A 23-Year-Old Female with Swelling of Her Parotid Region

Anna-Karoline Israel

A 23-year-old with hypertension, polycystic ovarian syndrome, and a history of a left parotid gland tumor status post resection 2 years ago presents to the head and neck clinic with recurrent swelling of the left parotid region. She recently moved to the area and has no specific information regarding her surgical and pathological history available. However, she believes the entire salivary gland was not resected. A CT scan of the neck reveals postoperative changes consistent with partial resection of the left parotid gland and masseter muscle with increased prominence of the soft tissue in the postoperative bed. Recurrent tumor cannot be excluded and an MRI is recommended.

CLINICAL PEARL

Polycystic ovary syndrome (PCOS) is one of the common endocrine illnesses in women of reproductive age with a prevalence ranging from 11% to 21%. It is characterized by chronic oligo- or anovulation, hyperandrogenism, and polycystic ovaries. PCOS is associated with several long-term health consequences such as infertility, obesity, hypertension, dyslipidemia, insulin resistance, and type II diabetes mellitus. Women with PCOS have an increased risk for endometrial cancer. The risk for breast and ovarian cancer is not increased in patients with PCOS. Some data further suggests an increased risk for kidney, colon, and brain cancer among patients with PCOS.

What is the cytology and histology of the normal salivary gland?

The major salivary glands are the paired parotid, submandibular, and sublingual glands. Further there are numerous minor salivary glands throughout the entire upper respiratory and digestive tract (lips, oral cavity, gingiva, floor of mouth, check, hard palate, soft palate, tongue, tonsillar area, oropharynx, larynx, trachea).

Histologically salivary glands are comprised of acini and a branching duct system. Acini can be serous, mucinous, or mixed and drain into the duct system. Serous acini are spherical with pyramid-shaped cells containing large basophilic zymogen granules, whereas mucous acini are tubular with round cells containing mucin (Fig. 17.1). Mixed acini are essentially mucous acini with crescent-shaped caps of serous cells (serous demilunes). The acini produce saliva, which is excreted and modified by the duct system and released into the oral cavity. The parotid gland is exclusively comprised of serous acini, the submandibular gland has a minor component of mucous acini, and the sublingual gland and minor salivary glands are predominantly comprised of mucinous acini.

CLINICAL PEARL

The salivary secretory unit consists of a terminal branched tubuloacinar structure composed exclusively of either serous or mucous secretory cells or a mixture of both types. In mixed secretory units where mucous cells predominate, serous cells often form semilunar caps called

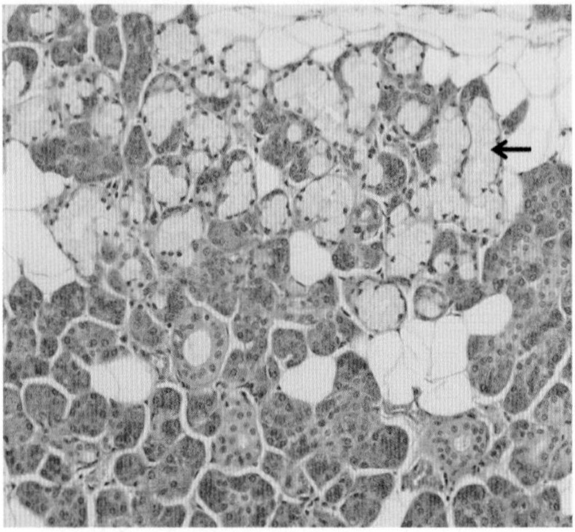

Fig. 17.1 Normal submandibular gland demonstrating granular, purple serous, and mucinous (arrow) acini (H&E, 200x).

serous demilunes surrounding the terminal part of the mucous acini. Myoepithelial cells embrace the secretory units; their contraction helps to expel the secretory product. The terminal secretory units merge to form small intercalated ducts, which are also lined by secretory cells. They drain into larger ducts called striated ducts, so named because of their striated appearance on light microscopy. The striations result from the presence of numerous interdigitations of the basal cytoplasmic processes of adjacent columnar lining cells. The serous cells secrete a fluid isotonic with plasma. In the striated ducts, ions are reabsorbed and secreted to produce hypotonic saliva containing less Na^+ and Cl^- and more K^+ and HCO_3^- than plasma. The mitochondria, which pack the basal processes, provide the energy for ion transport. Saliva contains water, mucins, α-amylase for initial digestion of carbohydrates, lysozyme to control bacterial flora, bicarbonate ions for buffering, antibodies, and the calcium and phosphate essential for healthy teeth. Approximately 150–1200 mL of saliva is produced in 24 hours.

What processes may cause swelling of salivary glands?

Swelling of salivary glands may be caused by trauma, viral and bacterial infections, autoimmune conditions, and benign and malignant neoplasms. Mucoceles are the most common lesion of salivary glands and are usually found on the lower lip. The pediatric and elder populations are most frequently affected. They result from blockage or rupture of a salivary gland duct. Mucus can dissect diffusely through soft tissues and induces a strong inflammatory response. The most common viral sialadenitis is mumps. Bacterial infections are most often secondary to sialolithiasis, which leads to *Staphylococcus aureus* infection. In addition, dehydration and decreased secretions may predispose to bacterial infections. Autoimmune conditions, such as lymphoepithelial sialadenitis (LESA), usually cause a bilateral and symmetric enlargement of salivary glands. Finally, benign and malignant neoplasms can cause swelling of major and minor salivary glands.

CLINICAL PEARL

The term *ranula* is being reserved for mucoceles that occur when mucus extravasates due to injury of the sublingual duct.

CLINICAL PEARL

Mumps is caused by the mumps virus, which belongs to the paramyxoviridae family. Mumps is transmitted through direct contact with respiratory secretions and has an incubation period of 12–25 days. The virus replicates in the upper respiratory tract and regional lymphoid tissue and disseminates systemically. It causes bilateral inflammation of parotid glands. Testes, pancreas, breast, brain, and spinal cord may be affected. Serum amylase is increased due to salivary gland or pancreatic involvement. Orchitis carries the risk of sterility.

Mumps is infectious 1–2 days before until 5 days after the onset of parotitis. In the pre-vaccination era, there were approximately 186,000 cases per year in the US (now 20–6,500 cases per year, depending on the amount of outbreaks).

CLINICAL PEARL

The key histologic findings of LESA are marked lymphoid infiltration and epimyoepithelial islands. LESA can be a manifestation of Sjögren syndrome, which is characterized by kerato-conjunctivitis, xerostomia, rheumatoid arthritis, and hypergammaglobulinemia. Lymphoid infiltrates are seen in major and minor glands as well as in lacrimal glands.

Case Point 17.1

The MRI shows diffuse signal enhancement in the previous tumor bed and recurrence is suspected. A fine-needle aspiration (FNA) is recommended, and the patient is scheduled for the procedure. The specimen is received for cytologic assessment. Cytologic preparations reveal clusters of intermediate and epidermoid cells. There are focal mucous cells. Keratinization is absent. There is abundant extracellular mucin present (Fig. 17.2).

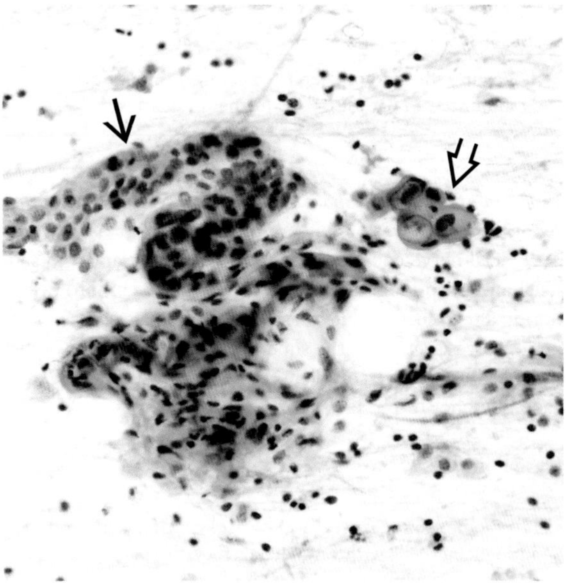

Fig. 17.2 The PAP-stained slide demonstrates intermediate cells (black solid arrow) and a cluster of mucus-containing cells (black open arrow). (From *ExpertPath*. Copyright Elsevier).

What resources could you utilize to establish a diagnosis?

Correlation of cytologic specimens with concurrent or previous surgical resection specimens pertinent to the suspected diagnosis can be helpful in establishing a diagnosis. This patient has a history of salivary gland swelling with resection of part of her parotid gland. Correlation of the past resection specimen and the current cytology specimen can help in determining if the disease processes are related. It is a good clinical practice to review pathology material, such as cytology slides, H&E slides, and special and immunohistochemical stains pertinent to a current case before further treatment is planned.

What is the utility of cytology in the workup of salivary gland neoplasms?

Cytology usually establishes a differential diagnosis and stratifies the findings and thus may aid in planning the follow-up and/or extent of surgery. Currently, the Milan System for Reporting Salivary Gland Cytopathology provides guidance on how to report salivary gland cytology. The sensitivity of salivary gland FNA ranges from 86% to 100%, and the specificity ranges from 90% to 100%.

CLINICAL PEARL

The Milan System for Reporting Salivary Gland Cytopathology was published in 2018 and promotes a standardized protocol on how to report findings in salivary gland FNAs. The system aids in treatment planning.

There are six main categories:

- Nondiagnostic
- Non-neoplastic
- Atypia of undetermined significance
- Neoplastic (benign and salivary gland neoplasm of uncertain malignant potential)
- Suspicious for malignancy
- Malignant

Case Point 17.2

Following the cytology report, a completion parotidectomy is scheduled. The resection specimen is submitted to pathology for further evaluation.

What complication is more likely in a re-resection compared with a primary resection of the parotid gland?

The facial nerve courses through the parotid gland and separates the parotid gland into a superficial and deep lobe. The facial nerve can be compromised during resection. This is more likely during a re-resection due to the formation of scar tissue and more superficial location of the facial nerve post resection of the superficial parotid lobe. In some situation the facial nerve needs to be sacrificed to achieve complete resection of the tumor. Adenoid cystic carcinoma is known to invade branches of the facial nerve frequently.

Case Point 17.3

Histologic sections reveal a salivary gland that is infiltrated by islands of epidermoid, intermediate and mucous cells with variable-sized cystic spaces and abundant mucin. There is a robust stromal reaction and some lymphocytic infiltrate surrounding the tumor islands (Figs. 17.3A–B).

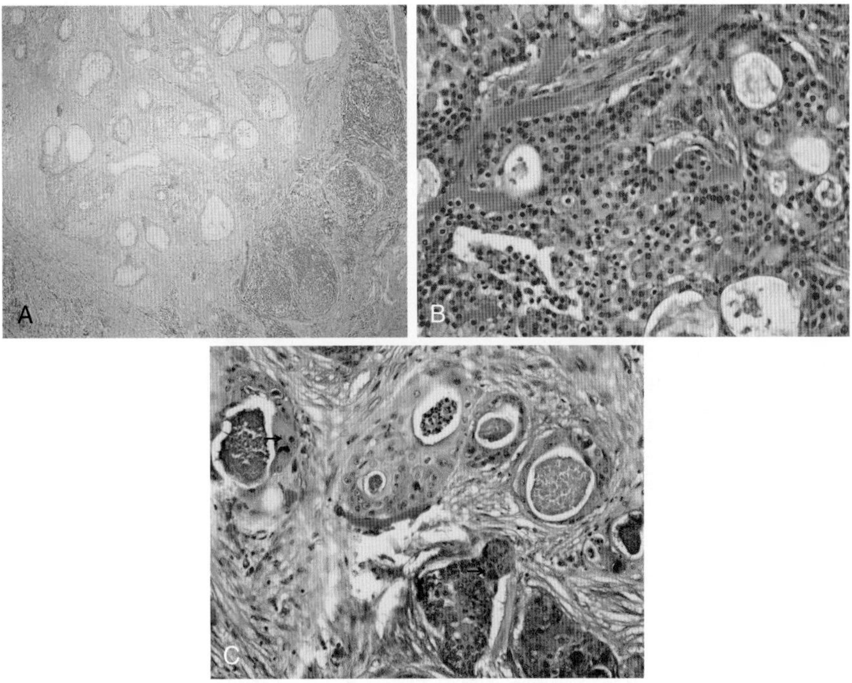

Fig. 17.3 (A) Mucoepidermoid carcinoma (H&E, 40x). (B) Mucoepidermoid carcinoma, (H&E, 100x).

What is the differential diagnosis and what ancillary studies can confirm it?

Salivary gland neoplasms are rare, accounting for less than 2% of all tumors. The annual incidence for malignant salivary gland tumors is 0.3–3/100,000. While the histology of the salivary glands is rather simple, they give rise to over 30 distinct neoplastic entities. Most commonly, neoplasms involve the parotid gland, and the vast majority of them are benign. In contrast, approximately 70%–90% of sublingual tumors are cancerous. The most common benign entity is pleomorphic adenoma, and the most common malignant entity in adults and children is mucoepidermoid carcinoma. Morphologic aspects are very crucial in diagnosing salivary gland neoplasms. An increasing amount of unique genetic alterations has been discovered for different entities. In addition to primary salivary gland neoplasms, metastatic tumors can occur in intraparotid or submandibular lymph nodes. In fact the most common tumor in the parotid and submandibular region is actually metastatic disease. Squamous cell carcinoma from the skin and upper aerodigestive tract and malignant melanoma are the most common entities. As noted, the differential diagnosis of salivary gland neoplasms is extensive, and the most common entities are further described (Tables 17.1 and 17.2; Fig. 17.4). This patent's tumor is composed of islands of epidermoid and intermediate cells with scattered mucocytes and variable sized cystic spaces and abundant mucin, therefore mucoepidermoid carcinoma is high on the differential. Mucicarmine and Kreyberg highlight mucocytes and mucin (see Fig. 17.3 C). Cytokeratin, p40 and p63 highlight epidermoid and intermediate cells.

What other differential diagnoses should you consider and rule out for the presented case?

Sialometaplasia, mucus extravasation reaction, and cystadenoma are benign entities that need to be considered when working up a case of mucoepidermoid carcinoma. Secretory carcinoma is a recently described low-grade malignant entity that shares some morphologic similarities with mucopepidermoid carcinoma. Salivary duct carcinoma is a high-grade malignancy that resembles ductal carcinoma of the breast morphologically and immunohistochemically (Table 17.3; Fig. 17.5).

TABLE 17.1 ■ **Most Common Benign Salivary Gland Neoplasms**

Entity	General Key Facts	Histologic Features	Cytologic Features	Ancillary Tests
Pleomorphic adenoma	Most common salivary gland neoplasm; affects mainly parotid gland; slow growing	Epithelial, myoepithelial, and mesenchymal differentiation; various architectural patterns (which named the entity); chondromyxoid, myxoid, or hyaline stroma; epithelial tissue may show spindle, clear cell, plasmacytoid, basaloid, squamous, or sebaceous differentiation	Clusters of epithelial cells with round-to-ovoid nuclei and delicate nuclear chromatin; atypia limited to single cells; fibrillar chondromyxoid stroma (deep purple on Diff-quick stain) presents as feathered edge that blends/surrounds epithelial/myoepithelial cells	Cytokeratin, p63, GFAP, S100, PLAG1(nuclear), and SMA show variable positivity; PLAG1 and HMGA2 rearrangements in 70%; cases with normal karyotype are often stroma rich (30%); overexpression of p53 may represent early malignant transformation
Warthin tumor	Second most common benign salivary gland tumor; exclusively involves parotid gland; may be bilateral in 10% of cases and multifocal; patients usually have a significant smoking history	Epithelial lining and lymphoid stroma; double layer of oncocytes lining papillary and cystic structures; mature lymphoid component with lymphoid follicles and germinal centers	Sheets of oncocytes; lymphocytes and proteinaceous (dirty) background	Positive for pancytokeratin; negative for S100, p63, calponin, GFAP, actin
Oncocytoma	Occurs most commonly in the parotid gland; 7th–9th decade; well demarcated from surrounding parenchyma and often has at least a partial capsule	Single nodule, distinct from surrounding parenchyma; variable pattern; composed exclusively of oncocytes	Oncocytes; absence of lymphocytes	Electron microscopy shows cytoplasms filled with mitochondria

GFAP, glial fibrillary acidic protein; HMAG2, high mobility group AT-hook 2; PLAG1, pleomorphic adenoma gene 1.

TABLE 17.2 ■ **Most Common Malignant Differential Diagnoses Of Mucoepidermoid Carcinoma**

Entity	General Key Facts	Histologic Features	Cytologic Features	Ancillary Tests
Acinic cell carcinoma	Second most common malignant salivary gland neoplasm; LG, but can undergo HG transformation; wide age range; slight female predominance; most common in parotid gland	Circumscribed, solitary, oval-to-round mass; solid, lobular, papillary-cystic and microcystic patterns; prominent zymogen granules; often associated with lymphoid infiltrate	Polygonal, monotonous cells with low N:C ratio and vacuolated cytoplasm; uniform, round, eccentric nuclei; minimal nuclear pleomorphism; stripped nuclei and lymphocytes in background	PAS-positive, diastase-resistant zymogen granules; IHC-positive for DOG-1
Squamous cell carcinoma	Most commonly metastatic	Cohesive clusters of eosinophilic cells with moderate-to-abundant cytoplasm and intercellular bridges; keratinization maybe present	Pleomorphic cells with high N:C ratio; epithelioid to spindly; keratinization appears orange on PAP stain	positive for p40
Adenocarcinoma, NOS	Most common in parotid gland; wide age range; diagnosis of exclusion	May have very little areas of specific salivary gland tumor morphology; three-tier grading system which evaluates ductal/tubular differentiation, pleomorphism, and mitoses	Atypical cells; lacks specific features	Limited utility
Adenoid cystic carcinoma	Peak incidence in 4th–6th decade; slight female predominance; tendency to invade nerves and often presents with facial nerve palsy	Three major histologic subtypes: tubular, cribriform, and solid; perineural invasion	Consists of epithelial and myoepithelial cells; uniform basaloid cells with high N:C ratio and scant cytoplasm surrounding acellular homogeneous basement membrane-like material; distinct separation of cells and amorphous material	Epithelial cells can be positive for CD117; t(6;9) chromosomal translocation resulting in MYB–NFIB fusion

HG, high grade; *IHC,* immunohistochemistry; *LG,* low grade; *N:C ratio,* nuclear-to-cytoplasmic ratio; *NOS,* not otherwise specified; *PAP,* papanicolaou.

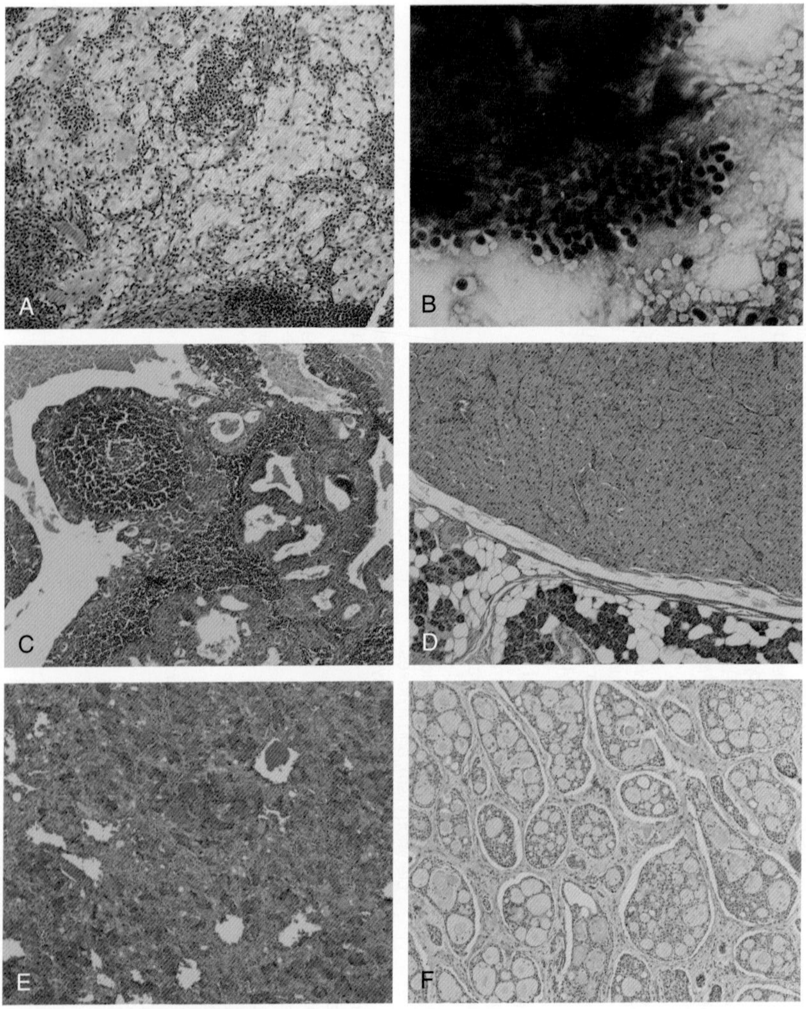

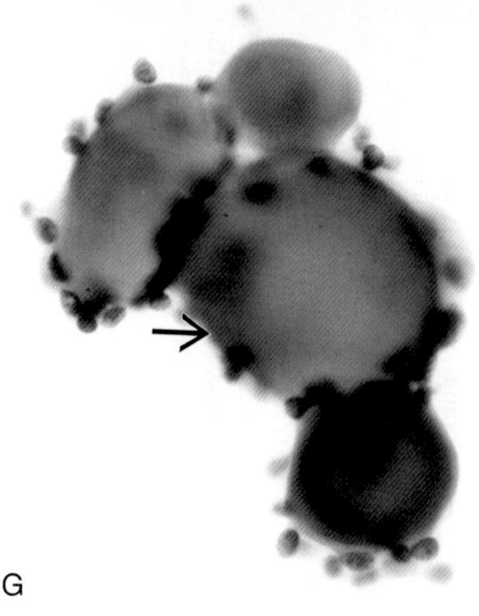

Fig. 17.4 (A) Pleomorphic adenoma (H&E, 100x). (B) Pleomorphic adenoma (Diff quick, 400x). (C) Warthin tumor (H&E, 100x). (D) Oncocytoma (H&E, 100x). (E) Acinic cell carcinoma (H&E, 100x). (F) Adenoid cystic carcinoma (H&E, 100x). (G) Adenoid cystic carcinoma (PAP, 100x). (G, from *ExpertPath*. Copyright Elsevier).

TABLE 17.3 ■ **Additional Differential Diagnoses for Mucoepidermoid Carcinoma**

Entity	General Key Facts	Histologic Features	Cytologic Features	Ancillary Tests
Benign				
Sialometaplasia	Inflammatory condition	Coagulative necrosis of salivary gland acini and squamous metaplasia of ductal structures; lobular architecture of salivary gland maintained; inflammatory infiltrate and mucin pools; pseudoepitheliomatous hyperplasia of overlying squamous epithelium	Overall benign cellular features	Usually not necessary
Mucous extravasation reaction	Common in pediatric population; most often in lower lip; mucocele or ranula	Mucin walled off by granulation tissue	Benign adjacent epithelium and ducts; oncocytic metaplasia maybe present	Usually not necessary
Cystadenoma	Most commonly in parotid gland; wide age range; female predeliction	Well circumscribed, variable encapsulated cystic spaces of varying number and sizes; cuboidal-to-columnar epithelial lining; papillary proliferation and oncocytes maybe present	Bland cytology	Usually not necessary
Malignant				
Salivary duct carcinoma	High-grade salivary gland malignancy; resembles ductal carcinoma of the breast	Unencapsulated, infiltrative tumor with rounded to irregular, solid, cystic or cribriform islands of tumor cells; Roman bridge architecture common; conspicuous comedonecrosis	Sheets of crowded, three-dimensional groups of overtly malignant cells; marked nuclear pleomorphism, anisonucleosis, and hyperchromasia; frequent mitosis; necrotic background	Positive for AR and Gata-3
Secretory carcinoma	Recently described low-grade salivary gland neoplasm; most commonly in parotid gland; occurs mostly in adults	Lesion with lobulated periphery and limited invasion; various patterns including cystic, tubular, follicular and papillary	Bland, cuboidal, polygonal cells with low N:C ratio occurring singly, or in tubular, follicular, or papillary groups; abundant vacuolated eosinophilic cytoplasm (apocrine-like); distinct nucleoli; absence of zymogen granules	Majority S100 and mammaglobin positive; t(12;15)(p13:q25) which leads to ETV6–NTRK3 fusion
Carcinoma ex Pleomorphic adenoma	Occur approximately a decade later than pleomorphic adenomas in the 6th and 7th decade; high-grade malignancy	Component of classic pleomorphic adenoma and carcinomatous component, most commonly salivary duct carcinoma or adenocarcinoma, NOS	Classic pleomorphic adenoma and high-grade component; diagnosis difficult to make on cytologic preparations alone	In carcinoma areas increased Ki-67 and AR positivity

NOS, not otherwise specified.

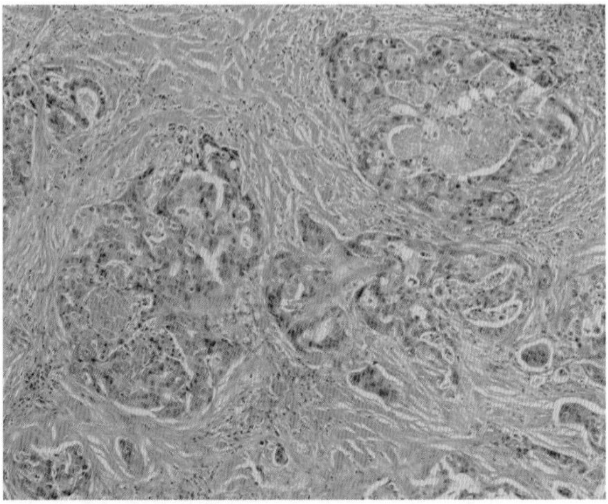

Fig. 17.5 Salivary duct carcinoma (H&E, 100x).

CLINICAL PEARL

Oncocytes are polygonal cells with abundant homogenous granular cytoplasm. They can occur in various organs and cancer types. There are often oncocytic variants of different cancers. They appear pink on H&E stain due to the abundance of mitochondria. Oncocytic metaplasia is a common phenomenon in salivary glands and most likely occurs in epithelial or myoepithelial cells. The cause for oncocytic metaplasia is not known, but it increases with age.

Case Point 17.4

Further histologic exam of this patient's completion parotidectomy revealed that the resection margins are negative for mucoepidermoid carcinoma. Metastatic mucoepidermoid carcinoma is identified in one out of four lymph nodes.

Intraoperatively facial nerve reconstruction with the greater auricular nerve was necessary. Postoperatively, she had a left marginal mandibular nerve weakness, but she could open her mouth to eat without difficulty. Furthermore, she could close her left eye completely.

The patient's case was discussed at the interdisciplinary tumor board, and adjuvant radiation therapy was recommended, which the patient completes. A year following the surgery, the patient complains about trismus at times, which sometimes causes difficulties with eating and speaking.

How is mucoepidermoid carcinoma treated?

The mainstay of treatment in mucoepidermoid carcinoma is complete surgical resection. Incomplete resection increases the risk of recurrence. Radiation therapy may be used in local recurrence and metastatic disease. Low-grade mucoepidermoid carcinomas have a good prognosis with a 5-year survival rate of 98%. About 55%–80% of high-grade tumors metastasize and have a poorer outcome (5-year survival of 65%). Grading of mucoepidermoid carcinoma is according to a three-tier system—low, intermediate, and high. Mucous cells become less apparent from low to high-grade and the solid component increases. In order to make a diagnosis of high-grade mucoepidermoid carcinoma, one or more of the following features needs to be present: nuclear anaplasia, necrosis, increased mitotic rate, perineural invasion, lymphovascular invasion, or bony invasion.

BEYOND THE PEARLS

- Proper orientation of any surgical specimen is essential for correct staging. If necessary, consult the surgeon and have them orient the specimen for you.
- CRTL1–MAML2 fusion is unique for mucoepidermoid carcinoma.
- Alcohol and tobacco are not risk factors for salivary gland neoplasms, except for Warthin tumor.
- More than 90% of salivary gland tumors arise in the parotid gland while 5% arise in the submandibular gland.
- Poor prognostic factors include postoperative recurrence, facial nerve paralysis, and high-grade tumor.
- Prior radiation increases the risk of developing pleomorphic adenoma.
- Salivary gland amyloidosis is usually secondary and involves the minor salivary glands.

References

Cibas ES, Ducatman BS. *Cytology: Diagnostic Principles and Clinical Correlates.* 4th ed. Philadelphia, PA: Elsevier/Saunders; 2014.

El-Naggar AK, Chan JKC, Grandis JR, Takata T, Slootweg PJ. *WHO Classification of Head and Neck Tumours.* 4th ed. WHO: 2017.

Faquin WC, Rossi ED, Baloch Z, et al. The Milan system for reporting salivary gland cytopathology. *Cancer Cytopathol.* 2017;125(10):757-766.

Goldblum JR, Lamps LW, McKenney JK, eds. *Rosai and Ackerman's Surgical Pathology.* 11th ed. Philadelphia, PA: Elsevier; 2018.

Gottschau M, Kjaer SK, Jensen A, Munk C, Mellemkjaer L. Risk of cancer among women with polycystic ovary syndrome: a Danish cohort study. *Gynecol Oncol.* 2015;136:99-103. doi:10.1016/j.ygyno.2014.11.012.

Kumar V, Abbas A, Aster J. *Robbins and Cotran Pathologic Basis of Disease.* Philadelphia, PA: Elsevier/Saunders; 2015.

Lester SC, French CA, Curtis SG. *Manual of Surgical Pathology.* 3rd ed. Philadelphia, PA: Saunders/Elsevier; 2010.

Mills SE. *Histology for Pathologists.* 4th ed. Philadelphia, PA: Lippincott Williams and Wilkins; 2012.

Wenig B. *Atlas of Head and Neck Pathology.* 3rd ed. Philadelphia, PA: Elsevier; 2016.

CASE 18

A 72-Year-Old Male with Pressure Sensation in His Face

Anna-Karoline Israel

A 72-year-old male with a personal medical history of coronary artery disease, hypertension, hyperlipidemia, seasonal allergies, and prostate cancer status post radical prostatectomy and coronary artery bypass several years ago presents to the clinical with a recently discovered nasal mass. He has trouble breathing through his nose and has constant rhinorrhea, which compromises his sleep and concentration during the day. His primary care physician suggested saline irrigation. He is unable to irrigate saline from one nostril to the other. His medications include flonase, claritin, aspirin, and ramipril.

His ENT exam reveals frond-like polypoid tissue in the anterior nasal cavity. A CT of the paranasal sinuses shows complete opacification of the right maxillary sinus and nasal cavity with extension of opacification to the nasopharynx, near-complete ethmoid opacification, and mild mucosa thickening of the inferior portion of the right frontal sinus is present, while the left paranasal sinuses remain clear (Fig. 18.1).

CLINICAL PEARL

Sino-Nasal Outcome Test (SNOT)-22 score

- Comprehensive assessment of 22 symptoms of chronic rhinosinusitis on a scale of 0–5 (0, no problem; 5, problem as bad as it can be)
- 22 symptoms assessed: need to blow the nose, nasal blockage, sneezing, runny nose, cough, post-nasal discharge, thick nasal discharge, ear fullness, dizziness, ear pain, facial pain/pressure, decreased sense of smell and taste, difficulty falling asleep, wake up at night, lack of good night's sleep, wake up tired, fatigue, reduced productivity, reduced concentration, frustration/restlessness/irritable, sadness, embarrassed
- Higher scores indicated more severe symptoms

What is your main differential diagnoses based on the clinical findings and imaging results?

The leading considerations in this clinical context are sinonasal inflammatory polyp, sinonasal papilloma, and less likely sinonasal carcinoma.

Case Point 18.1

The patient was referred to an ENT specialist who performed a biopsy of the nasal mass. Histologic sections show thickened, inverted squamoid epithelium with intraepithelial inflammatory cells and cysts with adjacent benign sinonasal mucosa (Fig. 18.2). In addition, there are fragments of edematous Schneiderian mucosa with thickened basement membrane and mixed inflammatory infiltrate (Fig. 18.3).

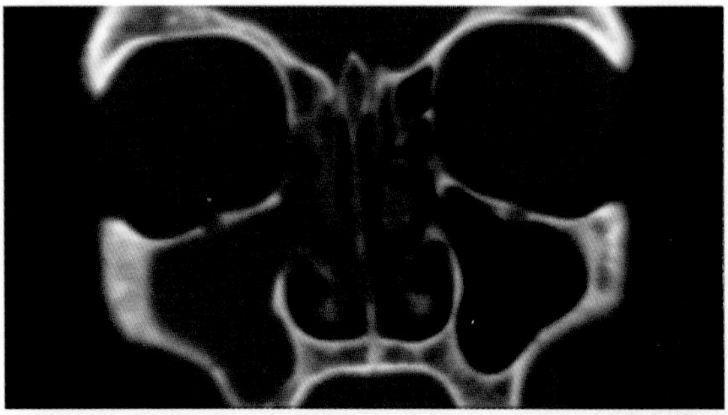

Fig. 18.1 A computed tomography scan of paranasal sinuses.

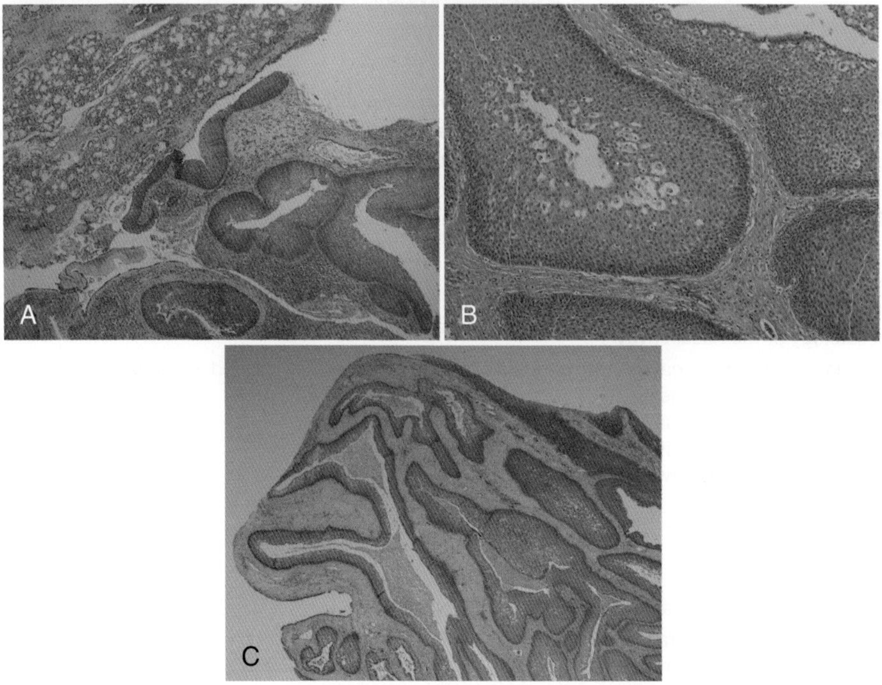

Fig. 18.2 (A) Inverted papilloma with adjacent benign sinonasal mucosa (H&E, 20x). (B) Inverted papilloma at higher power (H&E, 100x). (C) Inverted papilloma at lower power (H&W, 20x).

Following the biopsy, the patient undergoes endoscopic sinus surgery for complete removal of the mass as clinically indicated.

What are the gross pathology findings in nasal polypoid lesions?

You may receive multiple fragments of mucosa, soft tissue, and bone. Inflammatory polyps have a translucent and mucoid appearance. Sinonasal papillomas often have a tan-gray papillary, cauliflower-like, or warty appearance.

Based on the histologic findings of the biopsy and the endoscopic surgery, what is your diagnosis?

The histologic findings are consistent with sinonasal papilloma, inverted type, and sinonasal inflammatory polyp.

TABLE 18.1 ■ **Sinonasal Papillomas**

Type	Site/Location	Histologic Findings
Exophytic	Nasal septum	• Exophytic fibrovascular cores lined with well-differentiated stratified squamous epithelium and admixed mucocytes • Stroma with seromucinous glands
Inverted	Lateral nasal wall, paranasal sinuses, and rarely nasopharynx and middle ear	• Intact, inverted mucosa • Thickened squamoid epithelium and intrepithelial mucocytes • Intraepithelial cysts with mucin and neutrophils • Foci of cytologic atypia may be present • No seromucinous glands in stroma
Oncocytic	Lateral wall of nasal cavity, paranasal sinuses	• May have exophytic and endophytic patterns • Multiple layers of oncocytic epithelium (columnar cells with granular, eosinophilic cytoplasm)

What types of sinonasal papillomas exist and how are they differentiated?

Sinonasal papillomas are benign tumors that arise from the sinonasal (Schneiderian) mucosa and are categorized into three distinct types: inverted, exophytic, and oncocytic. The terminology reflects the differences in macroscopic and histologic appearance. While there is some overlap, they are considered separate entities based on the clinical and microscopic findings (Table 18.1).

BASIC SCIENCE PEARL

Histology of the nasal cavity

- Majority of nasal cavity and paranasal sinuses is lined by ciliated columnar epithelium (Schneiderian mucosa)
- Schneiderian mucosa is of ectodermal origin
- The nasal vestibule is lined by squamous mucosa
- The superior nasal wall is lined by olfactory mucosa

CLINICAL PEARL

Epidemiology of sinonasal papillomas

- <5% of sinonasal tract tumors
- Inverted type is the most common type.
- Oncocytic type is very rare.
- Generally affect middle-aged adults and are rare in children.
- Inverted and the exophytic types show a strong predilection for males (M:F = 3:1 for inverted papilloma; M:F = 10:1 for exophytic papilloma).
- Oncocytic papilloma affects males and females with equal likelihood.

CLINICAL PEARL

Clinical features of sinonasal polyps and sinonasal papillomas

- Unilateral nasal obstruction
- Rhinorrhea
- Facial pressure
- Headache
- Epistaxis is more commonly seen in sinonasal papillomas

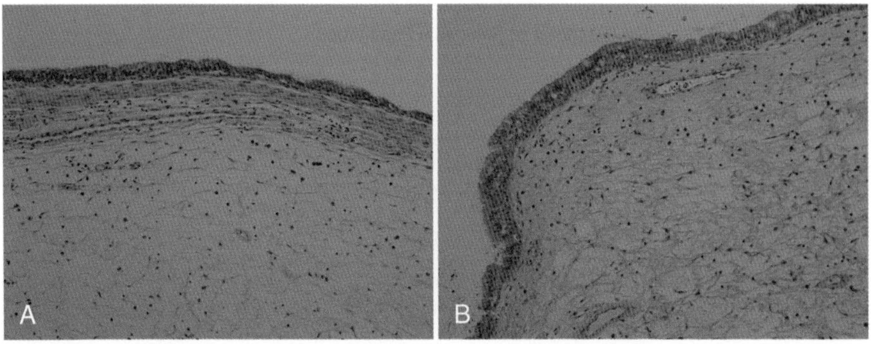

Fig. 18.3 (A and B) Sinonasal inflammatory polyp with markedly edematous stroma and mixed inflammatory cells including eosinophils (H&E, 100x).

What are the key features of sinonasal inflammatory polyp?

Sinonasal inflammatory polyps are very common and represent a non-neoplastic inflammatory swelling of the sinonasal mucosa. They have been associated with a variety of medical conditions including asthma, aspirin intolerance, cystic fibrosis, diabetes mellitus, and infections. Patients present with nasal obstruction, facial pressure or pain, headaches, and rhinorrhea. Sinonasal inflammatory polyps most commonly arise from the lateral nasal wall or the ethmoid sinus. Histologically, there is marked edema of the stroma underlying intact surface ciliated respiratory epithelium (Fig. 18.3A–B). The basement membrane is often thickened. Prominent vasculature with thickened vessel wall may be present. Seromucinous glands are absent. There is a mixed inflammatory infiltrate present, predominantly eosinophils, plasma cells, and lymphocytes. Secondary changes such as surface ulceration, fibrosis, infarction, and granulation tissue formation may occur.

What other mass-forming lesions need to be considered in this clinical scenario (Table 18.2)?

Rhinosporidiosis and sinonasal hamartomas, such as respiratory epithelial adenomatoid hamartoma, should be considered. In the younger male population, nasopharyngeal angiofibroma is a possibility. Malignant tumors of the nasal cavity, sinuses, and nasopharynx are uncommon, but squamous cell carcinoma and sinonasal adenocarcinoma are a possible differential diagnosis in this clinical scenario. Aggressive malignancies, such as sinonasal undifferentiated carcinoma, mucosal melanoma, NUT carcinoma, and extranodal NK/T-cell lymphoma, are very rare entities and often show a destructive growth pattern clinically and on imaging.

What is the treatment of sinonasal inflammatory polyps and sinonasal papillomas, and what is the prognosis?

Sinonasal inflammatory polyps may respond to treatment with topical and systemic steroid therapy and treatment of any underlying condition. In addition, surgical removal of polyp tissue is often performed. Approximately 50% of patients with sinonasal inflammatory polyps will have recurrence of the disease following surgery. Recurrence is more typical in patients with asthma and aspirin intolerance.

Sinonasal papillomas are treated with meticulous and complete surgical resection. They have an excellent long-term prognosis. However, they also recur frequently, up to 50%–60% for exophytic and inverted types. Carcinoma is present in approximately 2% of inverted papillomas.

TABLE 18.2 ■ **Differential Diagnosis of Sinonasal Papillomas**

Entity	General Facts	Histologic Features
Rhinosporidiosis	• Endemic in India, Sri Lanka, and Brazil; only sporadic in the US • Chronic infection with *Rhinosporidium seeberi* involving nasal cavity and nasopharynx • Treatment of choice is surgical excision	• Mucosal and submucosal cysts with innumerable endospores • Organisms can be highlighted with mucicarmine and periodic acid Schiff stain • Acute inflammation with giant cells when cysts rupture
Sinonasal hamartoma	• Includes respiratory epithelial adenomatoid hamartoma (REAH), seromucinous hamartoma (SH), chondroosseous and respiratory epithelial (CORE) hamartoma, and nasal chondromesenchymal hamartoma (NCH); • Occur commonly in the nasal cavity, particularly at the posterior septum; wide age range; • NCH more commonly in first 3 months of life	• REAH: glandular proliferation arising from the surface epithelium and growing inward/downward • SH: clusters and lobules of serous acini and tubules • CORE: feature of REAH with cartilaginous and osseous trabeculae • NCH: nodules of cartilage with varying differentiation
Nasopharyngeal angiofibroma	• Occurs in nasopharynx • Affects young males exclusively • Recurs in 20% of patients	• Disorganized, variable-sized vessels • Fibrous stroma with variable amounts of fine and coarse collagen fibers
Squamous cell carcinoma	• Occurs at older ager • Male predilection • More common in the maxillary sinus • Poor prognosis	• Epithelial cells with abundant pink cytoplasms and intercellular bridges • Keratinizing and nonkeratinizing types • P40 positivity
Nasopharyngeal carcinoma	• Keratinizing, nonkeratinizing and basaloid types • Nonkeratinizing associated with Epstein–Barr virus • Keratinizing type has poor prognosis	• Tumor cells with squamous differentiation and with or without keratinization, respectively
Sinonasal adenocarcinoma	• Intestinal, salivary gland and nonintestinal, nonsalivary gland types	• Resembles intestinal adenocarcinoma, salivary gland carcinomas, or neither

Case Point 18.2

Following the surgery, the patient recovers with no complications. His symptoms improve drastically and he is able to sleep soundly without difficulty breathing.

BEYOND THE PEARLS

- Sinonasal papillomas, particularly the inverted type, are frequently associated with low-risk human papillomavirus types 6 and 11.
- Oncocytic sinonasal papilloma show activated KRAS mutations.
- Nasopharyngeal angiofibroma is characterized by an activated β-catenin mutation.
- NUT midline carcinoma is a rare, aggressive, poorly differentiated carcinoma with squamous differentiation that occurs primarily in the midline and presents primarily at a young age. It is

genetically defined by a rearrangement of the NUTM1 gene. NUT immunohistochemistry highlights strong nuclear positivity.

- Sinonasal undifferentiated carcinoma is a rare, aggressive malignancy of unknown etiology with squamous and/or glandular differentiation.
- Necrotizing lesions of the nasal passages may be secondary to sinonasal inflammatory polyps or sinonasal papilloma. However, they may also be primary disease entities such as acute fungal infections or granulomatosis with polyangiitis.
- Invasive fungal rhinosinusitis refers to vessel invasive fungal disease and is a medical and surgical emergency that warrants immediate treatment. Immunocompromised patients are most commonly affected.

References

Kennedy JL, Hubbard MA, Huyett P, Patrie JT, Borish L, Payne SC. Sino-nasal outcome test (SNOT-22): a predictor of postsurgical improvement in patients with chronic sinusitis. *Ann Allergy Asthma Immunol.* 2013;111(4):246-251.e2. doi:10.1016/j.anai.2013.06.033.

Kumar V, Abbas A, Aster J. *Robbins and Cotran Pathologic Basis of Disease.* Philadelphia, PA: Elsevier/Saunders; 2015.

Thompson L, Bishop J. *Head and Neck Pathology.* 3rd ed. Philadelphia, PA: Elsevier; 2019.

Wenig B. *Atlas of Head and Neck Pathology.* 3rd ed. Philadelphia, PA: Elsevier; 2016.

CASE 19

A 57-Year-Old Man with Swelling of His Lip

Anna-Karoline Israel

A 57-year-old man with a medical history of hypertension, depression, and prediabetes presents to his primary care physician with a painful lesion of his lower lip. This started approximately 1 month ago with a pimple-like bump and quickly worsened with massive swelling and occasional bleeding. The patient presented to the emergency department a couple days ago where an incision and drainage was performed with no return of pertinent material. The patient denies fever, chills, or weight loss. He does not have a personal or family history of skin cancer. Physical examination shows an edematous lip with a raised crusted plaque. The patient is a long-term smoker and consumes alcohol socially.

What is your differential diagnosis based on the clinical history and physical exam?

The primary concern for the etiology of this lesion would be a neoplastic process, particularly a squamous cell carcinoma, considering that the patient is a long-term smoker. One would also want to rule out an infectious etiology from either viral (i.e., herpes simplex virus) or bacterial (*Staphylococci*) microorganisms. The differential diagnosis would also include a nonspecific inflammatory reaction to some prior injury (thermal injury, trauma).

Case Point 19.1

The patient is sent to a dermatology office for a consult, and a 4-mm skin punch biopsy is performed. Half of the specimen is send to microbiology for cultures and half is sent to surgical pathology histologic examination. The biopsy sections show a diffuse lymphocytic and histiocytic infiltrate throughout all levels of the dermis. Focally, this infiltrate is lichenoid and there are abundant plasma cells (Figs. 19.1–19.3).

What additional ancillary test would you request?

In terms of neoplastic etiologies, one could perform a cytokeratin stain to help exclude a subtle invasive carcinoma and lymphoid markers to help exclude a lymphoma, given the presence of an extensive inflammatory infiltrate. Stains for microorganisms could be helpful in the identification of an infectious agent as a cause for the lesion. Special stains for mycobacterial organisms (Fite, Acid fast bacteria—AFB), bacterial organisms (Brown and Brenn), and fungal organisms (Periodic acid Schiff—PAS and Grocott methamine Silver—GMS) are negative. Immunohistochemical stain for pancytokeratin (epithelial cell marker) is negative. CD3 and CD20 highlight a mixture of T and B cells, helping to exclude a lymphoid malignancy.

Case Point 19.2

An immunohistochemical stain against *Treponema pallidum* on the patient's biopsy reveals numerous spirochetes within the epidermis and focally in the dermis (Fig. 19.4).

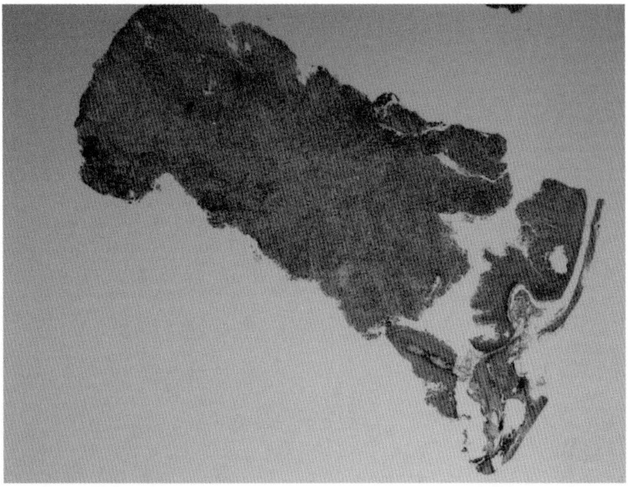

Fig. 19.1 Low-power view of 4-mm punch biopsy demonstrating a superficial and deep dermal lymphoplasmacytic infiltrate (H&E, 20x).

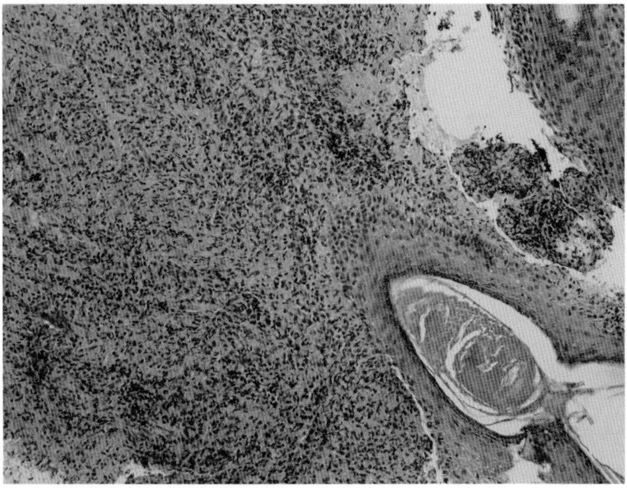

Fig. 19.2 Lymphoplasmacytic infiltrate at dermal–epidermal junction with focal lichenoid appearance (H&E, 100x).

CLINICAL PEARLS

Immunohistochemistry (IHC)

Pancytokeratin AE1/AE3 is a cytoplasmic stain. It targets the most common basic and acidic (high- and low-molecular-weight) cytokeratins, which are cytoskeletal proteins that belong to the family of intermediate filaments. Thus, it stains most epithelial cells.

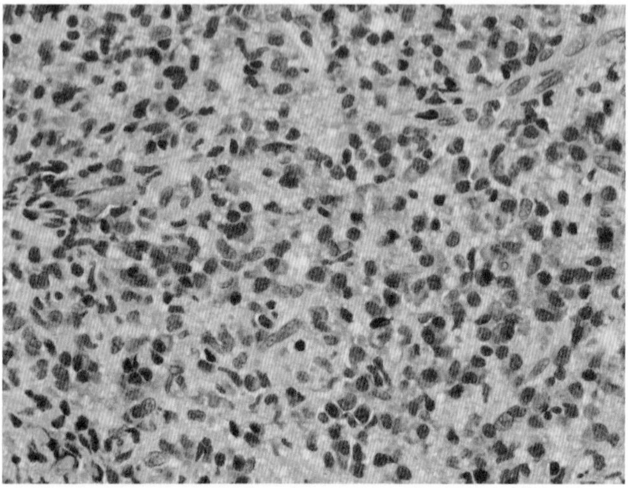

Fig. 19.3 Lymphocytic infiltrate with numerous plasma cells (H&E, 200x).

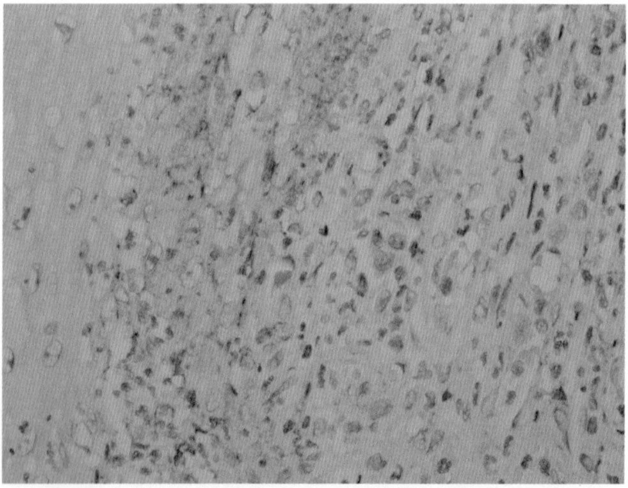

Fig. 19.4 *Treonema pallidum* immunohistochemistry demonstrating numerous spirochetes at the dermal–epidermal junction (*T. pallidum* 400x).

What additional special stain would have highlighted the organisms? Warthin–Starry is another stain that can be used; *T. pallidum* organisms appear as elongated, thin, rod-like structures.

Case Point 19.3

Based on the clinical history, physical examination, and histologic findings, the patient is rendered a diagnosis of primary syphilis infection.

What are the characteristics of the infectious agent of syphilis?

Syphilis is a sexually transmitted disease due to infection with the spirochete *T. pallidum*. Any sexually active individual can contract syphilis after unprotected anal, vaginal, or oral sex. Spirochetes are long, slender, motile, helically coiled gram-negative bacilli. *Leptospira* and *Borrelia* are also spirochetes. *T. pallidum* is extremely fastidious and fragile. It cannot be cultured in cell-free systems and is sensitive to disinfectants, heat, and drying.

What are the clinical stages of syphilis and how do these stages manifest?

Syphilis displays a variety of different clinical manifestations and occurs in stages (primary, secondary, tertiary, and congenital). Any stage can affect any site in the head and neck region.

Primary syphilis occurs upon initial contact with *T. pallidum*. The entrance of the organisms into the body causes the formation of single or multiple painless **primary chancres** 2–6 weeks after initial exposure. *T. pallidum* elicits a robust immune response of TH1 cells, macrophages, and plasma cells. This reduces the burden of disease but it is not completely adequate, as the spirochetes can disseminate and persist. The primary chancre heals with a stellate or nondescript scar. Without treatment, patients will progress to the secondary stage of the disease.

Secondary syphilis is caused by hematogenous and lymphatic dissemination of *T. pallidum* and strikes clinically as a "great imitator." It can affect virtually any part of the body. Often secondary syphilis manifests as widespread mucocutaneous maculopapular, scaly patches, or plaques that involve the oral cavity, palms of the hand, soles of the feet, extremities, and trunk. Further it can show a lichenoid rash, condyloma lata, "moth-eaten" alopecia, and hypomelanosis. It occurs usually 4–8 weeks after the primary chancre, but may present up to 6 months after the chancre heals.

Tertiary syphilis develops in 15%–30% of untreated patients and presents many years after the initial infection. It can involve aorta (cardiovascular syphilis), central nervous system (CNS; neurosyphilis), liver, bones, and testes. So-called "gummas" are present in 50% of cases. Other cutaneous presentations of tertiary syphilis are red-brown scaly nodules.

Latent syphilis is a term used for the symptom-free period between secondary and tertiary syphilis during which the patient has serologic proof of infection.

Congenital syphilis is caused by transplacental transmission of *T. pallidum* and may cause miscarriage, stillbirth, prematurity, low birth weight, or death shortly after birth. In the newborn it can cause various clinical manifestations (deformed bones, severe anemia, enlarged liver and spleen, jaundice, neurologic symptoms such as blindness or deafness, meningitis, and skin rashes.

CLINICAL PEARLS

Chancre: The word *chancre* is derived from French and means "little ulcer." It primarily refers to the primary manifestation of syphilis. The chancre most commonly occurs in the scrotum or penis of men (70%) and in approximately half of the cases on the vulva or cervix of women, but it can virtually affect any area of the head and neck. It can be up to several centimeters in diameter and presents as slightly elevated, firm, red, and ultimately erodes into a shallow-based ulcer.

CLINICAL PEARL

TORCH infections (Toxoplasmosis; Other—syphilis, varicella-zoster, parvovirus B19; Rubella; Cytomegalovirus; and Herpes) are the most common infections associated with congenital abnormalities. Generally, they cause mild maternal symptoms.

CLINICAL PEARL

Syphilis Epidemiology: The syphilis rate in the United States has been increasing since 2001. Its incidence was 9.5 cases per 100,000 population in 2017, which represents an increase of 10.5% compared with 2016 (8.6 cases per 100,000 population), and a 72.7% increase compared with 2013 (5.5 cases per 100,000 population).

Syphilis reporting started in 1941, and the lowest reported rate was in 2001. Syphilis incidence rates vary in different regions of the US, with the highest rates reported in the West and the lowest rates reported in the Northeast. Syphilis rates and increase in rates are substantially higher among men who have sex with men. However, rates among men who have sex with women and among women are steadily increasing as well, leading to a substantial increase in congenital syphilis. The Centers for Disease Control and Prevention reports that in 2017, there were a total of 918 reported cases of congenital syphilis, including 64 syphilitic stillbirths and 13 infant deaths, and the national rate was 23.3 cases per 100,000 live births.

What are the classic histologic findings of the different syphilis stages?

Histologically, the **primary chancre** shows ulceration in the center of the lesion. Acantholysis of the epidermis is often present at the periphery of the lesion. Neutrophils are often present within the epithelium. There are usually abundant lymphocytes and plasma cells at the base of the ulcer. Blood vessels show marked endothelial swelling (Fig. 19.5). Numerous spirochetes are usually present, especially near vessels and at the ulcer base.

Secondary syphilis shows several different histologic patterns (lichenoid, psoriasiform, and granulomatous). There are superficial and deep lymphohistiocytic infiltrates present. Neutrophils (especially in early lesions) and eosinophils may be present. Plasma cells and endothelial swelling may be absent.

Tertiary syphilis shows tuberculoid granuloma with or without caseation. Plasma cells and fibrosis are present, but spirochetes are usually not seen.

Congenital syphilis shows placental findings including the triad of enlarged hypercellular villi, proliferative fetal vascular changes, and acute or chronic villitis.

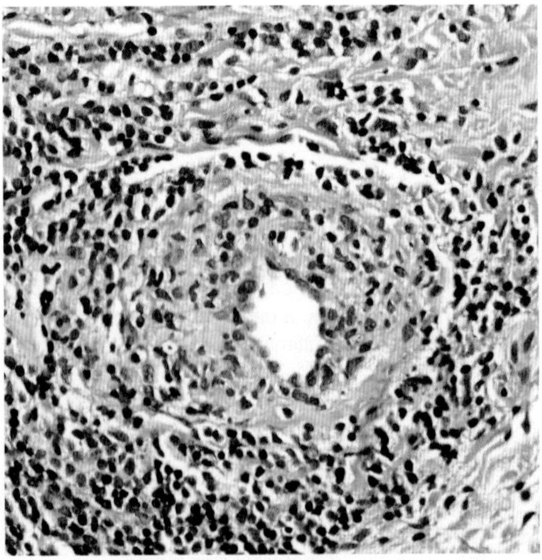

Fig. 19.5 Luetic vasculitis. (From *ExpertPath*. Copyright Elsevier).

CLINICAL PEARL

Luetic vasculitis: The term refers to endothelial swelling and proliferation with lymphocytes infiltrating vessels and associated fibrosis. This can occur at any syphilis stage.

Following the biopsy result, what should the patient be tested for?

Syphilis serology should be performed, including screening serology [venereal disease research laboratory (VDRL) and rapid plasma reagin (RPR)] and confirmatory testing fluorescent treponemal absorption, *T. pallidum* particle agglutination assay, or microhemagglutination assay. The patient should also be tested for other sexual transmitted diseases such as HIV, trichomonas, gonorrhea, and chlamydia.

CLINICAL PEARL

Syphilis Testing: *T. pallidum* can be highlighted with dark-field microscopy in scrapings from the base of a primary chancre. Serology is the mainstay of diagnosis, which includes non-treponemal and treponemal antibody tests. The VDRL and RPR tests measure antibody to cardiolipin, which is a phospholipid that is present in host tissue and *T. pallidum*. These non-treponemal tests become positive 4–6 weeks after infection, are nearly always positive in secondary syphilis, and become usually negative in tertiary syphilis. Treponemal antibody tests also become positive 4–6 weeks after infection but remain positive indefinitely even after successful treatment. The serologic response may be delayed, absent, or exaggerated in people that are coinfected with HIV.

Case Point 19.4

The patient's HIV test comes back nonreactive. The syphilis screen and confirmation are positive. The RPR screen is positive, and the RPR titer is 128.

What are your treatment recommendations?

The treatment of choice for all stages of syphilis is intramuscular benzathine penicillin. Doxycycline or tetracycline are alternative agents in patients allergic to penicillin.

Intravenous penicillin is recommended for patients with neurosyphilis due to poor penetration of benzathine penicillin into CNS.

CLINICAL PEARL

Jarisch–Herxheimer reaction: Antibiotic treatment in patients with high bacterial loads can cause a so-called cytokine storm, which is a massive release of endotoxins and manifests as high fevers, rigors, hypotension, and leukopenia. This can also be seen in other spirochetal disease such as Lyme disease. It can be easily mistaken for a drug reaction.

In addition to treating the patient, what else needs to be done?

The health department needs to be notified about this case. The health department will contact the patient and navigate the notification of sexual partners at risk and their medical assessment.

Case Point 19.5

Following treatment, the patient's symptoms resolve. Within 3 months, the RPR titer decreases to 16.

BEYOND THE PEARLS

- *T. pallidum* cannot be cultured.
- Polymerase chain reaction (PCR) can amplify bacterial DNA from infected tissue.
- IHC has a higher sensitivity in late stages than does PCR.
- The differential diagnosis for secondary syphilis is psoriasis, drug reaction, and lichenoid hypersensitivity reaction.
- The differential diagnoses for tertiary syphilis are neurodegenerative disorders.

References

CDC- Sexually Transmitted Disease Surveillance 2017. https://www.cdc.gov/std/stats17/2017-STD-Surveillance-Report_CDC-clearance-9.10.18.pdf.

Cornelissen CN, Fisher BD, Harvey RA. *Lippincott's Illustrated Reviews,ÄØ: Microbiology*. 3rd ed. Philadelphia, PA: Wolters Kluwer/Lippincott Williams & Wilkins Health; 2013.

Patterson JW, Hosler GA. *Weedon's Skin Pathology*. 4th ed. Edinburgh: Churchill Livingstone/Elsevier; 2016.

Rekhtman N, Baine MK, Bishop JA. *Quick Reference Handbook for Surgical Pathologists*. Cham, Switzerland: Springer; 2019.

Wenig BM. *Atlas of Head and Neck Pathology*. 3rd ed. Philadelphia, PA: Elsevier; 2016.

Breast

CASE 20

A 51-Year-Old Woman with a Breast Lump

Bradley M. Turner

A 51-year-old G0P0 woman presents to her primary care physician after noticing a "lump" in her right breast about 2 weeks ago. She thought it would go away, but it has not. Although she does not think that it is increasing in size, the lump is painful. She recently started an intensive exercise program and wonders if she might have injured herself. She has no significant past medical history; however, her maternal aunt has stage 3 breast cancer. The patient had not experienced menopause yet. The patient's temperature is 36.5°C (97.7°F), pulse rate is 90 beats per minute, respiration rate is 18 breaths per minute, and blood pressure is 104/69 mm Hg. The patient has a body mass index of 17.4 kg/m^2. Physical examination reveals a thin woman in no acute distress. Examination of the breasts reveals diffuse symmetrical "lumpiness" with a slightly more prominent "lumpy" area in the upper outer quadrant of the right breast. The slightly more prominent area is mildly tender, soft, movable, and regular. The remainder of the exam is unremarkable.

What are the causes of a palpable breast lump?

A palpable breast lump (a mass that can be felt) can be caused by both benign and malignant processes (Box 20.1). Most palpable breast masses are benign. On palpation, benign breast lumps are typically soft or cystic, mobile, and regular. Malignant breast lumps are typically characterized as hard, fixed, and irregular.

CLINICAL PEARL

Most palpable breast masses are benign.

What are the most common causes of breast masses or lumps?

The most common cause of a breast mass is normal tissue. The next most common cause is "fibrocystic change," including benign cysts (Fig. 20.1) and the benign neoplasm fibroadenoma (Fig. 20.2). Breast cysts are the most common cause of breast lumps in women aged between 35 and 50 years.

BOX 20.1 ■ Differential Diagnosis of a Palpable Breast Lump

Fibrocystic change	Scar
Abscess	Lactation adenoma
Fat necrosis	Pseudoangiomatous stromal hyperplasia
Infection	Benign tumor (lipoma, fibroadenoma)
Hematoma (trauma)	Malignant tumor

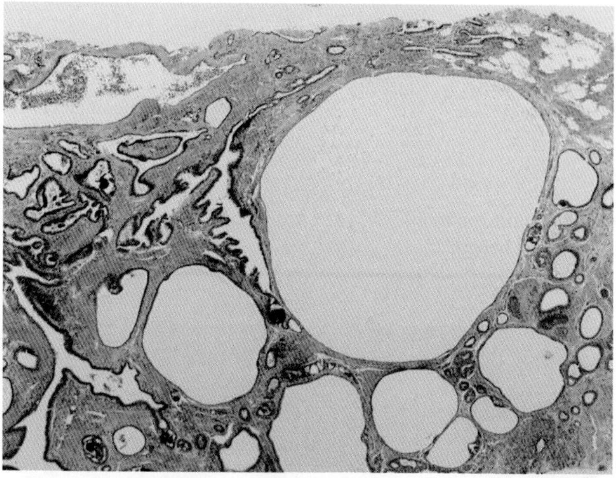

Fig. 20.1 Simple benign cysts of fibrocystic changes (H&E, 40x). Benign cysts lined by flattened epithelial cells. Multiple benign cysts can form a mass. Courtesy Dr. David Hicks, University of Rochester, Rochester, NY. Hicks DG, Lester SC. *Diagnostic Pathology: Breast*. 2nd ed. Philadelphia, PA. Elsevier; 2016. Section 5. Benign Epithelial lesions: Non-proliferative changes; pp. 96–99.

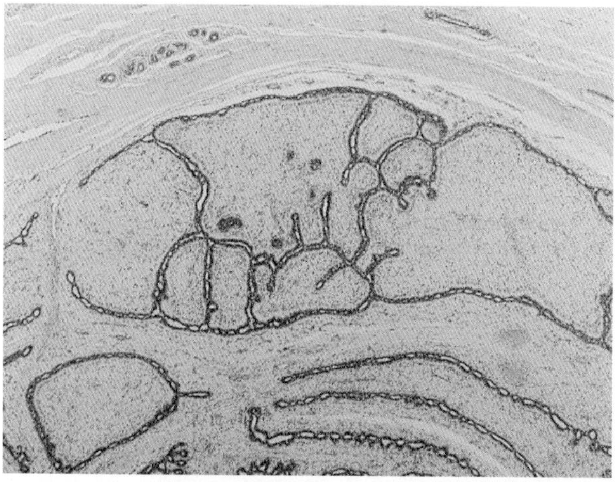

Fig. 20.2 Fibroadenoma (simple), intracanalicular pattern (H&E, 40x). Benign glandular epithelium in glands compressed and distorted by a benign stromal component. Notice the well-circumscribed borders. Courtesy Dr. David Hicks, University of Rochester, Rochester, NY (private collection).

CLINICAL PEARL

The most common cause of a breast mass is normal tissue.

What does the term "fibrocystic changes of the breast" mean?

The term "fibrocystic changes of the breast" encompasses a heterogeneous group of processes, and the description of the particular fibrocystic change or changes is more clinically useful. Fibrocystic changes can be further subclassified as non-proliferative and proliferative (Box 20.2; Figs. 20.3–20.7). While the risk of developing breast cancer associated with non-proliferative changes

BOX 20.2 ■ Classification of Fibrocystic Changes

Non-proliferative	Proliferative
Apocrine metaplasia	Fibroadenoma (complex)
Calcifications	Intraductal papilloma
Duct ectasia	Radial scar
Fibroadenoma (simple)	Sclerosing adenosis
Simple breast cysts (most common)	Florid usual ductal hyperplasia
Non-florid usual ductal hyperplasia	

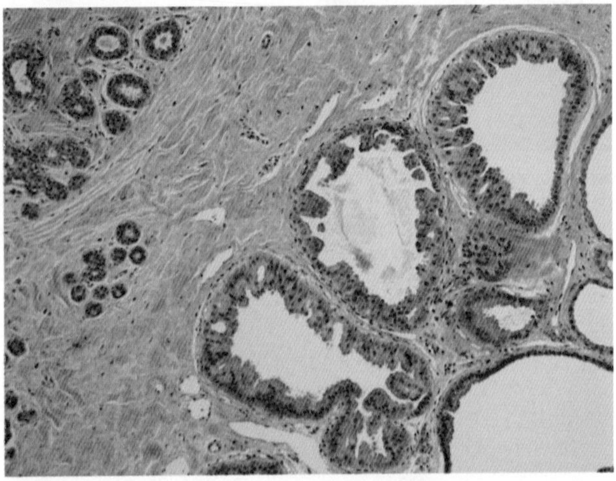

Fig. 20.3 Non-proliferative fibrocystic change: apocrine metaplasia (H&E, 40x). The epithelial cells show abundant eosinophilic cytoplasm and nuclei with prominent nucleoli. Courtesy Dr. David Hicks, University of Rochester, Rochester, NY (private collection).

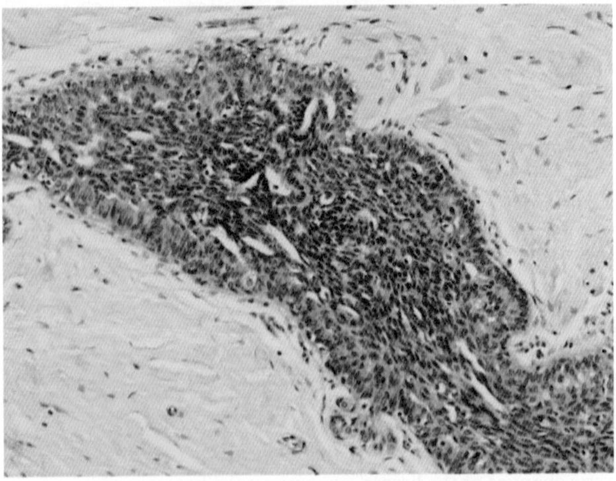

Fig. 20.4 Proliferative fibrocystic change: florid usual ductal hyperplasia (H&E, 200x). When florid, usual ductal hyperplasia is considered a proliferative fibrocystic change, with the associated risks. Note the varying sizes of the fenestrations and the compressed nuclei within cellular bridges, oriented in the same direction as the cellular bridges. Courtesy Dr. David Hicks, University of Rochester, Rochester, NY (private collection).

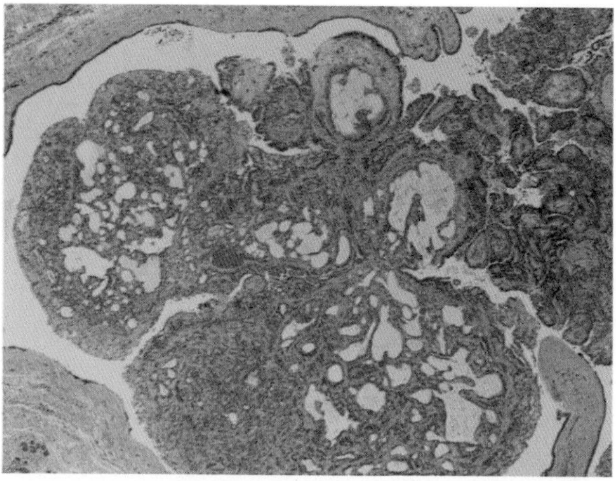

Fig. 20.5 Proliferative fibrocystic change: intraductal papilloma with florid usual ductal hyperplasia (H&E, 40x). Note the papillary fronds with fibrovascular cores and the florid usual ductal hyperplasia that fills the spaces between the papillae. Courtesy Dr. David Hicks, University of Rochester, Rochester, NY (private collection).

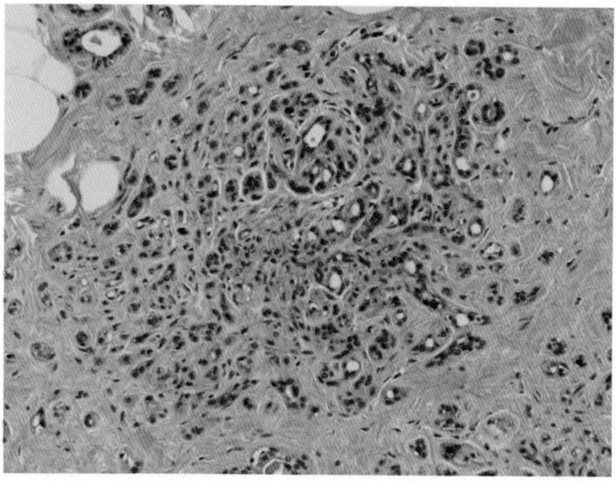

Fig. 20.6 Proliferative fibrocystic change: sclerosing adenosis (H&E, 200x). Sclerosing adenosis will often cause collapse of the duct lumen within fibrotic stroma, making it difficult to appreciate the myoepithelial cell layer. Immunohistochemistry for p63 will demonstrate retention of the myoepithelial cell layer in sclerosis adenosis. The myoepithelial cell will be absent in invasive carcinoma. Courtesy Dr. David Hicks, University of Rochester, Rochester, NY (private collection).

is comparable to the base line general population risk, there is a small increased risk of developing breast cancer in patients with proliferative fibrocystic change compared with the general population (relative risk: 1.5–2, lifetime 4%–6% increased risk).

CLINICAL PEARL

"Fibrocystic changes of the breast" may not be a clinically meaningful term to the treating physician, as this term encompasses a heterogeneous group of processes with different risks for the development of breast cancer.

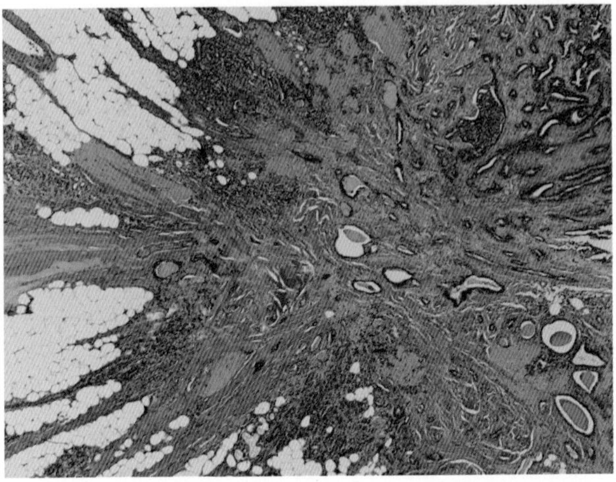

Fig. 20.7 Proliferative fibrocystic change: radial scar (H&E, 40x). The central area of stromal sclerosis with entrapped and distorted ducts is classic for this lesion, often described as an "architectural distortion" on mammographic imaging. A mass may be seen as well on imaging. The diagnosis of a radial scar on biopsy will likely result in surgical excision. Courtesy Dr. David Hicks, University of Rochester, Rochester, NY (private collection).

CLINICAL PEARL

There is a small increased risk of developing breast cancer in patients with proliferative fibrocystic changes compared with patients with non-proliferative fibrocystic changes.

CLINICAL PEARL

It may be more meaningful for the pathologist to list the specific fibrocystic change in descending order of importance with regard to their level of breast cancer risk.

What risk factors does this patient have for non-proliferative breast lesions?

Clinical factors associated with an increased risk of non-proliferative changes in this patient include late age at menopause, nulliparity, low body mass index, and a family history of breast cancer. Estrogen replacement therapy (not reported by this patient) is also associated with an increased risk of non-proliferative breast changes. Clinical factors associated with a decreased risk of non-proliferative breast changes include high parity, oral contraceptive use, physical activity, and tamoxifen (when used for breast cancer prevention).

CLINICAL PEARL

While estrogen replacement therapy is associated with an increased risk of non-proliferative breast changes, oral contraceptive use is associated with a decreased risk of non-proliferative breast changes.

Case Point 20.1

The patient is scheduled for an ultrasound, which shows a well-defined, oval, anechoic structure with a thin wall and internal echoes.

What findings on ultrasound are more consistent with benign breast changes?

Findings on ultrasound that are associated with benign breast changes include smooth and well-circumscribed lesions that are ellipsoid in shape with a thin echogenic capsule. The lesion should have three or fewer gentle lobulations and be hyperechoic, isoechoic, or mildly hypoechoic. The maximum diameter will typically be in the transverse plane.

Case Point 20.2

The radiologist reports the ultrasound findings as a complex cyst, and the patient is sent for a biopsy. On pathology review, the biopsy shows fibrous connective tissue lined by apocrine epithelium. Fluid and scattered secretory debris are present within the lumen of the cyst with associated microcalcifications. The patient is scheduled for a follow-up visit with surgery to discuss treatment options. The surgeon prescribes a trial of ibuprofen and acetaminophen; however, after several months, the patient returns with continued complaints.

What are the treatment options for "fibrocystic changes of the breast"?

Treatment options for "fibrocystic changes of the breast" are typically considered based on the type of fibrocystic change and on the presence and degree of symptoms. If symptoms are mild, no treatment may be needed. Medical treatment may include over-the-counter pain relievers, such as acetaminophen or nonsteroidal antiinflammatory drugs. Oral contraceptives may be considered based on data that suggest that oral contraceptives lower the levels of cycle-related hormones linked to fibrocystic breast changes. Patients with severe pain, particularly if associated with large cysts, may warrant surgical treatment. In patients who have symptomatic fluid-filled cysts, such as this patient, fine-needle aspiration may be used to drain the fluid from the cyst in an effort to relieve discomfort. Rarely, surgery may be needed to remove a persistent cyst that does not resolve after aspiration or to remove fibrocystic breast tissue that is persistently painful even after medical treatment.

CLINICAL PEARL

Treatment options for "fibrocystic changes of the breast" are typically considered based on the type of fibrocystic change, as well as the presence and degree of symptoms.

CLINICAL PEARL

Most patients with a diagnosis of "fibrocystic changes of the breast" will not require surgery; however, surgery may be required to remove fibrocystic breast tissue that is persistently painful after medical treatment.

Case Point 20.3

The patient is scheduled for surgery. The patient undergoes a needle-localized lumpectomy. The final pathology shows cystic apocrine metaplasia, florid usual ductal hyperplasia, duct ectasia, and microcalcifications.

BEYOND THE PEARLS

- The most common benign breast neoplasm is a fibroadenoma, a type of fibrocystic change in the breast.
- The etiology of fibrocystic changes in the breast may be related to excess hormonal stimulation and/or hypersensitivity of breast tissue.
- Fibrocystic change is a frequent finding and may be found in up to 60% of women of reproductive age.
- When used for breast cancer prevention, tamoxifen has been associated with a reduction in fibrocystic changes of the breast.

References

Abdull Gaffar B. Pseudoangiomatous stromal hyperplasia of the breast. *Arch Pathol Lab Med.* 2009;133(8): 1335-1338.

Bhanote M. Case 3. A 37-year-old female with a palpable breast mass. In: Dasgupta R, Kolaee RM, eds. *Medicine Morning Report: Beyond the Pearls.* Philadelphia, PA: Elsevier; 2017.

Calhoun BC. Core needle biopsy of the breast: an evaluation of contemporary data. *Surg Pathol Clin.* 2018;11(1):1-16.

Dabbs D. *Breast Pathology.* Philadelphia, PA: Elsevier Saunders; 2012.

Ellis IO. Intraductal proliferative lesions of the breast: morphology, associated risk and molecular biology. *Mod Pathol.* 2010;23(suppl 2):S1-S7. doi:10.1038/modpathol.2010.56.

Ferreira M, Albarracin CT, Resetkova E. Pseudoangiomatous stromal hyperplasia tumor: a clinical, radiologic and pathologic study of 26 cases. *Mod Pathol.* 2008;21(2):201-207.

Gokhale S. Ultrasound characterization of breast masses. *Indian J Radiol Imaging.* 2009;19(3):242-247.

Ha SM, Cha JH, Shin HJ, et al. Radial scars/complex sclerosing lesions of the breast: radiologic and clinicopathologic correlation. *BMC Med Imaging.* 2018;18(1):39.

Hicks DG, Lester SC. *Diagnostic Pathology: Breast.* 2nd ed. Philadelphia, PA. Elsevier; 2016.

Krings G, Bean GR, Chen YY. Fibroepithelial lesions; the WHO spectrum. *Semin Diagn Pathol.* 2017;34(5):438-452.

Ni YB, Tse GM. Pathological criteria and practical issues in papillary lesions of the breast—a review. *Histopathology.* 2016;68(1):22-32.

Schnitt SJ, Collins LC. *Biopsy Interpretation of the Breast.* Philadelphia, PA: Lippincott Williams & Wilkins; 2009.

Stone K, Wheeler A. A review of anatomy, physiology, and benign pathology of the nipple. *Ann Surg Oncol.* 2015;22(10):3236-3240.

Tan BY, Tan PH. A diagnostic approach to fibroepithelial breast lesions. *Surg Pathol Clin.* 2018;11(1):17-42.

Tatarian T, Sokas C, Rufail M, et al. Intraductal papilloma with benign pathology on breast core biopsy: to excise or not? *Ann Surg Oncol.* 2016;23(8):2501-2507.

Virk RK, Khan A. Pseudoangiomatous stromal hyperplasia: an overview. *Arch Pathol Lab Med.* 2010;134(7):1070-1074.

Vorherr H. Fibrocystic breast disease: pathophysiology, pathomorphology, clinical picture, and management. *Am J Obstet Gynecol.* 1986;154(1):161-179.

Vorherr H. Fibrocystic breast nondisease. *N Engl J Med.* 1985;312(19):1258-1259.

Wei S. Papillary lesions of the breast: an update. *Arch Pathol Lab Med.* 2016;140(7):628-643.

Wells CA, El-Ayat GA. Non-operative breast pathology: apocrine lesions. *J Clin Pathol.* 2007;60(12): 1313-1320.

CASE 21

A 46-Year-Old Woman with a Right Breast Mass and No Other Symptoms

Hasan Khatib

A 46-year-old woman presented to her primary physician at Comprehensive Breast Care Cancer with a main complaint of feeling a mass in her right breast. Past medical and surgical history is unremarkable, except cholecystectomy at age 35. Patient works as a manager in a local bank; she quit smoking 5 years ago and she drinks socially. Medications include only multivitamins. Upon physical examination, the patient's general appearance is within normal limits; she is alert and cooperative with no obvious stress. The patient's vital signs include a blood pressure of 121/82 mm Hg, pulse rate of 83 beats per minute, temperature of 36.3°C (97.3°F), and respiratory rate of 18 breaths per minute. Her height is 157.5 cm (5'2.01") and weight is 84.5 kg (186 lb 4.6 oz), with a body mass index (BMI) of 34.06 kg/m≤. The patient denies chest pain, headache, and vision changes.

A breast physical examination revealed an approximately 2.5-cm mobile, mildly tender mass above her nipple. She has never had any breast problems or breast surgery. She had her first mammogram at the age of 41 years, which was negative, and does regular breast self-examinations. There is no family history of breast cancer among her first-degree relatives; however, her paternal aunt was diagnosed with breast cancer at the age of 63. Patient's gynecologic history includes her first menstrual period at approximately 10 years of age, and her last period was a year ago. She is not currently taking any hormonal preparations and has never done so. She has never been pregnant.

What are the risk factors for breast cancers?

Breast cancer is the most common malignancy in women. According to World Health Organization (WHO), breast cancer accounts for 23% of all malignancy in women worldwide.

Breast cancer is a multifactorial disease, and the major risk factors are as follows:

- Age (most significant risk factor)
- Family history (BRCA1 and BRCA2 gene mutation)
- Early menarche, nulliparous, late age at first delivery
- Obesity (BMI) and menopausal status
- Physical activity (active lifestyle reduces breast cancer risk)
- Alcohol (moderate risk factor)

What are the most common signs and symptoms of breast cancer?

The most common signs and symptoms of breast cancer include a palpable mass (most common clinical sign), skin retraction or color changes, nipple inversion or discharge, and axillary lymphadenopathy (less common).

At what age does breast cancer screening start, and what imaging study is the method of choice?

Detection of breast cancer at an early stage plays an important role in determining patient prognosis and survival rate; therefore, all women at the age of 40 should start annual breast cancer screening tests that include physical examination and imaging study. If there is a family history of breast cancer (especially in first-degree relatives like mother or sister), breast annual screening should start 10 years younger than the age at which the relative was diagnosed with breast cancer.

Mammography is the baseline imaging method for the detection of breast cancer in women aged >40 years, and ultrasound is the method of choice for screening women aged <40 years.

Mammography and ultrasound are complementary imaging studies; they have an important role in determining the lesion size, shape, borders, extent, and presence of multifocal lesions.

Magnetic resonance imaging (MRI) is the most sensitive method for detecting breast cancer, but its use is confined to screening women at very high risk (e.g., carriers of mutations in the BRCA1 or BRCA2 genes) and also for local staging of certain breast cancers.

CLINICAL PEARLS

- Imaging studies define breast lesions shape, orientation, margin, lesion boundary, and echogenicity.
- Speculated, ill-defined mass without calcification is the classic appearance of breast cancer.
- Calcifications harbor only 19% risk of malignancy (according to WHO classification of breast tumors).

Case Point 21.1

Patient undergoes mammography that reveals a 3.5-cm well-defined lobulated mass surrounded by a lucent halo and with no microcalcifications (Fig. 21.1).

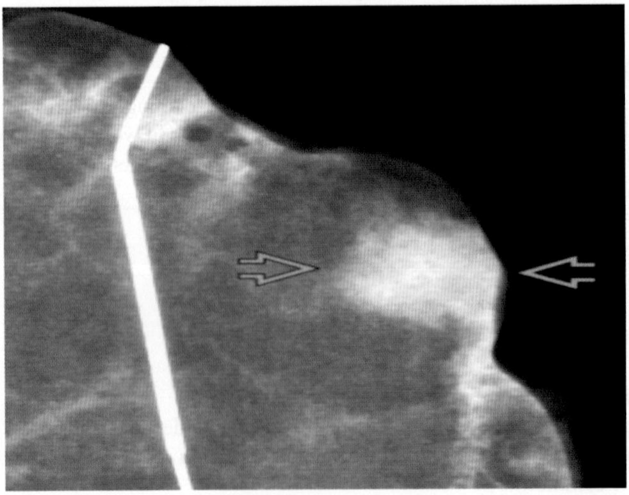

Fig. 21.1 Breast mammography with a 3.5-cm well-defined lobulated mass with no microcalcifications (arrows).

TABLE 21.1 ■ **Breast Imaging Reporting and Data System Categories**

Category	Definition	Result Interpretation
0	Additional imaging evaluation is needed	Not clear, possible abnormality
1	Negative	There is no significant abnormality to report
2	Benign	The most benign (noncancerous) breast findings visible on mammograms are as follows: • Simple cysts • Fibroadenomas • Fibrotic tissue • Calcifications: Small white dots on a mammogram, larger macrocalcifications are usually benign; on the other hand, tiny microcalcifications may be a sign of cancer.
3	Probably benign finding	Short-term interval follow-up suggested*
4	Suspicious abnormality**	Biopsy should be considered
5	Highly suggestive of malignancy	Appropriate action should be taken

*98% of this category lesions are benign, follow-up with repeat imaging in 6 months and regularly after that until the finding is known to be stable (usually at least 2 years). **This category is classified into **4A:** low suspicion of malignancy, **4B:** intermediate suspicion of malignancy, and **4C:** moderate concern of malignancy.

What are worrisome findings on imaging studies?

Breast mass, architectural distortion, and calcifications are the main suspicious findings on breast imaging studies. A standard system to describe mammogram findings and results, called the Breast Imaging Reporting and Data System (BI-RADS), is used, which consists of six categories (Table 21.1).

What is the reliable technique to sample radiological-proven worrisome breast lesion?

Percutaneous imaging-guided by ultrasound, stereotactic, or MRI-guided core needle biopsy is the standard procedure to sample suspicious breast lesions. Core needle biopsy is less invasive procedure than open surgery biopsy, with minimal scarring and complications (bleeding, bruising, and infection). Ultrasound-guided core needle biopsy is preferred due to following reasons: cost-effective technique, nonionizing radiation, and accessibility of difficult places, such as the axilla or the nipple.

Case Point 21.2

The necessity of breast lesion biopsy was discussed with the patient. The procedure was explained to the patient along with the possible procedure-related side effects and complications. Other alternative procedures were also mentioned in the discussion. The patient was sent for breast core needle biopsy. Patient underwent ultrasound-guided core needle biopsy. The biopsy reveals a biphasic lesion with arc-like epithelium-lined clefts embedded in cellular stroma (Fig. 21.2). The stroma displays mild atypia along with occasional mitotic figures (Fig. 21.3). The diagnosis of fibroepithelial lesion with cellular stroma is rendered.

Histological examination of breast lesion biopsy is the cornerstone for the definitive diagnosis; therefore, comprehension of normal breast histology is essential for accurate evaluation of breast specimens.

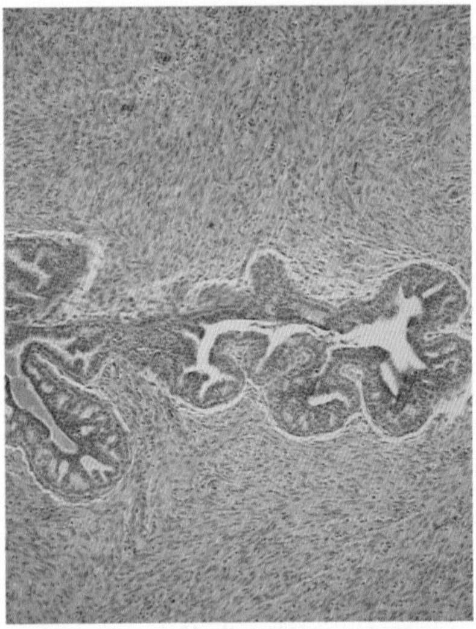

Fig. 21.2 Breast core needle biopsy biphasic lesion with arc-like epithelium-lined clefts embedded in cellular stroma (H&E, 200x).

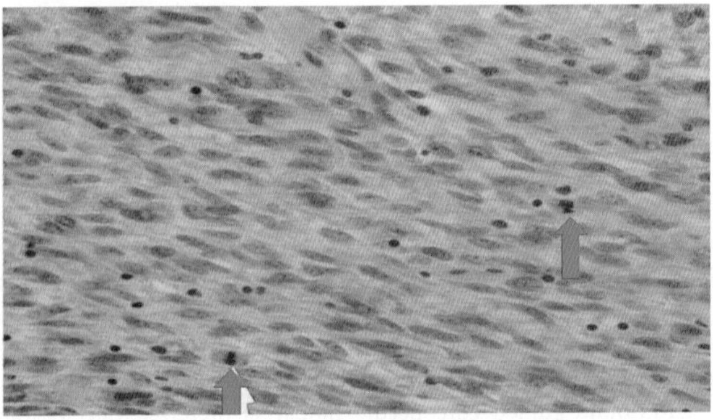

Fig. 21.3 Breast core needle biopsy occasional mitotic figures are also noted (arrows) (H&E, 400x).

The female breast consists of a series of ducts, ductules, and lobular acinar units (epithelial–myoepithelial) embedded within a stroma (mesenchyme) that is composed of varying amount of fibrous and adipose tissue. Mammary epithelial cells may show a wide range of metaplastic changes, including apocrine, clear cell, squamous, secretory, and mucinous metaplasia.

Breast neoplasms may originate from epithelial, myoepithelial, or stromal component. Neoplastic mammary epithelial cells may undergo genetic reprogramming, resulting in a change of morphology to spindle mesenchymal-like, squamous, and small cell in addition to other types of trans-differentiation, such as salivary gland, secretory, and clear cell differentiation.

What is the classification of breast tumors?

WHO classification of breast tumors is as following:

- **Epithelial tumors**
  - Invasive ductal carcinoma
  - Invasive lobular carcinoma

- **Epithelial–myoepithelial tumors**
  - Pleomorphic adenoma
  - Adenomyoepithelioma
  - Adenomyoepithelioma with carcinoma
  - Adenoid cystic carcinoma
- **Mesenchymal tumors**
  - Nodular fasciitis
  - Myofibroblastoma
  - Desmoid-type fibromatosis
  - Inflammatory myofibroblastic tumor
  - Benign vascular lesions: hemangioma, angiomatosis, atypical vascular lesions
  - Pseudoangiomatous stromal hyperplasia
  - Granular cell tumor
  - Benign peripheral nerve sheath tumors: neurofibroma, schwannoma
  - Lipoma, angiolipoma
  - Liposarcoma
  - Angiosarcoma
  - Rhabdomyosarcoma
  - Osteosarcoma
  - Leiomyoma
  - Leiomyosarcoma
- **Fibroepithelial tumors**
  - Fibroadenoma
  - Phyllodes tumor (PT)
    - Benign
    - Borderline
    - Malignant
  - Periductal stromal tumor, low grade
  - Hamartoma
- **Tumors of the nipple**
  - Nipple adenoma
  - Syringomatous tumor
  - Paget disease of the nipple
- **Malignant lymphoma**
- **Metastatic tumors**

What is the origin of breast spindle cell lesions?

Spindle cell tumors of the breast are less common than epithelial ones. The origin of breast spindle cell lesions is generally mesenchymal; some lesions also originate from epithelial and myoepithelial components. Breast spindle cell lesions can be composed purely of a mesenchymal element (monophasic) or of mixed mesenchymal and epithelial components (biphasic). Spindle cell lesions of breast can also arise from non-mammary-specific tissue, such as skin, smooth muscle, deep fascia, blood vessels, nerves, and other soft tissue elements. This in turn makes the spectrum of breast spindle cell lesion differential diagnosis wide ranging, from reactive process to aggressive malignant tumors.

What is the initial microscopic approach of breast spindle cell lesions?

The diagnosis of spindle cell lesions could pose interpretive challenges on core needle biopsy due to limited materials and overlapping histological feature between spindle cell entities. Therefore, it is important to recognize the characteristics and distinguishable histological features of each entity in order to render an accurate diagnosis and ensure appropriate management for the patient.

Evaluation of the following features of any breast spindle cell lesion is essential:

- **Lesion cellularity:** low-, moderate-, or high-cellular lesion
- **Lesion growth pattern:** fascicular, storiform, diffuse, or whirling
- **Lesion cytological and nuclear atypia:** benign, low-, or high-grade nuclear atypia
- **Lesion margins:** well-defined or infiltrative margins
- **Lesion components:** pure spindle cells or mixed with other cells, such as adipose tissue, muscle cells, inflammatory cells, and thick hyalinized collagen bundles.

It was found that initial categorization of breast spindle cell lesions into low-grade versus high-grade lesion (Box 21.1), in addition to classification of these lesions depending on predominant cell component (Box 21.2), is very useful in approaching the accurate diagnosis (Fig. 21.4; Tables 21.2 and 21.3).

CLINICAL PEARLS

- Some reactive spindle cell lesions of breast may display increased frequency of typical mitotic figures, such as nodular fasciitis.
- Necrosis is seen in high-grade lesions.
- Patient age, lesion size, location related to the skin and deep structures, growth rate, and clinical and radiological correlation is essential factors in evaluation of breast spindle cell lesions.

Case Point 21.3

The necessity of lesion resection was discussed with the patient. The patient underwent breast lumpectomy. The gross evaluation revealed a 2.7 × 2.7-cm ovoid fibroadipose mass with smooth surface and lobulated whorled cut surface without necrosis or hemorrhage (Fig. 21.5). The microscopic evaluation showed intracanalicular growth pattern with leaf-like stromal fronds projecting into stretched, arc-like epithelium-lined clefts. The stroma is cellular with mild atypia and high mitotic up to 8 per 10 HPF. Tumor borders are focally infiltrative; however, the margins are negative (Fig. 21.6). The diagnosis of borderline PT is rendered.

BOX 21.1 ■ Breast Spindle Cell Lesions Categorized Into Low- and High-Grade Neoplasms

Low-Grade Breast Spindle Cell Lesions

- Nodular fasciitis
- Pseudoangiomatous stromal hyperplasia
- Myofibroblastoma
- Desmoid fibromatosis
- Dermatofibrosarcoma protuberans
- Benign neural tumors
- Benign and borderline PT

High-Grade Breast Spindle Cell Lesions

- Spindle cell metaplastic carcinoma
- Malignant PT
- Sarcoma
- Metastasis

BOX 21.2 ■ Breast Spindle Cell Lesions Classification Depending on Predominant Cell Component

Lesions of Fibroblast Myofibroblast Origin

- Pseudoangiomatous stromal hyperplasia
- Fibromatosis
- Nodular fasciitis
- Myofibroblastoma
- Solitary fibrous tumor
- Fibrous scar
- Inflammatory myofibroblastic tumor

Lesions of Nerve Sheath Origin

- Neurofibroma
- Schwannoma

Lesions of Smooth Muscles Origin (Subareolar Smooth Muscle)

- Leiomyoma

Lesions of Epithelial/Myoepithelial Origin

- Adenomyoepithelioma
- Low-grade fibromatosis-like spindle cell metaplastic breast carcinoma

Breast Stromal Component

- Benign and borderline PT

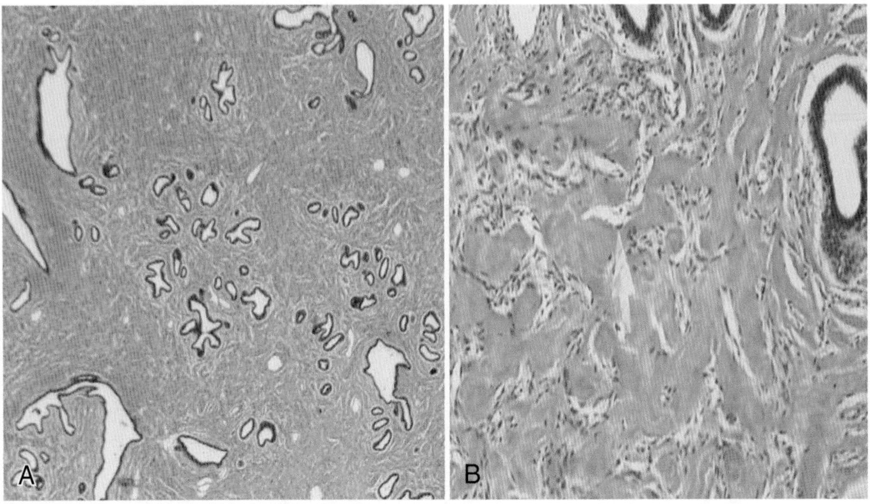

Fig. 21.4 (A) Pseudoangiomatous stromal hyperplasia (H&E, 200x). (B) Slit-like empty space lined by myofibroblasts with attenuated nuclei (arrow) (H&E, 400x).

PTs are classified into benign, borderline, and malignant. Table 21.4 illustrates the WHO classification criteria for PTs.

What is the prognosis and predictive factors for the patient?

Most PTs are benign. Local recurrence occurs in 10%–17% with benign PT, 14%–25% with borderline PT, and 23%–30% with malignant PT. Surgical margins, stromal overgrowth, atypia,

TABLE 21.2 ■ **Clinical, Radiological, and Pathological Features of Benign/Borderline Phyllodes Tumor (PTs), Pseudoangiomatous Stromal Hyperplasia (PASH), Myofibroblastoma, and Fibromatosis**

	Benign/Borderline PTs	PASH	Myofibroblastoma	Fibromatosis
Clinical features	Unilateral, firm, painless, lobulated mass not attached to skin in middle-aged women	Painless palpable mass Premenopausal women, incidental finding, localized mass or diffuse enlargement	Painless, well-defined, mobile slow-growing mass	Painless palpable mass and may associate with skin dimpling or retraction. Develops slowly and may exhibit local invasion in close proximity to the pectoralis.
Radiological features	Mammography: oval lobulated mass and may be surrounded by a lucent halo. Calcifications are rare Ultrasound: solid hypoechoic with moderate heterogeneity, and occasional internal microcystic areas MRI: oval lobulated mass with internal septations and rapid contrast enhancement	Mammography: partially or well-circumscribed mass without calcifications Sonographically well-circumscribed hypoechoic, avascular solid mass mimicking fibroadenoma. Solitary well-circumscribed mass or localized increase in stroma MRI: non-mass-like contrast enhancement	Mammography: well-circumscribed mass without calcifications or architectural distortion Ultrasound: hypoechoic heterogeneous mass with posterior attenuation MRI: may show isointense mass with homogenous or heterogeneous contrast enhancement may be seen	Mammography: spiculated irregular mass without calcifications mimicking malignant tumors Sonographically hypoechoic irregular mass with no significant vascularity MRI: irregular ill-defined heterogeneous mass with increased signal intensity
Gross and pathological features	Grossly: well-circumscribed, firm, bulging mass with gray whorled cut surface Hemorrhage and necrosis may be identified in large tumors Intracanalicular growth pattern with leaf-like stromal fronds projecting into stretched, arc-like epithelium-lined clefts PTs are classified into benign, borderline, and malignant (Table 21.4)	Well-defined, noncapsulated with firm rubbery homogenous lobulated cut surface Slit-like empty space lined by myofibroblasts, with attenuated nuclei resembling endothelial cells within a sclerotic collagenous hyalinized stroma (Fig. 21.4)	Grossly: well-circumscribed, lobulated tumor with rubbery consistency and yellow soft areas reflecting a fatty component Short fascicles of spindle cells interrupted by thick eosinophilic collagen bundles, can have variant histology	Ill-defined mass with white whorled trabeculated cut surface Long sweeping and intersecting fascicles of bland spindle cells with wavy nuclei within collagenous stroma Infiltrates and entraps adjacent breast lobules and fat Lymphocytes present often at periphery

Etiology	Some researchers hypothesize that they may develop secondary to fibroadenomas, given their genetic similarity	Increased progesterone receptor density and signaling result in proliferation of myofibroblasts which are arranged to form the pseudovascular channels Oral contraceptives in postmenopausal women	Occasional gynecomastia association	Rare disease and more common in women (female:male = 3:1). Unknown etiology Hormonal effect theory due to increased tumor size in pregnant women Sporadic or association with familial adenomatous polyposis, Gardner syndrome, previous trauma, or breast implants (reactive process)
Prognosis and management	PTs >3 cm are more likely to be malignant Wide local excision with negative margins	Recurrence rate is 13%–26% (WHO) Local recurrence may be related to incomplete resection Conservative management, surgical excision is rarely performed	Surgical resection No tendency for local recurrence	Recurrence in 20%–30% cases Complete surgical excision with free margins
Genetics	Wnt signaling pathway, upregulation of transcriptionally active beta-catenin and downstream effectors, such as cyclin D1	No known genetic correlation identified	Deletion of chromosome 13q14 by FISH Partial monosomy 13q in some cases	Beta-catenin gene activating mutations in 45% cases Mutations APC gene or 5q loss in 33% cases

APC, adenomatous polyposis coli; *FISH,* fluorescence in situ hybridization; *MRI,* magnetic resonance imaging; *WHO,* World Health Organization.

TABLE 21.3 ■ **Clinical, Radiological, and Pathological Features of Dermatofibrosarcoma Protuberans (DFSP), Nodular Fasciitis, and Neurofibroma (NF)/Schwannoma (SWN)**

	DFSP	Nodular Fasciitis	NF/SWN
Clinical features	Slow-growing, firm mass attached to skin, with skin tethering	Rapid-growing, painless mass (3–4 months)	Arise in the overlying skin or underlying chest wall
Radiological features	Mammography: dense mass without calcifications Ultrasound: oval mass lies parallel to the skin with heterogeneous echogenicity and posterior acoustic enhancement MRI: well-defined, broad-based mass inseparable from skin	Mammography: dense noncalcified spiculated mass with architectural distortion Sonographically: Poor defined hypoechoic mass with echogenic halo and central cystic changes MRI: avid contrast enhancement	Mammography: well-defined or irregular mass
Gross and pathological features	Firm gray-white cut surface in subcutaneous tissue without necrosis Storiform pattern of spindle cells in dermis invading into subcutis with characteristic honeycomb appearance. Low mitotic counts and without overt polymorphism	Well-defined mass with grey-white cut surface. Occasional central cystic changes Short fascicles of fibroblastic/myofibroblastic cells with vesicular nuclei and eosinophilic cytoplasm in a loose myxoid stroma, tissue culture-like appearance Mitosis figures may be frequent	NF: spindle cells with wavy nuclei, myxoid stroma, and shredded carrot-like collagen bundles and scattered mat cells SWN: alternating hypercellular and hypocellular areas of spindle cells with wavy nuclei, nuclear palisading, and hyalinized blood vessels
Etiology	Unknown etiology, some studies showed DFSP developed in injured skin by surgery or burn	Uncommon breast lesion and more frequent in females	Sporadic or syndromic in association with NF1
Prognosis and management	Wide local or via Moh's micrographic surgery excision with negative 2–4 cm margins Recurrence rate is up to 20%. Distant metastasis is extremely rare	Spontaneous regression with very infrequent recurrence	Benign behavior with rare local recurrence Malignant transformation in a setting of NF1 in 5%–10%
Genetics	Chromosomal translocation t(17;22) (q22;q13) COL1A1–PDGFB gene fusion	MYH9–USP6 gene fusion	Germline mutation in NF1 gene chromosome 17q11.2

NF1, neurofibromatosis.

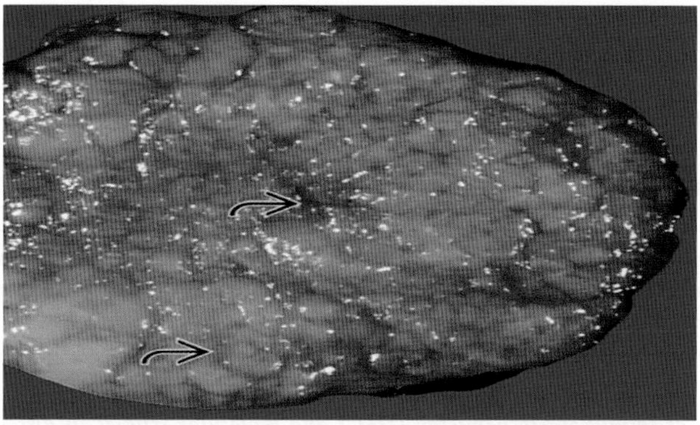

Fig. 21.5 Phyllodes tumor (PT): Gross appearance. PT typically appears circumscribed. The surface is tan and fleshy. The numerous small cleft-like slits correspond to areas of stromal overgrowth lined by epithelium (arrows).

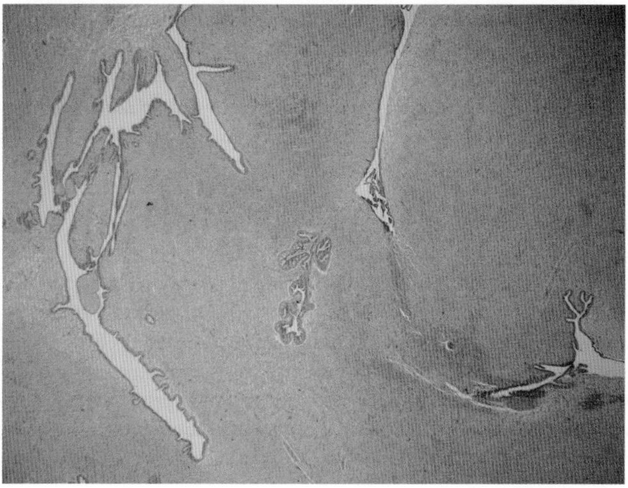

Fig. 21.6 Intracanalicular growth pattern with leaf-like stromal fronds projecting into stretched, arc-like epithelium-lined clefts. The stroma is cellular with mild atypia and high mitotic figures (H&E, 200x).

TABLE 21.4 ■ **World Health Organization Classification Criteria for Phyllodes Tumors (PTs)**

	PT		
Histological Features	**Benign**	**Borderline**	**Malignant**
Tumor border	Well-defined	Well-defined, focally irregular	Irregular
Stromal cellularity	Mild cellularity	Moderate cellularity	Diffuse marked cellularity
Stromal atypia	Mild or none	Mild or moderate	Marked
Mitotic activity	<5 per 10 HPF	5–9 per 10 HPF	≥ 10 per 10 HPF
Stromal overgrowth	Absent	Absent or focal	Frequent
Malignant heterologous elements	Absent	Absent	Occasional
Percentage (%)	60–75	15–20	10–20

necrosis, and mitotic activity are the histological features that possess predictive value for local recurrence. Local recurrence usually occurs within 2–3 years. Distant metastases have been reported in malignant PTs, with lungs and bones being the most common locations. Metastasis to axillary lymph nodes is rare.

Case Point 21.4

The patient is reassured. Despite negative margins, other histological features are worrisome; therefore, close follow-up visits are scheduled every 6 months for the first 2–3 years to ensure that there is no local recurrence.

What is the role of immunohistochemistry (IHC) and molecular studies in differentiating breast spindle cell lesions?

IHC and molecular studies play a very important role in differentiating spindle cell lesions (Table 21.5). Certain immunohistochemical stains can be positive in more than one entity; therefore, immunohistochemical stains should be applied as a panel to approach the correct diagnosis. See Fig. 21.7 for a simplified algorithmic approach to low-grade spindle cell lesions of the breast.

What is the differential diagnosis of high-grade spindle cell lesions of the breast?

The differential diagnosis of high-grade spindle cell lesions of the breast includes:

- Spindle cell metaplastic carcinoma
- Malignant PT
- Primary sarcoma
- Metastasis

Spindle cell metaplastic carcinoma is invasive carcinoma composed predominantly of malignant spindle cells arranged in short or long fascicles in a storiform growth pattern along with foci of epithelioid cells or squamous differentiation. Malignant heterologous elements such as chondroid (Fig. 21.8), osteoid, or rhabdomyoid may be present. Most of spindle cell metaplastic carcinomas are triple-negative breast cancer (negative for estrogen receptor, progesterone receptor, and human epidermal growth factor receptor 2). Spindle cell metaplastic carcinomas express keratin 5/6 and 14, EGFR, p63, and SMA. Lungs and brain metastasis is very common, and lymph node metastasis is less frequent.

Primary sarcomas are very rare. Angiosarcoma is the most common primary sarcoma that usually develops in the skin of women who undergo surgery and radiation therapy for breast cancer.

See Fig. 21.9 for a simplified algorithmic approach to high-grade spindle cell lesions of the breast.

CLINICAL PEARLS

In some cases, it may not be possible to render a definite diagnosis of breast spindle cell lesion due to a limited material on core needle biopsy. A list of differential diagnosis should be provided based on histological morphology and IHC studies. Discussion with clinicians and correlation with radiological findings will be a good aid in appropriate management to the patient.

TABLE 21.5 ■ **Immunohistochemistry and Molecular Profile of Breast Spindle Lesions and Differential Diagnosis**

	Fibrous scar	Nodular fasciitis	PASH	Myofibro-blastoma	Fibromatosis	DFSP	NF/SWN	BPT
CK	–	–	–	–	–	–	–	–/+
P63	–	–	–	–	–	–	–	–/+
	-							
SMA	+	+	+	+/–	+	–/+	+/– NF	–
Desmin	–	–	–/+	+	+/–	–	–	–
CD34	–	–	+	+	–	+/–	+/–NF	+
Nuclear β-catenin	–	–	–	–	+	–	–	+/–
S-100	–	–	–	–	–	–	+	–
Molecular studies		MYH9–USP6 gene fusion	Bcl2+, PR+. ER +/– CD31 – ERG –	Loss of RB expression Variable for Bcl-2, CD99 CD31 EMA ER & PR	CTNNB1 mutation	COL1A1–PDGFB gene fusion		Bcl2 + CD117+

BPT, benign and borderline phyllodes tumors; *DFSP,* dermatofibrosarcoma protuberans; *ER,* estrogen receptor; *NF,* neurofibroma; *PASH,* pseudoangiomatous stromal hyperplasia; *PR,* progesterone receptor; *SWN,* schwannoma.

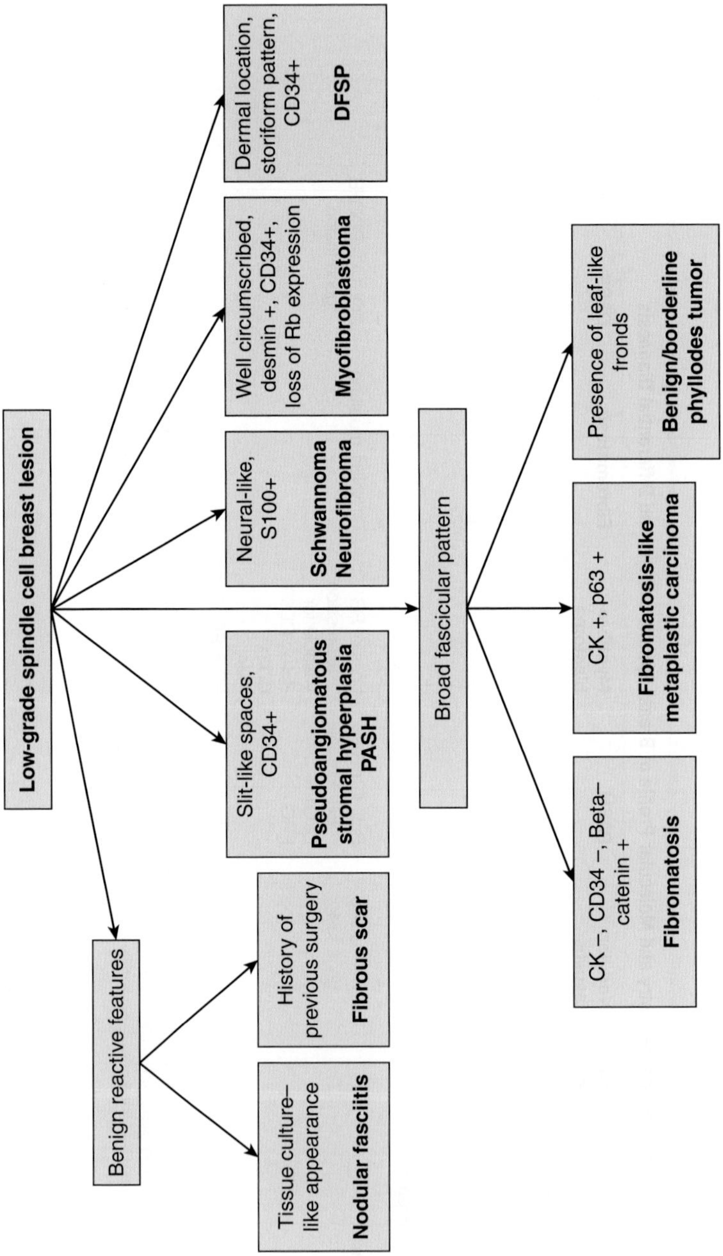

Fig. 21.7 Algorithmic approach to low-grade spindle cell lesions of the breast.

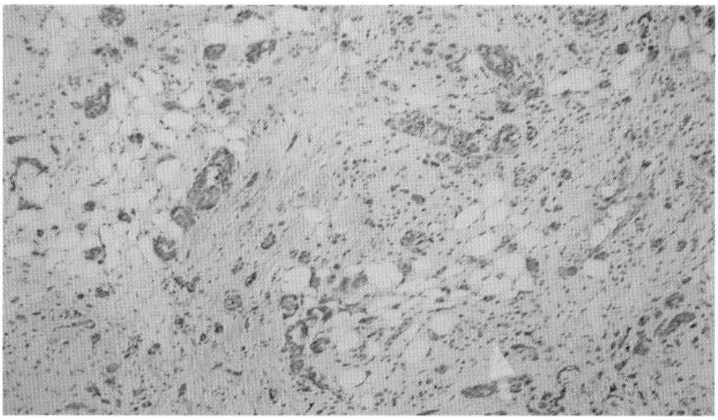

Fig. 21.8 Spindle cell metaplastic carcinoma with malignant heterogeneous chondroid elements (arrow) (H&E, 100x).

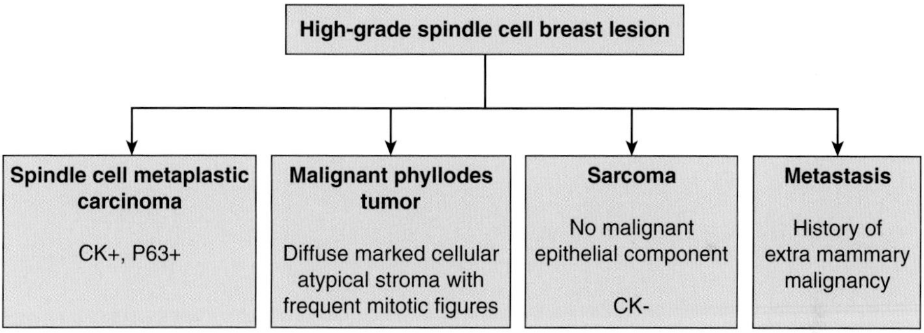

Fig. 21.9 Algorithmic approach to high-grade spindle cell lesions of the breast.

BEYOND THE PEARLS

- The origin of breast spindle cell lesions is generally mesenchymal; some lesions also originate from epithelial and myoepithelial components.
- Breast spindle cell lesions can be composed purely of a mesenchymal element (monophasic) or of mixed mesenchymal and epithelial components (biphasic).
- Initial categorization of breast spindle cell lesions into low-grade versus high-grade lesion is a helpful aid in approaching the accurate diagnosis.
- IHC and molecular studies play a very important role in differentiating spindle cell lesions.
- Immunohistochemical stains should be applied as a panel to approach the correct diagnosis.
- Spindle cell metaplastic carcinoma must be ruled out before rendering pathological diagnosis of breast spindle cell lesion.

References

American College of Radiology. *ACR BI-RADS® Atlas*. 5th ed. 2013.
Collins LC. Breast cancer screening guidelines. In: Mills SE, ed. *Histology for Pathologists*. 4th ed. 2012.
Hicks DG, Lester SC. *Diagnostic Pathology: Breast*. 2nd ed. Elsevier.

Lakhani SR, Ellis IO, Schnitt SJ. *WHO Classification of Tumours of the Breast.*

Orta LY, Beyda JN, Desman GT. Cutaneous/subcutaneous mesenchymal proliferations of the breast. *Semin Diagn Pathol.* 2017;34(5):470-478.

Rakha EA, Aleskandarany MA, Lee AHS, Ellis IO. An approach to the diagnosis of spindle cell lesions of the breast. *Histopathology.* 2016;68:33-44.

Taliaferro AS. Imaging features of spindle cell breast lesions. *AJR Am J Roentgenol.* 2017;209(2):454-464.

Tay TKY, Tan PH. Spindle cell lesions of the breast – An approach to diagnosis. *Semin Diagn Pathol.* 2017;34(5):400-409.

CASE 22

A 63-Year-Old Female Presenting for Annual Screening

Bradley M. Turner

A 63-year-old postmenopausal female presents for her annual screening mammogram. She gets screening mammograms on a yearly basis. She has no current complaints. She exercises daily and reports that she "watches her diet closely." She has a past medical history of atypical ductal hyperplasia (ADH) in the left breast 3 years ago and was treated with partial mastectomy, with no evidence of carcinoma on pathology. Her maternal grandmother died of breast cancer. The patient's temperature is 36.8°C (98.2°F), pulse rate is 75 beats per minute, respiration rate is 16 breaths per minute, and blood pressure is 132/89 mm Hg. Physical examination reveals a well-developed woman in no acute distress. Examination of the breasts reveals symmetrical breast tissue without evidence of any mass. The remainder of the exam is also unremarkable. An annual screening mammogram is performed. A density is noted in the left breast, BI-RADS-0[HD1], with recommendations for diagnostic testing. A diagnostic mammogram and ultrasound showed a suspicious spiculated density mass measuring 0.8 × 0.6 × 0.4 cm.

What is the epidemiology of invasive breast cancer (IBC)? Over 99% of breast cancers occur in women. The lifetime risk (LR) of developing IBC is approximately 3% for women without risk factors, increasing to over 80% depending on a woman's risk factors. The median age for a woman to develop IBC is 61 years. Approximately 43% of women with IBC are diagnosed after 65 years of age. Most breast cancer survivors (approximately 72%) are ≥60 years of age. The incidence of IBC for all women is estimated at 122.2 cases per 100,000 women. The mortality from breast cancer–related causes in the US is estimated at 22.6 deaths per 100,000 women.

CLINICAL PEARL

The LR of developing IBC is approximately 3% for women without risk factors.

CLINICAL PEARL

Approximately 20% of women with IBC are diagnosed prior to 50 years of age, with fewer than 10% of breast cancer survivors being <50 years of age.

What are the clinical risk factors associated with a diagnosis of breast cancer? Nonpathologic, clinical risk factors associated with a diagnosis of breast cancer are listed in Box 22.1. Age is an important risk factor, as >80% of new diagnoses occur after the age of 50. Mammographic density is a strong risk factor for breast cancer, with four to five times greater risk in women with density in >75% of their breast. Density of breast tissue is influenced by the patient's age, parity, body mass index, and menopausal status. Diet and obesity have been associated with a small increase in breast cancer risk, with exercise being associated with a small protective effect against risk. Factors associated with higher levels

BOX 22.1 ■ Nonpathologic Risk Factors Associated with a Diagnosis of Breast Cancer

Age	Family history
Breast density	Gender
Diet	Pregnancy
Estrogen exposure	Radiation exposure
Ethnicity	Screening

of estrogen and prolonged estrogen stimulation of breast epithelium, including early menarche, late menopause, nulliparity, late age at first live birth, and obesity in postmenopausal women, all increase the LR of developing breast cancer. Combination hormone replacement therapy (HRT) may be an acceptable alternative for treatment of moderate-to-severe menopausal symptoms in women up to age 59, or within 10 years of menopause; however, recent data from the Women's Health Initiative suggests that women who use combination HRT after menopause have a small but statistically significant increased risk of breast cancer more than a decade after they stop taking the pills. Data continues to support that estrogen-only HRT may be an option for women across all age groups who have previously had a hysterectomy. In fact, recent data from the Women's Health Initiative suggests that estrogen-only HRT can actually reduce the incidence and mortality of breast cancer. African-American women typically present at an earlier age of onset (median age 54), present at an earlier clinical stage, have more aggressive pathology, and have worse survival outcomes. Approximately 10% to 20% patients with breast cancer have a first-degree relative with breast cancer; women who have a first-degree relative with breast cancer have almost twice the risk of getting breast cancer as women who have no affected relatives. This risk increases as the number of first-degree relatives with breast cancer increases. Biologic gender is important to consider, as over 99% of breast cancers occur in biologic females. Pregnancy increases the risk of breast cancer in women aged over 35 years (a protective effect dominates in younger women), and cancers diagnosed during pregnancy or in the postpartum period are more likely to be of higher stage with a worse prognosis. Radiation exposure, particularly during adolescence, increases the risk of breast cancer inversely proportional to age and directly proportional to radiation dose. Screening mammography will increase the likelihood of being diagnosed with breast cancer while also maximizing the number of breast cancer deaths prevented. Although organizations differ on screening intervals, there is a general agreement that screening mammography should be offered to women aged 50–74 years.

CLINICAL PEARL

Although screening does not cause breast cancer, it increases the risk of being diagnosed with breast cancer.

What are the pathologic risk factors associated with a diagnosis of breast cancer? Pathologic risk factors associated with a diagnosis of breast cancer are listed in Box 22.2. A previous history of breast cancer is a significant risk factor for developing a recurrence or a second breast cancer. Proliferative-type benign breast disease (florid usual ducal hyperplasia intraductal papillomas, sclerosing adenosis, and radial scars) and columnar cell changes including flat epithelial atypia (Figs. 22.1 and 22.2) are associated with a relative risk of 1.5–2x compared with women without risk factors. Atypical lobular hyperplasia (ALH) (Fig. 22.3) and ADH (Fig. 22.4) are both associated with a relative risk of 4.5x compared with women without risk factors. This relative risk increases to 8x in patients with ALH that has pagetoid spread (Fig. 22.5). Lobular carcinoma in situ (LCIS) (Figs. 22.6 and 22.7) and ductal carcinoma in situ (DCIS) (Fig. 22.8) are both associated with a relative risk of 8–10x compared with women without risk factors. Approximately

BOX 22.2 ■ Pathologic Risk Factors Associated with a Diagnosis of Breast Cancer

- Previous history of breast cancer
- Proliferative breast changes
- Columnar cell changes
- Flat epithelial atypia
- ALH
- ADH
- LCIS
- DCIS
- Germline breast cancer susceptibility mutations

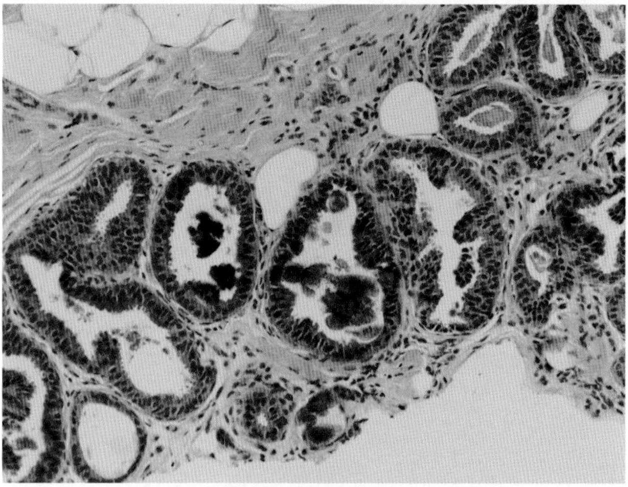

Fig. 22.1 Columnar cell change (H&E, 20x). Note the cystically dilated acini with secretions and calcifications. Calcifications are a frequent finding in columnar cell change. Cellular tufting can be seen. Courtesy Dr. David Hicks, University of Rochester, Rochester, NY (private collection).

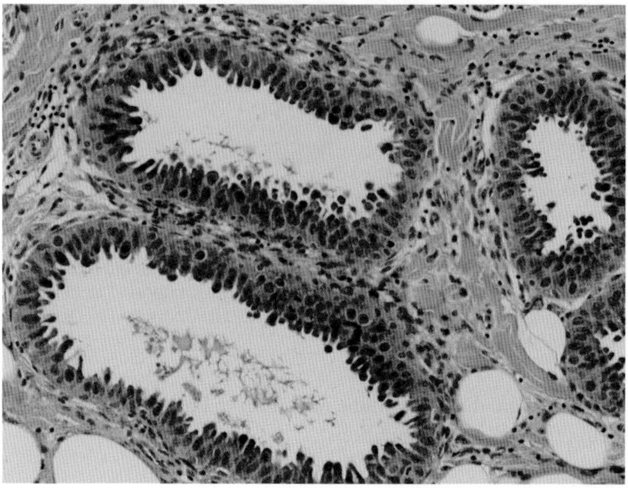

Fig. 22.2 Flat epithelial atypia (H&E, 20x). As with columnar cell change, cystically dilated acini with secretions, calcifications, and cellular tufting can be present in flat epithelia atypia (FEA); however, the acini in FEA have a more rounded configuration, and the nuclei are more monomorphic, appearing consistent with atypia. Courtesy Dr. David Hicks, University of Rochester, Rochester, NY (private collection).

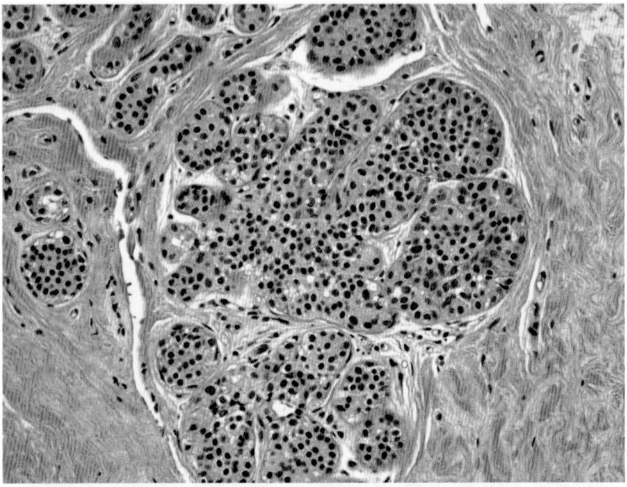

Fig. 22.3 Atypical lobular hyperplasia (H&E, 20x). Note the monomorphic proliferation of dyscohesive cells that only minimally distends the involved acini. Courtesy Dr. David Hicks, University of Rochester, Rochester, NY (private collection).

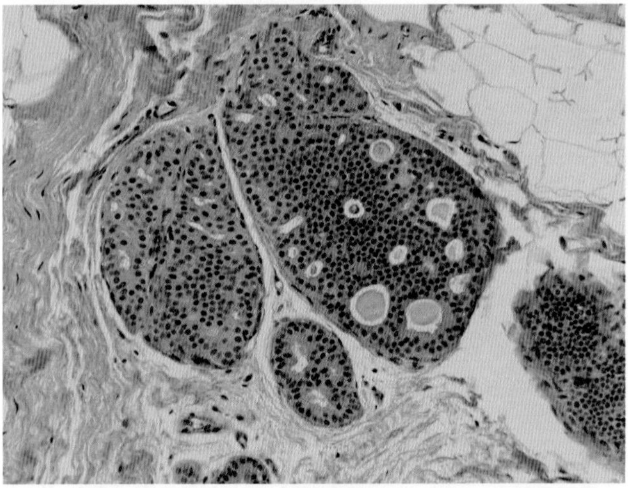

Fig. 22.4 Atypical ductal hyperplasia (H&E, 20x). Again note the monomorphic proliferation of cells; however, in atypical ductal hyperplasia, the cells are not dyscohesive, and the ducts are expanded with varying morphology including "rigid bridges," "round bridges," and or "irregular bridges." In difficult cases, e-cadherin may help to distinguish a lobular versus ductal origin (Fig. 22.9). Courtesy Dr. David Hicks, University of Rochester, Rochester, NY (private collection).

5%–10% of breast cancers are due to germline mutations in breast cancer susceptibility genes, the most prevalent being the BRCA1/2 mutations.

CLINICAL PEARL

Pathologic risk factors are associated with an increased risk for a subsequent diagnosis of breast cancer in both the breasts.

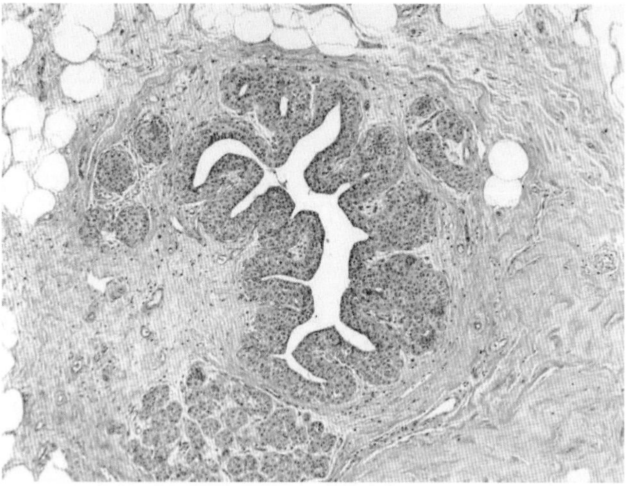

Fig. 22.5 Atypical lobular hyperplasia with pagetoid spread (H&E, 10x). Note the monomorphic proliferation of dyscohesive cells with duct involvement in a "clover leaf" pattern. Some pathologist would interpret this as lobular carcinoma in situ. Courtesy Dr. David Hicks, University of Rochester, Rochester, NY (private collection).

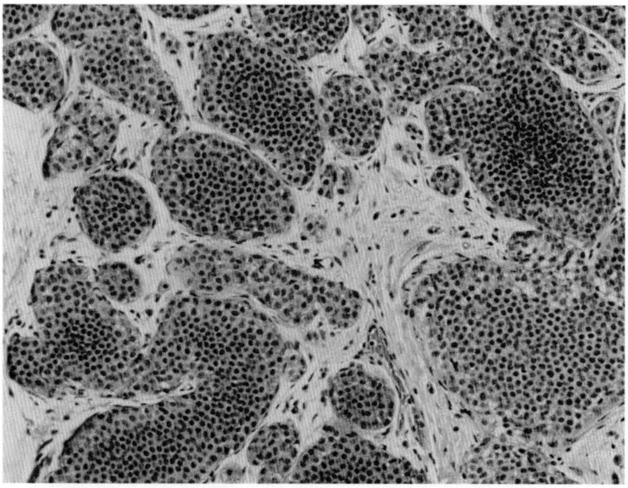

Fig. 22.6 Lobular carcinoma in-situ (H&E, 20x). Note the monomorphic proliferation of dyscohesive cells with rounded borders that distend and totally fill the acini. Courtesy Dr. David Hicks, University of Rochester, Rochester, NY (private collection).

CLINICAL PEARL

Women with a BRCA mutation have an increased LR (25%–85%) of developing breast cancer, depending on age and ethnic background.

CLINICAL PEARL

Risk models including but not limited to the Gail model and the Claus model may be helpful in assessing the patient's risk for breast cancer.

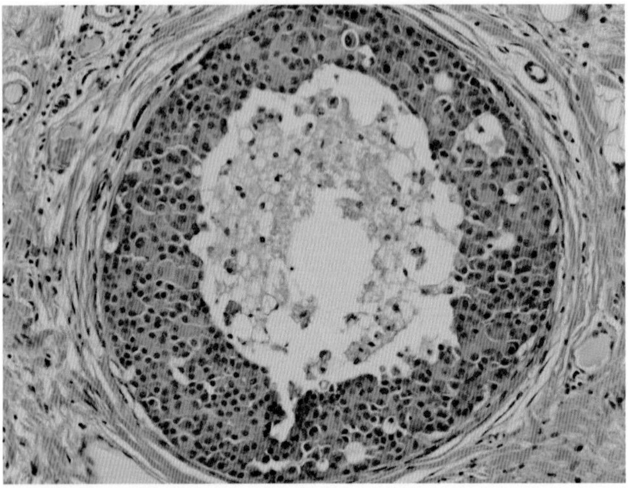

Fig. 22.7 Pleomorphic lobular carcinoma in-situ (H&E, 40x). This variant of lobular carcinoma in situ, with uncharacteristic heterogeneity of nuclear grade, can make it difficult to distinguish from ductal carcinoma in situ (Fig. 22.8). Courtesy Dr. David Hicks, University of Rochester, Rochester, NY (private collection).

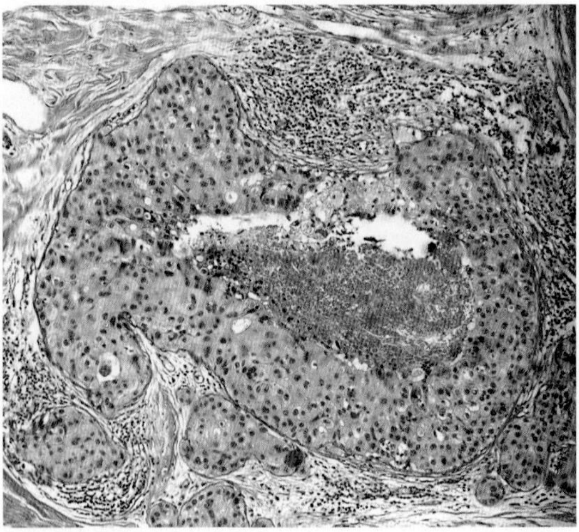

Fig. 22.8 Ductal carcinoma in-situ (H&E, 40x). The nuclear heterogeneity, cohesive cytology, irregular borders, and duct expansion with central necrosis favor a ductal origin. In difficult cases where a lobular origin is considered, e-cadherin can be helpful (Fig. 22.9). Courtesy Dr. David Hicks, University of Rochester, Rochester, NY (private collection).

What findings might be present in a patient with IBC? Patients with IBC may be asymptomatic with a nonpalpable mass (as in this case). Symptomatic patients may present with symptoms such as nipple discharge, skin changes, and breast asymmetry (Box 22.3). The most common symptom of breast cancer is a new lump or mass.

BOX 22.3 ■ Presenting Symptoms in Invasive Breast Carcinoma

Breast pain (rare)
Nipple discharge, changes in the breast skin (color changes, nipple excoriation, eczema, ulcers), and a palpable mass.
Breast asymmetry
Breast thickening
Color changes in the breast skin
Nipple excoriation, eczema, or ulceration
Palpable mass (most common)

CLINICAL PEARL

Breast pain without any other findings on physical examination is rarely a sign of carcinoma, and most women with carcinoma do not present with breast pain. Careful history to elicit the duration and frequency of the pain is important as cyclic breast pain may be related to menstrual cycle.

Breast pain and nipple discharge are rarely symptoms or signs of breast carcinoma; however, the likelihood of nipple discharge being secondary to carcinoma does increase with age. Most pathologic discharges are unilateral, bloody, and spontaneous. Other, more nonspecific symptoms that women with breast cancer present include general malaise, bony pain, and weight loss.

Case Point 22.1

The patient returns to the radiologist office for a follow-up ultrasound-guided biopsy. The specimen is submitted to pathology and shows a high-grade invasive ductal carcinoma, weakly estrogen receptor (ER) positive, progesterone receptor (PR) negative, and human epidermal growth factor receptor 2 (HER2) negative, with a proliferation index (Ki-67) of 50%.

What are the different types of "breast cancer"? Breast carcinoma is classified as either in situ or invasive (Figs. 22.6–22.8; Table 22.1). In situ means that the neoplastic cells are confined to the basement membrane of the duct they are in, whereas invasive means that they have passed through the basement membrane of the duct to infiltrate the surrounding tissues. The most frequent type of in situ breast carcinoma is DCIS (Fig. 22.8), which is considered a precursor of IBC, and accounts for 20%–25% of newly diagnosed breast cancers in the United States. LCIS (Figs. 22.6 and 22.7) is currently not considered a precursor of IBC but is associated with an increased long-term risk of bilateral IBC. At times, DCIS and LCIS may be difficult to distinguish from each other on the standard H&E slide. In more difficult cases, immunohistochemistry (IHC) for e-cadherin can be helpful, as it will stain positive in DCIS with a membrane pattern and will not typically stain LCIS (Fig. 22.9). Invasive ductal carcinoma of no special type (Fig. 22.10) accounts for approximately 75%–80% of IBCs. Invasive lobular carcinoma (Fig 22.11) accounts for about 10% of IBCs. The remaining 10%–15% of IBCs are classified into special histologic types based on specific morphologic features (Table 22.1; Figs. 22.12 and 22.13) that are typically associated with prognostic significance.

CLINICAL PEARL

DCIS is considered a neoplastic, **nonobligate** precursor of IBC.

TABLE 22.1 ■ **Morphologic Types of Carcinoma in situ and Invasive Carcinoma**

Morphologic types of carcinoma in situ	**Morphologic types of invasive carcinoma**
Ductal carcinoma in situ	Ductal carcinoma (no special type)
Lobular carcinoma in situ	Lobular carcinoma (classic and variant types)
Paget disease	Adenoid cystic carcinoma
Encapsulated papillary carcinoma	Apocrine carcinoma
Intracystic papillary carcinoma	Basal-like carcinoma
Solid papillary carcinoma	Carcinoma with extensive intraductal component Carcinoma with extramedullary features Carcinoma with medullary features Carcinoma with neuroendocrine features Carcinoma with osteoclast-like giant cells Cribriform carcinoma Inflammatory carcinoma Low-grade adenosquamous carcinoma Metaplastic carcinoma Micropapillary carcinoma Mucinous (colloid) carcinoma Papillary carcinoma Tubular carcinoma Tubulolobular carcinoma Secretory carcinoma

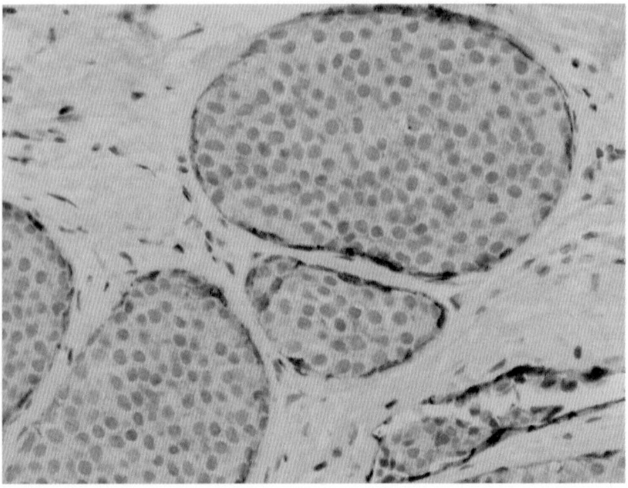

Fig. 22.9 Lobular carcinoma in situ (e-cadherin, 40x). Loss of e-cadherin in lobular carcinoma in situ. E-cadherin would stain positive in ductal carcinoma in situ. Courtesy Dr. David Hicks, University of Rochester, Rochester, NY (private collection).

What is the significance of ER, PR, HER2, and Ki-67 in breast cancer? ER is an intracellular steroid hormone receptor that interacts with the ligand estrogen, subsequently influencing a variety of hormonally responsive tissues, including breast tissue. ER is vitally important for regulating the expression of several genes that are important for both normal breast biology as well as breast cancer biology. Two forms of ER have been identified: ERα and ERβ. These two forms are the

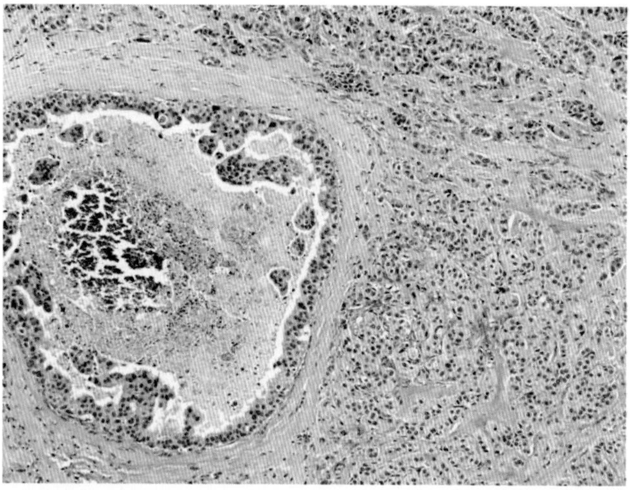

Fig. 22.10 Invasive ductal carcinoma, no special type (H&E, 10x). Atypical poorly formed nests of cells infiltrating the stroma characterize a typical invasive ductal carcinoma. The presence of an adjacent ductal carcinoma in situ is common. Courtesy Dr. David Hicks, University of Rochester, Rochester, NY (private collection).

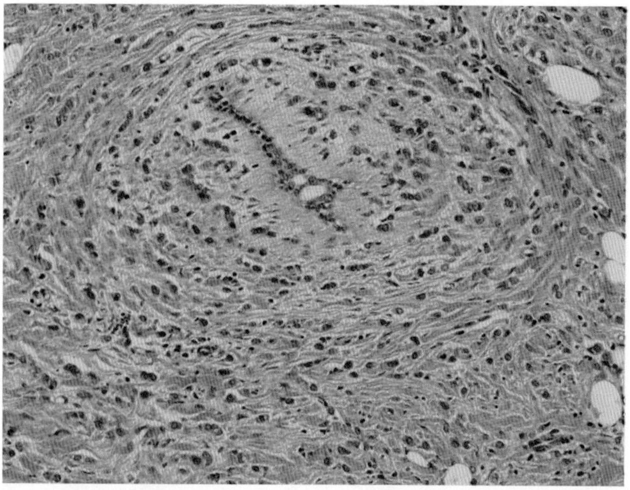

Fig. 22.11 Invasive lobular carcinoma (H&E, 20x). The pattern of single monomorphic cells infiltrating the stroma characterizes a classic invasive lobular carcinoma. Architectural variants of invasive lobular carcinoma exist and are likely to be of a higher grade. Courtesy Dr. David Hicks, University of Rochester, Rochester, NY (private collection).

products of two separate genes. ERα is the more relevant ER for IBC. ER expression in IBC is highly predictive of the clinical benefit associated with various antihormonal therapies that can be used in the adjuvant, metastatic, and neoadjuvant settings to treat IBC. Prospective clinical trials have shown that targeted hormonal treatment in ER-positive pre- and postmenopausal women significantly reduces breast cancer recurrence, resulting in improved patient survival.

PR is an intracellular steroid hormone receptor that is regulated by ER and activated by the ligand, progesterone. Human PR proteins exist as three different isoforms: PR-A, PR-B, and PR-C, transcribed from a single gene (unlike the isoforms of ER, which are transcribed from

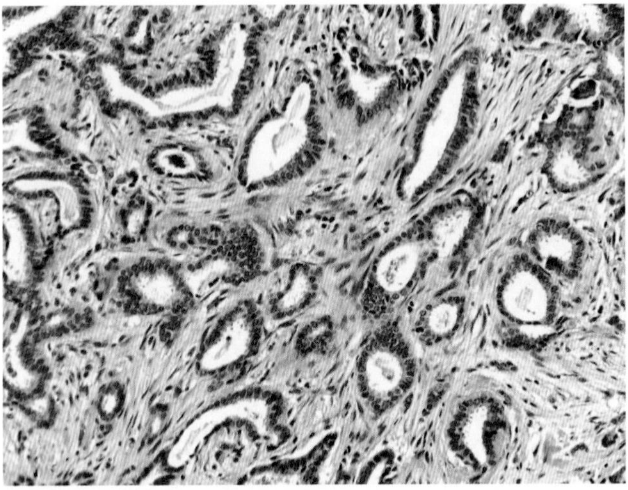

Fig. 22.12 Tubular carcinoma (H&E, 20x). The neoplastic ducts are well formed, with open lumina and low nuclear grade. Apical snouting is a characteristic feature. These tumors are a special histologic type that typically has a low metastatic potential and a favorable prognosis. Courtesy Dr. David Hicks, University of Rochester, Rochester, NY (private collection).

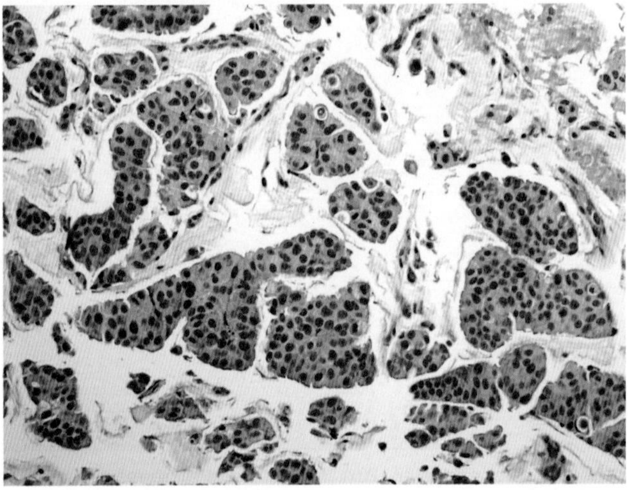

Fig. 22.13 Mucinous (colloid) carcinoma (H&E, 20x). Mucinous carcinoma, a special histologic type of invasive breast carcinoma, typically consists of invasive carcinoma in a background of mucinous fluid. Depending on the morphology and amount of background mucin, mucinous carcinoma can be characterized as pure, micropapillary, or mixed. This figure shows a micropapillary pattern. Courtesy Dr. David Hicks, University of Rochester, Rochester, NY (private collection).

different genes). Each PR isoform has some functional relation to the others. PR expression is an indicator of a functionally intact ER pathway; however, the evidence suggests that PR is not simply a passive marker of functional ER, but that the isoform ratio may influence tumor phenotype and patient outcome. PR also can be used to help predict the benefit from hormonal therapy. Clinical studies have confirmed that elevated total PR levels correlate with an increased probability of response to tamoxifen, longer time to treatment failure, and longer overall survival. PR may have significant prognostic value for breast cancer beyond that for ER alone.

HER2 is a member of the HER family of growth factor receptors, which participate in normal breast growth and development. The HER2 gene is located on chromosome 17. Amplification of HER2 gene in 15%–20% of IBCs results in overexpression of the HER2 protein at the membrane of the tumor cell, thereby dramatically increasing the likelihood of receptor activation and signaling. Overexpression of HER2 is responsible for more aggressive tumor biology and is associated with an increased likelihood of recurrence and mortality. Therapies that target the HER2 pathway are remarkably effective in both the metastatic, adjuvant and neoadjuvant settings in HER2-positive breast cancer patients, causing improvements in both disease-free and overall survival times.

Ki-67 is a nuclear protein associated with cellular proliferation. It has been shown that the Ki-67 nuclear antigen is expressed in certain phases of the cell cycle (S, G1, G2, and M phases), and that Ki-67 expression is a surrogate for tumor cell proliferation and mitotic activity. Ki-67 IHC can be used to assess the growth fraction of neoplastic cell populations. Mitotic activity is frequently increased in more aggressive breast cancers, and Ki-67 expression will typically be increased in those patients with increased mitotic activity.

At the turn of the 21st century, four significant groups of breast cancer subtypes were discovered using RNA expression profiling: luminal A (ER-positive, HER2-negative, with a Ki-67 less than 14%), luminal B (ER-positive, HER2-positive or ER-positive HER2 negative with a Ki-67 greater than or equal to 14%), HER2-overexpressing (ER- and PR-negative, HER2-positive), and basal-like (typically triple-negative). The intensity and percentage of ER, PR, HER2, and Ki-67 using IHC can be used to risk-stratifying patients into surrogates of these four groups (Table 22.2). Compared with the luminal A subtype, women with luminal B tumors and HER2 overexpressing breast carcinoma have roughly a twofold increased adjusted risk of breast cancer mortality. Women with triple-negative breast cancers have a poorer short-term prognosis than women with all the other subtypes.

CLINICAL PEARL

ER and PR are considered positive if there is at least 1% positive nuclear staining (Fig. 22.14).

CLINICAL PEARL

HER2 is considered positive if there is ≥10% complete membranous staining on IHC (Fig. 22.15).

TABLE 22.2 ■ **Breast Cancer Subtypes Based on Estrogen Receptor (ER), Progesterone Receptor (PR), Human Epidermal Growth Factor Receptor 2 (HER2), and Ki-67 Immunohistochemistry**

Immunohistochemistry	Luminal A	Luminal B	HER2	Triple-negative
ER	Positive	Positive	Negative	Negative
PR	Positive or Negative	Positive or Negative	Negative	Negative
HER2	Negative	Positive* or Negative**	Positive	Negative
Ki-67	<14%	Any***	Any***	Any***

*any Ki-67
**Ki-67 greater than or equal to 14%
***typically > 14%

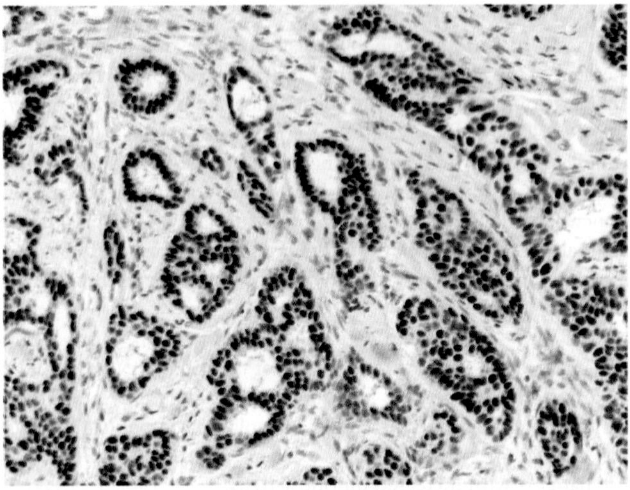

Fig. 22.14 Invasive ductal carcinoma (estrogen receptor, 20x). Positive staining for estrogen receptor immunohistochemistry. Courtesy Dr. David Hicks, University of Rochester, Rochester, NY (private collection).

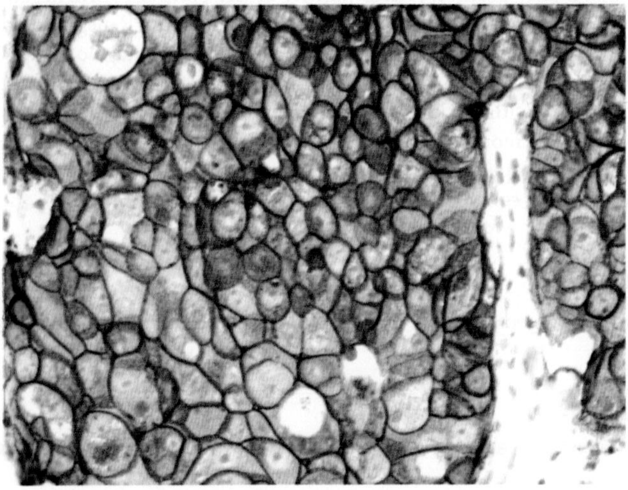

Fig. 22.15 Invasive ductal carcinoma (HER2, 20x). Positive staining for HER2 immunohistochemistry. Courtesy Dr. David Hicks, University of Rochester, Rochester, NY (private collection).

Case Point 22.2

The patient was scheduled for surgery and undergoes a partial mastectomy with sentinel lymph node biopsy. The final pathology reports a 1-cm, modified Scarff–Bloom–Richardson (SBR) score 8 of 9 (grade 3), infiltrating ductal carcinoma, with negative margins and with no evidence of lymph node involvement. The Rochester Modified Magee algorithm (RoMMa) score was 34, with an Oncotype DX® score of 37.

What is the significance of the modified SBR score? The modified SBR score is used to determine the Nottingham grade, which is prognostic for recurrence and outcome in breast cancer patients. The SBR score is based on the tumor morphology score (degree of tubular formation by tumor cells), nuclear grade score, and mitotic count score per 10 high-power fields. An SBR score of 3–5 has a low Nottingham grade (1) and is considered a well-differentiated cancer. An SBR score of 6 or 7 has an intermediate Nottingham grade (2). An SBR score of 8 or 9 has a high Nottingham grade (3) and is considered a poorly differentiated cancer. The SBR score and Nottingham grade are prognostic, and patients with higher SBR scores and Nottingham grades are at increased risk for breast cancer recurrence and worse outcomes.

What is the significance of the RoMMa and Oncotype DX® scores? Over the last decade, molecular approaches including multigene assays for predicting prognosis and treatment response have entered into the clinical arena of breast cancer care. Oncotype DX® is the most widely used of these multigene assays. Oncotype DX® (Genomic Health, Redwood City, CA, USA) is a 21-gene commercial quantitative reverse transcription–polymerase chain reaction-based assay (RTPCR) that has been shown to be prognostic and to be predictive of chemotherapy benefit in ER-positive lymph node-negative breast cancer patients. There is some evidence to suggest that the use of Oncotype DX® test can provide additional prognostic and predictive information in women with lymph node-positive breast cancer as well. Oncotype DX® uses an algorithm to calculate a recurrence score, giving the highest weight to proliferation (which includes Ki-67), followed by HER2, ER, and PR. The Oncotype DX® recurrence score is reported as a number that is divided into either low (<18), intermediate (18–30), or high (>30) recurrence risk categories. Oncotype DX® is an expensive test (current list price US$4620.00), and several studies have suggested that standard clinical, histopathologic, semiquantitative IHC, and biomarker data can provide information similar to that provided by the Oncotype DX® recurrence score. The average modified Magee equation is based on the new Magee equations (https://path.upmc.edu/onlineTools/mageeequations.html), which are available to the public free of charge. The average modified Magee equation. calculates a predicted recurrence score, which has been validated in an algorithm, RoMMa. The RoMMa score has been shown to correlate well with the Oncotype DX® recurrence score, and the RoMMa score independently predicts risk of breast cancer recurrence in ER-positive breast cancer patients. Using the information from the RoMMa in risk-stratifying ER-positive patients when Oncotype DX® is not available, or to identify cases where Oncotype DX® may not provide any additional significant clinical utility, can be helpful to clinicians in risk stratifying breast cancer patients, while providing significant cost savings for the health care system.

Case Point 22.3

Medical oncology recommends that the patient start anastrozole (1 mg daily) for at least 5 years. Further recommendations from medical oncology include a regimen of systemic chemotherapy to include dose-dense doxorubicin and cyclophosphamide, followed by paclitaxel (each given every 2 weeks for four cycles). Radiation oncology is consulted and recommends a regimen of radiation therapy to be performed over several weeks.

BEYOND THE PEARLS

- Breast cancer is the second most common cause of cancer mortality in women.
- The average LR of a woman getting breast cancer is approximately 12%, to over 80% in women with highly penetrant germline breast cancer susceptibility mutations.
- The LR of dying from IBC is approximately 2.7%.
- Approximately 1 in 10 women who have a screening mammogram will need further evaluation, and in most cases, additional testing will be negative for cancer.
- Pathology is the gold standard for diagnosing breast cancer.
- Approximately 70%–80% of breast carcinomas express ER.
- Approximately 15%–20% of patients with breast cancer will have amplification of the HER2 gene.
- In equivocal cases of HER2 IHC, HER2 in situ hybridization is the gold standard for determining a positive or negative result.
- BRCA1 is found on chromosome 17q21.
- BRCA2 is found on chromosome 13q12-13.
- **Prognostic factors** predict a patient's clinical course in terms of risk of disease recurrence and death and include lymph node metastasis, tumor size, American Joint Committee on Cancer stage, histologic grade, lymphovascular invasion, histologic type, HER2 status, and gene expression profile.
- **Predictive factors** predict likelihood that a patient will benefit from treatment and include ER and PR status, HER2 status, proliferative rate (indicated by the amount of mitotic activity and Ki-67 expression), and gene expression profile.
- Oncotype DX® (Genomic Health, Redwood City, CA, USA) is a 21-gene commercial quantitative RTPCR-based assay that has been shown to be prognostic and to be predictive of chemotherapy benefit in ER-positive lymph node-negative breast cancer patients.

References

Berry DA, Iversen ES, Gudbjartsson DF, et al. BRCAPRO validation, sensitivity of genetic testing of BRCA1/BRCA2, and prevalence of other breast cancer susceptibility genes. *J Clin Oncol.* 2002;20:2701-2712.

Bowman M, Neale AV. Family physicians improve patient health care quality and outcomes. *J Am Board Fam Med.* 2013;26:617-619.

Danforth DN. Disparities in breast cancer outcomes between Caucasian and African-American women: a model for describing the relationship of biological and nonbiological factors. *Breast Cancer Res.* 2013;15(3):208.

DeSantis C, Siegel R, Bandi P, Jemal A. Breast cancer statistics, 2011. *CA Cancer J Clin.* 2011;61:409-418.

DeSantis CE, Lin CC, Mariotto AB, et al. Cancer treatment and survivorship statistics, 2014. *CA Cancer J Clin.* 2014;64:252-271.

Edge S, Byrd DR, Compton CC, et al, eds. *AJCC Cancer Staging Manual.* 7th ed. Chicago: American Joint Committee on Cancer; 2009.

Griffin JL, Pearlman MD. Breast cancer screening in women at average risk and high risk. *Obstet Gynecol.* 2010;116(6):1410-1421.

Gurney EP, Nachtigall MJ, Nachtigall LE, Naftolin F. The Women's Health Initiative trial and related studies: 10 years later: a clinician's view. *J Steroid Biochem Mol Biol.* 2014;142:4-11.

Hartmann LC, Radisky DC, Frost MH, et al. Understanding the premalignant potential of atypical hyperplasia through its natural history: a longitudinal cohort study. *Cancer Prev Res (Phila).* 2014;7(2):211-217.

Hicks DG, Lester SC. *Diagnostic Pathology Breast.* Utah: Amirsys Publishing; 2012.

Inwald EC, Klinkhammer-Schalke M, Hofstädter F, et al. Ki-67 is a prognostic parameter in breast cancer patients: results of a large population-based cohort of a cancer registry. *Breast Cancer Res Treat.* 2013;139(2):539-552.

Jacobi CE, de Bock GH, Siegerink B, van Asperen CJ. Differences and similarities in breast cancer risk assessment models in clinical practice: which model to choose? *Breast Cancer Res Treat.* 2009;115(2):381-390.

Jemal A, Siegel R, Ward E, Hao Y, Xu J, Thun MJ. Cancer statistics, 2009. *CA Cancer J Clin.* 2009;59: 225-249.

Karami F, Mehdipour P. A comprehensive focus on global spectrum of BRCA1 and BRCA2 in breast cancer. *Biomed Res Int.* 2013;2013:1-21.

Lakhani SR, Ellis. IO, Schnitt, SJ, et al, eds. *WHO Classification of Tumours of the Breast.* Vol 4. Lyon, France: IARC press; 2012.

Mainiero MB, Lourenco A, Mahoney MC, et al. ACR appropriateness criteria breast cancer screening. *J Am Coll Radiol.* 2013;10:11-14.

Malone KE, Daling JR, Doody DR. Prevalence and predictors of BRCA1 and BRCA2 mutations in a population-based study of breast cancer in white and black American women ages 35-64 years. *Cancer Res.* 2006;66:8297-8308.

Parmigiani G, Chen S, Iversen ES, et al. Validity of models for predicting BRCA1 and BRCA2 mutations. *Ann Intern Med.* 2007;147:441-450.

Schnitt SJ, Collins LC. *Biopsy Interpretation of the Breast.* Philadelphia, PA: Lippincott Williams & Wilkins; 2009.

Shah R, Rosso K, Nathanson SD. Pathogenesis, prevention, diagnosis and treatment of breast cancer. *World J Clin Oncol.* 2014;5(3): 283-298.

Siegel R, Ma J, Zou Z, Jemal A. Cancer statistics, 2014. *CA Cancer J Clin.* 2014;64(1):9-29.

Turner BM, Gimenez-Sanders MA, Soukiazian A, et al. Risk stratification of ER positive breast cancer patients: a multi-institutional validation and outcome study of the Rochester Modified Magee algorithm (RoMMa) and prediction of an Oncotype DX® recurrence score < 26. *Cancer Med.* 2019;8(9):4176-4188.

Turner BM, Hicks DG. Breast cancer. In: Paulman P, Taylor RB, eds. *Family Medicine, Principles and Practice.* 7th ed. Germany: Springer; 2016.

Turner BM, Skinner KA, Tang P, et al. Use of modified Magee equations and histologic criteria to predict the Oncotype DX® recurrence score. *Mod Pathol.* 2015;28(7):921-931.

US Preventive Services Task Force. Screening for breast cancer: U.S. Preventive Services Task Force recommendation statement. *Ann Intern Med.* 2009;151(10):716-726.

CASE 23

A 70-Year-Old Male with a Mass Around His Nipple

Bradley M. Turner

A 70-year-old male presents to his primary care doctor after noticing a firm mass on his right breast around the nipple area. The mass does not hurt. He has no other complaints. He exercises daily and reports that he "watches his diet closely" since his heart attack about a year ago. He has a past medical history of myocardial infarction, atrial fibrillation, and depression. His medications include a baby aspirin, beta-blocker, ace inhibitor, and tricyclic antidepressant. His paternal grandmother died of breast cancer. The patient's temperature is 37.1°C (98.8°F), pulse rate is 95 beats per minute, respiration rate is 18 breaths per minute, and blood pressure is 157/95 mm Hg. The patient has a body mass index of 35.5 kg/m^2. Physical examination reveals a well-developed man in no acute distress. Examination of the breasts reveals slightly asymmetrical breast tissue with a palpable nontender 2–3-cm mass in the subareolar region of the right breast. The remainder of the examination is unremarkable. A diagnostic mammogram and ultrasound show a suspicious density behind the nipple, with associated calcifications, measuring 2.9 × 1.9 × 1.3 cm.

What is the epidemiology of male breast cancer?

Less than 1% of breast cancers occur in men. The median age for a man to develop invasive breast carcinoma is 67 years, slightly older than that for a woman (61 years). Approximately 2670 new cases of male breast cancer were reported in the US in 2019, with approximately 500 men dying from breast cancer–related causes that year. The incidence of male breast cancer has remained remarkably stable over time.

CLINICAL PEARL

The lifetime risk (LR) of developing and dying from male breast cancer in males without germline mutation is 0.12% (1 in 833) and 0.03% (1 in 3333), respectively.

What risk factors are associated with a diagnosis of male breast cancer?

Risk factors associated with a diagnosis of male breast cancer are listed in Box 23.1. Conditions associated with increased serum estrogen are a risk factor for male breast cancer and include liver disease, obesity, anti-androgen therapy for prostate cancer, and exogenous estrogen therapy. Conditions associated with decreased serum androgen are a risk factor for male breast cancer and include Klinefelter syndrome, testicular injury, testicular infertility, and occupational exposure to extreme high temperatures. Other than estrogen, exogenous agents associated with an increased risk for male breast cancer include digitalis, tricyclic antidepressants, marijuana, lavender oil, and tea tree oil. Similar to women, radiation exposure, particularly chest wall radiation, increases the risk of breast cancer. Similarly, a positive family history increases the risk of male breast cancer, and similar to women, the risk of breast cancer in men is increased in men who carry *BRCA1* and/or *BRCA2* mutations. Other germline mutations associated with male breast cancer include *CHEK2*, *PTEN*, and *TP53* mutations.

BOX 23.1 ■ Risk Factors Associated with a Diagnosis of Male Breast Cancer

Liver disease	Tricyclic antidepressants
Obesity	Marijuana
Anti-androgen therapy	Lavender oil
Exogenous estrogen therapy	Tea tree oil
Klinefelter syndrome	Chest wall radiation
Testicular injury	*BRCA* mutation carriers
Testicular infertility	Cowden syndrome (*PTEN* mutation)
Occupational exposure to extreme high temperatures	*CHEK2* mutation carriers
Digitalis	Li-Fraumeni syndrome *(TP53)*

CLINICAL PEARL

BRCA1 carries an LR of developing male breast cancer of approximately 1%–5%. The LR is higher in BRCA2 carriers, approximately 5%–10%.

What findings might be present in a male patient with breast carcinoma?

Male patients with breast carcinoma typically present with a painless firm mass, often located in the subareolar region, eccentric to the nipple. Fixation to the skin and/or the pectoralis muscle is common. A bloody nipple discharge is typically present in a majority of patients. Because of the relative rarity of male breast cancer and the absence of routine screening and/or examination, the diagnosis is often delayed, and these tumors are usually diagnosed at a higher stage compared with female breast cancer.

CLINICAL PEARL

Palpable lymph nodes are present in approximately 50% of male breast cancer patients.

Case Point 23.1

A core biopsy is performed and shows a papillary lesion with moderate atypia and associated calcifications. The tumor cells are strongly positive for estrogen receptor (ER) and progesterone receptor (PR), and negative for human epidermal growth factor receptor 2 (HER2), with Ki-67 of 5%. GATA3 was positive. Focal areas suspicious for invasion are reported.

What are the different types of male breast cancers?

As with female breast cancers, male breast cancers are classified as either in situ or invasive (Figs. 22.8–22.10). Ductal carcinoma in situ (DCIS) accounts for approximately 10% of male breast cancers (compared with 20%–25% of newly diagnosed female breast cancers in the United States), and there is a higher incidence of papillary DCIS (Fig. 23.1) in male breast cancer than in female breast cancer. It may be difficult to distinguish from a benign papilloma, particularly in cases when extensive sclerosing change is present. In difficult cases, immunohistochemistry for CK5 can be helpful (Fig. 23.2). Lobular carcinoma in situ (LCIS) (Figs. 22.6 and 22.9) is very rare in male patients. As with female breast carcinoma, invasive ductal carcinoma, no special type is the most common invasive male breast carcinoma. The second most common type of invasive breast carcinoma is lobular carcinoma in women and invasive papillary carcinoma in men (Fig. 23.3). Invasive lobular carcinoma along with other special types of mammary carcinoma may also be seen in male breast cancer, but they are generally uncommon.

CLINICAL PEARL

Male breast cancers are more likely to be larger and diagnosed at a higher stage than female breast cancers; however, the prognosis, when adjusted for number of positive axillary nodes, tumor size, and histologic grade, is similar in male and female breast cancer.

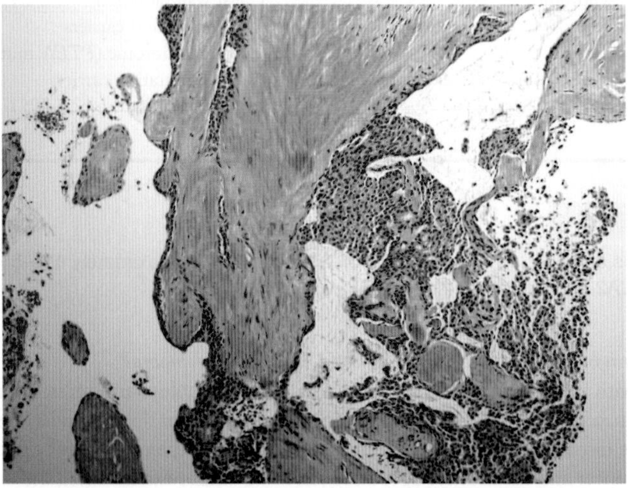

Fig. 23.1 Papillary ductal carcinoma in situ (H&E, 40x). Note the atypical cytology and extensive papillary architecture. The cell orientation is haphazard in intraductal papilloma (Fig. 20.5), whereas it is more uniform and perpendicular to the fibrovascular stalks in papillary ductal carcinoma in situ. (Courtesy Dr. David Hicks, University of Rochester, Rochester, NY.) (Private collection).

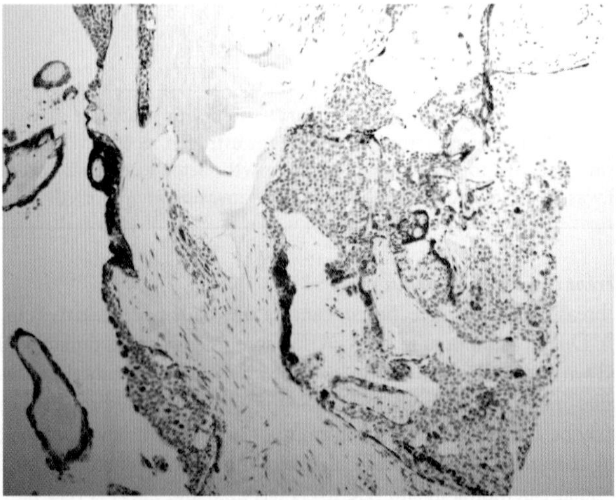

Fig. 23.2 Papillary ductal carcinoma in situ (CK5, 40x). In difficult cases, immunohistochemistry for CK5 can be helpful in distinguishing a benign papilloma from a papilloma with atypia. CK5 will have positive staining in a benign papilloma. Papillomas with atypia will not stain with CK5. Do not be confused by the positive staining in surrounding benign epithelium, which can occur in atypical papillary lesions. CK5 cannot distinguish an atypical papilloma from papillary ductal carcinoma in situ. (Courtesy Dr. David Hicks, University of Rochester, Rochester, NY.) (Private collection).

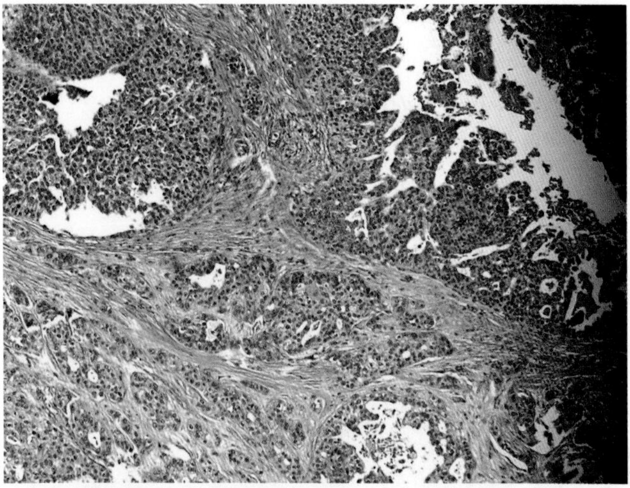

Fig. 23.3 Invasive papillary carcinoma (H&E, 100x). Note the infiltrative nests of papillae with fibrovascular cores adjacent to more well-circumscribed nests of papillary ductal carcinoma in situ.

What is the significance of ER, PR, HER2, and Ki-67 in male breast cancer?

The significance of ER, PR, HER2, and Ki-67 in breast cancer has already been discussed in the chapter on female invasive breast carcinoma, and the significance is similar in male breast cancer; however, breast cancer subtypes according to expression of ER, PR, and HER2 are different in male breast cancer. Male breast cancer is more likely to be of the luminal A or B subtype and less likely to be of the HER2 overexpressing or basal (triple-negative) subtype.

What is the significance of GATA3 in male breast carcinoma?

While a metastatic carcinoma to the breast is rare, it must be ruled out, particularly in men, as metastatic prostate or lung carcinoma would be much more likely. Expression of GATA3, ER, and PR would favor a breast primary.

Case Point 23.2

The patient underwent a total mastectomy with sentinel lymph node dissection. The final pathology reported a 3-cm, modified Scarff–Bloom–Richardson (SBR) score 6 (grade 2), invasive papillary carcinoma, with negative margins and no evidence of lymph node involvement. The Rochester Modified Magee algorithm score was 14, with an Oncotype DX® score of 17.

What is the treatment approach to patients with male breast cancer?

The treatment of male breast cancer is similar to that offered to female patients and includes a combination of surgical resection, followed by adjuvant therapy (endocrine therapy and/or chemotherapy and radiation therapy). The majority of male patients will undergo mastectomy and sentinel lymph node biopsy, as breast conservation is not generally relevant for cosmetic value. Adjuvant treatment decisions are based on American Joint Committee on Cancer stage, tumor grade, hormone receptor status, HER2 status, and in selected cases molecular testing, similar to female breast cancer patients.

What is the differential diagnosis of male breast carcinoma?

The differential diagnosis for male breast carcinoma is summarized in Box 23.2. Non-neoplastic enlargement of male breast tissue due to hyperplasia of epithelium and stroma (clinically gynecomastia, also known as fibroadenosis; Figs. 23.4 and 23.5) can be seen in infants, during puberty,

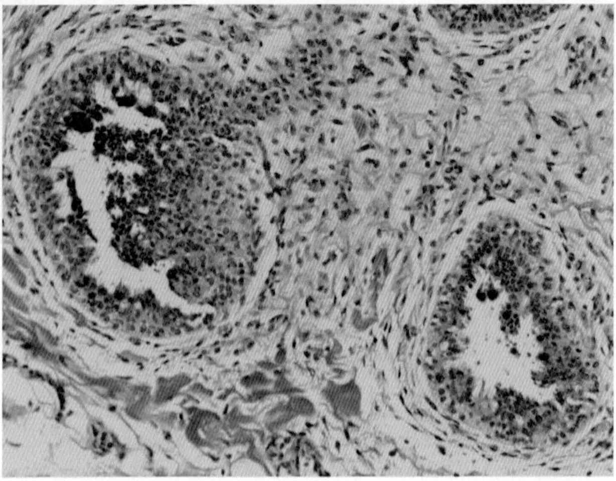

Fig. 23.4 Gynecomastia: Early active phase (H&E, 100x). The early active phase is characterized by loose hypercellular, myxoid, and edematous stroma. Inflammation may be present. (From Hicks DG, Lester SC. *Diagnostic Pathology: Breast*. 2nd ed. Philadelphia, PA. Elsevier; 2016. Section 4. Disorders of Development: Gynecomastia; pp. 80–83.)

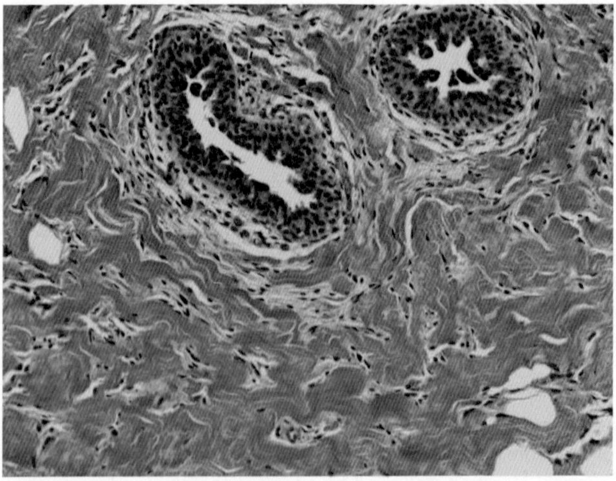

Fig. 23.5 Gynecomastia: Inactive fibrous phase (H&E, 100x). In later stages of gynecomastia, there is a gradual resolution of inflammation, with progressive fibrosis of the periductal stroma. (From Hicks DG, Lester SC. *Diagnostic Pathology: Breast*. 2nd ed. Philadelphia, PA. Elsevier; 2016. Section 4. Disorders of Development: Gynecomastia; pp. 80–83.)

BOX 23.2 ■ Differential Diagnosis of Male Breast Cancer

Gynecomastia
Myofibroblastoma
Metastatic cancer

or in the elderly. If gynecomastia is unilateral or asymmetric, there should be a higher suspicion for an associated carcinoma. Similar to invasive carcinoma, gynecomastia can present as a lesion behind the nipple, and can be mistakenly diagnosed on mammography when a carcinoma is truly present (Fig. 23.6). The clinical presentation of myofibroblastoma may overlap with male breast cancer (Fig. 23.7) as myofibroblastoma may present as a palpable breast mass in an elderly male. The histology of a uniform proliferation of CD34-positive (Fig. 23.8) and keratin-negative spindle-shaped myofibroblasts can help to distinguish a myofibroblastoma from an invasive carcinoma. The epithelioid variant of myofibroblastoma can closely mimic an invasive lobular carcinoma morphologically; in addition, these lesions will also express hormone receptors including ER, PR, and androgen receptor (AR). However, the cells are negative for cytokeratin, and a careful search for a spindle cells component to the lesion, which is frequently present, can be helpful in making this diagnostic distinction. Although metastatic tumor of the breast is rare, the diagnoses must be considered, particularly in men, as it can mimic primary breast cancer. Prostate and lung carcinoma metastases to the breast are more common in men than breast cancer and should always be considered in any breast cancer diagnosis in a male. A careful review and integration of the clinical history, imaging findings, and a search for an in situ component to the patient's tumor can be helpful in making this important diagnostic distinction.

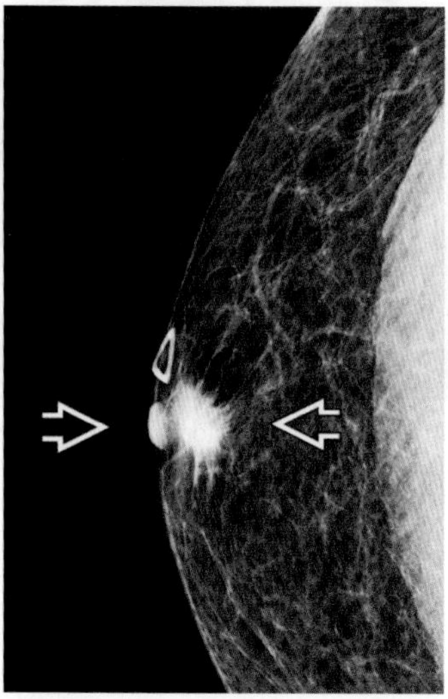

Fig. 23.6 Male breast cancer: Mammography. This breast cancer was initially mistaken for gynecomastia due to the location directly behind the nipple. Most male breast cancers are eccentrically displaced from the nipple. (From Hicks DG, Lester SC. *Diagnostic Pathology: Breast*. 2nd ed. Philadelphia, PA. Elsevier; 2016. Section 11. Unusual presentations of breast lesions: Breast carcinoma, male; pp. 660–663.)

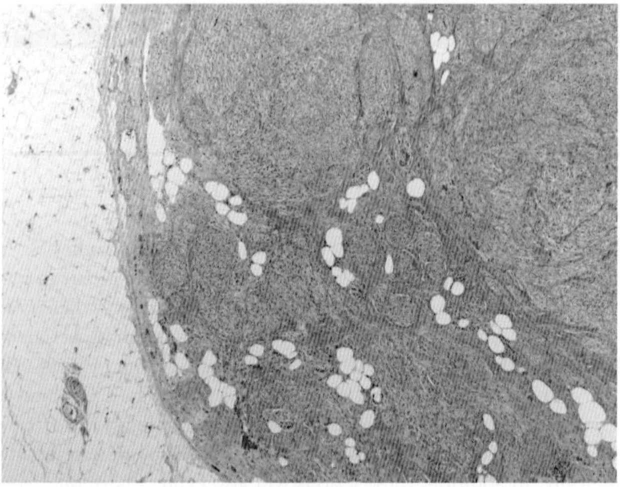

Fig. 23.7 Myofibroblastoma (H&E, 20x). Intersecting bundles of uniform spindle cells are separated by broad bands of hyalinized collagen. Notice the lack of mammary duct and lobular elements. (Courtesy Dr. David Hicks, University of Rochester, Rochester, NY.) (Private collection)

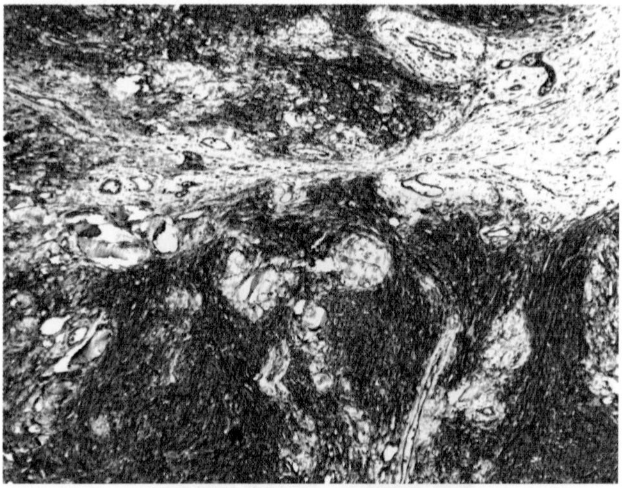

Fig. 23.8 Myofibroblastoma (CD34, 20x). Myofibroblastoma likely arises from CD34-positive mammary stromal cells and will typically show diffuse positive expression of CD34. (From Hicks DG, Lester SC. *Diagnostic Pathology: Breast*. 2nd ed. Philadelphia, PA. Elsevier; 2016. Section 7. Stromal lesions: Myofibroblastoma; pp. 518–525.)

Case Point 23.3

Medical oncology recommended that the patient start anastrozole (1 mg daily) for at least 5 years. The patient declined any further treatment.

BEYOND THE PEARLS

- Male breast cancer is histologically identical to female breast cancer.
- Approximately 15%–20% of male breast carcinoma patients have a family history of breast or ovarian carcinoma.
- While less than 4% of male breast cancer is BRCA1 associated, approximately 30% of patients with male breast cancer have a BRCA2 mutation.
- There is a 60%–75% chance that a family member of a male breast cancer patient will have a BRCA2 mutation.
- Male breast cancer patients have a 3%–8% chance of having Klinefelter syndrome.
- Most male breast carcinomas are either grade 2 (SBR score 6 or 7) or grade 3 (SBR score 8 or 9).
- Most male breast carcinomas are also AR-positive.

References

American Cancer Society. *Cancer Facts and Figures 2019*. Atlanta, GA: American Cancer Society; 2019.

American Cancer Society. *Key Statistics for Breast Cancer in Men*. 2019. Available at: https://www.cancer.org/cancer/breast-cancer-in-men/about/key-statistics.html.

Berry DA, Iversen Jr ES, Gudbjartsson DF, et al. BRCAPRO validation, sensitivity of genetic testing of BRCA1/BRCA2, and prevalence of other breast cancer susceptibility genes. *J Clin Oncol*. 2002;20:2701-2712.

DeSantis C, Siegel R, Bandi P, Jemal A. Breast cancer statistics, 2011. *Ca Cancer J Clin*. 2011;61:409-418.

DeSantis CE, Lin CC, Mariotto AB, et al. Cancer treatment and survivorship statistics, 2014. *CA Cancer J Clin*. 2014;64:252-271.

Edge SB, Byrd DR, Compton CC, Fritz AG, Greene FL, Trotti A, eds. *AJCC Cancer Staging Manual*. 7th ed. Chicago, IL: American Joint Committee on Cancer; 2009.

Hicks DG, Lester SC. *Diagnostic Pathology: Breast*. Utah: Amirsys Publishing; 2012.

Howlader N, Noone AM, Krapcho M, et al., eds. *SEER*Explorer. Breast Cancer Recent Trends in SEER Incidence Rates,* 2000-2016, by Race/Ethnicity. Bethesda, MD: National Cancer Institute; 2019. Accessed August 22, 2019. Available at: https://seer.cancer.gov/explorer/.

Howlader N, Noone AM, Krapcho M, Garshell J, Miller D, Altekruse SF, Kosary CL, Yu M, Ruhl J, Tatalovich Z,Mariotto A, Lewis DR, Chen HS, Feuer EJ, Cronin KA (eds). SEER Cancer Statistics Review, 1975-2011, National Cancer Institute. Bethesda, MD, https://seer.cancer.gov/archive/csr/1975_2011/, based on November 2013 SEER data submission, posted to the SEER web site, April 2014.

Jemal A, Siegel R, Ward E, Hao Y, Xu J, Thun MJ. Cancer statistics, 2009. *CA Cancer J Clin*. 2009;59:225-249.

Karami F, Mehdipour P. A comprehensive focus on global spectrum of BRCA1 and BRCA2 mutations in breast cancer. *Biomed Res Int*. 2013;2013:928562.

Lakhani SR, Ellis IO, Schnitt SJ, Tan PH, van de Vijver MJ, eds. *WHO Classification of Tumours of the Breast*. Vol 4. Lyon: IARC Press; 2012.

Parmigiani G, Chen S, Iversen Jr ES, et al. Validity of models for predicting BRCA1 and BRCA2 mutations. *Ann Intern Med*. 2007;147:441-450.

Schnitt SJ, Collins LC. *Biopsy Interpretation of the Breast*. Philadelphia, PA : Lippincott Williams & Wilkins; 2009.

Scott S, Morrow M. Breast cancer. Making the diagnosis. *Surg Clin North Am*. 1999;79(5):991-1005.

Shah R, Rosso K, Nathanson SD. Pathogenesis, prevention, diagnosis and treatment of breast cancer. *World J Clin Oncol*. 2014;5(3):283-298.

Siegel R, Ma J, Zou Z, Jemal A. Cancer statistics, 2014. *CA Cancer J Clin*. 2014;64(1):9-29.

Smith RA, Cokkinides V, Brawley OW. Cancer screening in the United States, 2009: a review of current American Cancer Society guidelines and issues in cancer screening. *CA Cancer J Clin*. 2009;59(1):27-41.

Smith RA, Saslow D, Sawyer KA, et al. American Cancer Society guidelines for breast cancer screening: update 2003. *CA Cancer J Clin*. 2003;53(3):141-169.

Tria Tirona M. Breast cancer screening update. *Am Fam Physician*. 2013;87(4):274-278.
U.S. Preventive Services Task Force. *Breast Cancer: Screening*. 2016. Available at: http://www.uspreventiveservicestaskforce.org/Page/Document/UpdateSummaryDraft/breast-cancer-screening. Accessed August 22, 2019.
US Preventive Services Task Force. Screening for breast cancer: U.S. Preventive Services Task Force recommendation statement. *Ann Intern Med*. 2009;151(10):716-726.

Genitourinary System

CASE 24

A 68-Year-Old Woman with a Renal Mass

Numbereye Numbere

A 68-year-old Caucasian woman comes to the clinic for follow-up of a right renal mass. She presented 3 weeks earlier at the emergency department with complaints of colicky right upper abdominal pain and nausea. An abdominal ultrasound (US) scan revealed a distended gallbladder with gallstones and an incidental right renal mass. A follow-up abdominal computed tomography (CT) scan revealed a 4.8-cm strongly enhancing mass in the inferior pole of the right kidney suspicious for renal cell carcinoma (RCC). A CT scan of the chest showed no evidence of metastatic disease. She underwent laparoscopic cholecystectomy for cholelithiasis and is now being followed up for the renal mass. She is currently asymptomatic. Her current medications include amlodipine for hypertension and atorvastatin for hyperlipidemia. She smokes one pack of cigarettes daily and drinks an average of two cans of beer per day. Her family history is noncontributory. Physical examination reveals obesity (body mass index 38 kg/m^2) and well-healed laparoscopic surgical incisions. Complete blood count, urinalysis, serum electrolytes, blood urea nitrogen (BUN), and creatinine are all within normal limits. She is informed of the diagnosis.

What is renal cell carcinoma?

RCC is a group of malignant tumors that arise from the renal tubular epithelium. Individual tumors have distinct clinical features, morphological characteristics, and genetic abnormalities. RCC makes up 2%–3% of all malignant tumors in adults and more than 90% of primary renal neoplasms. Its incidence varies among countries, with the highest rates in North America and Nordic nations. In 2018, there were approximately 65,340 new cases of RCC and 14,970 deaths due to RCC in the United States. Since 2008, a plateau in the national incidence of RCC has occurred in concert with a significant decrease in mortality that is mostly attributable to better control of risk factors, earlier diagnosis, and improved treatment options.

How are renal tumors classified? (Box 24.1)

This chapter will focus on some of the more common benign and malignant renal tumors. Unless otherwise stated, RCC refers to malignant tumors of renal tubular epithelium.

What are the clinical features and imaging findings of renal cell carcinoma?

RCC occurs most commonly in patients aged over 65 years with a 2:1 male-to-female ratio. Up to 60% of cases are discovered incidentally in patients investigated for unrelated conditions. When symptomatic, patients may complain of flank pain, flank tenderness, and gross hematuria. The oft-proclaimed triad of flank pain, swelling, and gross hematuria are uncommon, occurring in less than 10% of patients. Patients may be hypertensive at presentation. About one in four patients present with metastatic disease at the time of diagnosis with fever, unintentional weight loss, and fatigue. Metastases most frequently occur in lymph nodes, lung, liver, bone, adrenal gland, and brain. The occurrence of RCC in a young patient (≤46 years) should arouse suspicion of an autosomal dominant familial

BOX 24.1 ■ Classification of Common Renal Tumors

Renal Cell Tumors (Derived From Renal Tubular Epithelium)

- Benign
  - a. Papillary adenoma
  - b. Oncocytoma
- Malignant
  - a. Clear cell (conventional) renal cell carcinoma
  - b. Papillary renal cell carcinoma
  - c. Clear cell papillary renal cell carcinoma
  - d. Chromophobe renal cell carcinoma
  - e. Collecting duct carcinoma
  - f. Unclassified renal cell carcinoma

Metanephric Tumors

- Metanephric adenoma

Nephroblastic and Cystic Tumors Occurring Mainly in Children

- a. Nephroblastoma (Wilms tumor)
- b. Nephrogenic rests

Mesenchymal Tumors Occurring Mainly in Adults

- Benign
  - Angiomyolipoma
- Malignant
  - Epithelioid angiomyolipoma

Metastatic Tumors

variant and thus cue referral for genetic testing and counseling. Laboratory findings include polycythemia (4% patients), anemia (20%–40% patients), and hypercalcemia (3%–6% patients).

Imaging is performed when clinical suspicion for a renal tumor is aroused. Abdominal US scan is usually the first imaging procedure ordered. Renal CT scan is used to clarify suspicious ultrasonographic findings and to seek out metastatic spread of tumor. Magnetic resonance imaging (MRI) is used in place of CT scan in patients allergic to intravenous contrast, in pregnancy, in the evaluation of direct venous extension of tumor (Fig. 24.1), and in tumor surveillance. A percutaneous renal biopsy may be performed to diagnose radiologically indeterminate masses.

CLINICAL PEARL

Serum erythropoietin (EPO) is a tumor marker in RCC. Polycythemia due to the elaboration of EPO by tumor cells is a paraneoplastic feature of some benign and malignant renal tumors including RCC, metanephric adenoma, renal cysts, and hemangioma. Elevated serum EPO is associated with greater invasiveness and lower survival rates in patients with RCC.

CLINICAL PEARL

Malignant renal tumors, such as clear cell renal cell carcinoma and nephroblastoma, have a propensity for venous invasion and direct tumor extension (Fig. 24.1). The tumor may propagate to any level from the segmental renal veins, the main renal vein, the inferior vena cava, and the right atrium. Rarely venous invasion is seen in benign tumors such as oncocytomas. But unlike malignant tumors, venous invasion in oncocytomas is not associated with adverse clinical outcomes.

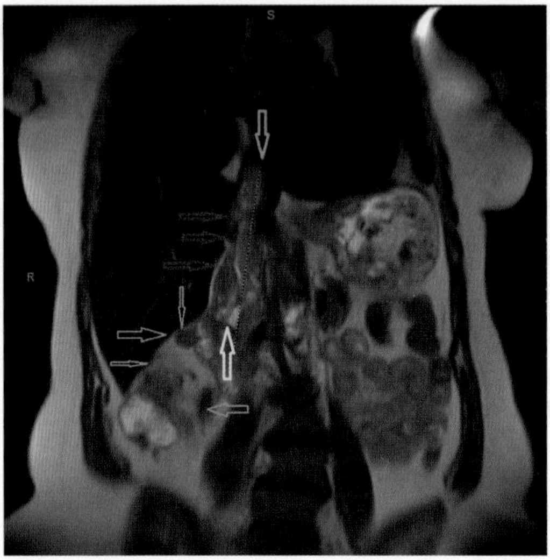

Fig. 24.1 This MRI image shows venous extension of a recurrent right renal cell carcinoma occurring years after a right radical nephrectomy. There is an extensive tumor thrombus arising from the superior right renal fossa (yellow arrow), extending superiorly within the inferior vena cava (red arrows), terminating at the cavoatrial junction (green arrow). Loops of bowel are also seen (blue arrows). The patient had previously undergone a left radical nephrectomy for a left-sided renal cell carcinoma.

Case Point 24.1

The patient is distraught about her diagnosis and asks what might have caused the tumor.

What are the risk factors for RCC?

Risk factors for RCC include smoking, hypertension, obesity, and chronic analgesic use; environmental exposure to certain chemicals (e.g., cadmium and trichloroethylene); a family history of renal cancer; and the presence of advanced kidney disease especially in patients who have been on dialysis for more than 3 years. In about 2% of cases, RCC occurs as a manifestation of inherited autosomal dominant disorders like von Hippel-Lindau (VHL) and Birt-Hogg-Dubé (BHD) syndromes.

What are the important molecular pathways in renal tumors?

Recent advances have provided several insights into the molecular alterations underlying renal neoplasms and their oncogenic signaling pathways. This understanding has enabled the design of more effective, targeted drug treatments aimed at key steps in the pathways. Some important hereditary renal cancer syndromes and their underlying molecular mechanisms are highlighted (Table 24.1).

The VHL Gene and the Hypoxia-Inducible Transcription Factor (HIF) Pathway

Mutations resulting in the inactivation of the *VHL* gene (3p25-26) occur in up to 86% of sporadic clear cell renal cell carcinomas (CCRCCs). About 40% of patients with the autosomal dominant VHL syndrome have CCRCC. The *VHL* gene product functions to target and degrade HIF. In the presence of inactivating *VHL* mutations and hypoxia (as exists in areas of

TABLE 24.1 ■ **Autosomal Dominant Hereditary Renal Cancer Syndromes**

Syndrome	Gene Name and Chromosome Location	Protein Product	Associated Renal Tumor	Other Features of the Syndrome
Birt-Hogg-Dubé syndrome	*FLCN* on 17p11.2	Folliculin	Oncocytoma; chromophobe RCC; hybrid oncocytoma/chromophobe RCC; CCRCC	Skin lesions, e.g., fibrofolliculomas, trichodiscomas, and acrochordons (skin tags); pulmonary cysts, pneumothorax
Hereditary papillary renal cancer	*MET* on 7q31	Receptor for hepatocyte growth factor	Type 1 papillary RCC	None
von Hippel-Lindau disease	*VHL* on 3p25-26	pVHL	CCRCC	CNS and retinal hemangioblastomas; pheochromocytoma, endolymphatic sac tumors of the middle ear, pancreatic neuroendocrine tumors
Hereditary leiomyomatosis and RCC	*FH* on 1q43	Fumarate hydratase	Type 2 papillary RCC	Leiomyomas and leiomyosarcomas of the uterus and skin
Tuberous sclerosis complex	*TSC1* on 9q34; *TSC2* on 16p13.3	Hamartin (TSC1); tuberin (TSC2)	Renal angiomyolipomas and cysts	Nervous system: cortical tubers, giant cell astrocytomas, retinal hamartomas Dermatologic: facial angiofibromas, fibrous forehead plaques, shagreen patches Others: subungual fibromas, cardiac rhabdomyomas, pulmonary lymphangioleiomyomatosis

CCRCC, clear cell renal cell carcinoma; *CNS,* central nervous system; *RCC,* renal cell carcinoma.

a rapidly growing tumor), HIF escapes VHL-mediated proteolysis and degradation. HIF thus accumulates in the cell and translocates to the nucleus where it increases transcription of genes that mediate tumor initiation, progression, and angiogenesis, e.g., the genes encoding vascular endothelial growth factor (VEGF), epidermal growth factor, platelet-derived growth factor, transforming growth factor alpha, and erythropoietin. A rich vascular network is characteristic of RCC; therefore, VEGF inhibitors such as pazopanib and sunitinib are used in the treatment of metastatic RCC.

The PI3K/Mammalian Target of Rapamycin (mTOR) Pathway

The mTOR pathway is downstream of the PI3K pathway and serves to regulate the expression of oncogenic proteins (e.g., HIF-1α, VEGF, cyclin D1, c-Myc). Inactivation of the mTOR pathway leads to inhibition of HIF-1α translation, among other outcomes. mTOR inhibitors (e.g., temsirolimus and everolimus) may be used to treat patients with metastatic RCC refractory to VEGF inhibitors or in patients with PI3K pathway alterations.

The Birt-Hogg-Dubé Syndrome

The autosomal dominant BHD syndrome is associated with benign skin tumors, lung lesions, and diverse benign and malignant renal neoplasms including CCRCC, oncocytoma, chromophobe RCC, and hybrid chromophobe RCC/oncocytoma. It is caused by the germline loss of function mutations in the tumor suppressor gene folliculin (*FLCN*, also known as *BHD*) on chromosome 17p11.2. The function of the folliculin protein is incompletely understood but is believed to play a role in diverse cellular pathways, including regulation of the mTOR pathway, intercellular adhesion, regulation of autophagy, and mitochondrial biosynthesis.

The Mesenchymal–Epithelial Transition (MET) Pathway

Hereditary papillary renal cell carcinoma (HPRCC) is an autosomal dominant condition associated with the development of bilateral and multifocal type 1 papillary RCC. HPRCC occurs due to germline mutations in the *MET* proto-oncogene located on chromosome 7q. *MET* encodes the receptor for hepatocyte growth factor (HGFR). A gain of function mutation in *MET* causes constitutive activation of HGFR by its ligand, leading to a protumorigenic state. Trisomy 7 is seen in 75% of sporadic papillary RCC (PRCC). *MET* mutation analysis is performed when HPRCC is suspected.

Genetic Alterations in Nephroblastoma (Wilms Tumor)

Nephroblastoma (WT) is associated with loss of function mutations in several tumor suppressor genes, including *WT1*, genes on the *WT2* locus, and *p53*. The precise tumorigenic mechanisms of these genetic alterations remain unknown. *WT1* (11p13) encodes the *WT1* transcription factor, which functions in renal and gonadal embryogenesis. The *WT2* gene locus (11p15.5) contains several genes, including *IGF2*, which undergo various combinations of genetic aberrations, including imprinting, duplication, and deletion to cause disease.

Case Point 24.2

The patient then asks if the disease could have been diagnosed earlier.

Due to an overall lack of benefit, screening for RCC is not recommended in asymptomatic individuals. Targeted screening with periodic imagining could be beneficial to patients with a hereditary predisposition or otherwise at increased risk (e.g., patients with a strong family history of RCC, patients on long term dialysis for end-stage renal disease, and patients with a history of prior irradiation of the kidney).

Case Point 24.3

The patient is scheduled for surgery in 2 weeks. A partial nephrectomy is performed, and the specimen is sent for histopathologic analysis.

What are the morphologic features of the various types of renal tumors?
Malignant tumors include CCRCC, PRCC, chromophobe RCC, and nephroblastoma. Benign tumors include oncocytoma and angiomyolipoma (AML).

Clear Cell Renal Cell Carcinoma

CCRCC is the most common (60%–70%) and most aggressive type of RCC. CCRCC exhibits high rates of local invasion, distant metastasis, recurrence, and mortality. The gross tumor is an unencapsulated soft, yellow, friable mass (Fig. 24.2A). Areas of cystic degeneration, hemorrhage, necrosis, and invasion of the renal vein are common. On histology, there is a nonpapillary, organoid arrangement of the tumor with division into lobules bordered by well-vascularized fibrous septa (Fig. 24.2B). The tumor cells are polygonal, and the cytoplasm may appear clear (due to abundant intracytoplasmic glycogen or lipid) or granular and eosinophilic (due to ample mitochondria).

Papillary Renal Cell Carcinoma

PRCC is the second most common type (10–20%) of RCC. PRCC is more frequently bilateral and multifocal than other types of RCC. The gross tumor is a circumscribed yellow-to-dark brown intracortical mass. A surrounding fibrous pseudocapsule (30% of cases) and areas of hemorrhage and necrosis may be seen. On microscopy, most tumors have a papillary architecture with foamy macrophages within fibrovascular cores that are lined by neoplastic epithelium (Fig. 24.3A). In 50% of cases, other architectural patterns including solid, trabecular, and tubular may coexist with areas of papillary growth. Psammoma bodies may be seen (Fig. 24.3B).

Chromophobe Renal Cell Carcinoma

Chromophobe RCC demonstrates a relatively better prognosis than other types of RCC. Macroscopically it is a circumscribed but unencapsulated light tan lobulated mass. A central scar and

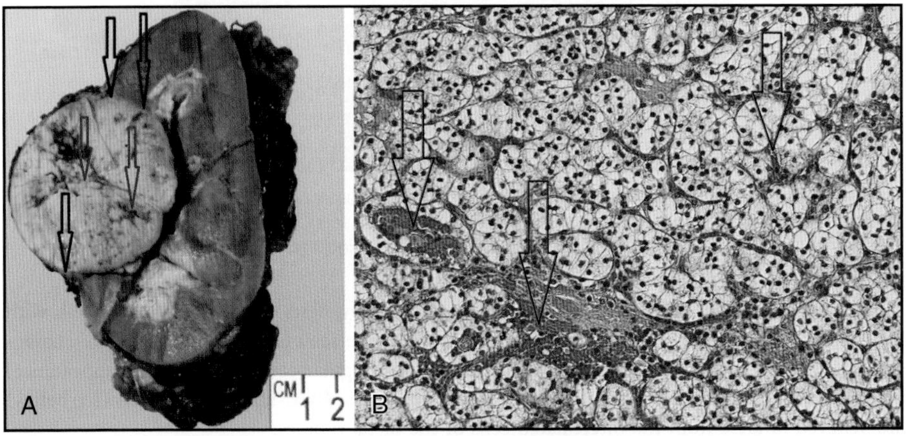

Fig. 24.2 (A) A radical nephrectomy specimen showing a clear cell renal cell carcinoma in the hilum of the kidney. The tumor is circumscribed (black arrows) but not encapsulated. The bright yellow appearance is due to the intracellular accumulation of glycogen and lipid. White-gray scars (red arrows) are present on the cut surface. (B) Under the microscope, the tumor cells of this clear cell RCC have clear cytoplasm and uniform small nuclei. The rich vascularity (black arrows) within the fibrous septa is a characteristic and useful feature in the differentiation from mimics, especially in the metastatic setting (H&E 200x).

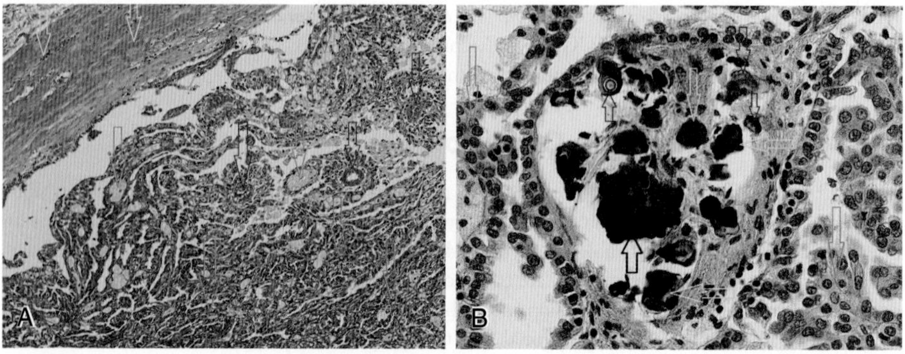

Fig. 24.3 (A) Papillary renal cell carcinoma (PRCC). Well-formed papillae with fibrovascular cores (red arrows) containing foamy macrophages (blue arrows) are seen. Other areas show tightly packed papillae (green arrows) imparting a more solid appearance. PRCCs may also have areas with other architectural configurations like solid, tubular, tubulopapillary, papillary-trabecular, and glomeruloid. Note the surrounding pseudocapsule of compressed fibrous and epithelial tissues (yellow arrows) (H&E 100x). (B) High-power view of psammoma bodies in a PRCC. Psammoma bodies are round, concentrically lamellated concretions of calcium that form from dystrophic calcification of tumor cells in the tips of papillae. A tight aggregate (black arrow), less tightly packed groups (yellow arrows), and individual forms (red arrows) are seen. Neoplastic cells of the PRCC (blue arrows) are seen in the background (H&E 400x).

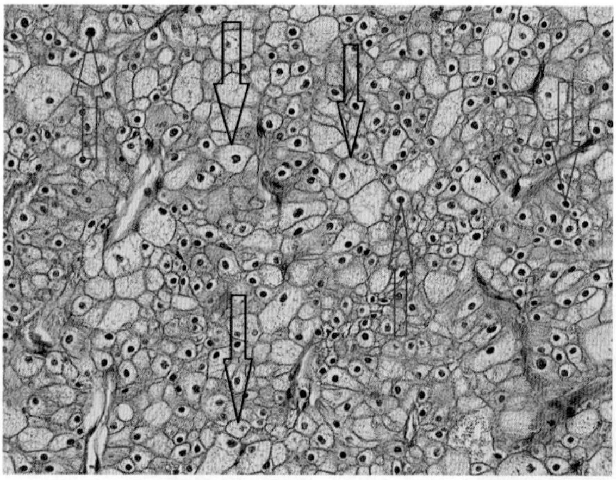

Fig. 24.4 Chromophobe renal cell carcinoma. Sheets of polygonal tumor cells containing an admixture of larger paler cells and smaller cells with greater cytoplasmic eosinophilia are seen. The cell membranes are well-defined (black arrows) and a corona of clear cytoplasm surrounds each raisinoid nucleus (blue arrows) (H&E 200x).

areas of necrosis are seen in 15%–20% cases. On microscopy, nests of polygonal tumor cells with pale eosinophilic cytoplasm and prominent cell borders are seen (Fig. 24.4). Nuclei are characteristically hyperchromatic and appear condensed with irregular contours (raisinoid appearance) and are surrounded by perinuclear halos. Both chromophobe RCC and oncocytomas (see below) are believed to arise from the intercalated cells of the distal tubules.

Nephroblastoma (WT)

WT accounts for 85%–90% of pediatric renal tumors. Majority of cases (90%) occur in patients aged ≤6 years. Most patients are brought to attention by a parent or caregiver as an asymptomatic

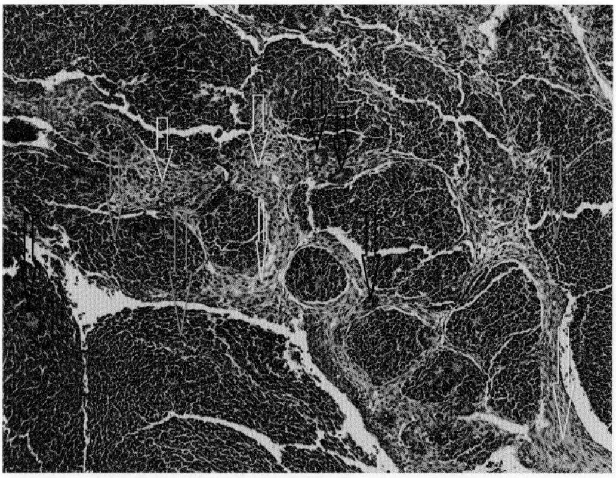

Fig. 24.5 Wilms tumor. A classic triphasic tumor with epithelial (black arrows), blastemal (green arrows), and stromal components (yellow arrows) is seen. The blastemal component is usually mitotically active (not discernible at this magnification). Biphasic or monophasic tumors also occur (H&E 100x).

flank or abdominal mass. About 20% of patients are symptomatic with abdominal pain, fever, loss of appetite, hematuria, anemia, or hypertension. WT is believed to occur from the malignant transformation of abnormally persistent embryonal renal cells (nephrogenic rests).

The gross tumor is a circumscribed friable, light gray mass. Five percent to 10% of tumors are bilateral and/or multifocal. Areas of hemorrhage, necrosis, or cystic degeneration may be present. Histologically, tumors most commonly recapitulate normal renal tissue with a mixture of epithelial, stromal, and blastemal components (Fig. 24.5). Biphasic or even monophasic tumors may occur.

WT is an aggressive neoplasm with metastatic spread most frequently to abdominal lymph nodes, lung, and liver.

Oncocytoma

Oncocytoma accounts for 4%–10% of renal epithelial tumors. Although benign, oncocytomas are important because differentiation from RCC can be challenging clinically, on imaging, and on microscopy. Grossly, oncocytoma is a circumscribed mahogany brown tumor. A central scar is present in up to one-third of cases. On histology, polygonal acidophilic cells with abundant granular cytoplasm and regular round nuclei are arranged in small nests and tubules within a myxoid or hyalinized stroma (Fig. 24.6).

Angiomyolipoma

AML is the most common benign renal tumor. AML is fittingly named for its composition of blood vessels, smooth muscle, and adipose tissue (Fig. 24.7). Most cases are sporadic, but up to 20% of cases occur in association with tuberous sclerosis or pulmonary lymphangioleiomyomatosis. The importance of AML lies in its differentiation from other renal neoplasms and the risk of clinically significant bleeding with increasing size.

Secondary Tumors

The kidney is an infrequent site of seeding of metastatic tumors. Potentially any malignant neoplasm could spread to the kidney, but the most commonly encountered secondary tumors are melanomas, and tumors of the lung, breast, gastrointestinal, and hematolymphoid systems.

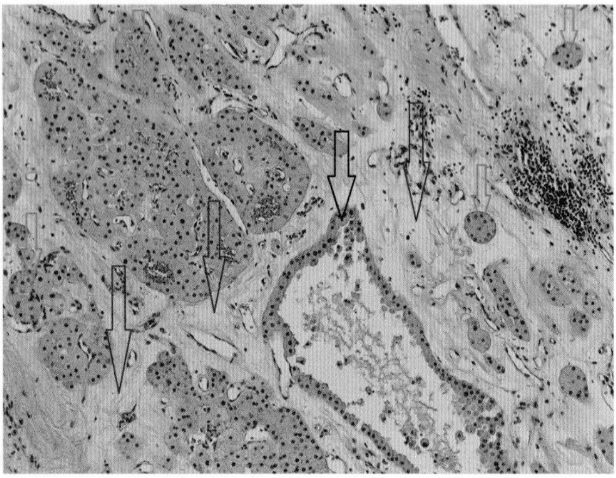

Fig. 24.6 Oncocytoma. Neoplastic cells form solid clusters (green arrows) and tubulocystic structures (black arrow) within a myxoid stroma (red arrows). The cells show abundant granular eosinophilic cytoplasm and round and uniform central nuclei (H&E 100x).

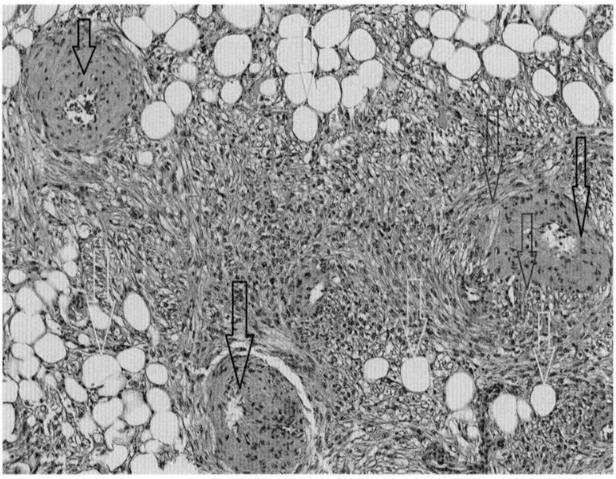

Fig. 24.7 Angiomyolipoma. The micrograph shows a prototypic triphasic tumor with vascular (black arrows), smooth muscle (green arrows), and adipocytic (yellow arrows) components. Radiation of smooth muscle from the wall of the blood vessels (blue arrows) is a characteristic feature of these neoplasms (H&E 100x).

What is the role of immunohistochemistry in the diagnosis of renal tumors?

Different renal neoplasms may demonstrate different immunohistochemical staining patterns that may help clarify the histologic subtype (Table 24.2).

Case Point 23.4

The patient presents for a follow-up 2 weeks after surgery. She feels well. Physical examination is unremarkable, except for well-healed surgical incision sites. Her complete blood count is normal. Her physician discusses the surgical pathology report, which states that the tumor is a stage I CCRCC. He also discusses her prognosis.

TABLE 24.2 ■ **Immunohistochemical Staining Patterns and Molecular Features of Common Renal Neoplasms**

Tumor	Immunohistochemical Profile	Cytogenetic/Molecular Features
Clear cell RCC	Positive for CAIX	3p deletion involving the VHL gene
Papillary RCC	Positive for CK7 and racemase; CAIX negative	Gain of chromosomes 3q, 7, 17, 12, 16, 20
Chromophobe RCC	Positive for CK7 (diffuse) and c-kit	Loss of chromosomes 1, 2, 6, 10, 13, 17, and 21
Oncocytoma	Positive for CK7 (patchy)	Loss of chromosomes Y and 1
Angiomyolipoma	Positive for melanoma markers: (HMB45 and Melan A), and muscle markers (actin and desmin). Negative for CKs	Genetic alterations in TSC1 (9q34) and TSC2 (16p13.3)
Nephroblastoma	Epithelial component positive for CK7, pax-8, and pax-2; blastemal and epithelial components positive for WT1; blastema may be positive for desmin.	WT1 (11p13) deletions or point mutations; WT2 (11p15) alterations; LOH for chromosomes 1p and 16q (associated with poor prognosis)

CK, cytokeratin; *LOH,* loss of heterozygosity; *RCC,* renal cell carcinoma; *WT,* Wilms tumor.

What are the prognostic factors in renal tumors?

Prognostic factors for RCC include the anatomic extent of disease as highlighted in the American Joint Committee on Cancer tumor-node-metastasis staging of RCC (Table 24.3). Other prognostic factors for RCC include the nuclear grade and the histologic type. Venous involvement, sarcomatoid or rhabdoid differentiation, histologic tumor necrosis, adrenal gland involvement, invasion of the urinary collecting system, and extension into the perinephric fat or renal sinus tissues are associated with poor outcomes in RCC.

Unfavorable prognostic factors in WT include age more than 2 years, diffuse anaplasia on histology, and loss of heterozygosity at chromosomes 1p and 16q.

How are renal tumors treated?

Management of renal cell carcinoma

Treatment options vary depending on several factors, including the size of the primary tumor, stage, and the presence of comorbidities. In patients fit enough for surgery, localized (stages I, II, and III) disease can be managed with resection of the tumor by either a radical or partial nephrectomy. Surgery is advised for multifocal disease. Periodic postresection surveillance with imaging should be performed. Tumors < 4 cm, especially those < 2 cm, have a low risk of spread; thus, although complete resection is preferred, nonsurgical treatment may be employed for these small lesions in patients who are not fit for surgery. Nonsurgical options include ablative procedures, such as cryoablation and radiofrequency ablation. Noninvasive approaches include tumor surveillance with serial CT scans and ultrasonograms. Unresectable locally advanced or systemic disease is managed with immunotherapeutic agents, molecularly targeted drugs, and radiotherapy.

Management of Nephroblastoma

The Childrens' Oncology Group guidelines recommend primary tumor resection before adjuvant chemotherapy, except in specific situations like synchronous bilateral disease. The specifics of drug therapy are guided by several factors, including the stage and status of unfavorable histologic factors. Agents utilized include actinomycin D, vincristine, cyclophosphamide, and etoposide. Targeted radiotherapy may be used for metastatic disease.

TABLE 24.3 ■ **American Joint Committee on Cancer Stage Grouping and Prognosis of Renal Cell Carcinoma**

Stage	Stage Grouping	Features	Prognosis
I	**T1, N0, M0**	The tumor is ≤7 cm and limited to the kidney (T1) without metastasis to regional lymph nodes (N0) or distant organs (M0).	Over 90% 5-year survival rate
II	**T2, N0, M0**	The tumor is >7 cm and is limited to the kidney (T2) without metastasis to regional lymph nodes (N0) or distant organs (M0).	75%–95% 5-year survival rate
III	**T3, N0, M0**	The tumor invades into a major vein (e.g., renal vein or vena cava) or into perinephric tissues, but not into the ipsilateral adrenal gland and not beyond Gerota's fascia (T3). There is no metastasis to regional lymph nodes (N0) or distant organs (M0).	59%–70% 5-year survival rate
	OR		
	T1 to T3, N1, M0	A primary tumor of any size which may extend outside the kidney, but not beyond Gerota fascia (T1, T2 or T3). There is metastasis to regional lymph nodes (N1), but no spread to distant lymph nodes or other organs (M0).	
IV	**T4, Any N, M0**	There is direct extension of the primary tumor beyond Gerota fascia or into the ipsilateral adrenal gland (T4). There may or may not be metastasis to regional lymph nodes (any N), but there is neither spread to distant lymph nodes nor distant organs (M0).	Median survival of 13 months (when treated with cytokines) or up to 29 months with treatment with newer molecularly targeted agents
	OR		
	Any T, Any N, M1	A primary tumor of any size, confined to the kidney or with direct extension outside the kidney (any T). There may or may not be metastasis to regional lymph nodes (any N). There is involvement of distant lymph nodes and/or other organs (M1).	

Management of Benign Tumors

Size and symptoms guide the management of AMLs. Tumors <4 cm are monitored with periodic imaging. Resection, embolization, or ablation is performed for larger or symptomatic tumors. Oncocytomas are cured by complete resection.

BEYOND THE PEARLS

- In CCRCC and PRCC, worse clinical outcomes are predicted by increasing nuclear grades. Nuclear grades 1-3 are defined by nucleolar prominence. Grade 4 tumors exhibit extreme nuclear pleomorphism, sarcomatoid and/or rhabdoid differentiation.
- Unclassified RCC is a diagnostic category comprised of primary malignant renal epithelial neoplasms that cannot be further classified into any of the recognized subtypes of RCC - they are distinguished for being distinguished. This motley ensemble features mixed tumors of multiple recognized subtypes, unclassified oncocytic neoplasms, and tumors with pure rhabdoid or sarcomatoid morphology.
- Syndromes associated with WT include the WAGR syndrome (WT, Aniridia, Genitourinary anomalies, and mental Retardation), Denys–Drash syndrome (WT, nephropathy, pseudo- or true hermaphroditism, and genital anomalies), and Beckwith–Wiedemann syndrome (embryonal tumors e.g., WT, macrosomia, hemihypertrophy, macroglossia, omphalocele, and visceromegaly).
- Paraneoplastic syndromes occur in 10% to 40% of patients with RCC. These include hypercalcemia (due to the elaboration of parathyroid hormone-related peptide), hypertension (due to

several mechanisms including, increased secretion of renin and polycythemia), polycythemia (due to the production of EPO), and Stauffer syndrome (hepatic dysfunction due to release of IL-6). Paraneoplastic syndromes may be the initial presentation of renal malignancies but are not necessarily markers of poor prognosis.

- Papillary adenomas are small tumors (≤5 mm) with morphologic similarity to PRCC. These indolent tumors do not progress to carcinoma. They are frequently seen in patients aged 65 years and older, in patients with acquired renal cystic disease, and in association with tobacco smoking. Like PRCC, papillary adenomas also show trisomy of chromosomes 7 and 17.
- PRCC is further classified into two groups: type 1 and type 2. Type 1 PRCC harbors a defining group of genetic alterations, e.g., gain of chromosome 7 and 17. Type 2 PRCC is characterized morphologically by cells with abundant pink cytoplasm and higher grade, pseudostratified nuclei. Unlike type 1 PRCC, type 2 PRCC does not have signature genetic alterations.
- Factors associated with poor prognosis in CCRCC include high Ki-67 proliferative index (>10%), low CAIX staining (≤85%), elevated serum levels of VEGF, high levels of HIF-1a expression, and loss of chromosomes 4p, 9p, and 14q.2. However, none of these factors is currently utilized in routine practice.

Case Point 24.5

No further treatment is administered. She is scheduled for a chest and abdominal CT scan in 6 months and a follow-up visit with the imaging results.

How are patients with RCC followed up?

Stage I disease: History and physical examination, urinalysis, serum BUN, and creatinine are performed at 6, 12, 24, and 36 months after tumor resection in all patients. Patients who had a partial nephrectomy undergo surveillance with abdominal CT or MRI at 6 months, followed by abdominal CT, MRI, or US at 12, 24, and 36 months. If a radical nephrectomy was performed, abdominal CT or MRI is performed at 6 months. Further follow-up and added surveillance with chest, central nervous system, bone, and pelvic imaging and laboratory tests are performed as clinically indicated.

Stage II–IV disease: History and physical examination, urinalysis, serum BUN, and creatinine are performed every 6 months for 5 years. Abdominal CT or MRI and chest CT are performed at 6 months. Following this, surveillance is with abdominal CT, MRI, or US and chest CT or radiograph every 6 months until 5 years. Further follow-up and added surveillance with central nervous system, bone, pelvic imaging, and laboratory tests are performed as clinically indicated.

References

Cao C, Bi X, Liang J, et al. Long-term survival and prognostic factors for locally advanced renal cell carcinoma with renal vein tumor thrombus. *BMC Cancer.* 2019;19;144.

Finley DS, Pantuck AJ, Belldegrun AS. Tumor biology and prognostic factors in renal cell carcinoma. *Oncologist.* 2011;16(suppl 2):4-13.

Haas NB, Nathanson KL. Hereditary renal cancer syndromes. *Adv Chronic Kidney Dis.* 2014;21;81-90.

Mills SE, Greenson JK, Hornick JL, Longacre TA, Reuter VE, Sternberg SS. Chapter 42: Adult renal tumors. In: *Sternberg's Diagnostic Surgical Pathology.* Philadelphia, PA: Wolters Kluwer Lippincott Williams & Wilkins; 2015.

Phelps HM, Kaviany S, Borinstein SC, Lovvorn HN, III. Biological drivers of Wilms tumor prognosis and treatment. *Children (Basel).* 2018;5:E145.

Saad AM, Gad MM, Al-Husseini MJ, Ruhban IA, Sonbol MB, Ho TH. Trends in renal-cell carcinoma incidence and mortality in the united states in the last 2 decades: A seer-based study. *Clin Genitourin Cancer.* 2019;17:46-57.e5.

CASE 25

A 63-Year-Old Male with Urinary Frequency and Gross Hematuria

Maria Cecilia D. Reyes

A 63-year-old male, current smoker, visited the outpatient urology clinic with complaints of urinary frequency at night and seeing blood in his urine. He has no known significant medical history and has not changed his exercise or diet program recently. He states that he has not experienced any physical trauma and has no pain on palpation of the lower pelvis. His cell counts with differential and chemistry panel are within normal limits. Gross hematuria is observed. His current vital signs are blood pressure of 140/79 mm Hg and pulse rate of 85 beats per minute. His urinalysis is positive for nitrites and blood, and urine protein is 100 mg/dL. The patient subsequently undergoes an ultrasound of the urinary bladder showing circumferential wall thickening.

What can be causes of hematuria?
The causes of hematuria may include urinary tract infection, medical renal disease, lithiasis, and urologic tumor.

CLINICAL PEARL

The American Urologic Association guideline for microhematuria is ≥3 red blood cells per high-power field. The causes of microhematuria and gross hematuria are similar.

What is the anatomy of the urinary bladder?
The urinary bladder is shaped like an inverted pyramid. The dome is the superior surface and is covered on the outside by peritoneum. The area in the base of the bladder between the ureteral orifices and the opening of the urethra is called the trigone (Fig. 25.1). The bladder neck is the distal portion of the bladder before it empties into the urethra. The layers of the urinary bladder include a mucosal urothelial lining, lamina propria, muscularis propria, and adventitia.

Case Point 25.1

The patient's urine specimen is collected and submitted to cytology for evaluation. The test preparation demonstrates large urothelial cells with irregular, hyperchromatic nuclei (Fig. 25.2). Some of the cells have a nuclear-to-cytoplasmic (N:C) ratio of >0.7.

What are the criteria for adequacy of urine specimens?
A volume cutoff of 30 mL is appropriate for unfixed voided specimens with a SurePath preparation. For bladder barbotage specimens, the criteria are based on the number of well-preserved, well-visualized urothelial cells per 10 high-power fields (Table 25.1). After the cytology specimen

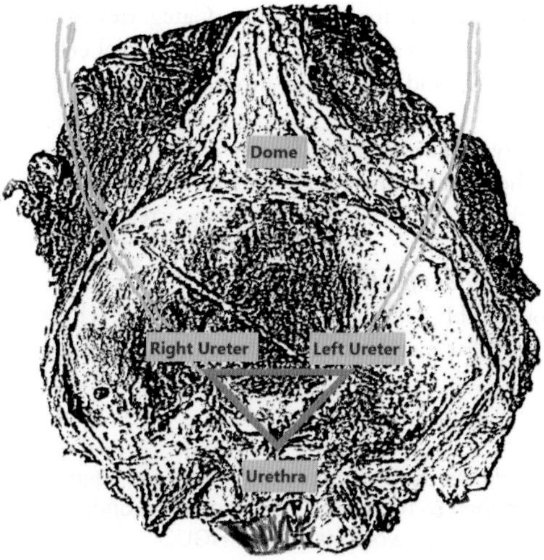

Fig. 25.1 Anatomy of the urinary bladder showing the dome, trigone (inverted triangle), ureters, and urethra.

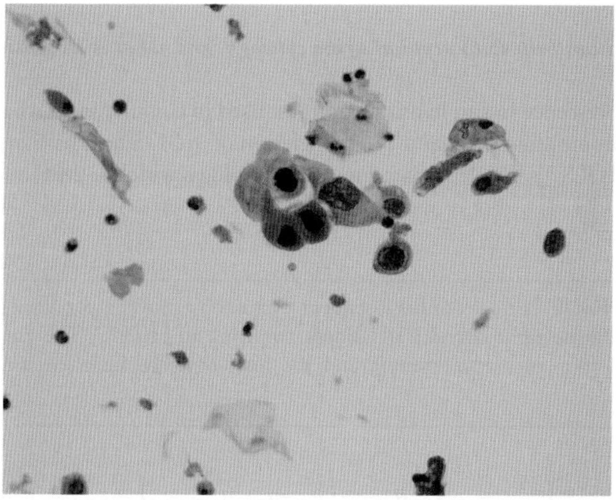

Fig. 25.2 Cells with high nuclear-to-cytoplasmic ratio, hyperchromasia, nuclear irregularity, and clumped chromatin (Pap 400x).

TABLE 25.1 ■ **Criteria for Adequacy in Bladder Washes**

Number of Well-Preserved, Well-Visualized Urothelial Cells per 10 High-Power Fields	Adequacy
>20	Satisfactory
10–20	Satisfactory but limited
<10	Unsatisfactory

is deemed adequate, it is evaluated for malignancy. Categories in urine cytology may include negative for high-grade urothelial carcinoma, atypical urothelial cells, suspicious for high-grade urothelial carcinoma (HGUC), and high-grade urothelial carcinoma.

What are the criteria for atypical urothelial cells on cytology?
Criteria for atypical urothelial cells on cytology include an N:C ratio of >0.5 and one of the following criteria: 1) hyperchromasia, 2) nuclear membrane irregularity, and 3) clumped chromatin.

What are the criteria for suspicious for HGUC?
The criteria for suspicious for HGUC include an N:C ratio >0.7, hyperchromasia (required), and one of the following: 1) nuclear membrane irregularity or 2) clumped chromatin.

CLINICAL PEARL

A quantity cutoff is sometimes used to differentiate between suspicious for HGUC and HGUC on cytology. Less than 5–10 atypical cells would fall under suspicious for HGUC and having at least 5-10 atypical cells would fall under HGUC.

What are the criteria for positive for HGUC?
The criteria for positive for HGUC include an N:C ratio of >0.7, hyperchromasia, clumped chromatin, and nuclear irregularity.

What ancillary test can help with atypical urine cytology, and what is its sensitivity for detecting HGUC?
UroVysion is a fluorescence in situ hybridization test used in conjunction with urine cytology that detects gains of chromosomes 3, 7, and 17 and deletion of 9p21. The sensitivity of UroVysion for the diagnosis of HGUC is 60% compared to urine cytology, which is 28%.

Case Point 25.2

A diagnosis of HGUC is made, and subsequent cystoscopy shows a papillary lesion measuring 8 × 5 × 3 cm on the right lateral wall. Biopsy confirms an HGUC. The patient undergoes a transurethral resection of bladder tumor, and the histologic specimen confirms a noninvasive HGUC (Fig. 25.3).

What are the differential diagnoses for flat and papillary lesions of the urinary bladder?

Flat Lesions

Flat urothelial hyperplasia is an increase in the thickness of urothelial mucosa compared with adjacent normal urothelium without atypia. It is seen in association with lithiasis, inflammatory disorders, papillary urothelial hyperplasia, dysplasia, carcinoma in situ (CIS), and low-grade papillary tumors. It is without malignant potential. No treatment is necessary if it is not associated with a urothelial neoplasm. It shares similar molecular abnormalities as low-grade papillary urothelial carcinomas, such as chromosome 9q deletions, and mutations in FGFR3 gene.

Flat urothelial dysplasia is a lesion with cytologic atypia that is considered to be preneoplastic, but these changes are insufficient for the diagnosis of CIS. The atypia can include loss of polarity and nuclear crowding. There is usually no denudation of the epithelium. Umbrellas cells are present; the atypia is present in the intermediate and basal cell layers. Mitotic figures are located basally when present. Aberrant expression of CK20 and overexpression of p53 and Ki-67

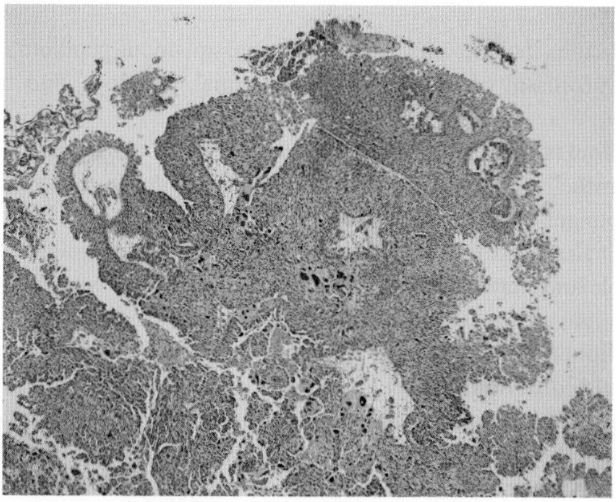

Fig. 25.3 Transurethral resection showing high-grade papillary urothelial carcinoma (H&E 40x) with large pleomorphic nuclei.

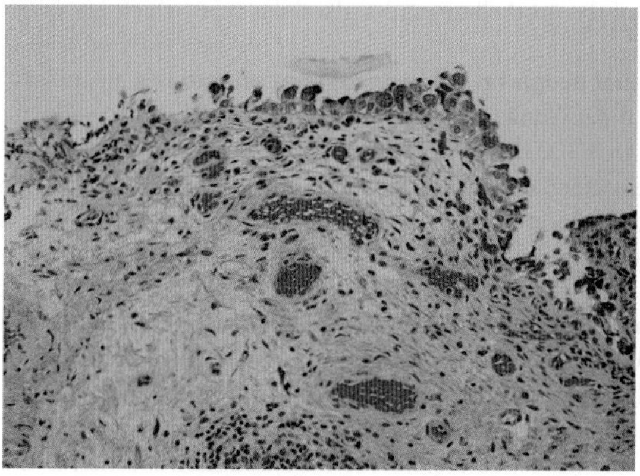

Fig. 25.4 Urothelial carcinoma in situ with adjacent area of denudation (H&E 200x). Nuclei are more than 5x the size of the stromal lymphocytes.

are helpful diagnostic clues. Patients with flat urothelial dysplasia require close follow-up for the development of urothelial CIS.

Urothelial CIS is composed of cells with severe atypia. It may or may not involve the full thickness of the urothelial lining and occurs during the fifth to sixth decade. Symptoms include hematuria, dysuria, frequency, or urgency. It is usually multifocal. Histologic features include crowding, loss of polarity, pleomorphism, and hyperchromatic nuclei enlarged to $\geq$ 5× the size of a stromal lymphocyte (Fig. 25.4). Normal urothelium has nuclei that are 2–3× the size of a stromal lymphocyte. CK 20 and P53 are diffusely positive throughout all layers of the urothelium in urothelial CIS, while CD44 staining is absent, which can be helpful in distinguishing urothelial CIS from reactive urothelial atypia. The current treatment for urothelial CIS is intravesicular Bacillus Calmette-Guérin (BCG) immunotherapy.

CLINICAL PEARL

A combination of diffuse positivity of CD20 throughout all layers of the urothelial and absent CD44 staining can help in the diagnosis of CIS.

Papillary Lesions

Papillary urothelial lesions includes urothelial papilloma, squamous papilloma, inverted papilloma, papillary urothelial neoplasm of low malignant potential, and low- and high-grade papillary urothelial carcinoma.

Urothelial papillomas are exophytic urothelial neoplasms consisting of papillary structures lined by a normal urothelial lining. These lesions have an incidence of 1%–4% bladder tumors. It usually occurs in younger patients, with a slight male predominance. Histologically, urothelial papillomas consist of slender papillary fronds lined by a normal urothelium. Superficial umbrella cells should be visible and may be prominent (Fig. 25.5). Mitotic figures are typically absent or rare. Cytoplasm can range from pale to eosinophilic to vacuolated.

Squamous papilloma is the squamous equivalent of urothelial papilloma. It occurs in elderly women and is not related to human papillomavirus.

Inverted papillomas are benign endophytic urothelial neoplasms involving the lamina propria. These lesions have a peak incidence between the sixth and seventh decade, with a male-to-female ratio of 7.3:1 and an association with smoking, chronic urinary bladder infection, and urinary tract obstruction. Most lesions are solitary. Grossly, it is sessile, pedunculated, or polypoid. Histologically, it has anastomosing cords and islands of normal urothelium invaginating downward into the stroma with minimal to no cytologic atypia (Fig. 25.6). There is a trabecular type, which originates from the basal cells of the urothelium, and a glandular type, which has overlapping features with cystitis glandularis.

Papillary urothelial neoplasm of low malignant potential is a papillary urothelial neoplasm resembling urothelial papilloma; however, there is increased thickness in the lining urothelium. These lesions occur in 3/100,000 individuals per year, usually in the lateral and posterior walls of the bladder near the ureteral orifices. It is a borderline tumor with minimal risk of recurrence and progression. It occurs predominantly in males at a mean age of diagnosis of 64.6 years. Biopsy sample shows discrete, slender papillae with thickened multilayered urothelium and minimal to no cytologic atypia (Fig. 25.7). The treatment of choice is transurethral resection.

Low-grade noninvasive papillary urothelial carcinoma is a papillary urothelial neoplasm that displays distinct architectural and cytologic variation but has an overall orderly appearance of the urothelium. These lesions have an incidence of 5/100,000 individuals per year. It has a male predominance with a mean age of diagnosis of 69.2 years. Invasion occurs in $<5\%$ of cases. It is usually a single lesion in most cases, and the most common location is the posterior or lateral walls of the bladder near the ureteral orifices. The lesion contains papillary fronds with nuclei that are enlarged but only have mild differences in shape (Fig. 25.8). Mitoses can be present in the

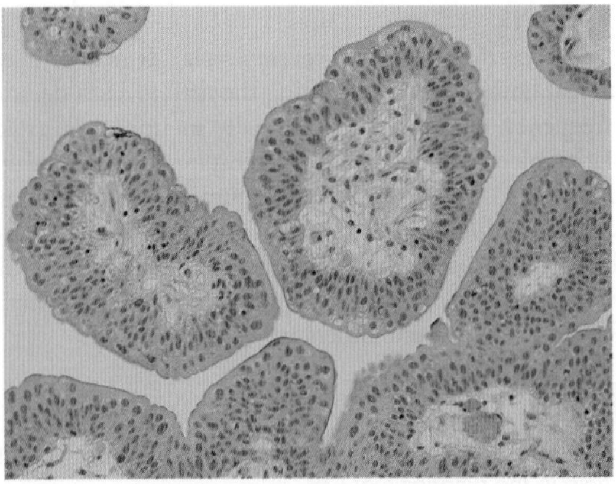

Fig. 25.5 Urothelial papilloma. Papillary fronds lined by normal urothelium with visible umbrella cells (H&E 200x).

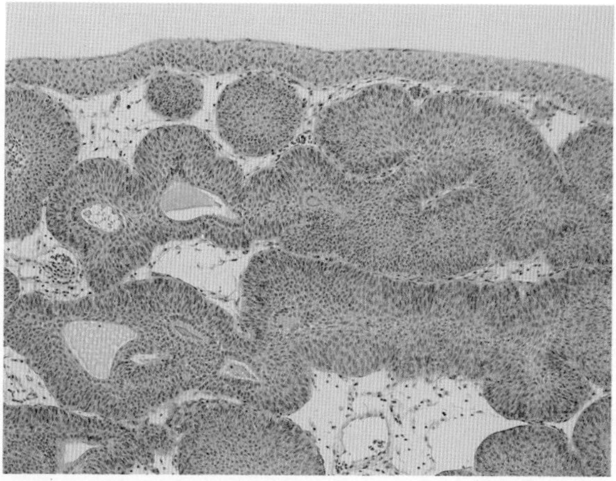

Fig. 25.6 Inverted papilloma showing a downward invagination of anastomosing normal urothelium (H&E 100x).

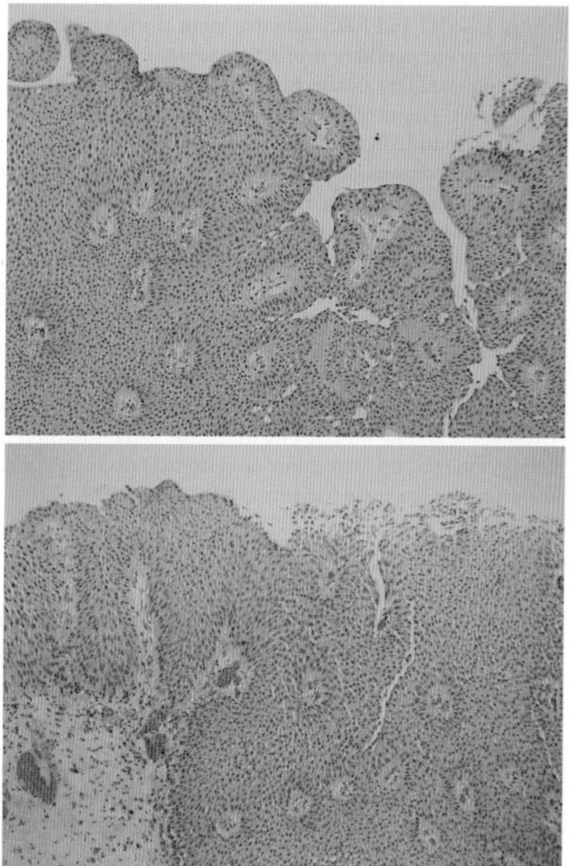

Fig. 25.7 Papillary urothelial neoplasm of low malignant potential showing papillary architecture (A, H&E x 100) and thickened urothelium with minimal cytologic atypia (B, H&E x 100).

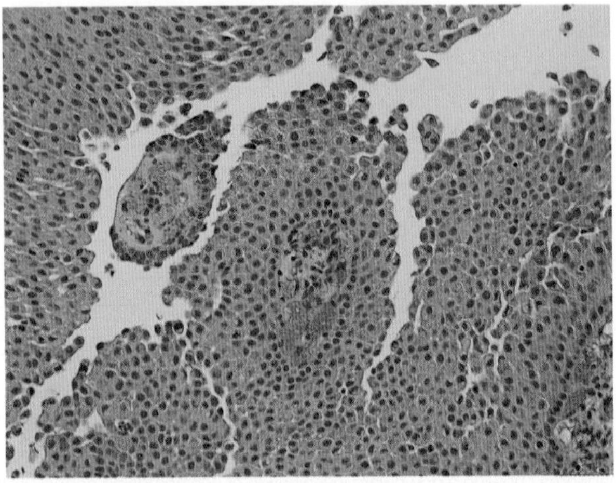

Fig. 25.8 Noninvasive low-grade papillary urothelial carcinoma with abnormal cellular polarization and nuclei with only mild differences in shape. (H&E 200x).

lower half of the urothelium. Low-grade papillary urothelial carcinoma is associated with mutations in FGFR3 and RAS. The treatment is transurethral resection.

High-grade papillary urothelial carcinoma is an exophytic growth with a disorderly lining epithelium, papillary architecture that is branching and fused, and cytoarchitectural abnormalities at low power. The neoplastic cells have clumped chromatin, moderately to markedly pleomorphic nuclei, and mitotic figures present at all layers of the urothelium. It has a high risk of progression to invasive carcinoma of 15%–40%. CIS and muscle-invasive bladder carcinomas are associated with mutations in TP53 or RB1.

Invasive urothelial carcinoma is a urothelial neoplasm that invades beyond the basement membrane into underlying structures. The usual demographic of the patient with invasive urothelial carcinoma is a male patient over 50 years old. The risk factors include cigarette smoking and exposure to aromatic amines and aniline dye. Chronic intake of medications with phenacetin is also a risk factor. Urothelial carcinoma can undergo divergent differentiation, squamous and glandular differentiation being the most common. Urothelial carcinoma can also have several variants, including nested, microcystic, micropapillary, lymphoepithelial-like, plasmacytoid, and sarcomatoid, among others. The treatment is transurethral resection with or without intravesical therapy, followed by cystectomy or cystoprostatectomy for muscle-invasive urothelial carcinoma. The prognosis for these patients is stage-dependent.

CLINICAL PEARL

The risk factors for urothelial carcinoma include cigarette smoking, exposure to aromatic amines and aniline dye, and chronic intake of phenacetin.

CLINICAL PEARL

Low-grade urothelial carcinomas are associated with mutations in FGFR3 and RAS where as muscle-invasive HGUC and urothelial CIS are associated with mutations in TP53 or RB1.

Squamous cell carcinoma of the urinary bladder accounts for 75% of bladder cancers where *Schistosoma haematobium* infection is endemic, such as in Egypt and parts of Africa. This diagnosis is reserved for pure squamous tumors.

Case Point 25.3

The patient undergoes six cycles of intravesical BCG therapy and surveillance cystoscopy.

After 1 year of surveillance, he develops a recurrence of urothelial carcinoma, this time muscle-invasive urothelial carcinoma (Fig. 25.9). Over 2 months, the patient completes four cycles of neoadjuvant cisplatin and gemcitabine. A month after completion of the neoadjuvant chemotherapy, the patient undergoes a robot-assisted radical cystoprostatectomy with lymph node dissection (Fig. 25.10). The tumor is staged as a pT3PN2.

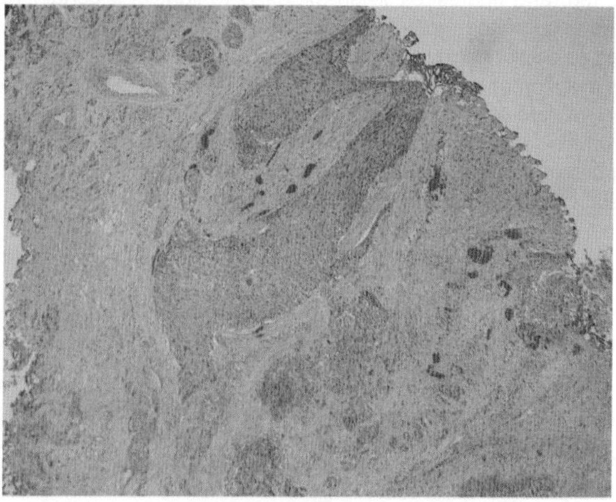

Fig. 25.9 Muscle-invasive urothelial carcinoma (H&E × 40).

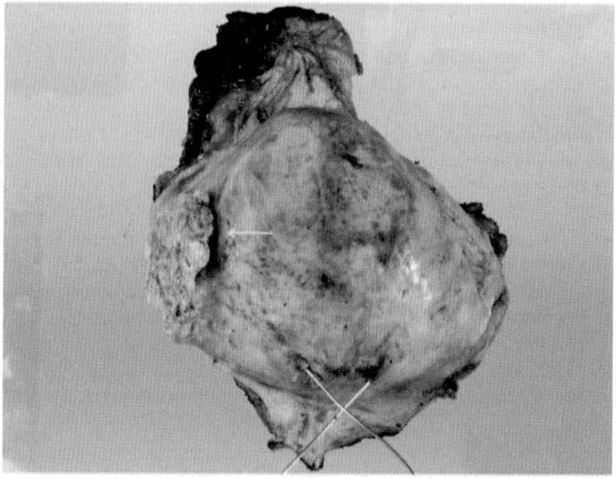

Fig. 25.10 Gross specimen showing an 8 × 5 × 3 cm tumor on the right lateral wall of the urinary bladder (arrow).

What is the staging of urothelial carcinoma?

The staging of urothelial carcinoma is based on the extent of invasion into the lamina propria, muscularis propria, perivesical soft tissue, and extravesical extension (Table 25.2).

Case Point 25.4

The patient continues to undergo surveillance (cystoscopy and urine cytology) at gradually increasing intervals.

BEYOND THE PEARLS

- Photodynamic diagnosis is the introduction of an exogenous photosensitizer to the body, such as 5-aminolevulinic acid or hexaminolevulinate, which is absorbed by the bladder surface, is excited, and fluoresces when exposed to light of a certain wavelength. These photosensitizers accumulate more in dysplastic or malignant cells than in normal cells and have been used to detect flat dysplastic epithelium and CIS.
- Progression to invasion of noninvasive HGUC is 15%–40%.
- The 5-year survival rate of a T1 lesion is 70%.
- Upper tract urothelial carcinomas account for less than 10% of bladder tumors.
- The more aggressive variants of urothelial carcinoma include micropapillary variant, sarcomatoid urothelial carcinoma, and nested variant.

TABLE 25.2 ■ **Pathologic Staging of Urothelial Carcinoma**

T	pTX: Primary tumor cannot be assessed pT0: No evidence of primary tumor pTa: Noninvasive papillary carcinoma pTis: Urothelial carcinoma in situ pT1: Tumor invades lamina propria pT2: Tumor invades muscularis propria pT2a: Tumor invades superficial muscularis propria (inner half) pT2b: Tumor invades deep muscularis propria (outer half) pT3: Tumor invades perivesical soft tissue pT3a: Tumor invades perivesical soft tissue microscopically pT3b: Tumor invades perivesical soft tissue macroscopically (extravesical mass) pT4: Extravesical tumor directly invades any of the following: prostatic stroma, seminal vesicles, uterus, vagina, pelvic wall, abdominal wall pT4a: Extravesical tumor invades directly into prostatic stroma, uterus, or vagina pT4b: Extravesical tumor invades pelvic wall, abdominal wall
N	pNX: Lymph nodes cannot be assessed pN0: No lymph node metastasis pN1: Single regional lymph node metastasis in the true pelvis (perivesical, obturator, internal and external iliac or sacral lymph node) pN2: Multiple regional lymph node metastasis in the true pelvis (perivesical, obturator, internal and external iliac or sacral lymph node metastasis) pN3: Lymph node metastasis to the common iliac lymph nodes
M (if present pathologically)	pM1: Distant metastasis pM1a: Distant metastasis limited to lymph nodes beyond the common iliacs pM1b: Non-lymph node distant metastases

Data from Paner, with original data from Amin, M., Edge, SB, Greene FL, et al, eds., AJCC Cancer Staging Manual, 8th Edition. 2017, New York, NY: Springer.

References

Amin, M.B., *Histological variants of urothelial carcinoma: diagnostic, therapeutic and prognostic implications. Mod. Pathol.* 2009. 22 Suppl 2: S96-S118.

Barkan GA, Wojcik EM, Nayar R, et al. The Paris system for reporting urinary cytology: the quest to develop a standardized terminology. *Acta Cytol.* 2016;60(3):185-197.

Blanco S, Raber M, Leone BE, Nespoli L, Grasso M. Early detection of urothelial premalignant lesions using hexaminolevulinate fluorescence cystoscopy in high risk patients. *J Transl Med.* 2010;8:122.

Bochenek K, Aebisher D, Międzybrodzka A, Cieślar G, Kawczyk-Krupka A. Methods of bladder cancer diagnostics - the role of autofluorescence and photodynamic diagnosis. *Photodiagnosis Photodyn Ther.* 2019;27:141-148.

Boorjian SA, Raman JD, Barocas DA. Evaluation and management of hematuria. In: Wein AJ, Kavoussi LR, Partin, AW, Peters, CA, eds. *Campbell-Walsh Urology*. Philadelphia, PA: Elsevier; 2016.

Cheng L, Lopez-Beltran A, MacLennan GT, Montroni R, Bostwick DG. Neoplasms of the urinary bladder. In: *Urologic Surgical Pathology Fourth Edition.*, Cheng L, MacLennan GT, Bostwick DG, Editors. Philaldephia, PA: Elsevier, 2020.

Deng F, Melamed J. Nonneoplastic diseases of the urinary bladder. In: Zhou M, Magi-Galluzi C, eds. *Genitourinary Pathology: Foundations in Diagnostic Pathology*. 2nd ed. Philadelphia, PA: Elsevier; 2015:138-180.

Guo A, Liu A, Teng X. The pathology of urinary bladder lesions with an inverted growth pattern. *Chin J Cancer Res.* 2016;28(1):107-121.

Inamura K. Bladder cancer: new insights into its molecular pathology. *Cancers (Basel)*. 2018;10(4):E100.

McKenney JK, Magi-Galluzzi C. Neoplasms of the urinary bladder. In: *Genitourinary Pathology: Foundations in Diagnostic Pathology*. 2nd ed. Zhou M, Magi-Galluzzi C, eds. Philadelphia, PA: Elsevier Saunders; 2015:181-250.

Mirza MT. *Hematuria*. In: Kellerman RD, ed. *Conn's Current Therapy 2020*. Philadelphia, PA: Elsevier; 2020.

Paner, GP, Zhou, M, et al. Protocol for the examination of cystectomy specimens from patients with carcinoma of the urinary bladder. In: *Cancer Protocol Templates*. College of American Pathologist (CAP); February 2020.

Rosenthal DL Wojcik EM, Kurtycz DF. *The Paris System for Reporting Urniary Cytology*. Springer; 2016.

Sassa N, Iwata H, Kato M, et al. Diagnostic utility of UroVysion combined with conventional urinary cytology for urothelial carcinoma of the upper urinary tract. *Am J Clin Pathol.* 2019;151(5):469-478.

Shah JB, Kamat AM. Fluorescence cystoscopy for nonmuscle invasive bladder cancer: is the honeymoon over for the blue light special? *Cancer.* 2011;117(5):882-883.

Solomon JP, Hansel DE. The emerging molecular landscape of urothelial carcinoma. *Surg Pathol Clin.* 2016;9(3):391-404.

Zhang XK, Wang YY, Chen JW, Qin T. Bladder papillary urothelial neoplasm of low malignant potential in Chinese: a clinical and pathological analysis. *Int J Clin Exp Pathol.* 2015;8(5):5549-5555.

CASE 26

A 34-Year-Old Male with Edema

Youssef Al Hmada

A 34-year-old male presents to his primary care physician with a complaint of swelling around his eyes and ankles. He has noticed that his urine looks "foamy." He has no significant past medical history and is on no known medications. He is married and works as a truck driver and has no significant history of smoking, drinking or illicit drug use. Physical examination shows periorbital edema, pitting edema in his ankles, blood pressure of 150/100 mm Hg, and heart rate of 65–70 beats per minute. The remaining physical examination is unremarkable. He is referred for a workup including basic metabolic panel, cell blood count, and urine analysis.

His initial panels of blood and urine workup show a blood albumin level of 2.1 g/dL (normal: 3.4–5.4 g/dL) and urine protein level of 5.1 g/day (normal: <80 mg/day). The cell blood count is within normal limits.

Due to his elevated urine protein levels, he is referred to a nephrologist for renal biopsy.

What are the four components of the kidney?
The kidney is composed of glomeruli, tubules, interstitium, and blood vessels. Kidney diseases can affect one or more of these components.

What does the glomerulus consist of?
The glomerulus consists of an anastomosing network of capillaries lined by fenestrated endothelium. Basement membrane separates the endothelium from the visceral epithelium (podocytes), whereas the parietal epithelium, situated on Bowman's capsule, lines the urinary space.

What is the difference between azotemia and uremia?
Azotemia is an elevation of blood urea nitrogen and creatinine levels, while *uremia* is the clinical manifestation and the systemic biochemical abnormalities caused by azotemia.

What are the symptoms of kidney disease (glomerulonephritis)?
Symptoms of kidney disease include hematuria (blood in urine), proteinuria (foamy urine), edema (swelling around eyes and ankles), and elevated blood pressure.

CLINICAL PEARL

The most common symptoms of kidney diseases include proteinuria, hematuria, and edema.

What is the difference between nephrotic and nephritic syndromes (Table 26.1)***?***
Symptoms of nephritic syndrome include hematuria and proteinuria (<3.5 g/day), whereas nephrotic syndrome is defined by the presence of heavy proteinuria (>3.5 g/day), hypoalbuminemia (<3 g/dL), and peripheral edema. Hyperlipidemia and thrombotic disease are also frequently observed.

TABLE 26.1 ■ **Clinical Syndromes in Glomerular Disease**

Nephrotic Syndrome	Nephritic Syndrome
Severe proteinuria (>3.5 g/day)	Proteinuria (<3.5 g/day)
Generalized edema	Hematuria
Hyperlipidemia	Hypertension
Lipiduria	Azotemia
Hypoalbuminemia (<3 g/dL)	Oliguria

CLINICAL PEARL

Lesions that manifest by nephritic syndromes have proliferation of the cells within the glomeruli and inflammatory cell infiltrate.

What are the primary glomerular diseases?

- Minimal change disease (most common in children)
- Focal segmental glomerulosclerosis
- Membranous nephropathy (MN)
- IgA nephropathy
- Acute postinfectious glomerulonephritis
- Membranoproliferative glomerulonephritis

What are the most common glomerulopathies secondary to systemic disease?

- Lupus nephritis
- Diabetic nephropathy
- Amyloidosis
- Glomerulonephritis secondary to multiple myeloma
- Henoch–Schönlein purpura
- Thrombotic microangiopathy

CLINICAL PEARL

The most common medical kidney disease in adults is focal segmental glomerulosclerosis.

CLINICAL PEARL

What is the most common kidney disease in children?

Minimal change disease.

CLINICAL PEARL

The pathologic findings of minimal change disease with both light microscopy and direct IF reveal no abnormalities, while EM shows uniform and diffuse effacement of podocytes.

CLINICAL PEARL

Patients with minimal change disease respond very well to a short course of corticosteroid therapy.

CLINICAL PEARL

SLE and medications are common causes of secondary MN.

What is the purpose of obtaining a renal biopsy?

The nephrologist uses the renal biopsy results to reach a diagnosis or to follow up a chronic disease with renal involvement, such as systemic lupus erythematosus (SLE).

How is the kidney biopsy processed?

The nephrologist examines the patient, and if necessary, a renal biopsy is sent to the pathologist to reach a definitive diagnosis. Two to four renal core biopsies are usually obtained. The pathologist triages these cores and evaluates the presence of glomeruli via a light microscope. A portion of the renal biopsy is sent for electron microscopy (EM) examination, a core or a portion of the core is saved for direct immunofluorescence (IF) examination, and the rest of the tissue is processed to be examined under the light microscopy with H&E stain.

How does the pathologist reach a diagnosis of renal disease?

The renal pathologist combines the light microscopic, direct IF, and EM findings. The pathology results should be correlated with the clinical findings.

Case Point 26.1

The patient's kidney biopsy shows MN stage 1. The patient is admitted to the hospital, and supportive care with chlorothiazide and benazepril is initiated.

MN

MN is one of the most common causes of the nephrotic syndrome in adults. Most cases are classified as primary (previously idiopathic). Antibodies to the M-type phospholipase A2 receptor (PLA2R), a major antigen expressed on podocytes, are specifically found in a high proportion of patients with primary (idiopathic) MN. Secondary MN is caused by other disorders.

CLINICAL PEARL

MN is characterized by subepithelial (spike and dome pattern) basement membrane deposits by EM.

What are the causes of secondary MN?

- Infections (e.g., chronic hepatitis B)
- Malignant tumors (e.g., melanoma)
- Autoimmune conditions (e.g., SLE)
- Drugs (e.g., captopril)
- Exposure to inorganic salts (e.g., gold)

CLINICAL PEARL

MN, SLE, and poststreptococcal glomerulonephritis are the common kidney diseases with basement membrane immune complex deposits.

What are the light microscopic, direct IF, and EM features of MN?

MN reflects the primary histologic change noted on light microscopy: glomerular basement membrane (GBM) thickening with little or no cellular proliferation (Fig. 26.1). Direct IF shows intense granular membranous deposits for IgG and C3 (Fig. 26.2). EM reveals subepithelial dense deposits with spikes formation (Fig. 26.3).

What is the treatment for primary MN?

The treatment focuses on the symptoms, such as hypertension, edema, and elevated blood cholesterol levels. No specific treatment is available for MN.

CLINICAL PEARL

There is no specific treatment for MN. The current treatment focuses on treating the symptoms.

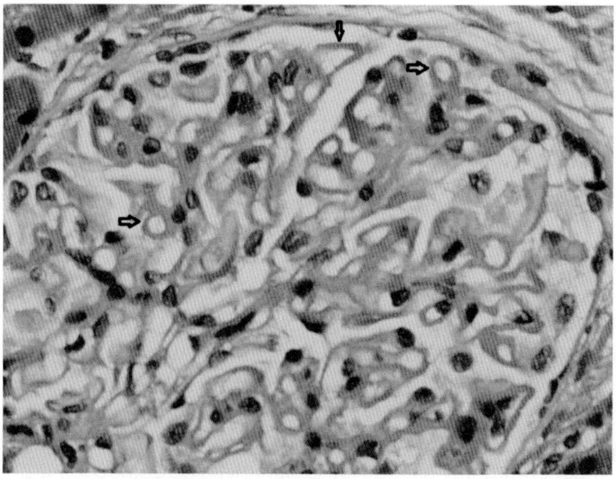

Fig. 26.1 Histopathology of membranous glomerulonephritis with diffuse thickening of glomerular basement membrane (arrows) (courtesy of Dr. Jack Lewin) (H&E, 400x).

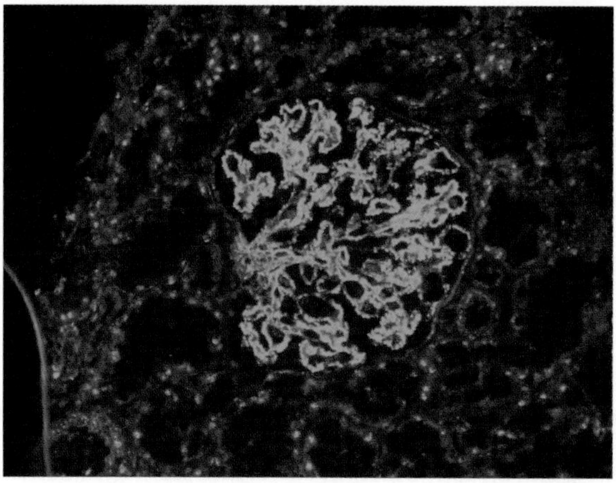

Fig. 26.2 Immunofluorescence for IgG shows granular global subepithelial positivity of the glomerular capillary walls.

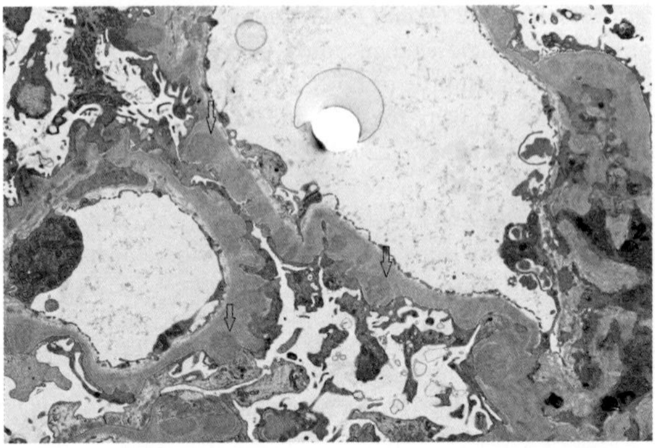

Fig. 26.3 Subepithelial and intramembranous electron dense deposits with intervening glomerular basement membrane spikes (arrows).

What is the treatment for secondary MN?

If the patient is on a medication that causes MN, it is crucial to stop the medication or switch to another medication. In case of a chronic disease (e.g., SLE), treating the underlying disease is the treatment of choice for secondary MN.

BEYOND THE PEARLS

MN is characterized by:

- Light microscopy: Diffuse thickening of the capillary wall with no cell proliferation
- Direct IF: Granular global subepithelial positivity for IgG and C3
- EM: Basement membrane subepithelial deposits (spike and dome pattern)

Acute poststreptococcal glomerulonephritis typically occurs 2–4 weeks after a Streptococcal infection, most commonly caused by B-hemolytic *Streptococci*. It presents with nephritic syndrome with elevated antistreptolysin O titers. IF demonstrates granular deposits of IgG, IgM, and C3 throughout the glomerulus.

Goodpasture syndrome occurs due to the production of antibodies directed against the basement membrane causing damage to the lungs and kidneys. IF shows a smooth and linear pattern of IgG and C3 in the GBM.

Rapidly progressive glomerulonephritis/Crescentic glomerulonephritis has a poor prognosis with progression to renal failure.

IgA nephropathy (Berger disease) is the most common glomerulonephritis in the world, characterized by recurrent hematuria. IF shows mesangial dipositive of IgA and C3.

Membranoproliferative glomerulonephritis affects the glomerular mesangium and basement membranes and has a variable clinical presentation. It is known to have a specific splitting of the basement membrane "tram track" appearance.

References

Beck LH Jr, Bonegio RG, Lambeau G, et al. M-type phospholipase A2 receptor as target antigen in idiopathic membranous nephropathy. *N Engl J Med.* 2009;361(1):11-21.

Fogo AB, Lusco MA, Najafian B, Alpers CE. AJKD atlas of renal pathology: membranous nephropathy. *Am J Kidney Dis.* 2015;66(3):e15-e17.

Hall CL, Jawad S, Harrison PR, et al. Natural course of penicillamine nephropathy: a long term study of 33 patients. *Br Med J (Clin Res Ed)*. 1988;296(6629):1083-1086.
Kumar V, Abbas A, Aster J. Kidney and its collecting system. In: *Robbins and Cotran Basic Pathology*. 9th ed. Philadelphia: Elsevier; 2013:517-549.
Rosenberg AZ, Kopp JB. Focal segmental glomerulosclerosis. *Clin J Am Soc Nephrol*. 2017;12(3):502-517.
Vivarelli M, Massella L, Ruggiero B, Emma F. Minimal change disease. C*lin J Am Soc Nephrol*. 2017;12(2):332-345.

Respiratory System

CASE 27

A 75-Year-Old Female with Shortness of Breath and Chest Pain

Jennifer J. Prutsman-Pfeiffer

A 75-year-old female is brought to the emergency department from a medical rehabilitation clinic where she is found on the bathroom floor complaining of sudden onset shortness of breath. She is nebulized twice without any relief of her dyspnea prior to being transported to another hospital emergency room for higher level of care. Her medical history includes a cerebrovascular accident in the past month with resultant right hemiparesis, obesity, congestive heart failure, peripheral vascular disease, hyperlipidemia, hypertension, gastroesophageal reflux disease, anxiety, and asthma. Medications include ciprofloxacin, hydrochlorothiazide, clopidogrel, losartan, valdecoxib, fluticasone propionate, albuterol, ranitidine, diazepam, clonidine, and docusate sodium. She is allergic to aspirin.

En route, she has severe respiratory distress and requires bag and mask ventilation. Upon arrival, she is hemodynamically unstable with hypotension, tachypnea, bradycardia, and hypoxia. Her respiratory status continues to deteriorate, and she is intubated. A chest x-ray shows no acute lung disease and her D-dimer level is greater than 2000 ng/mL. Despite advanced cardiac life support efforts, the patient is pronounced dead, and the family and healthcare team request an autopsy.

CLINICAL PEARL

D-dimer levels can be measured in a blood test to indicate if a blood clot is present. Alternative names for the test are fragment D-dimer or fibrin degradation fragment test. A high level of D-dimer indicates part of a protein that persists after a blood clot forms and begins breaking down. A D-dimer level of 500 ng/mL or higher is considered abnormal. Elevated D-dimer levels are associated with disseminated intravascular coagulation, DVT, and PE. Levels may be higher in people with other health issues including infection, heart attack (myocardial infarction), liver disease, cancer, and trauma.

An autopsy limited to the thorax is performed. The cause of death is pulmonary embolism (PE). Findings include a large saddle pulmonary embolus (Fig. 27.1) extending from the pulmonary trunk into the pulmonary vasculature of both lungs in the lobar, segmental, and subsegmental arteries. Additional diagnoses include cardiomegaly with ventricular dilatation and coronary artery disease. Microscopically, the thrombi are both acute and organized with adherence to the intimal wall of the vasculature (Fig. 27.2A and B). There is cardiac myocyte hypertrophy with interstitial fibrosis and focal contraction band necrosis. The patient's recent stroke and resultant immobilization places her at high risk for deep vein thrombosis (DVT); she has additional risks factors, given her hyperestrogenic state (obesity), and increased hemostasis due to congestive heart failure.

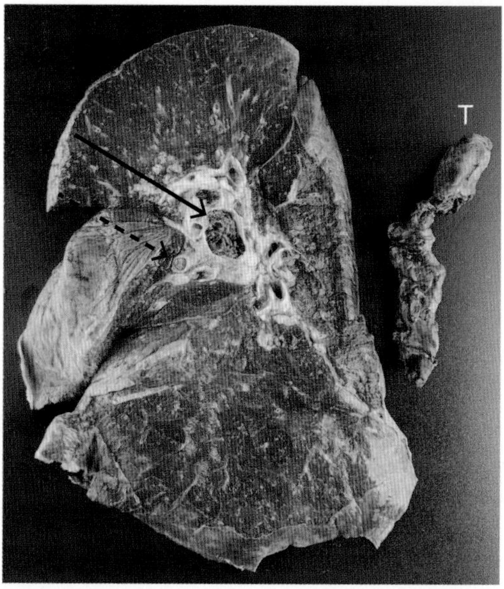

Fig. 27.1 Right lung sectioned in parasagittal plane lateral to hilum showing massive saddle pulmonary embolism in right main pulmonary artery with lines of Zahn (arrow) and organized thrombus occluding right middle lobar artery (dashed arrow); saddle portion of thrombus (T) removed from pulmonary artery bifurcation.

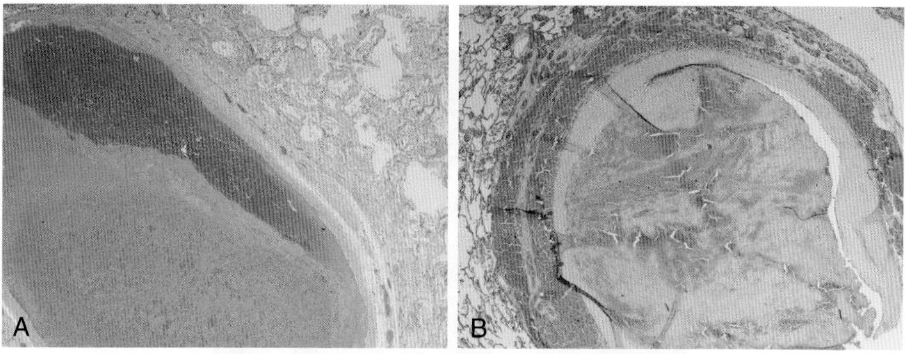

Fig. 27.2 Pulmonary thromboemboli. (A) Acute thrombus (H&E 20x). (B) Organized thrombus with attachment to vessel wall (H&E 20x).

What is thrombosis?

Thrombosis is an intravascular blood clot. The most common location is a DVT of the leg or large veins of the pelvis. Indwelling venous lines are another source of thrombi formation (Fig. 27.3), commonly found in the superior vena cava or right atrium of the heart with central venous lines and in arteriovenous fistulas in hemodialysis patients. Thromboses are characterized by lines of Zahn—alternating layers of platelet/fibrin and red blood cells and attachment to the vessel wall (Figs. 27.4 and 27.2B). A thrombus can be distinguished from a postmortem blood clot by both of these features. Acute thrombi may not have attachment to the vessel wall or established lines of Zahn due to their temporal recency (Fig. 27.5A and B; Fig. 27.2A). The major risk factors for

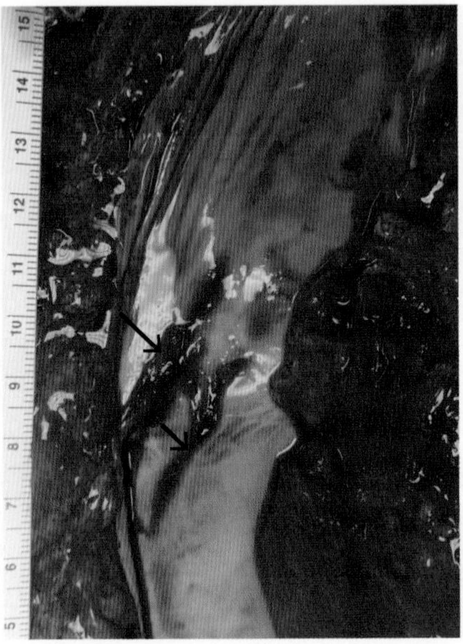

Fig. 27.3 Inferior vena cava with linear attached mural thrombus (arrows) at the level of renal vein, apparent after removal of left groin venous extracorporeal membrane oxygenation cannula at autopsy.

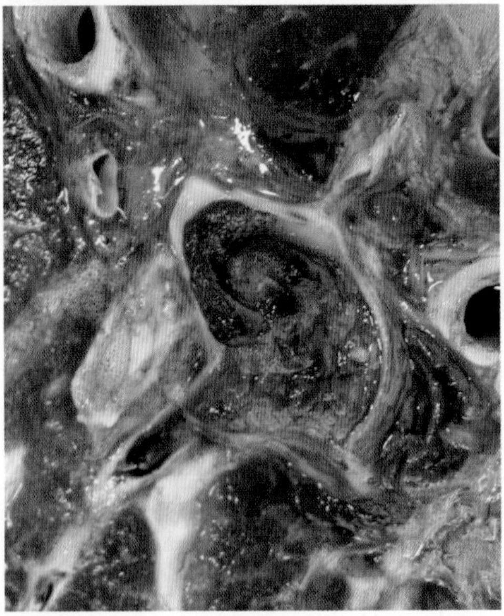

Fig. 27.4 Pulmonary embolism at right main pulmonary artery with lines of Zahn, alternating layers of red cells, and white cells and fibrin.

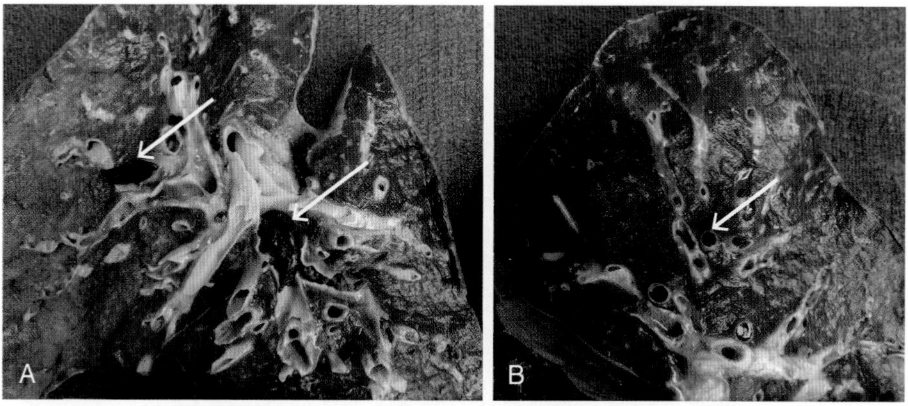

Fig. 27.5 Acute pulmonary emboli. (A) Left lung hilum with recent organized thrombi not adherent to lobar vessel walls (arrows). (B) Right lung upper lobe with recent gelatinous thrombi distending segmental pulmonary arteries (arrow). Image courtesy of Bennett Wilson, DO.

thrombosis are collectively known as the Virchow triad: disruption of blood flow (stasis/turbulence), endothelial cell damage (atherosclerosis, vasculitis, high levels of homocysteine), and a hypercoagulable state. Patients who have undergone recent surgery, have sustained a hip fracture, or are inactive due to paralysis are at increased risk for thrombosis.

What is an embolism?

An embolism is an intravascular solid, gaseous, or liquid mass that travels and occludes downstream vessels; a thromboembolism is a blood clot that dislodges. Emboli are not always formed from blood clots and can originate from other types of material, a category designated as nonthrombotic: atherosclerotic plaque fragments, bone marrow, fat molecules, air/gas, amniotic fluid, infected material, foreign substances, or tumor. Thromboemboli in pulmonary arteries almost always originate from deep veins of the lower extremity.

CLINICAL PEARL

Atherosclerotic embolus occurs when atherosclerotic plaque material dislodges from the intima of an artery. Common consequences of atherosclerotic plaque embolism are transient ischemic attack (stroke) or myocardial infarction (heart attack).

CLINICAL PEARL

Bone marrow fragments and associated elements can escape into the blood from the bone marrow when long bones are traumatically fractured during aggressive cardiopulmonary resuscitation efforts or during bone surgery (Fig. 27.6).

CLINICAL PEARL

Fat may be introduced into the systemic circulation during surgical procedures such as liposuction and fat grafting. Fat is an element of the bone marrow and may be seen in relation to bone marrow embolus. There are occasions when lipids are liberated from other sources, such as patients with hepatic steatosis and subsequent necrosis due to alcohol abuse (Fig. 27.7A and B).

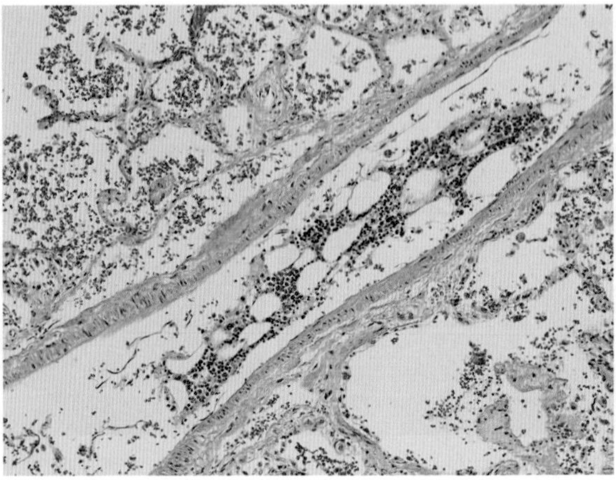

Fig. 27.6 Bone marrow embolism in pulmonary vasculature (H&E 100x).

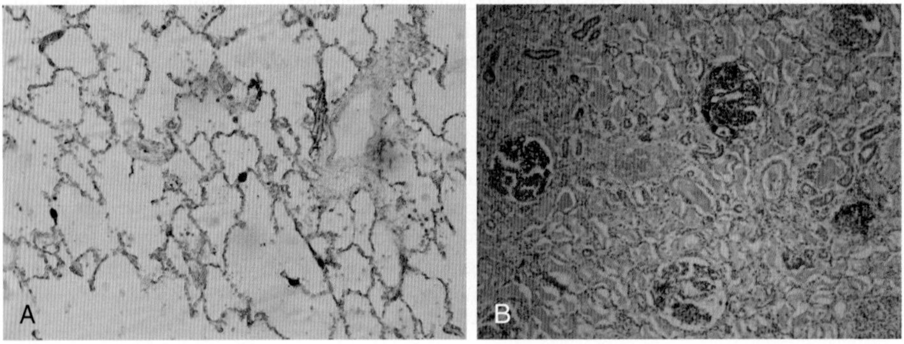

Fig. 27.7 Systemic fat embolism. (A) Lung with intracapillary fat globules (Oil Red O stain 40x). (B) Kidney with numerous fat globules in glomerular capillaries and scattered peritubular capillaries (Oil Red O stain 100x).

CLINICAL PEARL

Air bubbles may form emboli if a catheter in one of the large veins (central veins) is inadvertently opened to air. Air emboli may also form when a vein is operated on to remove a blood clot. Laparoscopic surgery carries a risk as air is pumped into abdomen. An additional risk is underwater diving and rapid ascent to the surface (decompression sickness, nitrogen gas precipitates out of blood, also known as "the bends"). Diagnosis is made by imaging studies.

CLINICAL PEARL

Amniotic fluid containing squamous cells and keratin debris from fetal skin may enter the maternal venous circulation during a complicated labor and delivery and can result in an embolus (Fig. 27.8). Amniotic fluid embolization is a rare occurrence immediately postpartum, following an abortion, after amniocentesis or abdominal/uterine trauma.

CLINICAL PEARL

Infected material may form emboli and travel to the lung, also known as septic emboli. Causes include intravenous drug use, certain heart valve infections as vegetations, and inflammation of a vein with blood clot formation and infection (septic thrombophlebitis).

CLINICAL PEARL

A foreign substance can be introduced into the bloodstream by intravenous injection of ground inorganic substances (pills or other particulates) by drug users. The material can form emboli and travel to the lung. In microscopy, the material is visible in a hematoxylin and eosin stain and may be more prominent under polarized light (Fig. 27.9A and B). Surgically, bone cement may occasionally enter the bloodstream after a procedure called vertebroplasty; silicone injected for body augmentations or cosmetic procedures has been demonstrated to embolize.

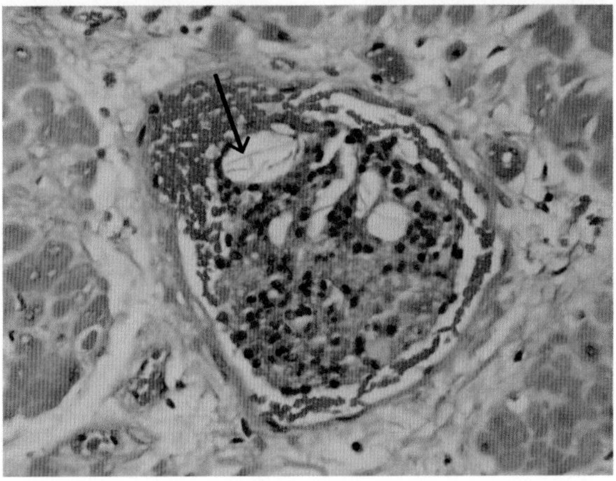

Fig. 27.8 Amniotic fluid embolism with fetal squamous cells (arrow) in wall of uterus of a recently delivered deceased patient (H&E, 200x). Image courtesy of Stewart Cramer, MD and Philip Katzman, MD.

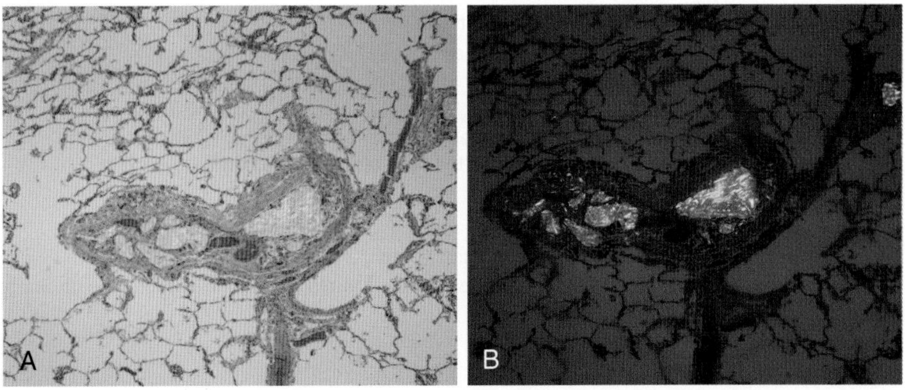

Fig. 27.9 Left upper lung lobe, chronic pulmonary foreign body embolization consistent with intravenous injection of crushed pills (A) H&E 40x, (B) birefringent foreign material, H&E stain 40x with polarization.

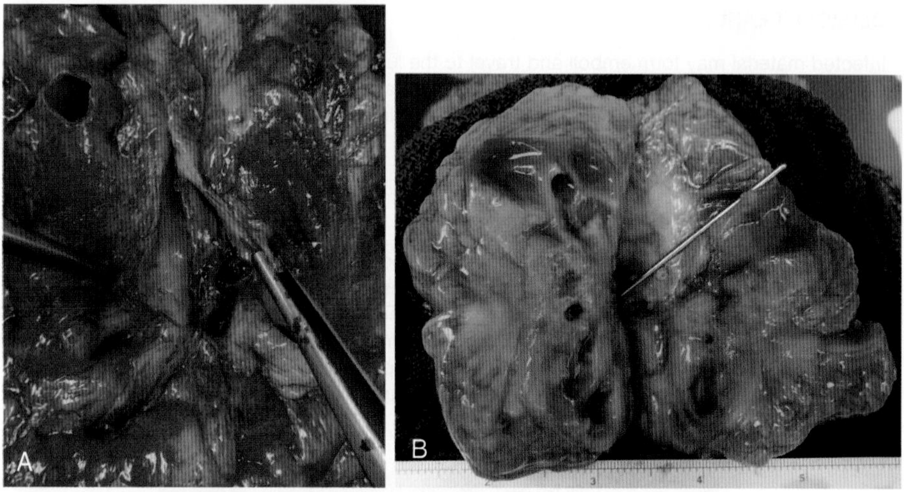

Fig. 27.10 (A) Tumor thrombus of right renal vein extending from (B) right kidney with tumor (urothelial carcinoma), metal probe in ureteropelvic junction.

CLINICAL PEARL

Tumor embolus occurs as direct intravascular tumor extension usually into a vein and has the highest proclivity in Wilms tumor, renal cell carcinoma, adrenal cortical carcinoma, and hepatocellular carcinoma. The presence of tumor embolus markedly worsens prognosis (Fig. 27.10A and B). Alternatively, cancer cells in clumps may break free into the circulation to form tumor emboli and settle at distant sites resulting in metastases.

What is a PE?

A PE originates as a DVT of the lower extremity, often in immobilized individuals, involving the femoral, iliac, or popliteal veins. Once a clot dislodges, it travels a route through the inferior vena cava (IVC) to the right atrium of the heart, over the tricuspid valve, through the right ventricle, and into the pulmonic arterial system. Pulmonary emboli are clinically silent because the lung has a dual blood supply from pulmonary and bronchial arteries, especially in cases of small emboli that resorb. Pulmonary emboli are named after the anatomic location in the pulmonary circulation and are saddle, lobar, segmental, or subsegmental.

CLINICAL PEARL

Emboli can originate from thrombi in the upper extremity or neck veins, in which case the travel route is from the superior vena cava to the right atrium of the heart.

PE affects primarily adults, and more men than women. There are about 350,000 cases yearly worldwide and more than 50,000 deaths per year in the United States. PE is the cause of death in 10% of acute hospital deaths of adults.

What is a saddle embolus?

A saddle embolus is a massive pulmonary thromboembolus of the main pulmonary arterial trunk at the bifurcation. The term “saddle” arises from the placement of the embolus across the bifurcation into both right and left main pulmonary arteries. The thrombus is typically large, snake-like, and unstable. Patients with saddle embolus are at risk for sudden hemodynamic collapse.

What are the risk factors for PE?

Risk factors for PE are trauma, hypercoaguable states, lupus anticoagulant, Factor V Leiden mutation, prothrombin mutation, protein C/S deficiency, carcinoma, Trousseau's syndrome, heart failure, oral contraceptives, pregnancy, immobilized medical or surgical patients, and older age.

CLINICAL PEARL

Risk factors for developing DVT

Trauma or injury (broken bones)

Hypercoagulable state: numerous causes including medications, postoperative period, pregnancy, phospholipid antibodies and blood, cancer, elevated homocysteine levels, inherited protein deficiencies

Inherited clotting disorders

Protein C and/or protein S deficiency: congenital condition, inherited thrombophilia; may also be acquired

Prothrombin mutation: also called factor II mutation, form of inherited thrombophilia

Lupus anticoagulant

Factor V Leiden mutation

Antiphospholipid syndrome

Trousseau's syndrome: recurrent episodes of vessel inflammation due to thrombophlebitis (blood clot) that appear in different locations of the body over time

Carcinoma

Oral contraceptives

Pregnancy or recent parturition

Heart failure

Older age

Surgical or medical patients who are immobilized

Long periods of sitting or lying down

What are the symptoms of PE?

About 50% of DVTs are asymptomatic, and 60%–80% of pulmonary emboli are clinically silent. Symptoms of PE include shortness of breath, hemoptysis (less frequently), pleuritic chest pain, and pleural effusion. Clinically, the symptoms of PE may be nonspecific. Patients may range in presentation from asymptomatic to sudden death.

CLINICAL PEARL

Temporal presentation of PE

Acute: immediate signs and symptoms after obstruction of pulmonary vasculature

Subacute: symptoms develop days or weeks after obstruction of pulmonary vasculature

Chronic: symptoms develop over many years; chronic thromboembolic pulmonary hypertension

Often there is little to no warning of a large, fatal PE. Sudden death occurs when 60% or more of the pulmonary circulation is obstructed by embolus. Scenarios of individuals who develop DVTs are long-distance truck drivers, those on long airline flights, and those who have undergone recent surgery and are nonactive or bedridden. The presentation of a large, fatal PE is sudden onset of shortness of breath and a feel of impending doom. Bystanders report the individual is fine, complains of the symptoms, and collapses. Sudden death can occur with a large saddle embolus that blocks both left and right main pulmonary arteries. A large pulmonary artery with significant occlusion can cause death due to electromechanical dissociation with rhythm but no pulse, or cause acute cor pulmonale due to localized increased resistance to blood flow, pulmonary hypertension, and right-sided heart failure.

What is pulmonary infarction?

An infarction occurs when a segmental or subsegmental pulmonary artery is occluded by a thrombus. The infarction results in a wedge-shaped subpleural region of tissue that becomes consolidated, congested, and firm with hemorrhage into alveoli and edema (Fig. 27.11). Within 24–48 hours, the extravasated red cells break down into hemosiderin, and necrosis of the alveolar walls and parenchyma result in infarction. The infarcted area is replaced by fibrosis and scarring after a few weeks (Fig. 27.12A).

Pulmonary infarction occurs in a minority of patients with PE; in patients with healthy lungs, the hemorrhage resolves prior to necrosis and the infiltrate clears, never forming an infarction. A good predictor of infarction is preexisting cardiopulmonary disease.

Cavitation of the infarction is more common when the infarction is 4 cm or greater in diameter, and tends to occur in the right lung apical or posterior upper lobe or apical segment of lower lobe. Hemorrhagic infarction can occur in any lobe (Fig. 27.12B).

Abscess formation is linked to larger infarctions where there is coexisting diseased lung tissue (congestion or atelectasis) and infection or sepsis present elsewhere in the body. The mean time to cavitation for an infected pulmonary infarction is reported to be 18 days.

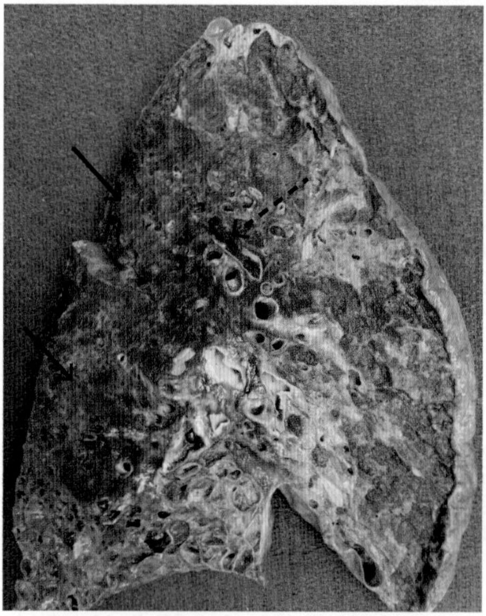

Fig. 27.11 Left lung with interstitial fibrosis, sarcoidosis, saccular, and cylindrical bronchiectasis. Wedge-shaped infarction of upper lobe and apical lower lobe (arrows), pulmonary embolism of upper lobe lobar artery (dashed arrow).

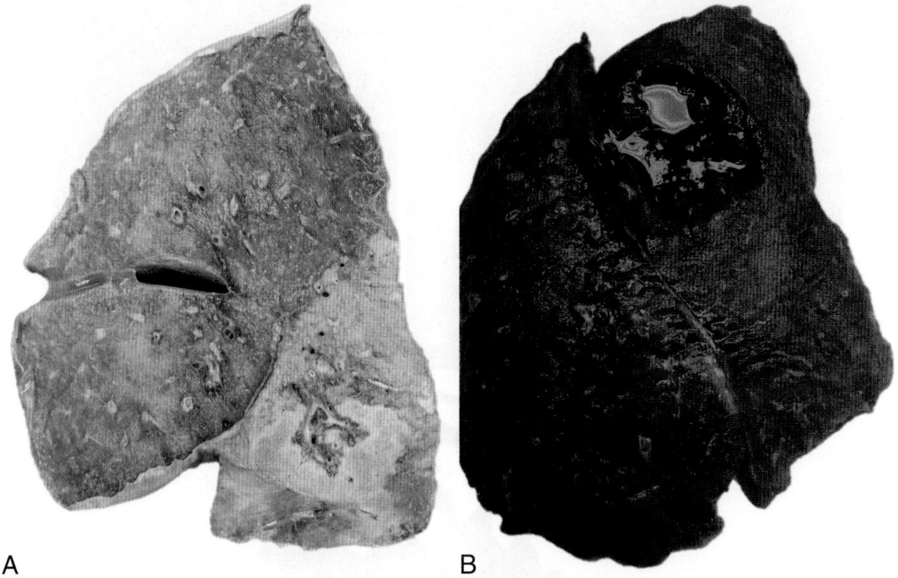
A B

Fig. 27.12 (A) Right lung, with extensive chronic organizing infarct involving the entire right lower lobe. Photo credit: Chelsea Milito, MD. (B) Left upper lobe of lung with 7 × 6 × 2 cm hemorrhagic cavitated infarct suggestive of septic infarct. Surrounding consolidated parenchyma with bronchopneumonia.

How is PE diagnosed?

Pulse oximetry, chest x-ray, electrocardiogram, and arterial blood gas measurements are initial diagnostic tests to exclude other diagnoses. Tests most useful for diagnosing or excluding PE include D-dimer blood test (if elevated, PE suspected), computerized tomographic angiography to show vascular filling defects in the lung (Fig. 27.13A and B), ventilation/perfusion lung scan evaluates circulation of blood and perfusion of air in the lungs, Doppler ultrasound of the lower extremity can detect DVT, and duplex ultrasound (scan and then compress leg veins; if veins do not completely compress, a thrombus may be present). Echocardiography may be useful to identify PE on the way to the lung, indicating a clot in transit.

How is PE treated?

In patients with known recurrent DVTs, an IVC filter (also known as umbrella filter or Greenfield filter) can be surgically placed in the vessel to break up and disperse large clots. The IVC filter looks like the metal frame portion of an umbrella and has thin sharp hooks at the ends to attach to the intima of the vena cava (Fig. 27.14). Occasionally, the IVC filter may not keep a firm attachment and may migrate within the vessel to be found in unsuspecting places, anywhere along the vena cava and even in the heart or lungs. An additional surgical approach for treatment is embolectomy (Fig. 27.13C).

Other treatments for PE are preventative including compression stockings for the legs to discourage the development of lower extremity thrombosis, anticoagulants, or thrombolytic medications.

What is the prognosis for PE?

Patients may shower the lungs with small emboli that resolve completely or leave signs of emboli past in recanalization of previously involved blood vessels (Fig. 27.15A and B). Adverse outcomes that are associated with PE include recurrent thromboembolism, chronic thrombotic pulmonary hypertension, and death.

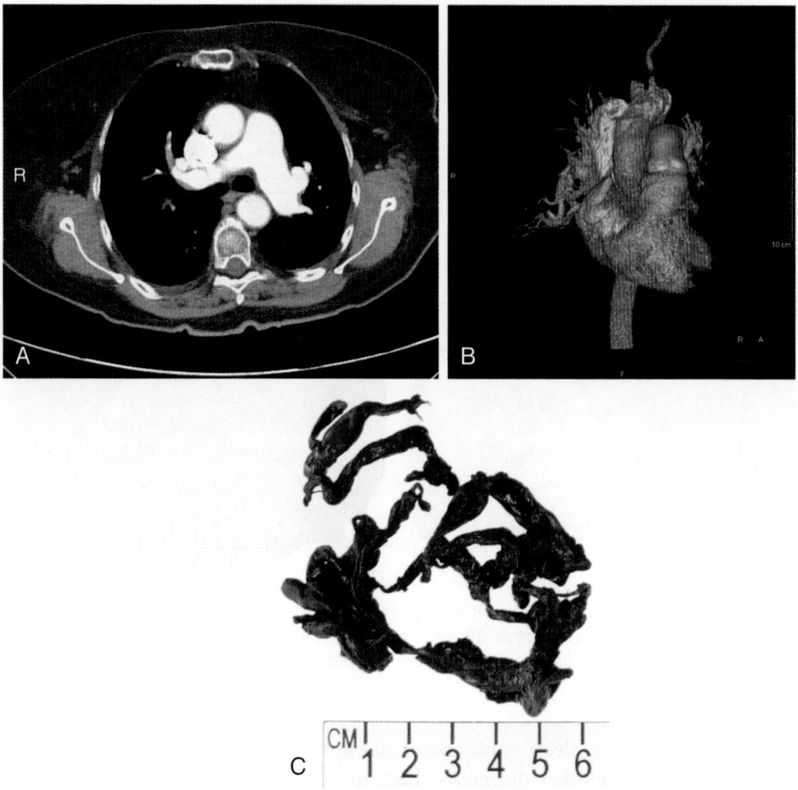

Fig. 27.13 (A) Chest computed tomography angiogram showing saddle pulmonary embolism with extension to lobar, segmental, and subsegmental pulmonary arteries. (B) Three-dimensional computed tomography reconstruction. (C) Embolectomy specimen with laminated, tortuous bifurcations.

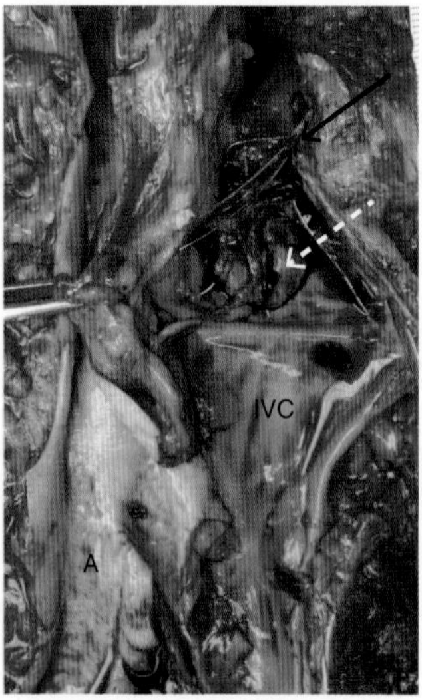

Fig. 27.14 Inferior vena cava (IVC) opened demonstrating metal umbrella filter (arrow) holding back thrombosis (dashed arrow). Intima of abdominal aorta (A).

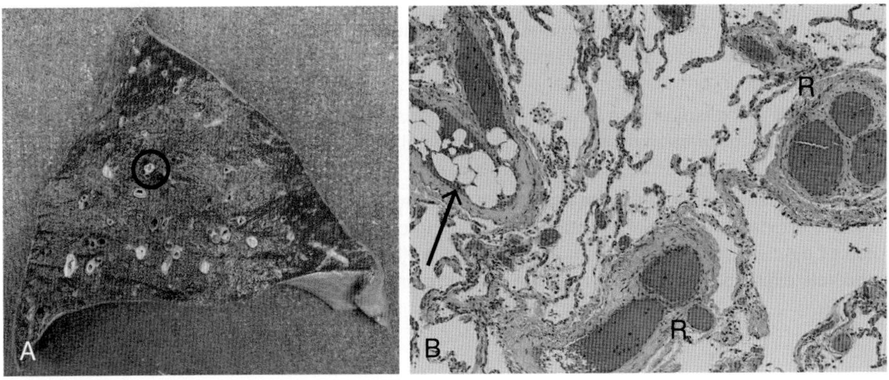

Fig. 27.15 (A) Right lower lobe of lung with recanalization of artery after resolved pulmonary embolism (circle). (B) Recanalization (R) of pulmonary vasculature and fat embolism (arrow) (H&E 100x).

BEYOND THE PEARLS

The Wells score system and Pulmonary Embolism Rule-Out Criteria (PERC) rule are used by clinicians to assess the chance that acute PE is preset.

Wells Score System DVT Probability:

Paralysis, paresis, or recent orthopedic casting of lower extremity (1 point)
Recently bedridden (>3 days) or major surgery within past 4 weeks (1 point)
Localized tenderness in deep vein system (1 point)
Swelling of entire leg (1 point)
Calf swelling 3 cm greater than other leg (measured 10 cm below the tibial tuberosity) (1 point)
Pitting edema greater in the symptomatic leg (1 point)
Collateral nonvaricose superficial veins (1 point)
Active cancer or cancer treated within 6 months (1 point)
Alternative diagnosis more likely than DVT (Baker's cyst, cellulitis, muscle damage, superficial venous thrombosis, post phlebitic syndrome, inguinal lymphadenopathy, external venous compression) (–2 points)
DVT Risk Score Interpretation

- 3 to 8 points: high probability of DVT
- 1 to 2 Points: moderate probability of DVT
- –2 to 0 Points: low Probability of DVT

PERC: presence of these criteria in a clinically low-risk patient suggests testing for PE is not indicated:

- Age < 50 years
- Heart rate < 100 beats per minute
- Oxygen saturation ≥ 95%
- No prior DVT or PE
- No unilateral leg swelling
- No estrogen use
- No hemoptysis
- No surgery or trauma requiring hospitalization within the past 4 weeks

Fat embolism syndrome (FES) is a rare but potentially fatal syndrome where fat is released into the circulatory system. The classic triad of presentation are hypoxemia, neurologic disturbances, and petechial rash (none of these features are specific for FES). The syndrome is most commonly associated with long bone or pelvic fracture, but may occur as a result of surgical trauma in orthopedic surgery. Treatment is supportive therapy while FES resolves.

Paradoxical embolism occurs when embolic material from the venous circulation passes through a patent foramen ovale or other anatomical shunt and into the arterial circulation; common result is cerebral ischemic event (stroke).

Microembolism occurs when the emboli are so small that they are able to pass from the pulmonary arterial to pulmonary venous circulation through the lungs and eventually to the left side of the heart. This mechanism is supported by the finding of embolized material in the systemic circulation in the absence of a patent foramen ovale.

References

Dalen JE. Pulmonary embolism: What have we learned since Virchow? Natural history, pathophysiology, and diagnosis. *Chest*. 2002;122(4):1440-1456.

Kirchner J, Obermann A, Stückradt S, et al. Lung infarction following pulmonary embolism: A comparative study on clinical conditions and CT findings to identify predisposing factors. *Fortschr Röntgenstr*. 2015;187:440-444.

Koroscil MT, Hauser TR. Acute pulmonary embolism leading to cavitation and large pulmonary abscess: a rare complication of pulmonary infarction. *Respir Med Case Rep*. 2016;20:72-74.

Sweet PH III, Armstrong T, Chen J, Masliah E, Witucki P. Fatal pulmonary embolism update: 10 years of autopsy experience at an academic medical center. *JRSM Short Rep*. 2013;4(9):1-5.

CASE 28

A 64-Year-Old Male with Progressive Shortness of Breath

Stefania Pirrota ■ Lucas Cruz ■ Raj Dasgupta

The patient is a 64-year-old-man who is referred to a pulmonologist by his primary care doctor for evaluation of symptoms of progressive shortness of breath. The patient has noticed his symptoms for several years, initially only feeling short of breath with great exertion, but it is now present with minimal movements around his home. He can no longer speak in full sentences while doing a simple task such as folding laundry due to the sensation of inability to catch his breath. In addition to the shortness of breath, he reports a daily cough productive of whitish sputum, which has also been present for over a year. He denies any associated fevers, chills, night sweats, chest pain, or palpitations, but has noticed generalized fatigue and weight gain. The patient's past medical history includes coronary artery disease, requiring percutaneous intervention in the past, as well as type 2 diabetes mellitus, hypertension, and hyperlipidemia. He reports compliance with all of his prescribed home medications, which include aspirin, clopidogrel, atorvastatin, metformin, and lisinopril. He is an active smoker of about half a pack of cigarettes daily and has been smoking for the past 40 years. The patient has lived his whole life in upstate New York, denies any recent travel, and denies any significant alcohol or recreational drug use. He is self-employed as a deli owner but is planning on retiring soon, as his dyspnea is interfering with his ability to perform his job. He denies any family history of lung or heart disease.

What is the most likely cause of this patient's symptoms of progressive dyspnea and chronic, productive cough?

Dyspnea is defined by the American Thoracic Society as a subjective experience of breathing discomfort of varying intensity due to multiple physiological, psychological, and social factors. Our patient's complaints could be the result of a wide variety of pathologies, but his medical history, description of his symptoms, and risk factors suggest underlying chronic obstructive pulmonary disease (COPD) is the likely culprit (Table 28.1).

The Global Initiative for Chronic Obstructive Lung Diseases (GOLD) has defined COPD as a disease state characterized by chronic respiratory symptoms and airflow limitation that is not fully reversible and is usually the result of repeated exposures to toxic particles or gases. The disease states of COPD include emphysema, chronic bronchitis, and/or small airways disease. According to the Centers for Disease Control and Prevention, COPD is the fourth leading cause of death in the United States, responsible for 161,374 deaths in 2016 alone.

Dyspnea is the predominant symptom of COPD, the driving reason patients seek medical attention, and the predominant cause for patient disability. Patients often describe a sensation of air hunger, inability to catch their breath, increased work of breathing, or even chest tightness.

CLINICAL PEARL

Activities that require significant arm activity at or above shoulder level result in increased sensation of dyspnea in patients with COPD. Conversely, activities that allow for the arms to be rested/braced on a stationary object are better tolerated (e.g., walking while pushing a shopping cart).

TABLE 28.1 ■ **Differential Diagnosis for Patients Presenting with Cough, Sputum Production, Progressive Dyspnea, or Signs of Airflow Limitation**

Diagnosis	Features Shared with COPD	Features Differing From COPD
Asthma	Dyspnea, wheezing, airflow limitation	• Younger age of onset • Associated with atopic history • Airflow limitation less severe and REVERSIBLE • Less sputum production • Increased steroid responsiveness
Bronchiectasis	Dyspnea and sputum production	• Larger volume of sputum production • Associated with repeated bacterial infections • Bronchial dilation and wall thickening
Congestive heart failure	Dyspnea	• Chest imaging demonstrates pulmonary edema • PFTs do not demonstrate obstructive pattern
Bronchiolitis obliterans	Obstructive pattern on PFTs	• Submucosal fibrosis leads to narrowing of bronchiolar lumen • Develops after lung or bone marrow transplant • Can be associated with IBD or CTD
Diffuse panbronchiolitis	Obstructive pattern on PFTs	• Involves both the upper and lower respiratory tracts • Associated with sinus disease • Predominantly seen in Far East/Japanese populations

COPD, chronic obstructive pulmonary disorder; *CTD*, connective tissue disease; *IBD*, inflammatory bowel disease; *PFT*, pulmonary function testing.

In addition to dyspnea, chronic cough is often an early symptom of COPD. Cough may be nonproductive or productive, and will vary in intensity, frequency, and severity. Chronic bronchitis is a clinical condition defined as regular sputum production for 3 or more months in 2 consecutive years. Chronic bronchitis typically affects the large airways. Emphysema is a diagnosis based on morphologic and radiographic features that demonstrate the destruction of the gas-exchanging airspaces (the acini, which include the respiratory bronchioles, alveolar ducts, and alveoli), resulting in their permanent enlargement. These two disease states usually coexist, but may also occur individually, and both are associated with cigarette smoke exposure.

Emphysema is generally classified by its anatomic distribution within the lung parenchyma, with either centriacinar or panacinar distribution of pathology (Fig. 28.1).

Risk factors for COPD include, most commonly, cigarette smoke exposure, but also other environmental exposures and host predisposing factors (Table 28.2).

Case Point 28.1

The patient now presents to you in pulmonary clinic and confirms the above history. On examination, his vital signs include a temperature of 37.16°C (98.8°F), heart rate of 91 beats per minute, blood pressure of 118/70 mm Hg, respiration rate of 22 breaths per minute, and oxygen saturation of 91% on room air. In general, he is an obese man, appears comfortable at rest, mucus membranes are moist, no evidence of jugular venous distention, and heart sounds demonstrate regular heart rate and rhythm. Lung exam is significant for prolonged expiratory phase of ventilation with fine expiratory wheezing appreciated diffusely. Extremities demonstrate no clubbing, cyanosis, or edema.

Initial laboratory investigations including complete blood count, comprehensive metabolic profile, D-dimer, troponins, B-type natriuretic peptide, and arterial blood gas are all within normal limits. He then undergoes a chest radiograph (CXR), computed tomography (CT) of the chest, and pulmonary function testing for further evaluation. Spirometry demonstrates reduced forced expiratory capacity in 1 second (FEV_1), as well as reduced ratio of FEV_1 to forced vital capacity (FVC) (Fig. 28.2). CXR demonstrates increased lung volumes and flattened diaphragms bilaterally, consistent with lung hyperinflation (Fig. 28.3). CT of the chest demonstrates a significant reduction of parenchymal lung markings (Fig. 28.4).

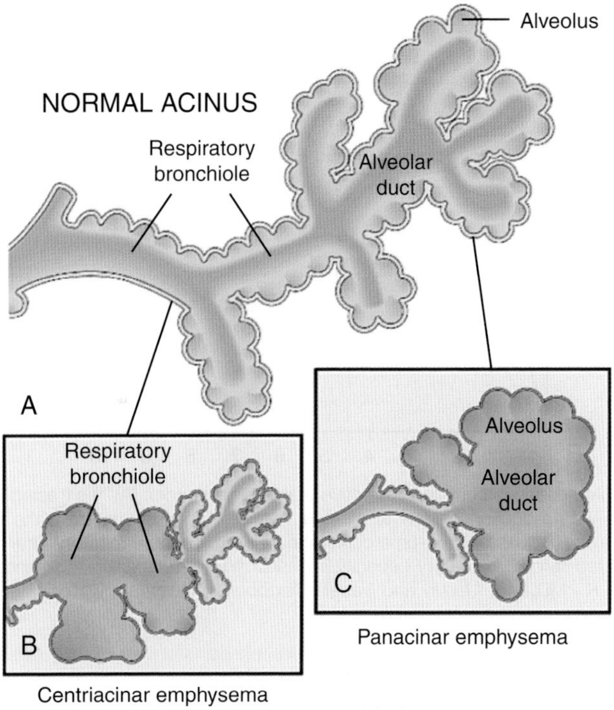

Fig. 28.1 (A) Normal acinar unit containing the respiratory bronchioles (RB), alveolar ducts, and terminal alveolus. (B) Depiction of centriacinar emphysema, in which the more proximal airways are affected and the distal airway is spared. (C) Panacinar emphysema, in which the acinus is uniformly enlarged from RB to alveolus. (Kumar, V., Abbas, A. K., Aster, J. C., & Perkins, J. A. (2018). *Robbins basic pathology* (Tenth edition.). Philadelphia, Pennsylvania: Elsevier. Fig. 13.5).

TABLE 28.2 ■ **Risk Factors for the Development of Chronic Obstructive Pulmonary Disorder**

Risk Factor	Description
Tobacco smoking	Accelerates decline in FEV_1 in dose–response relationship
Indoor air pollution	Biomass fuel for cooking and heating; secondhand tobacco smoke exposure
Occupational exposures	Inhalation of organic and inorganic dusts, chemicals, or fumes
Outdoor air pollution	Particulate air pollution exposure results in increased circulating levels of segmented and band PMNs, monocytes, and cytokines
Genetic factors	Severe deficiency of AATD
Asthma and airway hyper reactivity	Chronic asthma can lead to irreversible airflow limitation

AATD, alpha-1 antitrypsin deficiency; *FEV_1,* forced expiratory capacity in 1 second; *PMN,* polymorphonuclear neutrophils.

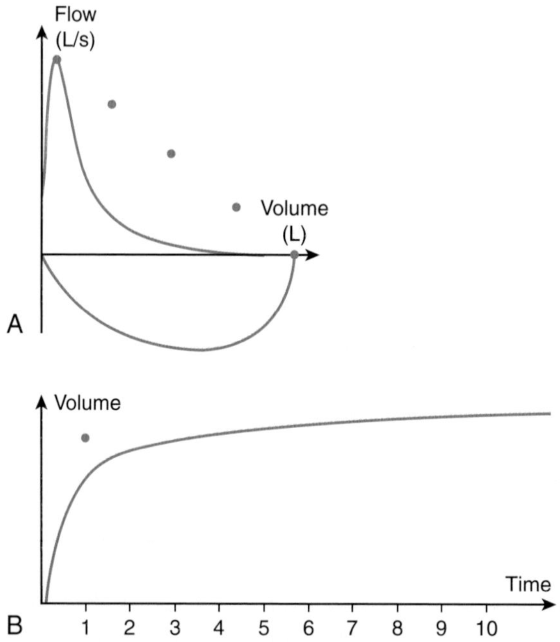

Fig. 28.2 Flow–volume loop in chronic obstructive pulmonary disorder. (A) The tracing shows a concave flow–volume loop with reduction of flow at all lung volumes. The dots indicate the expected flow at various lung volumes. (B) The volume–time curve shows a prolonged expiratory time. The dot demonstrates the predicted forced expiratory capacity in 1 second. (COPD: Clinical Diagnosis and Management Han, Meilan K., MD, MS, *Murray and Nadel's Textbook of Respiratory Medicine*, 44, 767-785.e7. Figure 44-3).

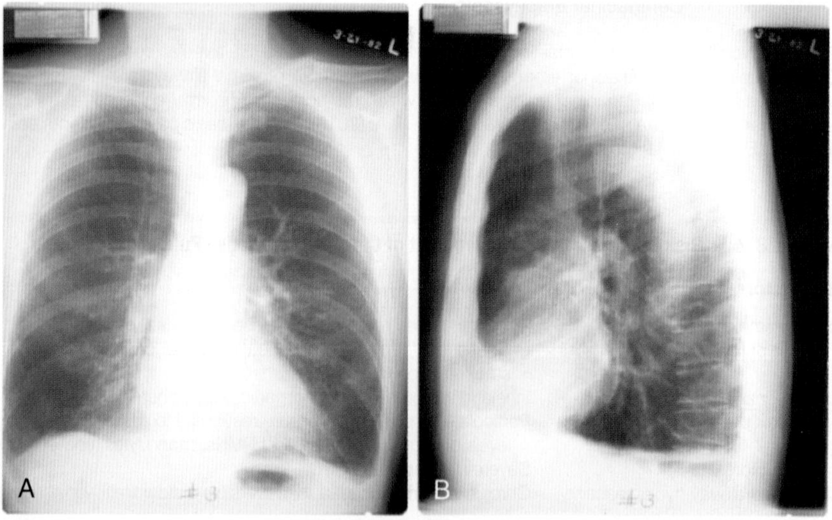

Fig. 28.3 Chest radiograph demonstrating severe obstructive pulmonary disease, with hyperinflated lungs and flattened diaphragms. (A) Posteroanterior view. (B) Lateral view. (Chronic Obstructive Pulmonary Disease. Weinberger, Steven E., MD, MACP, FRCP, *Principles of Pulmonary Medicine*, 6, 93-112. Figure 6.9).

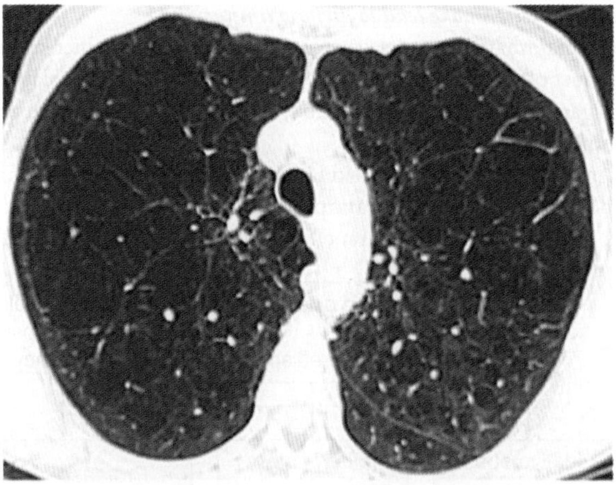

Fig. 28.4 Computed tomography chest imaging demonstrating upper lobe predominant centrilobular emphysema. (Hyperlucent Thorax Reed, James C., MD, *Chest Radiology: Patterns and Differential Diagnoses*, 22, 304-317), (COPD: Clinical Diagnosis and Management. Han, Meilan K., MD, MS, *Murray and Nadel's Textbook of Respiratory Medicine*, 44, 767-785.e7).

How is the diagnosis of COPD established?

COPD should be considered in the differential for any patient who presents with complaints of chronic, progressive dyspnea and productive cough in the setting of the appropriate risk factors. However, in addition to the history, establishing the diagnosis of COPD requires spirometry-confirmed airflow limitation, as demonstrated by a post-bronchodilator FEV/FVC ratio <0.70. Imaging studies will demonstrate classic patterns of hyperinflation and parenchymal lung destruction, but are not necessary in establishing the diagnosis or in guiding the management of COPD.

GOLD classifies COPD based on the degree of airflow obstruction present on spirometry testing (Table 28.3).

TABLE 28.3 ■ **The Global Initiative for Chronic Obstructive Lung Diseases (GOLD) Classification of Chronic Obstructive Pulmonary Disorder Based on Degree of Airflow Limitation**

GOLD Stage	Severity	Spirometry
0	At risk	Normal, but with chronic cough/sputum production
1	Mild	$FEV_1/FVC < 0.7$ and $FEV_1 \geq 80\%$ predicted
2	Moderate	$FEV_1/FVC < 0.7$ and $50\% \leq FEV_1 < 80\%$ predicted
3	Severe	$FEV_1/FVC < 0.7$ and $30\% \leq FEV_1 < 50\%$ predicted
4	Very Severe	$FEV_1/FVC < 0.7$ and $FEV_1 < 30\%$ predicted OR $FEV_1 < 50\%$ predicted and respiratory failure/cor pulmonale

FEV_1, forced expiratory capacity in 1 second; *FVC,* forced vital capacity.

How does exposure to cigarette smoke lead to airflow limitation?

In COPD, chronic inflammation results in structural changes that increase as disease severity worsens. COPD is most often caused by an abnormal response to the inhalation of toxic particles and gases, such as cigarette smoke or air pollution, resulting in a destructive process that persists well after the exposure has ceased.

Inhalation of cigarette smoke results in oxidative stress, the recruitment of inflammatory cells and mediators to the lung, and a protease–antiprotease imbalance, leading to a destruction of the extracellular matrix (ECM) of the lung parenchyma and alveolar cells (Figs. 28.5 and 28.6).

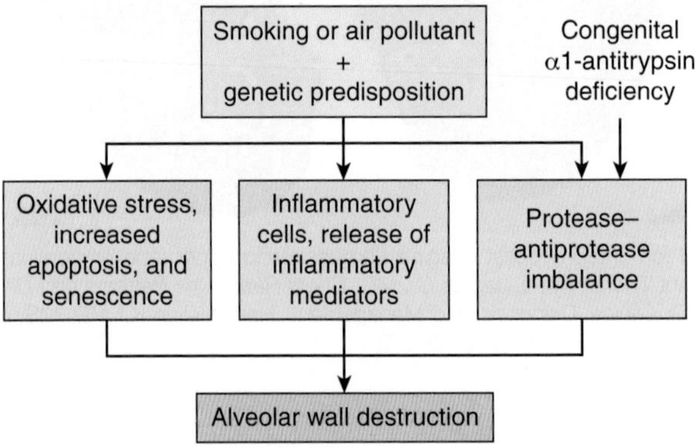

Fig. 28.5 The pathogenesis of alveolar wall destruction in emphysema. (Kumar, V., Abbas, A. K., Aster, J. C., & Perkins, J. A. (2018). *Robbins basic pathology* (Tenth edition.). Philadelphia, Pennsylvania: Elsevier.)

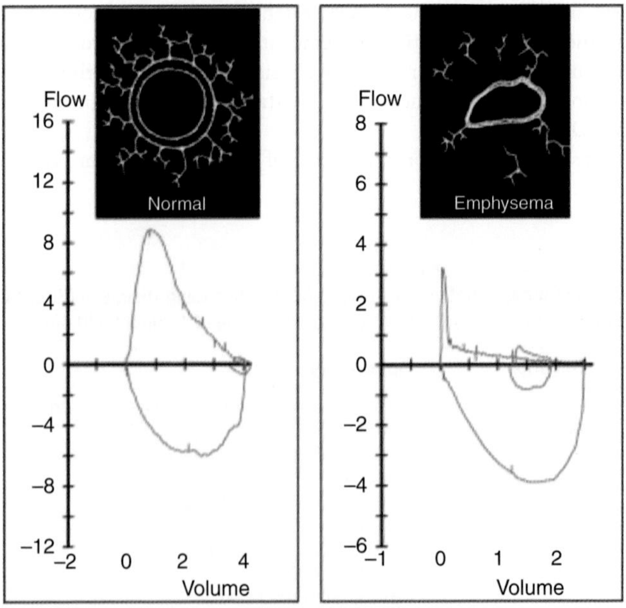

Fig. 28.6 Normal flow–volume loop on the left, with a schematic insert depicting a medium-sized airway, embedded in normal alveolar tissue, providing radial traction resisting airway collapse until the end of exhalation when lung volume is low. The flow–volume loop on the right demonstrates a severe obstructive defect, with a schematic insert depicting a medium-sized airway prone to premature collapse at the beginning of exhalation when lung volume is still high, secondary to decreased radial traction. (Pulmonary function testing. Landsberg, Judd W., MD, *Clinical Practice Manual for Pulmonary and Critical Care Medicine*, Chapter 3, 22-35. Fig. 3.3)

CLINICAL PEARL

Inflammatory mediators such as matrix metalloproteinase-9, leukotriene B4, interleukin-8, and tumor necrosis factor-α attract macrophages, neutrophils, and lymphocytes to the lung, thereby amplifying the inflammatory process, as these cells then release additional inflammatory mediators, proteases, and reactive oxygen species.

CLINICAL PEARL

The predominant mechanism for the airflow limitation seen in emphysema lies in the protease–antiprotease imbalance. Respiratory bronchioles, which are normally held open by the elastic recoil of the surrounding alveolar tissue, collapse due to the loss of elastic tissue in the walls of the alveoli. This results in the classic airflow obstruction seen on spirometry flow–volume loops (Fig. 28.6).

Loss of the ECM of the alveolar cells results in apoptosis of the structural cells of the lung. As cells and their ECM are destroyed, the airspaces coalesce into larger accumulated alveolar spaces, thereby reducing the effective surface area for gas exchange (Fig. 28.7). In centriacinar emphysema, this destruction predominantly occurs in the respiratory bronchioles and alveolar ducts, whereas panacinar emphysema results in destruction of the entire acinar unit (Figs. 28.8–28.10).

Alpha-1 antitrypsin (A1AT) disease is a clinical condition that manifests when there is a genetic deficiency in the enzyme A1AT. A1AT is encoded by a gene located on chromosome 14 and is a major inhibitor of proteases within the body. When absent (Z allele mutation), the protease–antiprotease balance is disrupted in a similar manner to that described earlier; however, patients typically do not carry a history of cigarette exposure, and A1AT disease often results in lower lobe–predominant, panacinar emphysema.

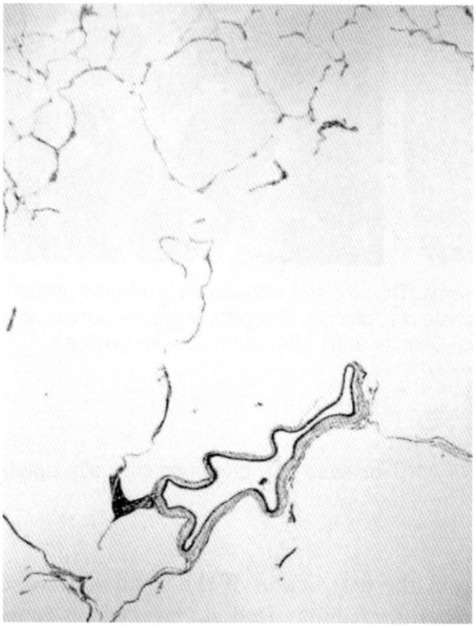

Fig. 28.7 Emphysema showing bronchiolar collapse due to loss of alveolar attachments. (Diseases of the conductive airways. Corrin, Bryan, MD FRCPath, *Pathology of the Lungs*, Chapter 3, 91-134. 2011, Elsevier Limited.)

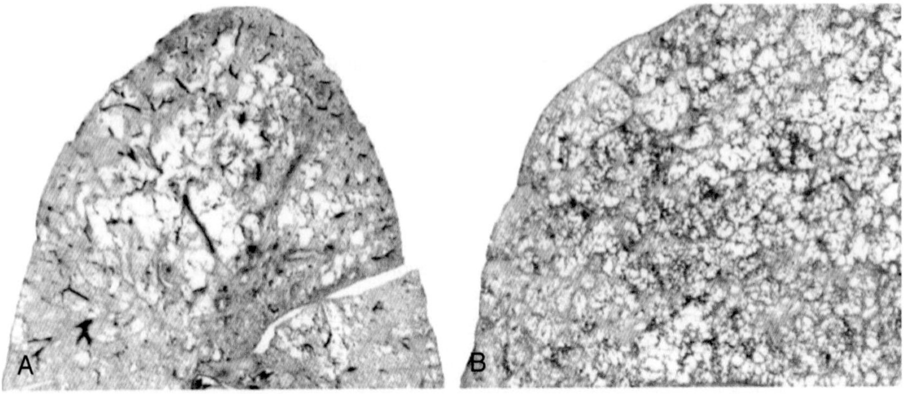

Fig. 28.8 Gross section prepared from the whole lung demonstrating centriacinar emphysema with peripheral sparing (A) and panacinar emphysema that more evenly affects the entire acinus (B). (Nonneoplastic Pathology of the Large and Small Airways. Barbareschi, Mattia, MD, *Practical Pulmonary Pathology: A Diagnostic Approach*, 9, 299-334.e9).

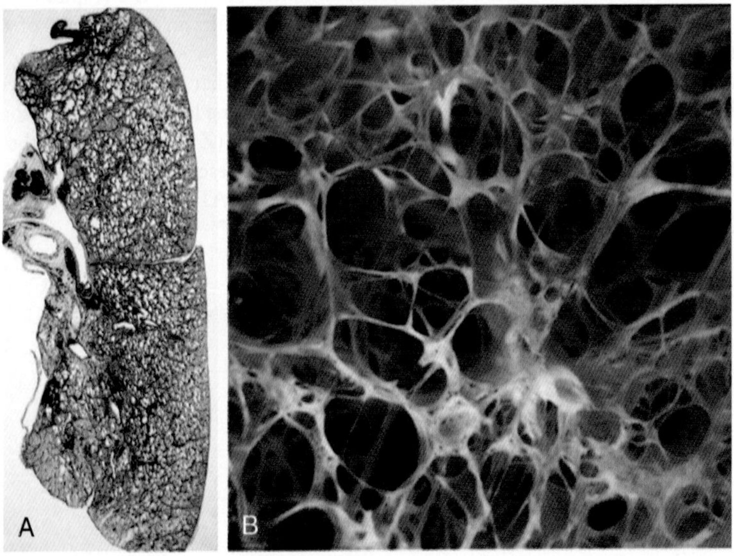

Fig. 28.9 Panacinar emphysema. The whole of lung acinus is affected uniformly. (A) Paper-mounted whole lung section. (B) Barium sulphate precipitation. (Diseases of the conductive airways Corrin, Bryan, MD FRCPath, *Pathology of the Lungs*, Chapter 3, 91-134. 2011, Elsevier Limited.)

CLINICAL PEARL

The enzyme deficiency of A1AT disease only becomes clinically significant in patients homozygous for the Z allele.

In addition to aiding in the destruction of the small airways, cigarette smoke also induces damage to the large and medium-sized airways, which generally manifests with the symptoms of chronic bronchitis. The noxious irritants attract chronic inflammatory cells,

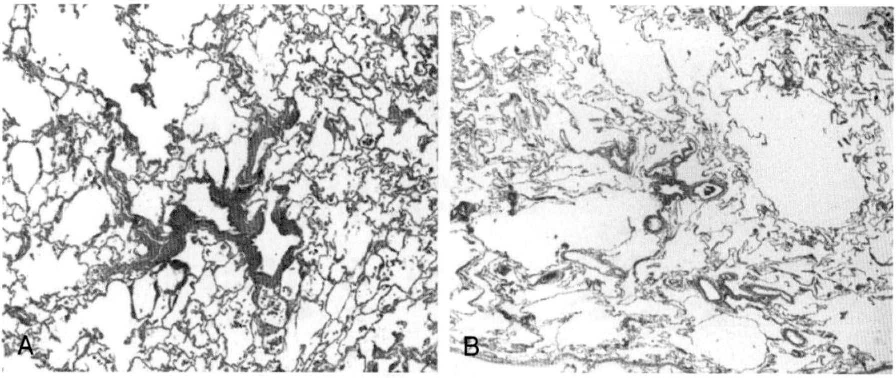

Fig. 28.10 Emphysema. The type and severity of emphysema may be difficult or impossible to determine on histopathologic grounds. (A) Here, centriacinar emphysema is seen with dilation of the airspaces surrounding the bronchiole. (B) By contrast, panacinar emphysema features a more diffuse airspace dilation. (Nonneoplastic Pathology of the Large and Small Airways. Barbareschi, Mattia, MD, *Practical Pulmonary Pathology: A Diagnostic Approach*, 9, 299-334.e9. Figure 9.55).

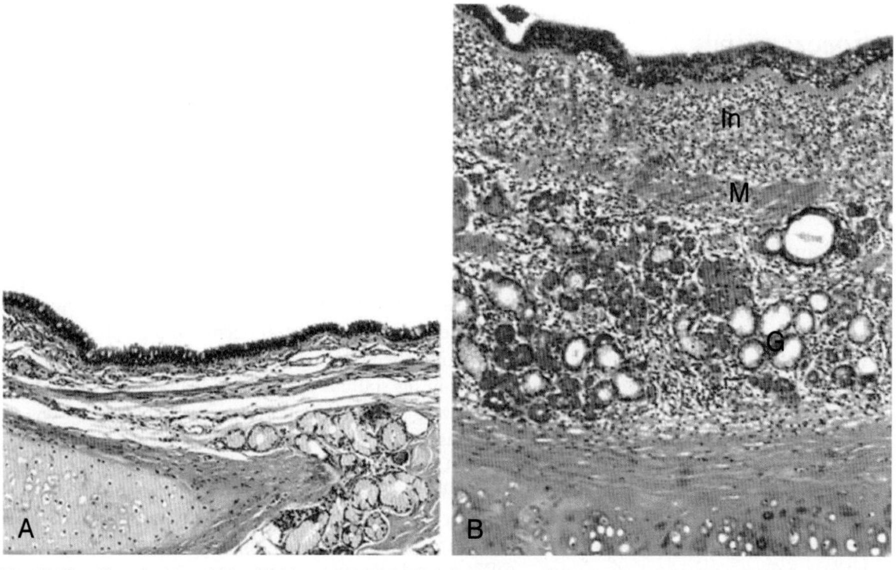

Fig. 28.11 Chronic bronchitis. (A) Normal bronchial wall. (B) Bronchial wall in chronic bronchitis demonstrating inflammatory cells (In), mucosal smooth muscle hypertrophy (M), and hypertrophy of the mucus glands or goblet cells (G). (Respiratory System. O'Dowd, Geraldine, BSc(Hons), MBChB(Hons), FRCPath, *Wheater's Pathology: A Text, Atlas, and Review of Histopathology*, 12, 133-149.e8. Fig. 12.9).

which invade the submucosa of the bronchial tree. There is also marked hypertrophy of the smooth muscle of the bronchiolar wall. Most significantly, there is an increase in the size and number of goblet cells in the trachea and bronchial tree. Cilia are destroyed and replaced by mucus secreting goblet cells, resulting in both mucus hypersecretion as well as impaired mucociliary clearance, manifesting as a chronic, productive cough in these patients (Figs. 28.11 and 28.12).

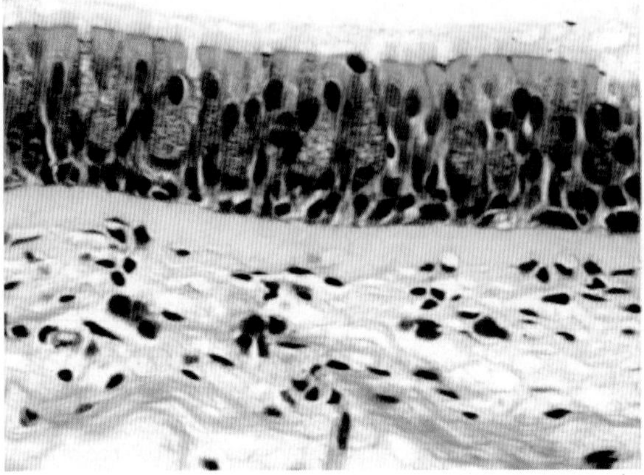

Fig. 28.12 Chronic bronchitis demonstrating replacement of ciliated cells with goblet cells. (Respiratory System. O'Dowd, Geraldine, BSc(Hons), MBChB(Hons), FRCPath, *Wheater's Pathology: A Text, Atlas, and Review of Histopathology*, 12, 133-149.e8).

CLINICAL PEARL

Macrophages and neutrophils accumulate in the respiratory bronchiole, so the bronchoalveolar lavage (BAL) fluid cell count from a smoker will usually demonstrate >95% macrophages and 1%–2% neutrophils, both of which are not normally present in nonsmokers' BAL sample.

Case Point 28.2

The diagnosis of GOLD stage 3 COPD was established for this patient based on his symptoms and spirometry results. You have ensured that he is up to date with influenza and pneumococcal vaccinations and have begun to address the goal of smoking cessation. Unfortunately, over the past 1 week, the patient has experienced an increase in his sputum production, change in the quality of his sputum, and increased symptoms of wheezing. He is also reporting intermittent fevers and chills and significantly worsened dyspnea. On assessment in your office, the patient's vital signs are significant for temperature of 38.22°C (100.8°F), heart rate of 105 beats per minute, blood pressure of 140/86 mmHg, respiratory rate of 32 breaths per minute, and oxygen saturation of 87% on room air. His examination is significant for diffuse inspiratory and expiratory wheezing present on lung auscultation, as well as tachycardia and tachypnea. You advise that he must be admitted for management of an acute COPD exacerbation.

What are the defining features of an acute COPD exacerbation?

A COPD exacerbation is defined by the GOLD initiative as "an acute worsening of respiratory symptoms that results in the need for additional therapy." Acute exacerbations are often triggered by an inciting factor, most commonly an acute bacterial/viral infection; by an exposure to a new environmental irritant; or, in some cases, no obvious trigger may be identified at all. During an exacerbation, there is a reduction in the expiratory flow, leading to increased air trapping and hyperinflation, resulting in the sensation of increased dyspnea. In addition, increased airway inflammation results in worsened ventilation and perfusion mismatching, sometimes leading to new or worsened hypoxemia or hypercarbia.

CLINICAL PEARL

Rhinovirus is the most commonly isolated viral cause of COPD exacerbations. Exacerbations tend to be more severe when associated with viral infections than other triggers, resulting in longer duration of symptoms and higher hospitalization rates.

CLINICAL PEARL

Eosinophils can be found in increased concentrations in the airways, lung parenchyma, and circulating blood in the setting of an acute COPD exacerbation, especially in the setting of a viral infection.

How do you treat an acute COPD exacerbation?

Treatment of an acute exacerbation is dependent on the severity of the patient's symptoms (Table 28.4).

The mainstay of treatment for all acute COPD exacerbations includes inhaled ß-agonists, usually given concomitantly with short-acting antimuscarinic agents. If indicated, antibiotics can be used and should cover the most common bacterial triggers for COPD exacerbations, including *Streptococcus pneumonia, Haemophilus influenza,* and *Moraxella catarrhalis*, as well as atypical bacteria. Systemic glucocorticoids are often indicated in moderate to severe exacerbations, especially in patients requiring hospitalization.

CLINICAL PEARL

Systemic glucocorticoid administration has been shown to decrease the hospital length of stay and the frequency of recurrent exacerbations in patients who required hospitalization for their exacerbation.

In addition to the above therapies, treatment of patients hospitalized for an acute COPD exacerbation should also include supplemental oxygen if they present with hypoxia, and noninvasive positive pressure ventilatory support (NIPPV) in patients presenting with hypercarbic respiratory failure (arterial partial pressure of carbon dioxide >60 mm Hg). Invasive ventilatory support should only be reserved for those patients who have failed initial therapies resulting in ongoing hypoxic and/or hypercarbic respiratory failure.

CLINICAL PEARL

Early use of NIPPV has been shown to reduce the hospital length of stay, need for invasive mechanical ventilation, and mortality.

TABLE 28.4 ■ **Treatment Guidelines for Acute Chronic Obstructive Pulmonary Disease Exacerbations**

Severity	Symptoms	Treatment
Mild	Increased dyspnea, sputum production	SABD +/– SAMA therapy
Moderate	Above symptoms with associated fevers, chills, malaise	SABD, SAMA therapy, and antibiotics +/– oral corticosteroids
Severe	Moderate to severe respiratory distress; hypoxia or hypercarbia; abnormal CXR	SABA, SAMA, antibiotics, oral corticosteroids, and usually hospitalization

CXR, chest radiograph; *SABD,* short-acting bronchodilator; *SAMA,* short-acting muscarinic antagonist.

Case Point 28.3

The patient was hospitalized for his acute COPD exacerbation. Infectious investigation had revealed *S. pneumoniae* lobar pneumonia. He was started on scheduled albuterol and ipratropium inhaled nebulizer treatments every 4 hours, as well as prednisone 60 mg orally daily and levofloxacin 750 mg daily. He initially required supplemental oxygen via nasal cannula, but this was weaned off by hospital day 3. He was discharged home on hospital day 5, with plans to complete a 7-day antibiotic and oral corticosteroid course. He continues his ongoing attempts to quit smoking.

References

Broaddus VC, Mason RJ. *Murray & Nadel's Textbook of Respiratory Medicine.* 6th ed. Philadelphia, PA: Elsevier Saunders; 2016.

Corrin B, Nicholson AG, Burke MM, Rice A. *Pathology of the Lungs.* 3rd ed. Edinburgh, New York: Churchill Livingstone/Elsevier; 2011.

Fauci AS. *Harrison's Principles of Internal Medicine.* 17th ed. New York: McGraw-Hill Medical; 2008.

Kumar V, Abbas AK, Aster JC, Perkins JA. *Robbins Basic Pathology.* 10th ed. Philadelphia, PA: Elsevier; 2018.

Landsberg JW. *Manual for Pulmonary and Critical Care Medicine.* Philadelphia, PA: Elsevier; 2018.

Leslie KO, Wick MR, Leslie KO. *Practical Pulmonary Pathology: A Diagnostic Approach.* 3rd ed. Philadelphia, PA: Elsevier; 2018.

O'Dowd, O'Dowd G. *Wheater's Pathology.* 6th ed. Philadelphia, PA: Elsevier; 2020.

Reed JC. *Chest Radiology: Patterns and Differential Diagnoses.* 7th ed. Philadelphia, PA: Elsevier; 2018.

Singh D, Agusti A, Anzueto A, et al. Global strategy for the diagnosis, management, and prevention of chronic obstructive lung disease: the GOLD science committee report 2019. *Eur Respir J.* 2019; 53(5):1900164.

Tejada-Vera B, Chong Y, Lu L, Sutton PD. *Leading Causes of Death: United States, 1999–2016.* National Center for Health Statistics; 2018.

Weinberger SE, Cockrill BA, Mandel J. *Principles of Pulmonary Medicine.* 7th ed. Philadelphia, PA: Elsevier; 2019.

CASE 29

A 70-Year-Old Male with a History of Increased Shortness of Breath

Moises J. Velez ■ Jennifer J. Prutsman-Pfeiffer

An active 70-year-old male with a history of multiple pneumonias presented to a pulmonologist for cough and increased shortness of breath. He works in the dairy industry and is involved in sampling milk from farms. He also raises chickens and has been exposed to dust from barns. He has a family history of idiopathic interstitial lung disease (ILD). He recently started oxygen and underwent a high-resolution computed tomography (HRCT) scan of the chest, which demonstrated scattered and diffuse bilateral ground glass opacities, bilateral interlobular septal thickening, and bilateral traction bronchiectasis with questionable honeycombing (concerning for cystic airspaces with fibrosis). The radiologic findings are compatible with ILD.

What is ILD?

ILD is a general term for a broad category of lung disorders that lead to varied histologic patterns of lung injury or remodeling that affect the lung parenchyma and alveoli. Some individuals may have a genetic predisposition to developing ILD.

What are the causes of ILD?

In genetically susceptible individuals, progressive ILD may be caused due to collagen vascular disease (CVD; e.g., rheumatoid arthritis [RA], scleroderma, polymyositis, and Sjögren's syndrome), exposure to certain agents such as silicosis, berylliosis, asbestosis, smoking, chemicals, certain medications, and environmental fungi and molds (hypersensitivity pneumonitis [HP]). Some cases may be sporadic or idiopathic. If there is no clear etiology, the term idiopathic interstitial pneumonia is appropriate. ILD may show a familial distribution. Bird fancier's lung is a type of HP caused by exposure to organic avian protein found in feathers and bird droppings. Farmer's lung is a type of HP caused by exposure to thermophilic *Actinomyces* and *Aspergillus* species.

CLINICAL PEARL

Upregulation of transforming growth factor β1 (TGF-β1) ligands are observed in ILD. TGF-β regulates multiple cellular processes including suppression of epithelial cells, fibroblast activation, and extracellular matrix organization. Additional mediators of fibrosis include fibroblast growth factor, platelet-derived growth factor, and vascular endothelial growth factor.

What are examples of ILD?

ILDs comprise a broad category with 200–300 or even more lung diseases. ILDs with known etiologies include HP, pneumoconiosis (silicosis, berylliosis, and asbestosis), CVD-induced ILD, and drug toxicity. Major idiopathic (unknown etiology) ILDs (Box 29.1) include idiopathic pulmonary fibrosis (IPF; Fig. 29.1A–C), respiratory bronchiolitis with ILD (Fig. 29.2), desquamative interstitial pneumonia (Fig. 29.3), acute interstitial pneumonia (histologically manifests as diffuse alveolar damage and is an idiopathic version of acute respiratory distress syndrome) (Fig. 29.4A–C, cryptogenic organizing pneumonia, and idiopathic nonspecific interstitial pneumonia (NSIP; Fig. 29.5).

CLINICAL PEARL

Acute and subacute HP typically shows a cellular bronchiolocentric pattern (surrounding airways) of inflammation with poorly formed granulomas. NSIP and UIP patterns of lung injury may also be observed in chronic or fibrotic HP (Selman). RA-associated ILD may manifest with a UIP (most common) or NSIP pattern of lung injury.

BOX 29.1 ■ Major Idiopathic Interstitial Pneumonias Recognized by the American Thoracic Society/European Respiratory Society Classification

Major Idiopathic Interstitial Lung Diseases

- Idiopathic pulmonary fibrosis (IPF)
- Respiratory bronchiolitis with interstitial lung disease (RB-ILD)
- Desquamative interstitial pneumonia (DIP)
- Acute interstitial pneumonia (AIP)
- Cryptogenic organizing pneumonia (COP)
- Idiopathic nonspecific interstitial pneumonia (I-NSIP)

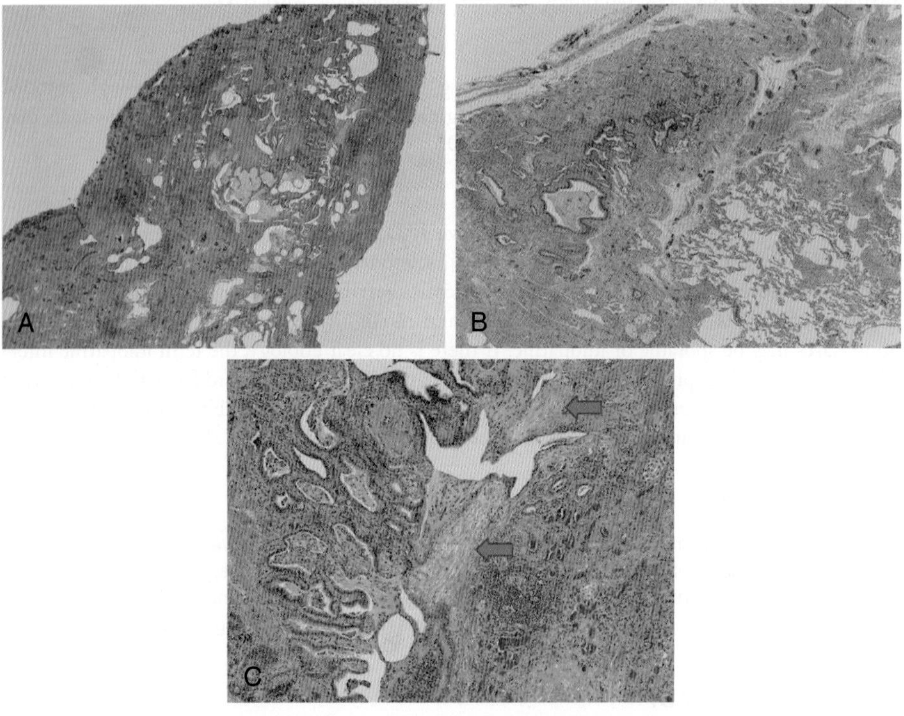

Fig. 29.1 (A) Lower lung lobe exhibiting complete architectural replacement of normal alveolar parenchyma by fibrosis and peribronchiolar metaplasia (PBM). Cystic air spaces are noted. The findings are compatible with usual interstitial pneumonia (UIP) pattern and honeycomb lung (H&E 20x). (B) Subpleural fibrosis and PBM adjacent to relatively normal lung architecture in a patient with idiopathic pulmonary fibrosis (IPF; H&E 40x). (C) Subpleural fibrosis and PBM in a patient with IPF/UIP pattern of injury. Note the fibroblastic foci (arrows) at the edge of the fibrotic parenchyma (H&E 100x).

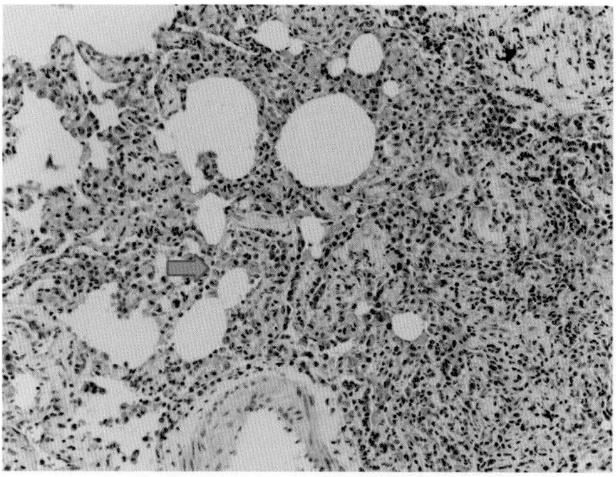

Fig. 29.2 Scattered pigmented macrophages (arrow) and cystic air spaces in the background of a dense lymphoplasmacytic infiltrate and interstitial fibrosis in a patient with respiratory bronchiolitis with interstitial lung disease (RB-ILD; H&E, 200x).

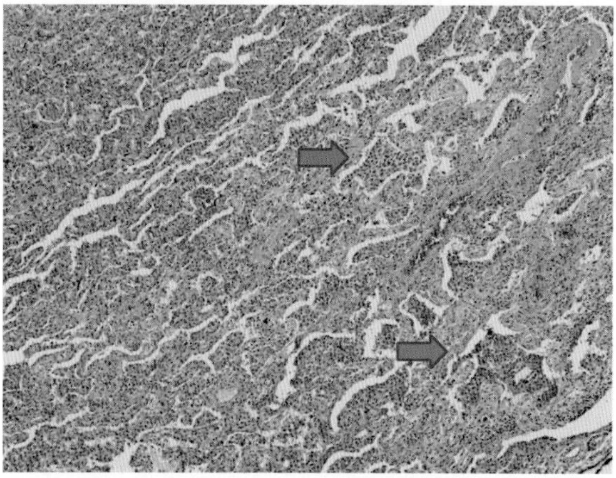

Fig. 29.3 Diffuse intra-alveolar macrophages (arrows) in a patient with desquamative interstitial pneumonia (DIP; H&E, 100x).

How do you make a diagnosis of ILD?

Diagnosis requires gathering pertinent clinical history and evaluation including serologic studies to evaluate for exposures (e.g., HP panel), autoimmune disease, review of medications, and a chest HRCT scan for radiologic correlation. In the absence of a clear radiologic and clinical correlation, a lung biopsy (generally a wedge resection) may be helpful to evaluate for patterns of lung injury. Cryobiopsies is a new emerging modality to obtain tissue for histologic evaluation. The pathologic diagnosis requires correlation with a chest HRCT (inspiratory, expiratory, and prone HRCT imaging) with consideration of a detailed clinical history. A multidisciplinary approach and consensus discussion will help narrow the diagnosis.

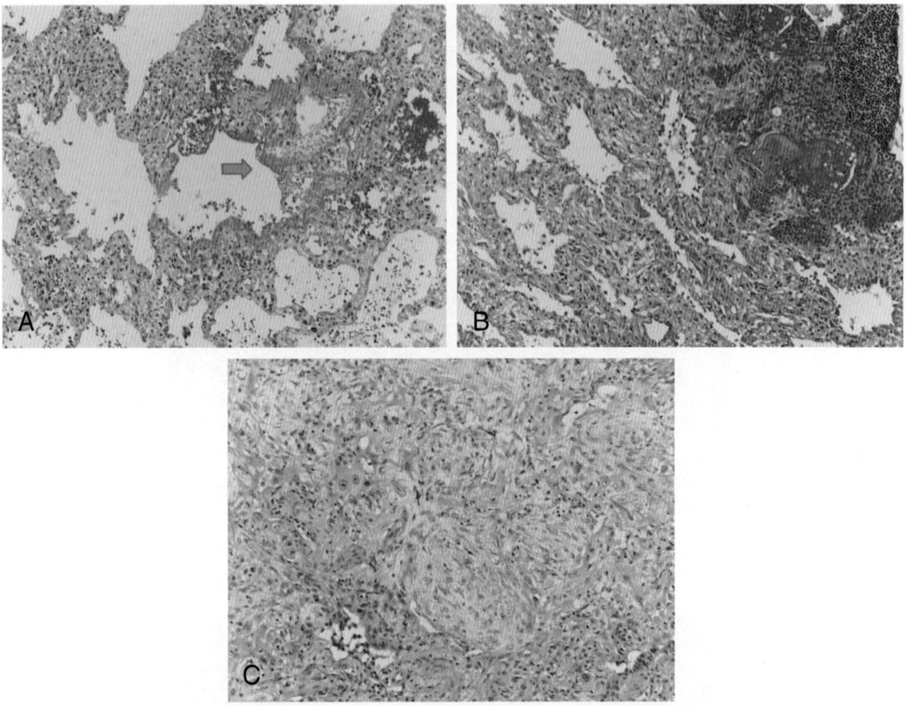

Fig. 29.4 (A) Alveolar injury characterized by hyaline membrane (arrow) formation, consistent with diffuse alveolar damage (DAD) pattern of injury (H&E, 200x). (B) Alveolar hyaline membrane formation on the left and adjacent squamous metaplasia to the right (H&E, 200x). (C) Alveoli filled with loose myxoid fibroblastic proliferations, consistent with organizing pneumonia (OP) pattern. Hyaline membranes were identified within other lung fields. The findings of hyaline membranes and OP are compatible with DAD, organizing phase (H&E, 200x).

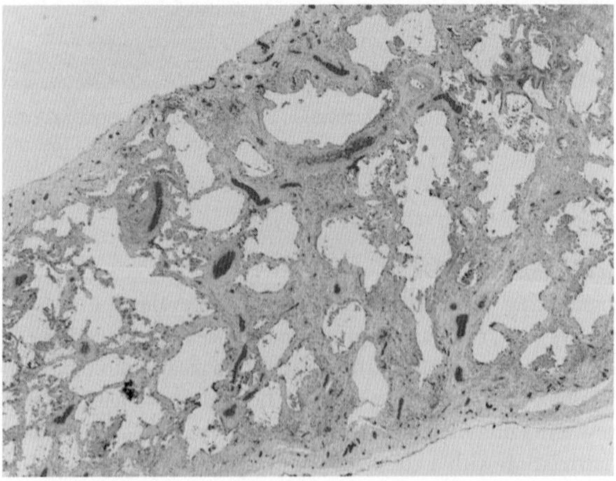

Fig. 29.5 Relatively retained lung architecture or air spaces with interstitial fibrosis and a cellular inflammatory infiltrate. The histologic findings are best in keeping with nonspecific interstitial pneumonia pattern (NSIP; H&E, 40x).

CLINICAL PEARL

An HP panel or serum precipitin testing for specific environmental antigens (including fungi and theromophilic actinomycetes) may help guide clinical practice. Chemical HP (typically following occupational chemical exposure) and hot-tub HP (due to non-tuberculosis mycobacteria) are due to different antigens.

Case Point 29.1

Pulmonary function tests showed severe reduction in the first second of forced expiratory volume and forced vital capacity, typical of restrictive lung disease. He has been receiving prednisone without improvement. The HP panel was negative despite his considerable exposure to thermophilic actinomyces in the barn. Given his worsening condition despite treatment and questionable honeycomb lung on HRCT, he underwent an open lung biopsy of the right upper and lower lung lobes for histologic evaluation of his ILD. Histologic sections showed interstitial fibrosis with extensive architectural remodeling or honeycombing and areas of normal lung (Fig. 29.6). A bronchiolocentric or airway-centered pattern of injury was seen (Fig. 29.7). Fibroblastic foci composed of loose myxoid connective tissue are seen. Subpleural fibrosis is identified. There is also mucus plugging and peribronchiolar metaplasia. The organizing pneumonia is primarily seen in the lower lobe. In less fibrotic areas, a bronchiolocentric distribution is seen. Intra-alveolar giant cells with cholesterol clefts are present (Fig. 29.8). Grocott's methenamine silver (GMS) staining is negative for fungal organisms.

The pattern of lesions raises the differential diagnosis of chronic HP, drug toxicity, infection, asbestosis, CVDs, or an idiopathic process. However, in this case both the radiologic (HRCT) and pathologic features are against IPF.

CLINICAL PEARL

The radiologic findings of IPF are lower lobe predominant ground-glass opacities with reticulation, traction bronchiectasis, and honeycombing (remodeling of lung architecture histologically characterized by, cystic spaces with fibrosis and areas of relatively normal lung which is compatible with a UIP pattern).

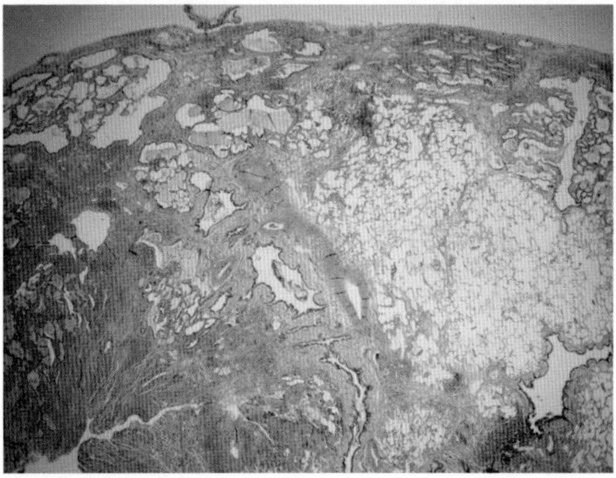

Fig. 29.6 Interstitial fibrosis with extensive architectural remodeling or honeycombing (left of the image) and areas of normal lung (right of the image) (H&E, x1.25).

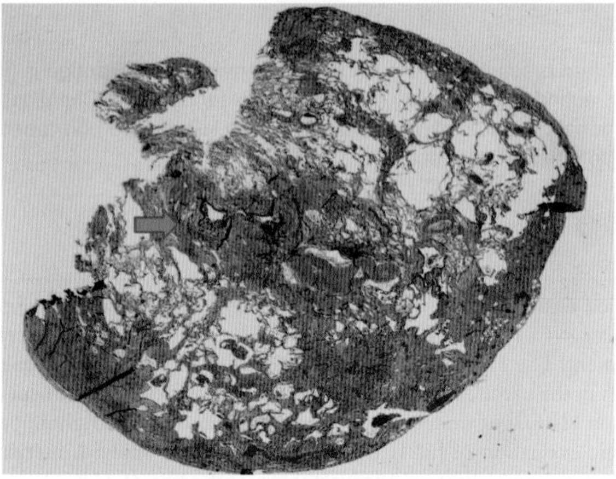

Fig. 29.7 Subpleural and bronchiolocentric (arrow) distribution of fibrosis and cellular injury in a patient with chronic hypersensitivity pneumonitis (H&E, 20x).

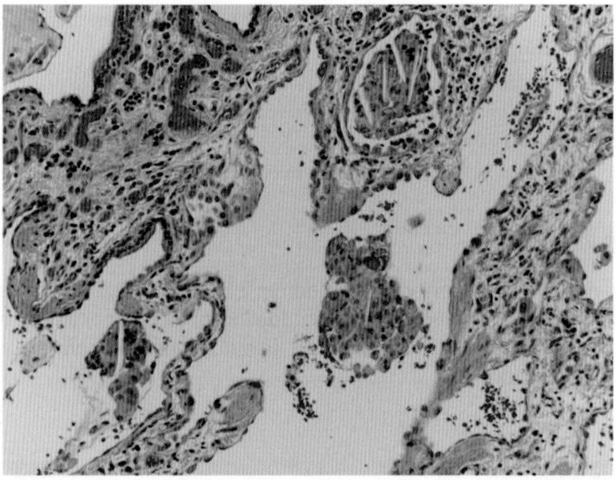

Fig. 29.8 Intra-alveolar giant cells with cholesterol clefts in a patient with chronic hypersensitivity pneumonitis (H&E, 200x).

CLINICAL PEARL

The most common radiologic findings of NSIP include peripheral, lower lobe predominant ground-glass opacities with reticulation, traction bronchiectasis, and pulmonary volume loss.

Case Point 29.2

The histology and negative GMS stain do not suggest a fungal etiology. Serology was negative for rheumatoid factor (RF) and antinuclear antibodies (ANAs). The bronchiolocentricity and presence of intra-alveolar giant cells, along with the history of multiple airborne exposures in a

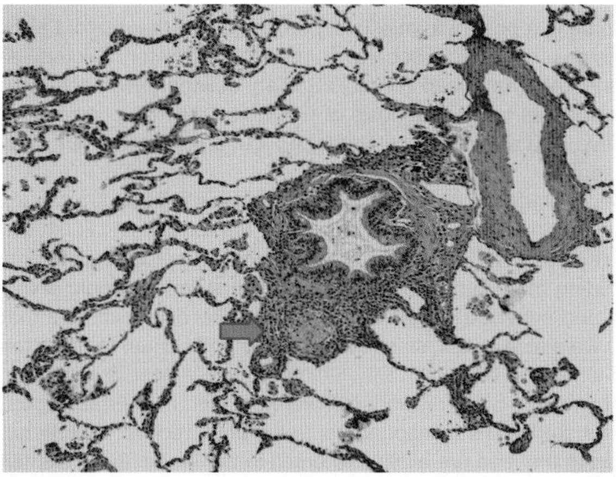

Fig. 29.9 Bronchiolocentric poorly formed non-necrotizing granuloma (arrow) with a cellular inflammatory infiltrate in a patient with hypersensitivity pneumonitis (H&E, 100x).

farm setting, raises concern for HP. Based on the history of exposures, morphology, and radiological findings, this is best characterized (pathologically) as a bronchiolocentric fibrosing and cellular interstitial pneumonia with a usual interstitial pneumonia (UIP) pattern that is most compatible with chronic HP despite the absence of granulomas (Fig. 29.9).

CLINICAL PEARL

Granulomas may be absent in up to one-third of cases of HP.

CLINICAL PEARL

The NSIP and UIP patterns of injury may be seen in both CVDs and HP. Therefore, honeycombing (UIP pattern) can be present microscopically with these conditions. Cellular and fibrotic forms of NSIP exist, with the latter showing poor treatment response. NSIP may also be idiopathic. UIP pattern predicts a worse prognosis in patients with RA-associated ILD.

Case Point 29.3

ANA and RF were ordered and found to be negative. Given the clinical, radiologic, and pathologic findings, the consensus diagnosis was chronic HP. The patient was continued on steroids, and avoidance or decreasing the risk of exposures was strongly recommended.

BEYOND THE PEARLS

- Silicosis is caused by exposure to silica (silicon dioxide) and can be seen in occupational exposures such as miners, sandblasters, and metal grinders; the lungs may show nodular fibrosis.
- Berylliosis is caused by exposure to beryllium, which may be in the aerospace industry with nuclear reactors; lungs may show granuloma formation.

- Caplan syndrome is a pneumoconiosis accompanied by rheumatoid arthritis.
- Refer to the American Thoracic Society/ European Respiratory Society/ Japanese Respiratory Society and Latin American Thoracic Society collaborative consensus clinical practice guidelines for updates in the diagnosis of IPF which discuss clinical manifestations, diagnostic modalities, and diagnostic criteria for IPF. An official document is available at https://www.thoracic.org.
- There was a high incidence of ILD in people who were exposed to the dust cloud after the collapse of the World Trade Center buildings on September 11, 2001. The dust cloud was a complex mixture of environmental pollutants, including products of combustion of jet fuel, pulverized building materials, asbestos, cement dust, microscopic shards of glass, silica, heavy metals, and numerous organic compounds. Recovery workers that arrived after the initial collapse were also at risk, since the materials and human remains removed from lower Manhattan to either the New York City Office of the Medical Examiner or the staging area at Fresh Kills Landfill in Staten Island, NY, were covered in the hazardous material after the dust and debris settled. First responders, volunteers, recovery workers, and people who lived or worked in the area are eligible to enroll in the World Trade Center Health Program, housed under the U.S. Department of Health and Human Services and administered by the National Institute for Occupational Safety and Health, Centers for Disease Control and Prevention. The program covers the additional locations of the Pentagon and Shanksville, PA. For more information visit: https://www.cdc.gov/wtc

References

Barratt SL, Creamer A, Hayton C, Chaudhuri N. Idiopathic pulmonary fibrosis (IPF): an overview. *J Clin Med.* 2018;7(8):E201.

Fenoglio CM, Reboux G, Sudre B, et al. Diagnostic value of serum precipitins to mould antigens in active hypersensitivity pneumonitis. *Eur Respir J.* 2007;29(4):706-712.

Fjällbrant H, Akerstrom M, Svensson E, Andersson E. Hot tub lung: an occupational hazard. *Eur Respir Rev.* 2013;22(127):88-90.

Kim EJ, Collard HR, King TE Jr. Rheumatoid arthritis-associated interstitial lung disease: the relevance of histopathologic and radiographic pattern. *Chest.* 2009;136(5):1397-1405.

Kligerman SJ, Groshong S, Brown KK, Lynch DA. Nonspecific interstitial pneumonia: radiologic, clinical, and pathologic considerations. *Radiographics.* 2009;29(1):73-87.

Kronborg-White S, Folkersen B, Rasmussen TR, et al. Introduction of cryobiopsies in the diagnostics of interstitial lung diseases—experiences in a referral center. *Eur Clin Respir J.* 2017;4(1):1274099.

Li J, Cone JE, Brackbill RM, Giesinger I, Yung J, Farfel MR. Pulmonary fibrosis among world trade center responders: results from the WTC health registry cohort. *Int J Environ Res Public Health.* 2019;16(5):E825.

Lynch DA. Lung disease related to collagen vascular disease. *J Thorac Imaging.* 2009;24(4):299-309.

Man MA, Man SC, Motoc NŞ, Pop CM, Trofor AC. Fatal hypersensitivity pneumonitis after chemical occupational exposure. *Rom J Morphol Embryol.* 2017;58(2):627-634.

Millon L, Roussel S, Rognon B, et al. Aspergillus species recombinant antigens for serodiagnosis of farmer's lung disease. *J Allergy Clin Immunol.* 2012;130(3):803-805.e6.

Mueller-Mang C, Grosse C, Schmid K, Stiebellehner L, Bankier AA. What every radiologist should know about idiopathic interstitial pneumonias. *Radiographics.* 2007;27(3):595-615.

Saito A, Horie M, Nagase T. TGF-β signaling in lung health and disease. *Int J Mol Sci.* 2018;19(8):E2460.

Selman M, Pardo A, King Jr TE. Hypersensitivity pneumonitis: insights in diagnosis and pathobiology. *Am J Respir Crit Care Med.* 2012;186(4):314-324.

Talbert JL, Schwartz DA, Steele MP. Familial interstitial pneumonia (FIP). *Clin Pulm Med.* 2014;21(3):120-127.

Wu M, Gordon RE, Herbert R, et al. Case report: lung disease in World Trade Center responders exposed to dust and smoke: carbon nanotubes found in the lungs of World Trade Center patients and dust samples. *Environ Health Perspect.* 2010;118(4):499-504.

CASE 30

A 59-Year-Old Male with Productive Cough

Lucas Cruz ■ Peter Chung ■ Raj Dasgupta

A 59-year-old male is referred to a pulmonologist by his primary care doctor for 2 months of persistent productive cough with white and occasionally blood-tinged sputum. He has low-grade fevers and shortness of breath on exertion. His wife reports that he has had significant weight loss since the onset of symptoms. He has a history of diabetes mellitus type 2 and diabetic nephropathy that led to chronic kidney disease and a kidney transplant 3 years ago. His current medications include prednisone, tacrolimus, and mycophenolate. He reports adherence to his medication regimen. He is up-to-date on his vaccinations, including influenza and pneumococcal vaccines. On further questioning, the patient has lived in California his entire life and has no recent travels. He has no sick contacts and no known exposures to tuberculosis (TB). He is a retired accountant and his lifelong hobby has always been playing golf. He denies alcohol and drug usage. He has never smoked and does not recall any other relevant exposures.

What are the main causes of pulmonary infection in immunocompetent and immunosuppressed patients?
Our patient's complaints could be due to a wide variety of diagnosis. Although noninfectious etiologies are possibilities and need to be considered, the constellation of his symptoms in the setting of immunosuppression raises the concern for infectious causes.

Pneumonia, in broad terms, is defined as an infection of the lung parenchyma (as opposed to bronchitis, in which the infection is located predominantly in the airways). A useful clinical classification considers the chronicity (acute, subacute, or chronic), the setting (community or nosocomial), and the underlying immune status of the patient (immunocompetent or immunocompromised). Such a focused approach facilitates in narrowing the differential diagnosis.

CLINICAL PEARL

Most pulmonary infections are caused by the following groups of pathogens: viruses, bacteria (typical or atypical), mycobacteria, and fungi (endemic or opportunistic).

Viral infections: Common community-acquired viral pneumonias (such as those caused by influenza virus, respiratory syncytial virus, adenovirus, and human metapneumovirus) typically have an acute presentation with a viral prodrome and are often self-limiting. However, they can be more severe in certain situations, such as in patients with underlying immunosuppression or pregnancy. A simple viral infection can be sometimes followed by a superimposed bacterial pneumonia. Some viruses are notable for causing pneumonias specifically in immunocompromised hosts, such as cytomegalovirus (Fig. 30.1), leading to a significant disease that requires targeted antiviral therapy.

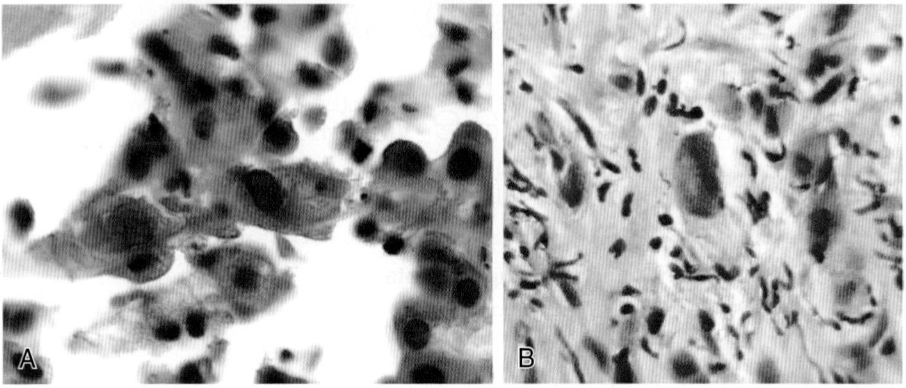

Fig. 30.1 Cytomegalovirus (CMV) pneumonia: (A) CMV inclusions in an alveolar cell. (B) Post-therapy CMV inclusion with smudging and eosinophilia. (From Ivanovic, M. Transplantation-related lung pathology. In *Pulmonary Pathology: A Volume in the Series Foundations in Diagnostic Pathology*, Second Edition, 499-513.e1. FIG. 24.14.).

CLINICAL PEARL

One of the mechanisms of superimposed bacterial pneumonia is the direct effect of viral infections on decreasing the size of the cells, leading to cilia loss in the pulmonary epithelia. This predisposes to bacterial infections. The most common bacteria seen in these cases are S. pneumoniae, S. aureus, and methicillin-resistant S. aureus. (Treanor JJ. Influenza (including avian influenza and swine influenza). In: *Principles and Practice of Infectious Diseases*, 8th ed, Bennett JE, Dolin R, Blaser MJ (Eds), Elsevier Saunders, Philadelphia 2015. p. 2000.)

Bacterial infections: *Streptococcus pneumoniae* (also called pneumococcus) is still considered the most common cause of community-acquired bacterial infections. *Haemophilus influenzae*, *Moraxella catarrhalis*, and *Mycoplasma pneumoniae* are also common culprits. *Staphylococcus aureus* can also be seen, especially as secondary bacterial pneumonia following viral respiratory infections. Among the agents of nosocomial pneumonia, methicillin-resistant *S. aureus* is of special consideration as well as drug-resistant gram-negative bacteria, such as *Pseudomonas aeruginosa*, *Klebsiella pneumoniae*, *Escherichia coli*, and *Serratia marcenscens*. Infections with these organisms usually have an acute or a subacute presentation, and they respond to short courses of antibiotics, provided no other underlying predisposing factor exists. Other less common bacteria such as *Actinomyces* and *Nocardia* species usually cause chronic infections and are of concern especially in the immunocompromised individuals (Fig. 30.2).

CLINICAL PEARL

Nosocomial pneumonia is defined as a pneumonia that occurs 48 hours or more after hospital admission and does not appear to be incubating at the time of admission.

CLINICAL PEARL

Lobar pneumonias are classically described in terms of four macroscopic stages of inflammatory response: congestion, red hepatization, gray hepatization, and resolution (Fig. 30.2).

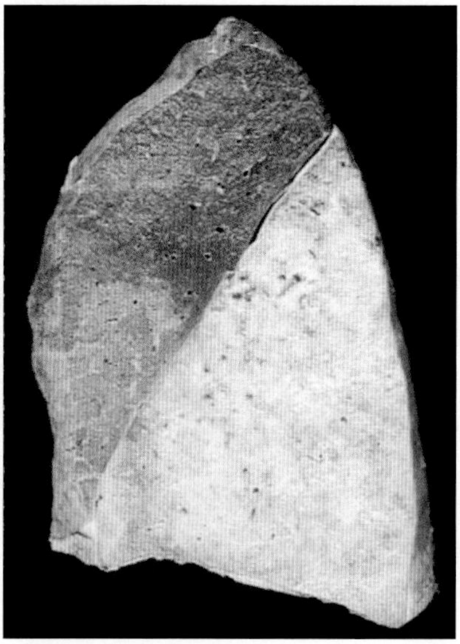

Fig. 30.2 Lower lobe consolidation representing pneumonia with gray hepatization. (From Kumar V, Abbas, AK, Aster JC. *Robbins Basic Pathology*, Tenth Edition. 2017. Fig. 13.30).

CLINICAL PEARL

Species of Nocardia and Actinomyces appear as filamentous gram-positive branching rods. They can be differentiated by the fact that Nocardia exhibits acid-fast staining and grows under aerobic conditions, while Actinomyces does not exhibit acid-fast staining and grows under anaerobic conditions.

Mycobacterial infections are usually subdivided into TB and non-tuberculous mycobacteria (NTM). They tend to have a chronic, protracted course and require prolonged courses of treatment that may not be completely effective in eradication. TB can affect any individual, especially those with risk factors for the disease, but it tends to be more prevalent and more severe in immunosuppressed patients. Among the NTM, *Mycobacterium avium* complex (MAC) is especially prevalent, with a tendency to affect patients with prior underlying lung disease such as chronic obstructive pulmonary disease or underlying bronchiectasis (Fig. 30.3).

CLINICAL PEARL

There is a significant concern regarding the development of drug resistance among mycobacteria. Therefore, treatment regimens include multiple agents. The typical initial treatment for TB includes rifampin, isoniazid, ethambutol, and pyrazinamide. For MAC infections, initial regimen includes azithromycin (or clarithromycin), rifampin, and ethambutol. Regardless of the initial selection, it is important to tailor the therapy depending on antibiotic sensitivities reported by the microbiology laboratory.

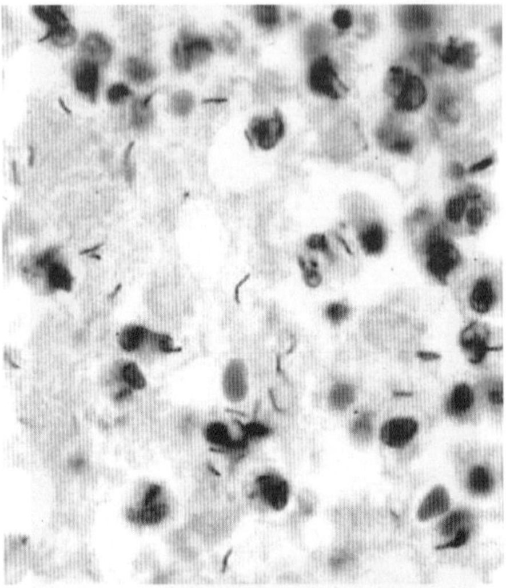

Fig. 30.3 Acid-fast bacilli (Ziehl–Neelsen stain): Mycobacterium tuberculosis. (From McCullough AE, Leslie, KO. *Practical Pulmonary Pathology: A Diagnostic Approach*, Third Edition. Philadelphia, PA: Elsevier. 2018. Figure 7.15).

Fungal infections affecting the lung can be caused by various organisms that can be either restricted to a specific geographical distribution (endemic) or ubiquitous and affecting mostly immunocompromised patients (opportunistic). Among the endemic fungal infections in North America, the most commonly seen are histoplasmosis, coccidioidomycosis, and blastomycosis (Fig. 30.4). These agents tend to cause chronic and often asymptomatic infections in immunocompetent hosts. They may remain latent for years and do not always require antifungal treatment. If the host becomes immunosuppressed, these agents may disseminate throughout the body and cause clinically significant disease. On the other hand, the opportunistic fungi are often ubiquitous in the environment and do not typically cause infection in immunocompetent patients. They are of significant concern in patients with impaired immunity and can have a wide range of presentations, from chronic to acute life-threatening infections. The main opportunistic pulmonary fungal infections are aspergillosis, mucormycosis, cryptococcosis, pneumocystis jirovecii pneumonia (PCP).

CLINICAL PEARL

The endemic fungi are considered thermally dimorphic. They grow as mycelium in lower temperatures in nature (around 25°C) but undergo morphogenesis into yeasts or spherules at higher temperatures, similar to those seen in the human body (around 37°C).

CLINICAL PEARL

Opportunistic fungi can be divided into those that appear as yeast (unicellular existing as single rounded or elongated cells), such as Candida and Cryptococcus, or as mold (multicellular filamentous fungi), such as Aspergillus and Mucor.

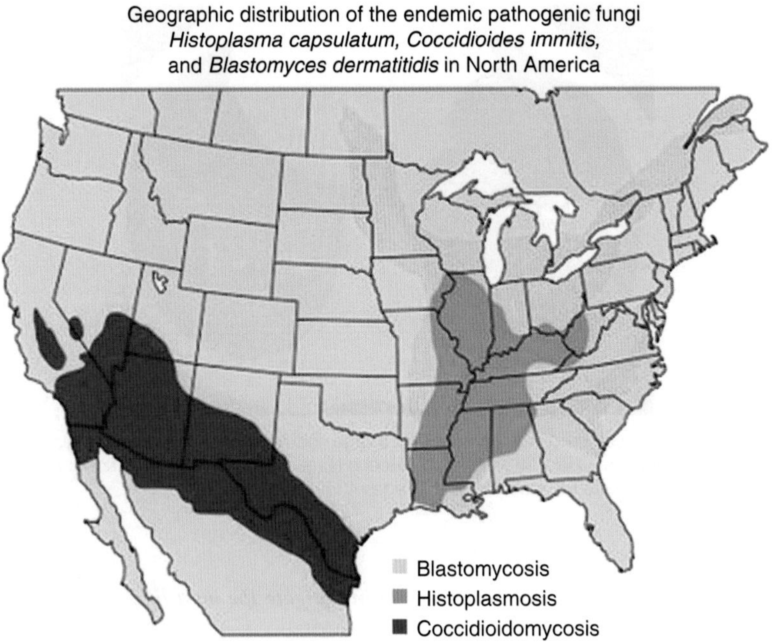

Fig. 30.4 Endemic mycoses. (From Nosanchuk, JD. Endemic mycoses. In: *Murray & Nadel's Textbook of Respiratory Medicine*, Sixth Edition. Elsevier; 646-660.e11. Figure 37-1).

CLINICAL PEARL

Pulmonary infections due to candida are exceedingly rare. Isolates from the respiratory tract almost always indicate colonization and do not require antifungal therapy.

The patient in our case exhibits subacute to chronic symptoms and has underlying immunosuppression, as he is taking medications to prevent rejection from his kidney transplantation. This particular presentation makes etiologies such as typical bacteria and common viruses less likely to be responsible for his symptoms. Instead, there is a high suspicion for infections that commonly affect immunocompromised patients that tend to have a more protracted course, especially fungi (endemic and opportunistic), mycobacteria, and Nocardia.

Case Point 30.1

Initial laboratory investigations including complete blood count, comprehensive metabolic profile, D-dimer, troponins, and B-type natriuretic peptide were within normal limits. Chest radiograph revealed right lower lobe (RLL) nodular opacity and computed tomography (CT) of the chest performed afterwards revealed large RLL nodule with surrounding halo of ground glass attenuation (Fig. 30.5).

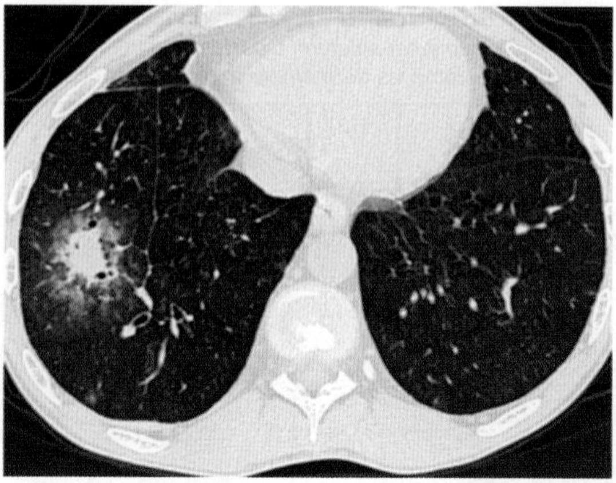

Fig. 30.5 Halo sign: Axial computed tomography with a large nodule surrounded by ground glass attenuation in the right lower lobe. (From Chabi ML, Goracci A, Roche N, et al. Pulmonary aspergillosis. *Diagnostic and Interventional Imaging*, Volume 96, Issue 5, 2015, Pages 435-442, Figure 9.).

What other noninvasive tests can be ordered to investigate the most likely causes of patient's presentation?

The information provided by initial laboratory tests and imaging was useful to rule out other noninfectious diagnosis. Further ancillary testing should be directed at refuting or confirming our hypotheses. As infectious etiologies are being considered, it is usually recommended to obtain cultures of relevant sites. In this case, obtaining samples of sputum for regular bacterial culture, fungal cultures, and acid-fast bacilli (AFB) stain and culture (useful for mycobacteria as well as *Nocardia* and *Actinomyces*) would be essential. Blood cultures (including fungal blood cultures) should be obtained as well.

Other noninvasive testing can be ordered specifically for fungal infections. 1,3-beta-D-glucan is a cell wall component of many fungi, and commercial tests are available to help in the diagnosis of different fungal infections including aspergillosis, candidiasis, and PCP. Galactomannan is a cell wall component of Aspergillus species and tends to be more specific for these organisms. It can be tested in the serum or in specimens obtained from bronchoalveolar lavage, although the latter would require the patient to undergo a bronchoscopic procedure. Serum levels are more commonly elevated in cases of invasive aspergillosis; therefore, a negative result may not exclude other more chronic presentations of the disease.

Additional tests for other fungal etiologies can be found in Table 30.1.

CLINICAL PEARL

1,3-beta-D-glucan testing is typically negative in patients with mucormycosis or cryptococcosis.

CLINICAL PEARL

The most common causes of false-positive results of 1,3-beta-D-glucan are: hemodialysis with cellulose membranes, intravenous immunoglobulin, use of albumin, and infections with bacteria that contain cellular beta-glucans, such as P. aeruginosa.

TABLE 30.1 ■ **Most Commonly Used Noninvasive Testing for Pulmonary Fungal Infections**

	Noninvasive Tests	Comments
Aspergillosis	Serum 1,3-Beta-D-glucan, Serum or BAL galactomannan, BAL PCR	Serum galactomannan more specific than 1,3-Beta-D-glucan but most commonly positive in invasive aspergillosis
Mucormycosis	No widely used noninvasive testing	Serum 1,3-Beta-D-glucan, and galactomannan are typically negative which is useful in differentiating from aspergillosis
Cryptococcosis	Serum cryptococcal antigen	Antigen testing is more sensitive in immunocompromised patients
Histoplasma capsulatum	Serum and urine histoplasma antigen, serological antibody testing	Antigen testing is more sensitive in cases of diffuse pulmonary disease, whereas serological testing is typically more useful for localized disease.
Coccidioidomycosis	Serological testing for anticoccidioidal antibodies	Anticoccidioidal complement fixing antibody concentrations in excess of 1:16 are associated with severe disease
Blastomycosis	Serum and urine antigen, serological antibody testing	Antigen and serological antibody testing are less useful than for other fungal infections due to higher rates of cross reactivity.
PCP	LDH, Serum 1,3-Beta-D-glucan	Elevated LDH is useful in HIV-infected patients but less specific in other populations. Serum 1,3-Beta-D-glucan can be elevated in other fungal infections.

BAL, bronchoalveolar lavage; HIV, human immunodeficiency virus; LDH, lactate dehydrogenase; *PCP, Pneumocystis* pneumonia; *PCR,* polymerase chain reaction.

CLINICAL PEARL

The most common causes of false-positive results of serum galactomannan are cross reactivity with other fungal infections such as Histoplasma species, among others. In the past, there were reports of false-positive results in patients being treated with intravenous piperacillin-tazobactam, but this is no longer a problem with current preparations of the drug.

Case Point 30.2

Further testing was performed. Sputum cultures, sputum AFB culture, sputum fungal culture, and blood cultures were negative. Serum 1,3-beta-D-glucan and serum galactomannan were positive. Antigen and serological testing for histoplasmosis, cryptococcosis, and coccidioidomycosis were negative.

What would be the next appropriate diagnostic test in order to confirm a pulmonary fungal infection as a cause of this patient's symptoms?

The elevated serum 1,3-beta-D-glucan is highly concerning for fungal etiology for the patient's presentation, as is the positive serum galactomannan. The fact that the cultures are negative does not exclude the diagnosis, as the sensitivity can be low and highly dependent on the quality of the specimen provided by the patient. Therefore, there is no definitive diagnosis at this point, and obtaining a sample of the large nodule seen on the CT scan is appropriate.

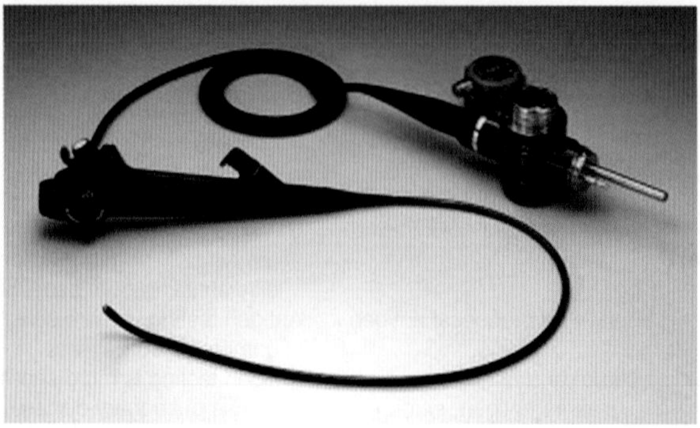

Fig. 30.6 Flexible bronchoscope. (Courtesy of Olympus Corporation. Vachani, Anil, Clinical Respiratory Medicine, Chapter 11, 154-173).

This can be performed with a transbronchial biopsy during a flexible bronchoscopy procedure. In this procedure, a bronchoscope (Fig. 30.6) is introduced into the patient's airways under visualization with a camera located at the tip of the scope. Once the desired lung segment is reached, biopsy samples of the airways or the parenchyma can be obtained. The samples obtained can be sent directly for staining and visualization by pathologists and for cultures in the microbiology laboratory.

Case Point 30.3

The patient underwent a bronchoscopy with transbronchial biopsy. Pathology result revealed septated hyaline hyphae with dichotomous acute angle (45°) branching. It also revealed hyphal invasion of tissue.

What are the main characteristics and morphologic features of fungal infections involving the lungs?
Table 30.2 summarizes the main histopathological characteristics of the most common pulmonary fungal infections.

TABLE 30.2 ■ **Histopathologic Characteristics of Common Fungal Infections in the Lung**

	Histopathology of Fungus
Aspergillus spp.	Narrow septated hyaline hyphae with dichotomous acute angle (45°) branching (Fig. 30.7)
Mucormycosis	Broad hyphae with rare septations and approximately right angle (90°) branching (Fig. 30.8)
Cryptococcus spp.	Round narrow-based yeast with clear halo on H&E (Fig. 30.9)
Histoplasma capsulatum	Small, uniform, oval, narrow-based yeast (Fig. 30.10)
Coccidiodes spp.	Large thick-walled spherules typically containing endospores (Fig. 30.11)
Blastomyces dermatitidis	Round, uniform broad-based yeast with thick walls (Fig. 30.12)
Pneumocystis jirovecii	Narrow-based budding yeast resembling "crushed ping-pong balls" (Fig. 30.13)

H&E, hematoxylin and eosin stain.

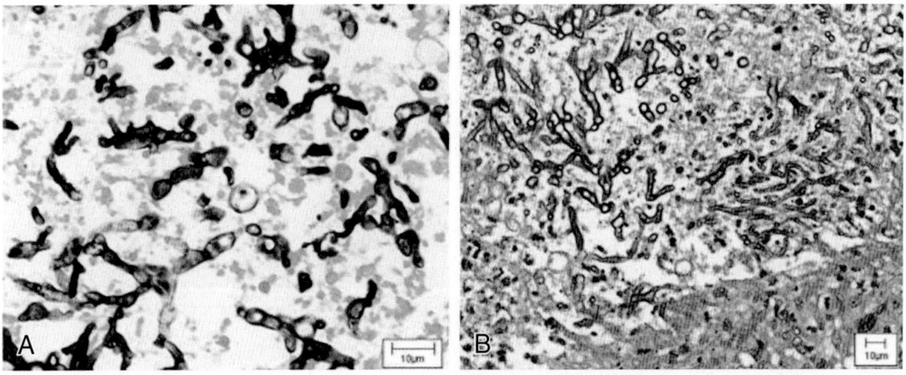

Fig. 30.7 Aspergillus: (A) Gomori methenamine silver stain and (B) Hematoxylin and eosin stain demonstrating branching septated hyphae. (From B.J. Webb, J.E. Blair, S. Kusne, R.L. Scott, D.E. Steidley, F.A. Arabia, and H.R. Vikram. Concurrent Pulmonary Aspergillus fumigatus and Mucor Infection in a Cardiac Transplant Recipient: A Case Report. Fig 3).

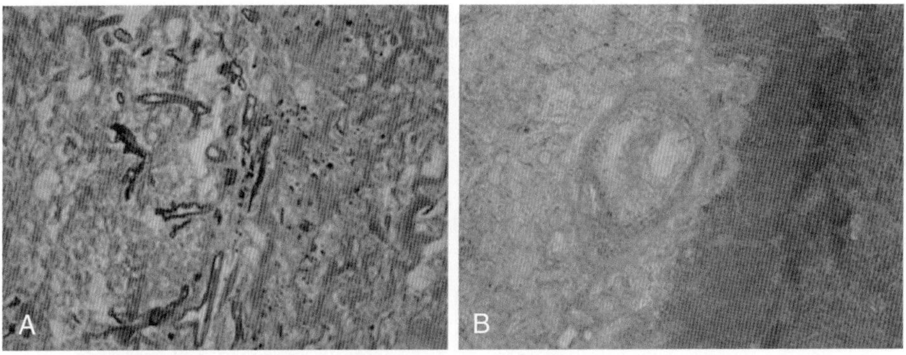

Fig. 30.8 Mucormycosis: (A) Infarcted lung with broad, ribbon-shaped hyphal structures. (B) Infarcted lung with angioinvasive fungal organisms (Surgical Treatment of Multifocal Pulmonary Mucormycosis. Mills, Sara E.A., BA, *Annals of Thoracic Surgery*, Volume 106, Issue 2, e93-e95).

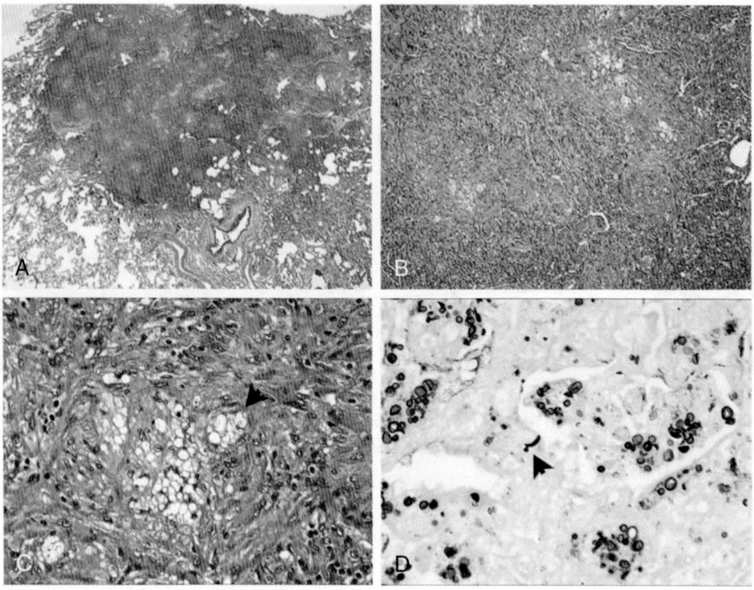

Fig. 30.9 Cryptococcus neoformans: (A) Nodular process within alveoles of lung parenchyma. (B) Nodules composed of proliferating fibroblasts and chronic inflammatory cells representing organizing pneumonia. (C) Clusters of varying size of round and oval structures (arrow) within organizing pneumonia. (D) Narrow-based budding (arrow) under Grocott methenamine silver stain. (A.C. Roden, A.N. Schuetz / *Seminars in Diagnostic Pathology* 34 (2017) 530-549).

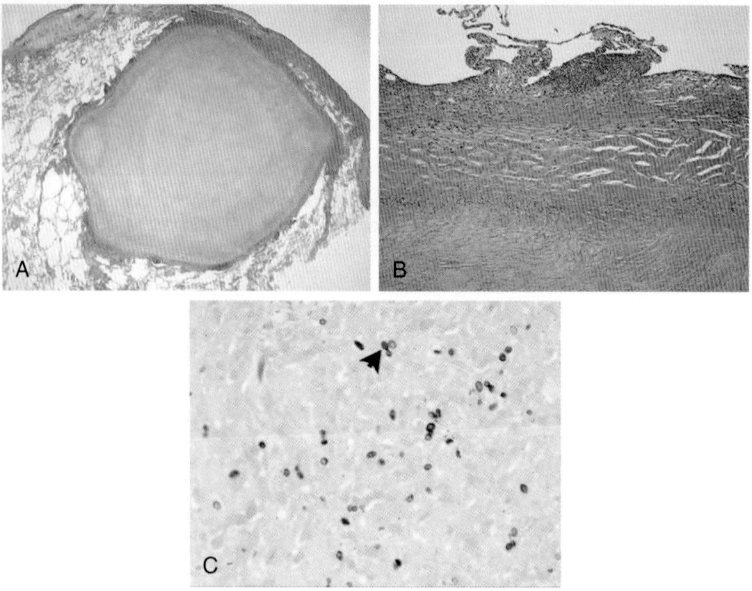

Fig. 30.10 Histoplasma capsulatum: (A) Necrotizing granuloma with a large area of central necrosis. (B) Layering and rims by hydralized fibrosis and chronic inflammation. (C) Clusters of small oval fungal yeasts with narrow-based budding (arrow) within the necrosis. (A.C. Roden, A.N. Schuetz / *Seminars in Diagnostic Pathology* 34 (2017) 530-549).

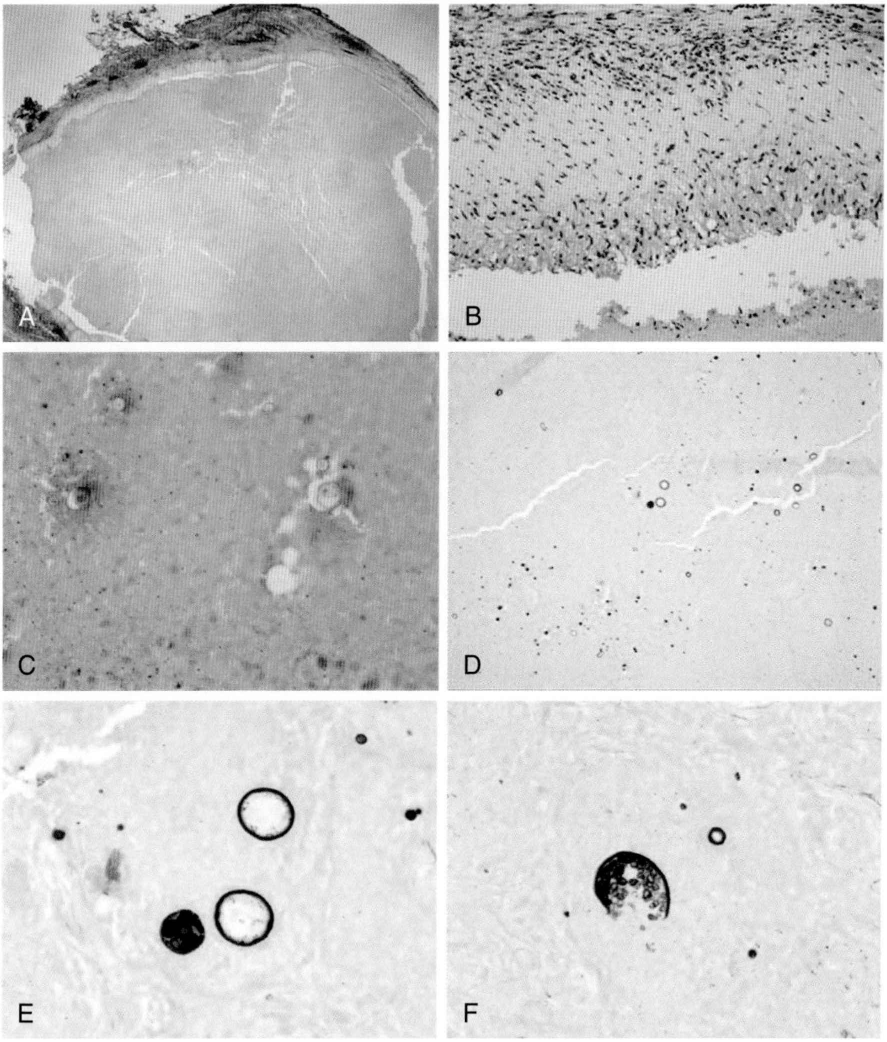

Fig. 30.11 Coccidioides spp.: (A) Necrotizing granuloma. (B) Rims by epithelioid histiocytes. (C) Multiple large spherules under high magnification. (D) Scattered large and small microorganisms within necrosis. (E) Microorganisms characterized by spherules with contained and expelled endospores. (F) Ruptured spherule releasing endospores. (A.C. Roden, A.N. Schuetz / *Seminars in Diagnostic Pathology* 34 (2017) 530-549).

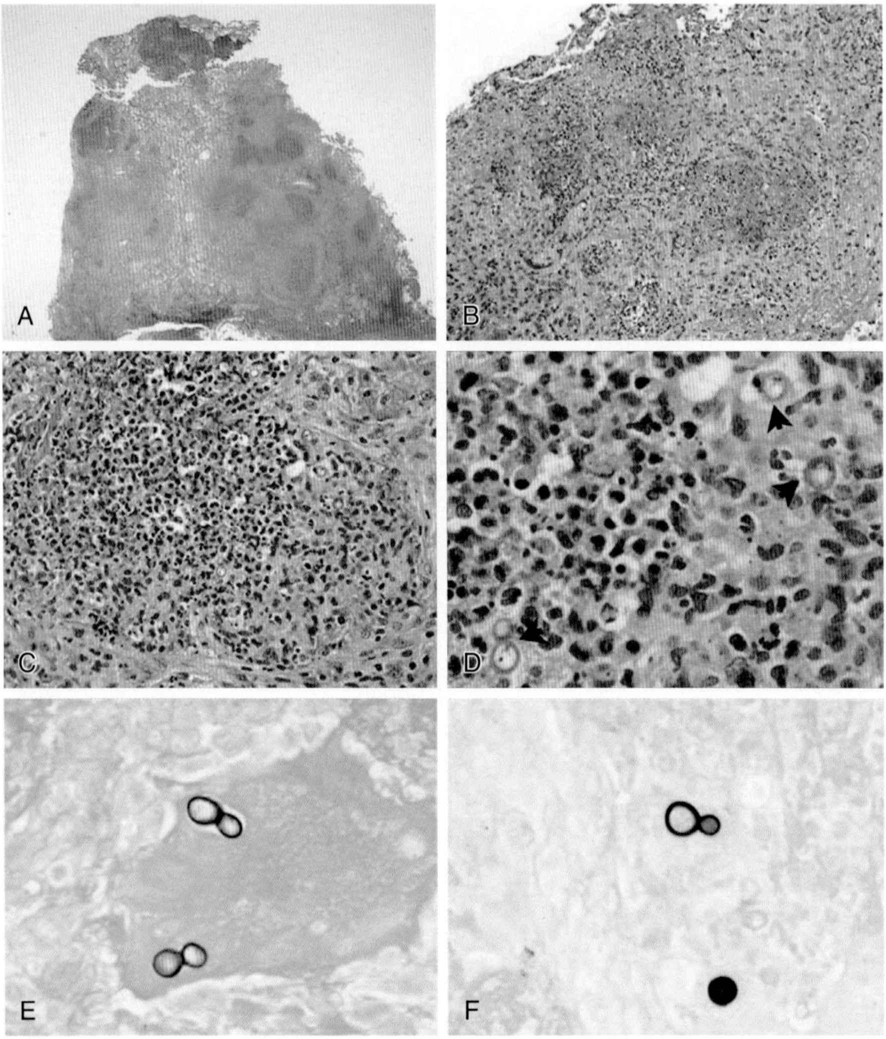

Fig. 30.12 Blastomyces dermatitidis: (A) Multinodular lesion in the lung at low magnification; (B) Illdefined necrotizing granuloma at high magnification. (C) Central necrosis comprising neutrophils and debris representing suppurative granulomas. (D) Large fungal organisms (arrows). (E) and (F) Broad-based budding. (A.C. Roden, A.N. Schuetz / *Seminars in Diagnostic Pathology* 34 (2017) 530-549).

CLINICAL PEARL

The Grocott methenamine silver stain is most useful to identify fungal organisms in tissues.

CLINICAL PEARL

Infections with Aspergillus can present with a wide variety of clinical syndromes depending on the host's immune status and other underlying predisposing conditions. See Fig. 30.14 for a summary of the most common presentations and their underlying predisposing features.

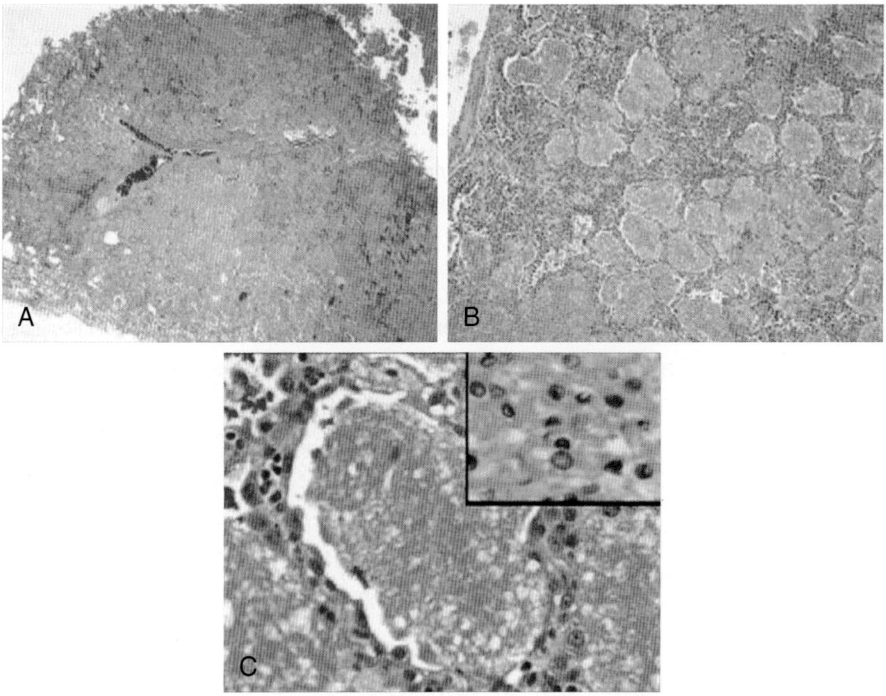

Fig. 30.13 Pneumocystis jirovecii: (A) Alveolar filling process at low magnification. (B) Alveolar filled with pink material. (C) Frothy pink intra-alveolar material at high magnification, showing typical oval, crescent, and helmet-shaped nonbudding organism. (A.C. Roden, A.N. Schuetz / *Seminars in Diagnostic Pathology* 34 (2017) 530-549).

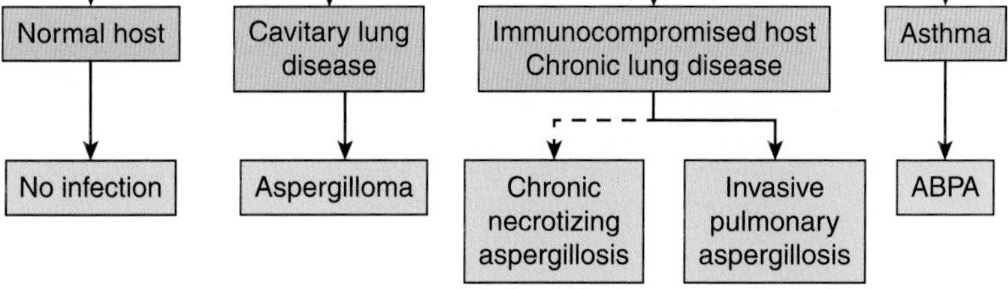

Fig. 30.14 ABPA: Allergic bronchopulmonary aspergillosis. (Aspergillosis. Handa, Sajeev, D., *Ferri's Clinical Advisor* 2019, 142-144.e1).

Case Point 30.4

A diagnosis of chronic necrotizing aspergillosis was made based on the histologic findings as well as the clinical presentation.

What are the recommended treatment agents for pulmonary fungal infections?

The most commonly recommended first-line regimens for pulmonary fungal infections are summarized in Table 30.3.

TABLE 30.3 ■ **Recommended First-Line Treatments for Most Common Pulmonary Fungal Infections**

	Recommended Treatment	Comments
Aspergillosis	Invasive aspergillosis: IV voriconazole or IV liposomal amphotericin B. Severe cases may require addition of IV micafungin or caspofungin. Chronic necrotizing aspergillosis: Voriconazole. May need induction with IV liposomal amphotericin B in severe cases. ABPA: treatment mainly with cortiscosteroids. Itraconazole can be used as steroid-sparing agent. Aspergilloma: no indication for routine antifungal treatment. Surgical resection may be considered depending on symptoms.	Reversal of immunosuppression should be done when possible. Surgical resection may be an option in cases of aspergillomas or chronic necrotizing disease.
Mucormycosis	Initial therapy with IV amphotericin B. Can be transitioned to posaconazole or isavuconazole after initial response.	Surgical debridement of the infectious source frequently necessary.
Cryptococcosis	Localized pulmonary disease: Fluconazole or itraconazole. CNS or disseminated disease: Induction with IV amphotericin B and flucytosine, maintenance with fluconazole or itraconazole.	Secondary prophylaxis with fluconazole in HIV-infected patients is continued after treatment is completed until CD4 count is >200/μL.
Histoplasma capsulatum	Symptomatic mild pulmonary infection: itraconazole. Moderate or severe pulmonary infection: Induction with IV amphotericin B with possible adjunctive corticosteroids. Maintenance with itraconazole. Progressive disseminated infection: Induction with IV amphotericin B. Maintenance with itraconazole.	Some presentations of histoplasmosis require no antifungal therapy, including asymptomatic mild pulmonary infection, broncholithiasis, or fibrosing mediastinitis.
Coccidioidomycosis	Limited pulmonary infection: no therapy usually needed in immunocompetent hosts. In case of immunosuppression, treatment with fluconazole or itraconazole. Disseminated disease: Treatment with fluconazole or itraconazole. Induction with IV amphotericin B may be required in severe cases. Meningitis: fluconazole or itrazonazole for life. Intrathecal amphotericin B may be required.	Anticoccidioidal complement fixing antibody concentrations in excess of 1:16 in an indicator of severe disease.
Blastomycosis	Mild to moderate disease: itraconazole. Life-threatening severe blastomycosis or meningeal infection: induction with IV amphotericin B and maintenance with itrazonazole or fluconazole.	Corticosteroids may be considered as an adjunct in case of severe gas-exchange abnormalities.

TABLE 30.3 ■ **Recommended First-Line Treatments for Most Common Pulmonary Fungal Infections** (Continued)

	Recommended Treatment	Comments
PCP	Trimethoprim plus sulfamethoxazole are considered first-line treatment. Alternatives include atovaquone, pentamidine, and primaquine plus clindamycin.	Adjunctive corticosteroids are recommended in patients with moderate to severe disease (PaO_2 on room air <70 mm Hg or alveolar-arterial oxygen gradient >35).

ABPA, allergic bronchopulmonary aspergillosis; CNS, central nervous system; HIV, human immunodeficiency virus; IV, intravenous; PCP, pneumocystis jirovecii pneumonia.

Case Point 30.5

The patient was started on oral therapy with voriconazole. He had improvement in his symptoms over the following weeks, and a follow-up CT of the chest was performed after 6 months of therapy. It revealed a complete resolution of the previously observed pulmonary abnormalities.

BEYOND THE PEARLS

- Allergic bronchopulmonary aspergillosis is a hypersensitivity reaction in response to colonization of the airways with Aspergillus that occurs almost exclusively in patients with asthma or cystic fibrosis. The mainstay of treatment is corticosteroids, but itraconazole is often added as a steroid-sparing agent.
- *Cryptococcus neoformans* has a wide distribution worldwide and is considered an opportunistic fungus. *Cryptococcus gattii* is endemic in tropical and subtropical regions, but in North America, it is classically seen in British Columbia, Canada, and Pacific Northwest of the United States. *C. gattii* infection has been associated with exposure to certain trees such as eucalypts. Unlike *C. neoformans*, it tends to affect individuals without predisposing immunodeficiency.
- Some fungi, especially Cryptococcus and Cocciodiodes, have strong tendency to involve the central nervous system (CNS). In these cases, a lumbar puncture is performed to rule out CNS involvement, especially in cases of disseminated disease.
- Mucormycosis is an infection caused by fungi from the order Mucorales. The fungi genera most commonly found in human infections are Rhizopus, Mucor, and Rhizomucor.
- Aside from typical immunosuppressing conditions and medications, uncontrolled diabetes mellitus predisposes to mucormycosis infection.
- The most common clinical presentation of mucormycosis is rhino–orbital–cerebral infection. A black eschar is classically seen in the affected areas, which is a result of tissue necrosis and vascular invasion by the fungus. This is a life-threatening condition with high mortality rates. Treatment involves aggressive surgical debridement and prolonged antifungal therapy.

References

Chabi ML, Goracci A, Roche N, Paugam A, Lupo A, Revel MP. Pulmonary aspergillosis. *Diagn Interv Imaging*. 2015;96(5):435-442.

Handa S. Aspergillosis. In: Ferri FF, *Ferri's Clinical Advisor 2020*. Philadelphia, PA; Elsevier; 2020:152-154.e1

Ivanovic M, Husain AN. 24-transplantation-related lung pathology. In: Zander DS, Farver CF, eds. *Pulmonary Pathology*. 2nd ed. Philadelphia, PA: Elsevier; 2018:499-513.e1.

Kumar V, Abbas A, Aster J. *Robbins Basic Pathology*. 10th ed. Philadelphia, PA: Elsevier; 2017.

McCullough AE, Leslie KO. Lung infections. In: Leslie KO, Wick MR, eds. *Practical Pulmonary Pathology: A Diagnostic Approach*. Philadelphia, PA: Elsevier; 2018.

Mills SE, Yeldandi AV, Odell DD. Surgical treatment of multifocal pulmonary mucormycosis. *Ann Thorac Surg*. 2018;106(2):e93–e95.

Nosanchuk JD. Endemic mycoses. In: Broaddus VC, Mason RJ, Gotway MB, eds. *Murray and Nadel's Textbook of Respiratory Medicine*. Elsevier; 2016:646-660.e11.

Roden AC, Schuetz AN. Histopathology of fungal diseases of the lung. *Seminars in Diagnostic Pathology*. 2017;34(6):530-549.

Vachani A, Haas AR, Sterman DH. Bronchoscopy. In: Spiro SG, Silvestri GA, Agustí A, eds. *Clinical Respiratory Medicine*. 4th ed. Philadelphia, PA: Elsevier; 2012:154-173.

Webb BJ, Blair JE, Kusne S, et al. Concurrent pulmonary *Aspergillus fumigatus* and mucor infection in a cardiac transplant recipient: a case report. *Transplant Proc*. 2013;45(2):792-797.

CASE 31

A 79-Year-Old Woman with a Pulmonary, Right Upper Lobe Mass

Moises J. Velez

A 79-year-old woman with a history of hypertension and diverticular bleed presented to the emergency department following a syncopal episode that prompted a workup. High-resolution computed tomography (HRCT) of her chest revealed a predominately ground-glass and partially solid pulmonary right upper lobe mass measuring 3.1 × 1.5 cm (Fig. 31.1A). She denied further syncopal episodes or dizziness. She has never smoked cigarettes and regularly attends aerobics class, twice a week for an hour daily. She denies weight loss, loss of appetite, fever, chills, headaches, chest pain, recent infection, and shortness of breath. A subsequent positron emission tomography (PET)/CT study showed low-grade FDG uptake, suspicious for a neoplastic lesion. A tissue biopsy was recommended. No evidence of hypermetabolic lymphadenopathy, distant metastasis, or peripheral lesions was seen on PET/CT.

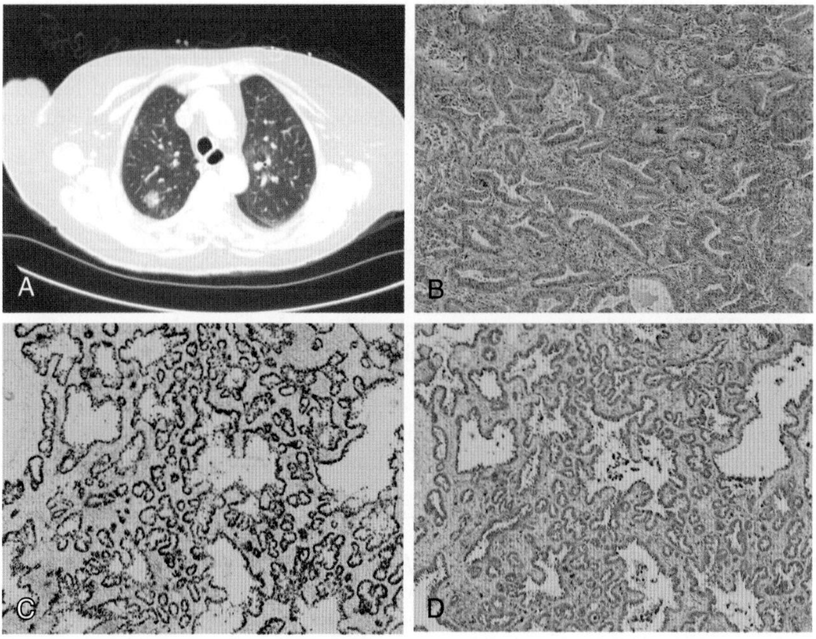

Fig. 31.1 (A) High-resolution computed tomography scan showing a partially solid, right upper lobe peripheral mass. (B) Tumor cells arranged in an invasive acinar pattern of growth (H&E, 200x) (C) Nuclear positivity with thyroid transcription factor-1 (200x) (D) Cytoplasmic positivity with napsin A (Napsin A, 200x).

TABLE 31.1 ■ **Differential Diagnosis for a Solitary Solid Pulmonary Nodule on High-Resolution Computed Tomography**

Neoplastic	Non-Neoplastic
• Pulmonary non–small cell carcinoma • Carcinoid tumor • Lymphoma • Metastatic tumor (typically bilateral nodule)	• Organizing pneumonia • Fibrosis • Necrotizing and non-necrotizing granulomas • Rheumatoid nodule • Pulmonary chondroid hamartoma

TABLE 31.2 ■ **Differential Diagnosis for Ground-Glass Opacities on High-resolution Computed Tomography**

Neoplastic	Non-Neoplastic
• Adenocarcinoma in situ • Minimally invasive adenocarcinoma • Pulmonary non–small cell carcinoma • Lymphoma	• Organizing pneumonia • Infection • Fibrosis • Acute lung injury • Interstitial lung disease • Drug toxicity

What are the possibilities for a solid pulmonary nodule identified on chest HRCT?

The possibilities include organizing pneumonia, fibrosis, granuloma, and a neoplasm including carcinoid tumor, carcinoma, lymphoma, and metastatic disease. Commonly, metastatic disease presents with bilateral lung nodules (Table 31.1).

What are the possibilities for pulmonary ground-glass opacities identified on chest HRCT?

The possibilities include organizing pneumonia, infection, fibrosis, interstitial lung disease, acute lung injury or acute respiratory distress syndrome, a neoplastic process, and drug toxicity (Table 31.2).

Case Point 31.1

The patient underwent video-assisted thoracoscopic surgery. The left upper lobe wedge resection demonstrated a tan-red ill-defined nodule measuring 2.2 cm in greatest diameter. Hematoxylin and eosin (H&E)-stained slides reveal tumor cells with a predominant acinar pattern of growth (Fig. 31.1B). Tumor cells were seen growing along the alveolar wall. Intra-alveolar tumor cell clusters or tufts lacking a fibrovascular core are present. The tumor did not invade through the elastic layer of the visceral pleura. The periphery of the tumor did not reveal intra-alveolar spreading of tumor cells. Immunohistochemical studies showed that the tumor cells were diffusely positive for thyroid transcription factor-1 (TTF-1) and napsin A, which is supportive of a lung primary (Fig. 31.1C and D).

What are some differential diagnoses of primary pulmonary non–small cell lung cancer (NSCLC)?

The differential diagnoses of primary pulmonary NSCLC are broad and not limited to squamous cell carcinoma, keratinizing and non-keratinizing subtypes, adenocarcinoma including mucinous and non-mucinous subtypes, carcinoid tumors, and large cell neuroendocrine carcinoma (LCNEC). While this is not a comprehensive list, it includes the most commonly encountered subtypes.

CLINICAL PEARL

Cancer staging was developed by the UICC and AJCC for the purpose of defining how much cancer is present within the body. Cancer is staged using the UICC/AJCC (currently Eighth Edition) TNM classification. T describes the tumor size, N defines regional lymph node involvement, and M describes metastatic disease if present. The pathologic stage is described on pathology reports using the UICC/AJCC TNM classification.

What are the histologic subtypes of primary pulmonary adenocarcinoma?

Lung adenocarcinoma has five predominant subtypes. Lung tumors can have one subtype or a combination of two or more. The lepidic pattern shows tumor cells growing along the alveolar wall (Fig. 31.2A). Lepidic growth is a noninvasive pattern by definition. The acinar pattern is defined by a glandular pattern of growth (Fig. 31.1B). Cribriform pattern at this time is a subtype of acinar pattern defined by back-to-back glands with well-formed luminal structures (Fig. 31.2B). Histologic differentials of cribriform pattern of growth include neuroendocrine tumors with rosette-like structures. The papillary pattern is an invasive growth pattern defined by tumor cells and stroma architecturally showing papillae with a fibrovascular core (Fig. 31.2C). The micropapillary pattern is an invasive growth pattern defined by tumor cells clusters arranged in frond-like structures that lack a fibrovascular core (Fig. 31.2D). The solid pattern is an invasive growth pattern defined by solid sheets of tumor cells (Fig. 31.2E).

CLINICAL PEARL

The histologic subtypes of adenocarcinoma have prognostic implications and are Grade 1: lepidic, Grade 2: acinar, and papillary and Grade 3 (worse prognosis: micropapillary, solid, and cribriform pattern corresponding to well, moderate, and poorly differentiated subtypes, respectively).

What is spread through air spaces (STAS)?

STAS is a recently described pattern of invasion in NSCLC. As described in the 2015 World Health Organization classification, STAS is defined as micropapillary clusters, solid nests, or single cells spreading within air spaces beyond the edge of the main tumor (Fig. 31.3). A ring-like pattern of STAS has also been described. STAS is associated with increased local regional recurrence in patients who undergo sublobar resection for stage 1 disease. At this time, the presence of STAS is an optional data element recorded in surgical pathology reports/protocol as recommended in the American Joint Committee on Cancer (AJCC) Eighth Edition of the cancer staging manual. STAS should not be incorporated into the total tumor size.

How do you define adenocarcinoma in situ (AIS)?

AIS is an adenocarcinoma with a pure lepidic pattern measuring 3 cm or less.

How do you define minimally invasive adenocarcinoma (MIA)?

MIA is an adenocarcinoma, with a predominant lepidic pattern measuring 3 cm or less, with an invasive component measuring 0.5 cm or less.

CLINICAL PEARL

On radiology, AIS and MIA typically present as pure ground-glass and ground-glass/partially solid opacity measuring >0.5 cm, respectively.

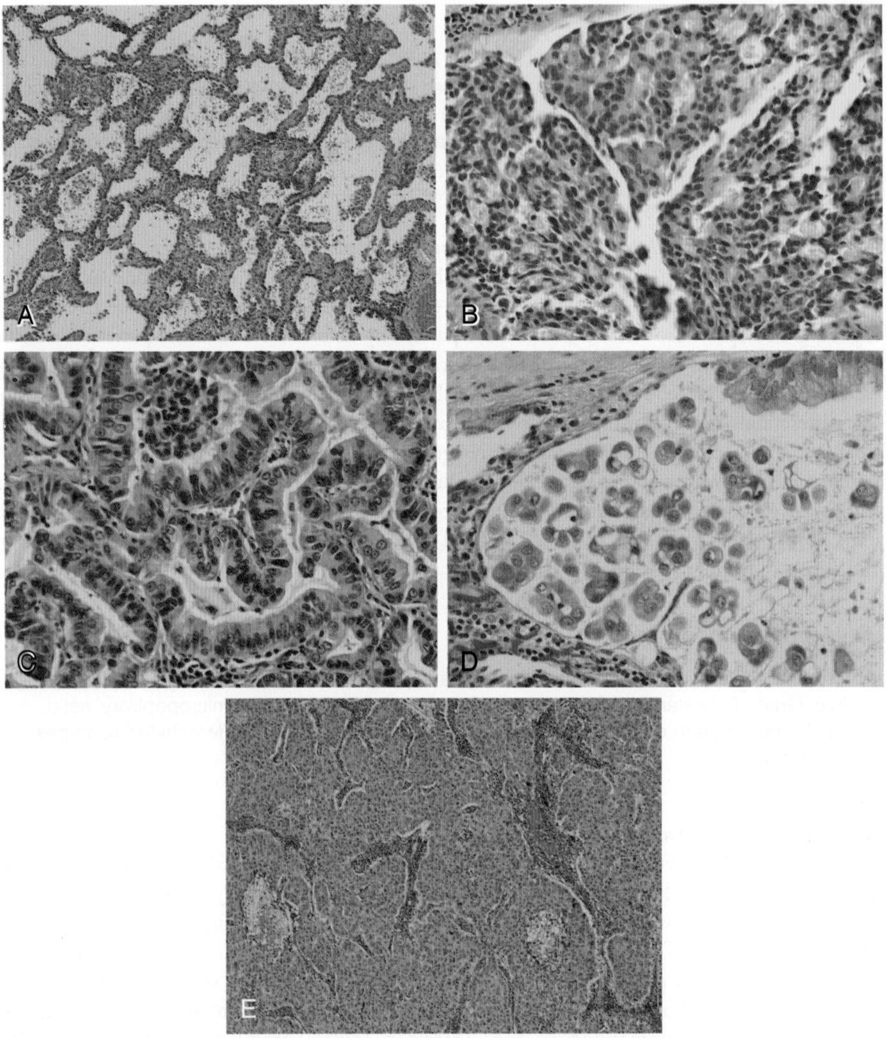

Fig. 31.2 (A) Lepidic pattern, characterized by tumor cells proliferating along the alveolar walls (H&E. 100x), (B) Cribriform pattern, characterized by back-to-back glands with well-formed luminal structures (H&E, 400x), (C) Papillary pattern, characterized by papillae with a fibrovascular core (H&E, 400x), (D) Micropapillary pattern, characterized by frond-like clusters which lack a fibrovascular core (H&E, 400x), (E) Solid pattern, characterized by sheets of tumor cells (H&E, 100x).

What histologic features, if present, exclude AIS and MIA?

Tumor necrosis, STAS, lymphovascular invasion, and visceral pleural invasion (invasion beyond the pleural elastic layer) exclude the diagnosis of AIS and MIA.

CLINICAL PEARL

AIS and MIA, if completely resected, should have a 5-year, 100% disease-free and recurrence-free survival.

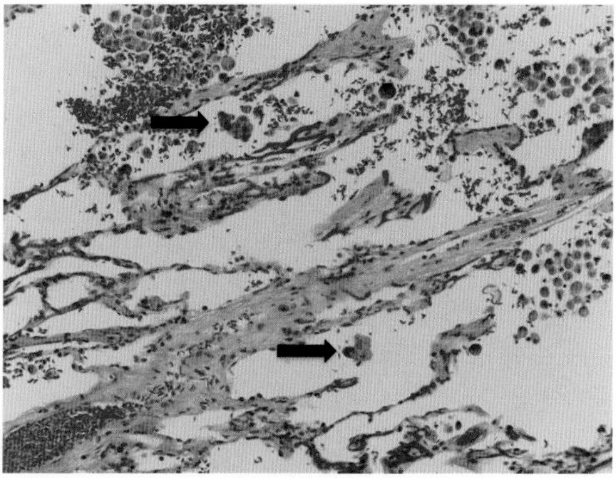

Fig. 31.3 Tumor spread through air space (STAS; arrows), beyond the tumor edge (H&E, 200x).

How do you define atypical adenomatous hyperplasia (AAH)?

AAH is a localized proliferation of atypical or monotonous pneumocytes that typically appear cuboidal, show a pure lepidic pattern of growth, and measure less than or equal to 0.5 cm.

Case Point 31.2

The patient was diagnosed with non-mucinous adenocarcinoma with acinar (75%), micropapillary (5%), and lepidic (20%) patterns. Lymph nodes were submitted for staging and were not involved. The total tumor size was 2.2 cm; however, the invasive tumor size was calculated by excluding the percentage of the lepidic component (noninvasive growth pattern) and multiplying the sum of the invasive percentages by the total tumor size: 0.8×2.2 cm = 1.76 cm. The pathologic stage as determined by using the invasive tumor size in non-mucinous subtypes of adenocarcinoma is pT1b, pN0 [Union for International Cancer Control (UICC)/AJCC Eighth Edition].

CLINICAL PEARL

In non-mucinous subtypes of adenocarcinoma, the invasive tumor size is thought to better correlate with prognosis and is used to determine the tumor size (T). The invasive tumor size is not calculated for mucinous subtypes of adenocarcinoma.

What are the immunohistochemical profiles and molecular genotypes for the following subtypes of adenocarcinoma?

Invasive mucinous adenocarcinoma (IMA) is a distinct subtype of pulmonary adenocarcinoma composed of columnar cells that lack cilia and show basally oriented nuclei and abundant apical mucin proliferating along the alveolar walls (Fig. 31.4). Careful examination often reveals an invasive pattern of growth with desmoplastic stroma. The tumor cells in IMA typically lack nuclear expression with TTF-1 and napsin A and may be positive with cytokeratin 7, as well as for CDX-2, a marker for intestinal differentiation. IMA are typically associated with KRAS mutations and often lack mutations for EGFR, ALK, and ROS1. A small subset of IMAs may show CD74–NRG1 fusions.

The non-mucinous adenocarcinoma subtype typically shows nuclear expression with TTF-1 and cytoplasmic staining with napsin A. Both TTF-1 and napsin A expression support adenocarcinoma

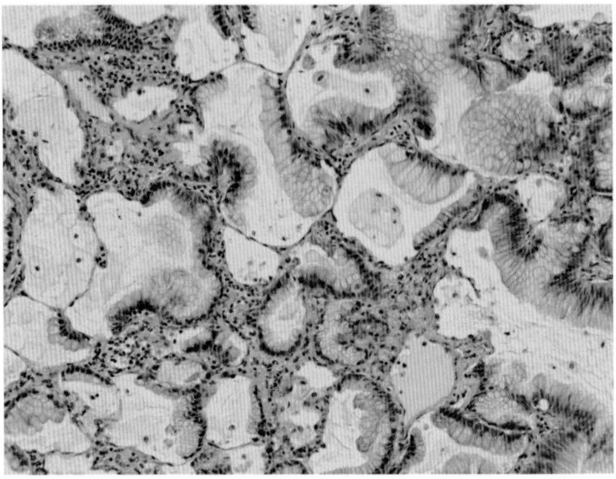

Fig. 31.4 Invasive mucinous adenocarcinoma composed of columnar cells with basally oriented nuclei and abundant apical mucin (H&E, 400x).

differentiation; however, positivity may be seen in pulmonary neuroendocrine tumors as described below. Non-mucinous adenocarcinoma may show oncogenic driver mutations including EGFR, ALK, and ROS1 rearrangements.

What molecular testing is considered standard-of-care for adenocarcinoma?
Sequencing for EGFR, and testing for ALK and ROS1 gene rearrangements.

Case Point 31.3

Immunohistochemistry was performed on representative sections of the tumor (formalin-fixed paraffin-embedded tissue). The tumor cells showed reactivity with TTF-1 and napsin A, which supports a lung primary adenocarcinoma. P40, a marker for squamous cell carcinoma, was negative. Molecular and cytogenetic studies were ordered. An in-frame deletion in exon 19 in the EGFR gene was detected. The mutation identified is associated with a good response to EGFR tyrosine kinase inhibitors (TKIs) gefitinib and erlotinib. Given her clinical stage (stage IA2) and complete resection, the patient is currently undergoing observation.

CLINICAL PEARL

EGFR mutations are most common in never-smokers and in women more than men. ALK gene rearrangements in adenocarcinoma are associated with never- or light smokers. Patients tend to be younger. ROS1 similarly has been associated with light to never smoking history, female sex, and non-Asian ethnicity.

CLINICAL PEARL

TKIs as the first-line treatment show a benefit in NSCLC harboring EGFR mutations (exon 19 deletion and L858R mutation within exon 21), ALK, and ROS1 gene rearrangements. T790M (within exon 20) mutations occur following treatment with a first-line TKI, such as gefitinib and erlotinib, and confer resistance to therapy. In this setting, treatment with a third-line TKI (osmiertinib) may be useful. Targeted therapy with TKIs is also available for NSCLC harboring BRAFV600E mutations, as well as RETS gene rearrangements and MET Exon 14 mutations.

What are the immunohistochemical characteristics and histologic criteria for the diagnosis of typical carcinoid tumor?

Typical carcinoid tumor is a low-grade neuroendocrine tumor composed of solid or trabecular proliferation of bland epithelioid or spindled cells with round to oval nuclei with fine chromatin, which lacks necrosis and shows a mitotic count of <2 mitosis per 2 mm^2 (Fig. 31.5A). Typical carcinoid is often centrally located and is commonly negative for TTF-1. Peripheral carcinoid tumors often show positivity with TTF-1. Tumor cells are positive for pancytokeratin, synaptophysin, chromogranin (Fig. 31.5B), and CD56. Ki67 (MIB-1) is recommended on small biopsies and is often helpful in resection specimens. In typical carcinoid tumors, Ki67 shows a proliferative index of less than or equal to 5% (Fig. 31.5C).

What are the immunohistochemical characteristics and histologic criteria for the diagnosis of atypical carcinoid tumor?

Atypical carcinoid tumor is an intermediate-grade neuroendocrine tumor composed of bland epithelioid or spindled cells with round to oval nuclei with fine chromatin, which shows a mitotic count of 2–10 mitosis per 2 mm^2 and/or necrosis (may be punctate necrosis). Ki67 is recommended on small biopsies and is often helpful in resection specimens. In atypical carcinoid tumors, Ki67 shows a proliferative index up to 20%. Atypical carcinoid is often centrally located, and the immunohistochemical profile parallels that of a typical carcinoid tumor.

CLINICAL PEARL

Generally, the distinction between typical and atypical carcinoid tumor requires a resection specimen for complete evaluation of the tumor.

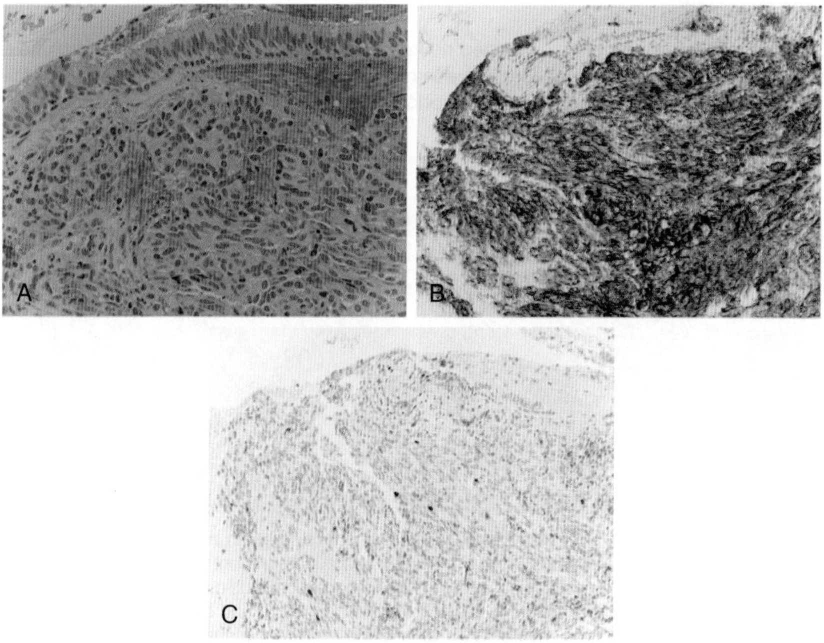

Fig. 31.5 (A) Typical carcinoid tumor, characterized by bland epithelioid and spindled cells with eosinophilic cytoplasm, and round to oval nuclei with fine chromatin (H&E, 400x). (B) Typical carcinoid tumor showing cytoplasmic positivity for chromogranin A (H&E, 200x). (C) Typical carcinoid tumor with a proliferative index (Ki67) less than 5% as seen by rare nuclear positivity in the tumor cells (H&E, 200x).

What are the immunohistochemical characteristics and histologic criteria for the diagnosis of small cell carcinoma (SCC)?

SCC is a high-grade neuroendocrine carcinoma composed of sheets of small basophilic cells with a scant amount of cytoplasm (Fig. 31.6A) and may show necrosis, apoptotic bodies, nuclear molding, crush artifact, and a mitotic count of over 10 mitotic figures (median 80) per 2 mm^2. Ki67 is recommended on small biopsies and is often helpful in resection specimens (SCC is not commonly excised) and shows a proliferation index of at least 50% (commonly over 90%). SCC is often positive for TTF-1 and shows immunoreactivity with pancytokeratin, synaptophysin, chromogranin, and CD56. Napsin A is negative in SCC.

CLINICAL PEARL

Immunohistochemistry for Ki67 (MIB-1) is recommended on small biopsies to help differentiate between carcinoid tumors and high-grade neuroendocrine carcinomas.

What are the immunohistochemical characteristics and histologic criteria for the diagnosis of LCNEC?

LCNEC is a high-grade neuroendocrine carcinoma composed of large cells with ample cytoplasm, vesicular chromatin, and prominent nucleoli (Fig. 31.6B). Solid, trabecular, and glandular-like proliferation with rosette-like structures and peripheral palisading may be seen. Geographic necrosis is often present; however, this may not be apparent on a small biopsy. Ki67 is recommended on small biopsies and is often helpful in resection specimen and shows a proliferation index of at least 40% (commonly over 80%). LCNEC is often negative for TTF-1 and shows immunoreactivity with pancytokeratin, synaptophysin, chromogranin, and CD56. Uncommonly, napsin A can be focally positive.

CLINICAL PEARL

INSM1 and ASCL3 are recently described neuroendocrine immunohistochemical markers that may be helpful in the distinction between neuroendocrine carcinomas and adenocarcinoma, especially when neuroendocrine morphology is present and other neuroendocrine markers are negative.

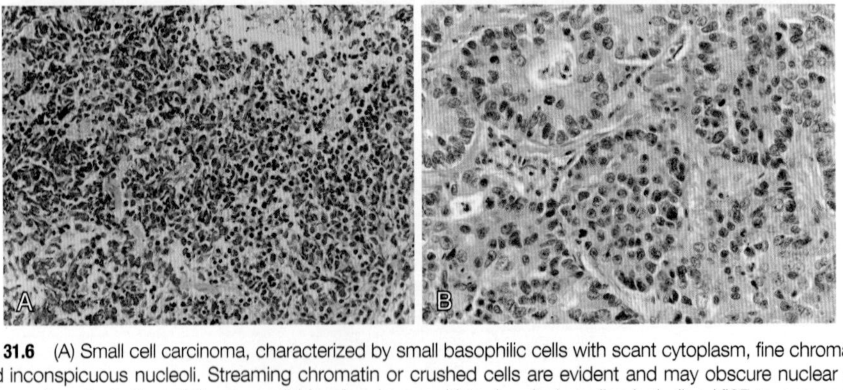

Fig. 31.6 (A) Small cell carcinoma, characterized by small basophilic cells with scant cytoplasm, fine chromatin and inconspicuous nucleoli. Streaming chromatin or crushed cells are evident and may obscure nuclear assessment and mitotic activity on small biopsies. Immunohistochemical studies including Ki67 to access the proliferation index will help confirm the diagnosis of small cell carcinoma and differentiate from other mimics including carcinoid tumors. (B) High magnification of large cell neuroendocrine carcinoma, characterized by peripheral palisading, rosette-like structures, brisk mitotic activity and nuclei with vesicular chromatin. Nucleoli are prominent. Immunohistochemical studies including Ki67 are recommended, particularly on small biopsies to help confirm the diagnosis (H&E, 400x).

BEYOND THE PEARLS

- Data shows that prognosis correlates with the invasive tumor size in non-mucinous adenocarcinoma. The UICC/AJCC Eighth edition lung cancer protocol has adopted this rule for the examination of specimens from lung primary non-mucinous adenocarcinoma.
- Refer to the College of American Pathologist (CAP) lung cancer protocol template for updates in lung cancer staging: https://www.cap.org/protocols-and-guidelines/cancer-reporting-tools/cancer-protocol-templates
- Molecular guidelines are reviewed every 4 years or earlier in the event of publication and high-quality evidence (3). Refer to CAP/IASLC/AMP website for current updates in molecular testing guidelines and relevant clinical information: https://www.jto.org/article/S1556-0864(17)33071-X/fulltext
- Lung cancer is the leading cause of cancer worldwide. Immunotherapy has emerged as an effective treatment modality in patients with lung cancer, and triggers the innate immune system to recognize and defend against cancer cells. Programmed death-ligand 1 (PD-L1) immunohistochemical testing has emerged as standard-of-care in the evaluation of PD-L1 ligand expression. Currently, drugs that target PD-L1 and its receptor programmed cell death protein 1 are commercially available.

References

Butnor KJ, Beasley MB, Dacic S, et al. *Protocol for the Examination of Specimens from Patients with Primary Non-Small Cell Carcinoma, Small Cell Carcinoma, or Carcinoid Tumor of the Lung.* 2017. Available at: https://documents.cap.org/protocols/cp-thorax-lung-2017-protocol-4003.pdf.

Lindeman NI, Cagle PT, Aisner DL, et al. Updated molecular testing guideline for the selection of lung cancer patients for treatment with targeted tyrosine kinase inhibitors: guideline from the College of American Pathologists, the International Association for the Study of Lung Cancer, and the Association for Molecular Pathology. *Arch Pathol Lab Med.* 2018;142(3):321-346.

Travis TD. *World Health Organization Classification of Tumours of the Lung, Pleura, Thymus and Heart.* 4th ed. Lyon Cedex, France: International Agency for Research on Cancer; 2015.

CASE 32

An 86-Year-Old Male with Cough and Dyspnea on Exertion

Jennifer J. Prutsman-Pfeiffer ■ Moises J. Velez

An 86-year-old male presents to his primary care physician with a 3-week history of coughing with no hemoptysis and occasional expectoration of thick clear phlegm. The cough is worse in the morning and when lying on his back. An office electrocardiogram shows an arrhythmia, and he is advised to go to the emergency department. He is healthy with relatively unremarkable medical history. He is a former smoker with a 30-pack-year history, having quit his habit of 1 pack per day 30 years ago. He enjoys drinking one or two Manhattan cocktails daily and has no recreational drug history. He is married, has children and grandchildren, and splits his time between southern and northern states during the year. He enjoys traveling, playing golf, and is retired from Eastman Kodak.

His blood pressure is 156/84 mm Hg, heart rate is 50–60 beats per minute, respiratory rate is 16–21 breaths per minute, and oxygen saturation is 90%–94% on room air. Chest x-ray shows a right pleural effusion and interstitial edema (Fig. 32.1A). All laboratory values are within normal limits.

Given the dyspnea with exertion, right pleural effusion, and interstitial lung changes, he is diagnosed with acute congestive heart failure. The patient receives enoxaparin sodium for anticoagulation. A thoracentesis drains 2 L of fluid, and analysis reveals an exudative pleural effusion. A computed tomography (CT) scan of the chest with contrast shows severe hyperinflation of the lower lung fields, pulmonary scarring with subpleural honeycombing bilaterally, and a small right pleural effusion (Fig. 32.1B). The heart is of normal size. There are no hilar masses or central pulmonary emboli. Fluid cytology following a thoracentesis indicates a strong suspicion of malignancy. The overall recommendation from the northern and southern health care providers is consultation from thoracic surgery.

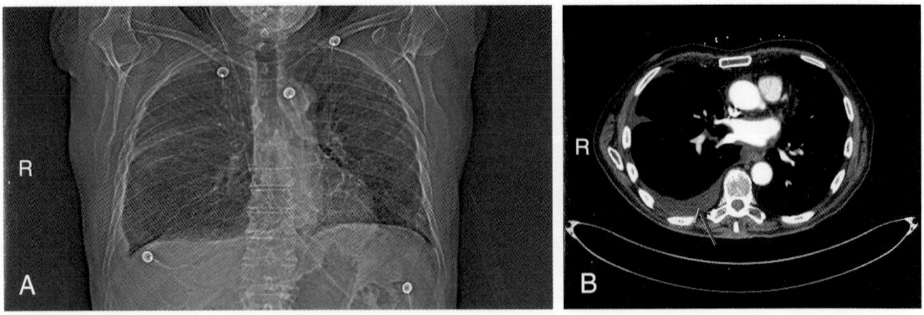

Fig. 32.1 (A) Chest x-ray showing right pleural effusion and interstitial edema. (B) Chest computed tomography with contrast showing severe hyperinflation of the lower lung fields, pulmonary scarring with subpleural honeycombing bilaterally, and a small right pleural effusion (arrow).

What is a pleural effusion?

A pleural effusion is a condition of excess fluid collecting in the thoracic cavity between the visceral pleura lining the cavity and parietal pleura covering the lungs. The normal amount of pleural fluid is 10–20 mL. Fluid can be transudative with an increased hydrostatic pressure and decreased plasma oncotic pressure (heart failure, cirrhosis with ascites) or exudative with increased capillary permeability resulting in exudation of fluid (pneumonia, cancer, pulmonary embolism, viral infection, tuberculosis).

Physical symptoms of a pleural effusion include shortness of breath and chest pain, or there may be no symptoms at all. Physical examination may reveal dullness to percussion and decreased breath sounds on the side of the effusion. Pleural effusions are diagnosed by chest x-ray or chest CT. A blunted costophrenic angle indicates an effusion; normally 175 mL will cause this appearance but it may take up to 500 mL. Very large pleural effusions opacify portions of the hemithorax and can cause mediastinal shift, or cause complete opacification of the hemithorax (effusions greater than 4 L) and mediastinal shift to the contralateral side.

Thoracentesis should be done to initially diagnose the cause of the effusion and in patients who have pleural fluid >10 mm in thickness on CT. Patients who do not generally require thoracentesis are those who have heart failure with symmetric pleural effusions and no chest pain or fever; these patients can have diuresis and thoracentesis avoided unless the effusion persists for more than 3 days. Pleural fluid should be sent to pathology for cytologic evaluation and to exclude a malignant effusion.

CLINICAL PEARL

Thoracentesis is performed using ultrasonographic guidance, increasing the yield of fluid and decreasing the risk of pneumothorax or puncture of the intra-abdominal region

Pleural fluid analysis is performed to diagnose the cause of the effusion first by visual inspection, and then sent to the laboratory for general chemistry, microbiology, and cytology histologic studies.

If etiology remains unclear, CT angiography is indicated to diagnose possible pulmonary emboli, pulmonary infiltrates, pulmonary, or mediastinal lesions.

Findings suggestive of cancer or tuberculosis may require bronchoscopy or thoracoscopy with CT or ultrasound guidance.

What is malignant mesothelioma (MM)?

MM is a malignant neoplasm of mesothelial cells that line the serous cavities of the body.

CLINICAL PEARL

Mesothelium cells line serous cavities of the body to include parietal pleura, peritoneum, pericardium, and tunica vaginalis. Pleural mesothelioma is most common.

MM is highly associated with occupational or passive asbestos exposure. Patients present with recurrent pleural effusions (right sided 60% of the time), progressive shortness of breath, chest pain (possibly unilateral), cough, malaise, fever, myalgia, and weight loss.

The pulmonary pathology begins as diffuse interstitial fibrosis of the lower lobe of lung, resulting in progressive dyspnea, which may be complicated cor pulmonale and secondary pulmonary hypertension. There is usually a prolonged latency period (over 15 years) after exposure to asbestos or erionite fibers in dust or particulates. Recent studies with high-resolution microscopic imaging and animal models have revealed mechanisms of interaction between the pathogenic particulate fibers and the mesothelial cells; cells undergo chronic injury, prolonged states of

TABLE 32.1 ■ **Types of Asbestos with Physical and Biological Properties and Uses**

Type	Physical/Biological Properties	Uses
Chrysotile	Serpentine fibers Fragments into short fibrils Unstable in acidic environments Clearance half-life in humans is weeks to months	Commercial applications: flooring, walls, ceilings, roof materials
Amphiboles Amosite Crocidolite	Straight, long, needle-like fibers (>8 µm in length and <0.25 µm in diameter) Resistant to fragmentation	Many commercial applications
Tremolite Anthophyllite Actinolite	Resistant to chemical dissolution Clearance half-life in humans is decades (or never)	Contaminate intrusions in other mineral ore deposits (vermiculite, talc)

inflammation that activate the inflammasome, which in turn cascades to a unique tumor proliferating microenvironment.

Studies have not showed a linear dose/response, so no lower amount of dust exposure is considered safe. Occasionally, mesothelioma may be idiopathic or occur in the absence of asbestos exposure. The incidence of MM is rising worldwide. The age-adjusted mortality rate is 4.9 per million, and mean age at death is 70 years. The incidence of mesothelioma in men is 3.6 times higher than that in women.

What is asbestos?

Asbestos is a naturally occurring silicate mineral, broadly classified into two main groups with different physical properties, and subsequent varying biological effects. There are six types of asbestos (Table 32.1). Asbestos exposure causes asbestosis (mesothelioma) when dust and asbestos fibers are inhaled. Chrysotile fibers are a magnesium silicate that has a serpentine form and breaks into smaller fibrils that are easily digested and dissolved by macrophages. Amphibole asbestos (amosite, crocidolite, tremolite, actinolite, anthrophyllite) cleave into long fibrous fibrils with relatively parallel sides (length, 8 µm; diameter, 0.25 µm) resistant to fragmentation and do not dissolve. The biopersistence of fibers within the lung is a significant determinant of the pathogenicity.

Asbestos has been used for many years for its properties of high tensile strength, durability, and chemical and heat resistance in thousands of products from the 1920s to 1970s. Current use of asbestos persists in vehicle parts (brake pads, clutches, gaskets) where protection is needed from friction, fire, or heat; insulation; construction materials (roofing tiles, corrugated sheeting, prefabricated cement); fireproof clothing (firefighters, glassblowers); and potting soils (contaminated vermiculite—silicate material found in close proximity to asbestos deposits).

In 1989, a ban on asbestos was implemented by the Environmental Protection Agency (EPA). A federal court overturned the ban on products that had a historical use of asbestos (Table 32.2). The court upheld the EPA ban for new uses of asbestos. The continued concern lies in older homes and structures built prior to the 1980s, and any time asbestos containing materials are degraded or disturbed through remodeling.

Asbestos exposure is a serious occupational hazard for a wide range of workers involved in maintenance, construction, plumbing, welding, machinists, pipefitters, and other similar trades.

Exposure to asbestos dust is compounded by poor ventilation and inappropriate personal protective equipment. Passive exposure is also a concern to people working in a building where asbestos is being disturbed. Even family members are at risk for "take-home" asbestos exposure from the dust that unknowingly settles on a worker's clothing, shoes, hair, and skin.

TABLE 32.2 ■ **Common Asbestos Products**

Consumer products	Talcum powder, stove mats, fume hoods, fertilizer, potting soil*, ironing board covers, iron rests, crockpots, hair dryers
Automotive*	Brake pads and linings, clutch linings, transmission parts
Electrical*	Furnaces, heating ducts, wires, cables and insulation, valves, pumps, boilers
Construction*	Insulation, plaster, cement, caulk, adhesives, roofing, shingles, siding, floor tiles
Fireproofing and fire protection*	Fire blankets, gloves, clothing, fire doors
Military	Navy ships, barracks, boiler and engine rooms

*Historical use of products exempted from 1989 environmental protection agency ban.

What is erionite?

Erionite is a naturally occurring silicate mineral (zeolite) found in volcanic ash that has been altered by groundwater and weathering. Erionite can have a fibrous form, with physical properties and health effects similar to those of amphibole asbestos (1970s exposure-induced mesothelioma in Turkey). Erionite deposits are also found in the sedimentary rocks of the western United States and mainly pose a hazard in the form of dust liberated from disturbed deposits and gravel roads. Exposure to this dust produces pathogenic effects similar to mesothelioma.

CLINICAL PEARL

Erionite is a silicate mineral of the zeolite group that has physical properties and health effects similar to those of asbestos and causes mesothelioma.

Are there any other causes of mesothelioma?

In a small group of patients diagnosed with mesothelioma, an exposure to asbestos cannot be identified. In these cases, recent studies have reported a link to other causes of secondary primary mesothelioma to include organic chemicals, man-made fibers, chronic inflammation, viruses (Simian virus 40), or irradiation for cancer therapy treatments.

What is the relationship to smoking?

Smoking is not a risk factor for mesothelioma; however, there is a synergistic effect of smoking and mesothelioma where smokers are more likely to develop asbestos-related lung cancer.

What are other pleural or lung-based diseases to consider in the differential diagnosis?

Other diseases in the differential diagnosis include atypical mesothelial hyperplasia, fibrous pleurisy, and synovial sarcoma.

How is MM diagnosed?

Diagnosis of MM at an early stage is difficult due to the disease typically in an advanced stage when symptoms appear. Diagnosis of MM is challenging, since direct pleural biopsy may be difficult to obtain and pleural fluid cytology cannot properly classify the histologic category. Cytospin analysis of large volume pleural fluid can increase the diagnostic accuracy. MM is typically diagnosed by tissue biopsy and less commonly by cytology. The appropriate morphology, immunohistochemical profile, and clinical and radiologic presentation may contribute to the appropriate diagnosis regardless of asbestosis exposure. Immunohistochemical markers expressed in MM include calretinin, cytokeratin (CK) 5 or CK5/6, WT1, and podoplanin (D2-40). Markers typically negative in MM and positive in carcinomas include claudin 4, MOC31,carcinoembryonic antigen, Ber-EP4, B72.3, TTF-1, and napsin A. Nuclear expression of BAP-1 can be lost in MM (predominately in the epithelioid subtype of MM); however, retained nuclear expression of BAP-1 does not exclude the diagnosis of MM. Malignancy can be confirmed histologically by an invasive growth pattern. Lung adenocarcinoma typically express carcinoma markers including TTF-1 and napsin A. In rare, equivocal cases where the diagnosis of MM cannot be established with immunohistochemistry, electron microscopy, and homozygous p16 deletion established by fluorescent in situ hybridization may be helpful. Sarcomatoid MM more commonly than epithelioid MM shows homozygous p16 deletion. However, homozygous p16 deletion is nonspecific and may be identified in sarcomatoid carcinoma. Electron microscopy studies are recommended if immunohistochemistry is unclear or unavailable.

CLINICAL PEARL

Mesothelioma diagnostic procedures:

Thoracentesis and pleural fluid cytology (cytospin block preparation)
CT-guided needle biopsy of pleural tissue
Video-assisted thoracoscopy surgery with direct visualization and biopsy of pleura
Open thoracotomy

Case Point 32.1

The patient is evaluated by thoracic surgery for his pleural effusion concerning for malignancy. He mentions that he has been exposed to asbestos throughout his life but did not directly work with it. He is scheduled for pulmonary function tests and a positron emission tomography (PET)/CT scan.

A PET scan is an imaging test to visualize tissues and organs with a radioactive drug (tracer), typically fludeoxyglucose F18 to show metabolic activity, and to better visualize body structures. In some instances, this scan can detect disease before it shows up on other imaging tests.

Case Point 32.2

The PET/CT scan showed a large right pleural effusion with leftward mediastinal shift, hypermetabolic standard uptake value (SUV 7) areas of pleural thickening (up to 1.6 cm) in the right hemithorax with areas of prominent nodularity, a 1.7 × 1.2 cm hypermetabolic (SUV 6) nodule along the right major fissure, and a hypermetabolic (SUV 4) 1.0 cm short-axis right paratracheal lymph node concerning for metastasis (Fig. 32.2A and 32.2B). Again, this is likely a mesothelioma. A baseline pulmonary function test is performed.

What is the treatment for mesothelioma?

Treatment for mesothelioma involves some combination of chemotherapy, radiation therapy, and surgery in low-staged cases (malignant pleural mesothelioma is the only type that has a formal staging system).

CLINICAL PEARL

Treatment for mesothelioma
- Induction chemotherapy with pemetrexed and cisplatin
- Surgery: Pleurectomy-decortication, palliative pleurectomy, or extrapleural pneumonectomy
- Pleural effusion management: Talc poudrage (pleurodesis) or pleural catheter

Long-term survival is improved by chemotherapy and radiotherapy

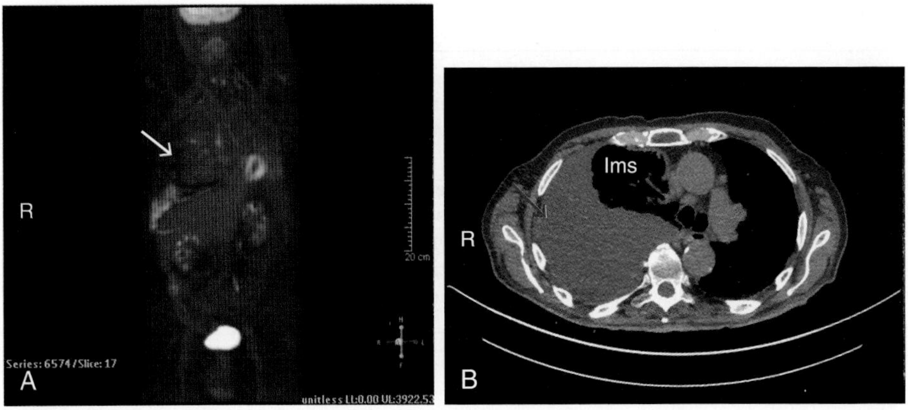

Fig. 32.2 (A) A positron emission tomography scan with large right pleural effusion (dark area outlining lung, arrow) hypermetabolic areas of pleural thickening in the right hemithorax with areas of prominent nodularity, a 1.7 × 1.2 cm hypermetabolic nodule along the right major fissure, hypermetabolic 1 cm short-axis right paratracheal lymph node concerning for metastasis. (B) A computed tomography scan showing large right pleural effusion (arrow) and leftward mediastinal shift (lms).

Case Point 32.3

The patient has worsening dyspnea over the next month, with sharp positional right-sided chest pain. Drainage of his 2000 mL of pleural effusion (Fig. 32.3A) brings some relief to his dyspnea. Cytology of the fluid reveals atypical mesothelial proliferation; however, definitive diagnosis of mesothelioma is not verified.

CLINICAL PEARL

Pleural fluid cytology:

Cannot assess invasion
Most useful in diagnosis of epithelioid variant

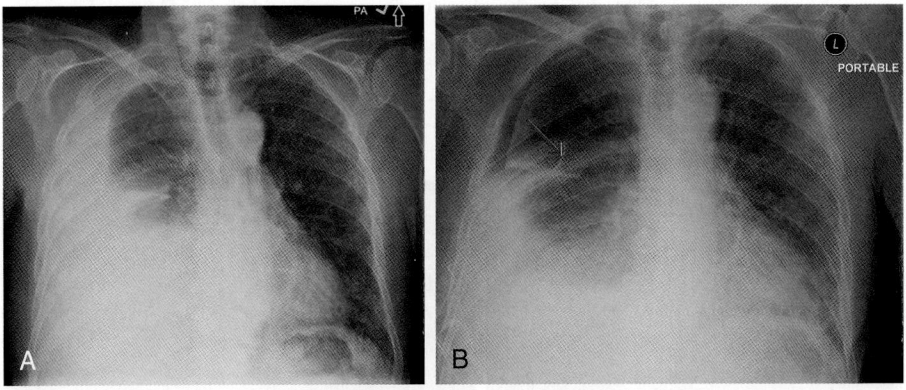

Fig. 32.3 (A) Chest x-ray showing increased right pleural effusion (opaque white region) with increasing right middle and lower lobe atelectasis. Peripheral interstitial opacities in left lung represent combination of emphysema pulmonary fibrosis. Mediastinum is shifted toward left. (B) Chest x-ray with small right lateral and apical pneumothorax with right-sided pleural catheter in place (arrow), right-sided pleural effusion markedly reduced.

Case Point 32.4

The patient sees an oncologist for treatment options and is informed that he is not a candidate for surgery, talc chemical pleurodesis (due to high output of fluid), or radiation therapy. The patient did not want chemotherapy and elects for palliative care at home.

Over the next week, he has worsening chest pain and rapid accumulation of pleural fluid. He has insertion of an indwelling pleural catheter, where 1700 mL serous fluid is removed and sent for cytology, again reporting atypical mesothelial proliferation, with recommendation of tissue biopsy. After the procedure, a chest x-ray shows good expansion with a small right lateral and apical pneumothorax and visualization of the pleural catheter with a moderate remaining pleural effusion, and marked peripheral reticular markings suggestive of fibrotic changes (Fig. 32.3B).

Case Point 32.5

The patient has home nursing visits thrice a week, and 300–800 mL of fluid is drained at each visit. He has lost 15 pounds over 3 months. The fluid accumulation is progressive; within several weeks, up to 700–1000 mL fluid is drained at each visit.

After 2 months, the patient presents to the emergency department with dehydration, hypotension, and dyspnea. The patient continues to decline and is placed on home hospice care. Within a week, the patient returns to the emergency department with syncope and increased fatigue. He has rapid decline over 2 days and dies with his family present. The family requests an autopsy to confirm mesothelioma diagnosis, since the patient did not have a biopsy.

What are the gross and histologic features of MM?

Mesothelioma results in plaque-like tumor studding (Fig. 32.4A and 32.4B) or complete encasement of the lungs and pleural surfaces; the disease may be unilateral (Fig. 32.5).

Case Point 32.6

The autopsy finds extensive white fibrotic thickened visceral pleura adherent to the parietal surface of the lung, and rind of tumor surrounding the pleural surface of the right lung (Fig. 32.6A and 32.6B). Hilar lymph nodes are positive, and the pleural catheter is in situ. The cause of death is reported as metastatic MM of right pleural cavity. Diagnosis is epithelioid MM with bilateral intrapulmonary and nodal metastases.

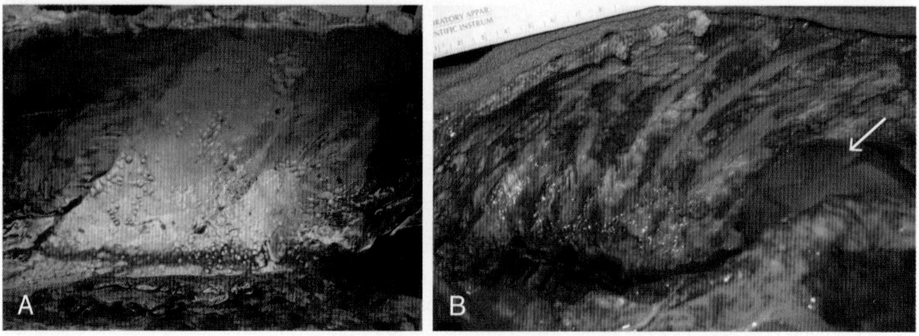

Fig. 32.4 (A) Left thoracic cavity with smooth and nodular visceral pleural plaque formation. (B) Left thoracic cavity with sporadic nodular plaque formation; arrow indicates diaphragm.

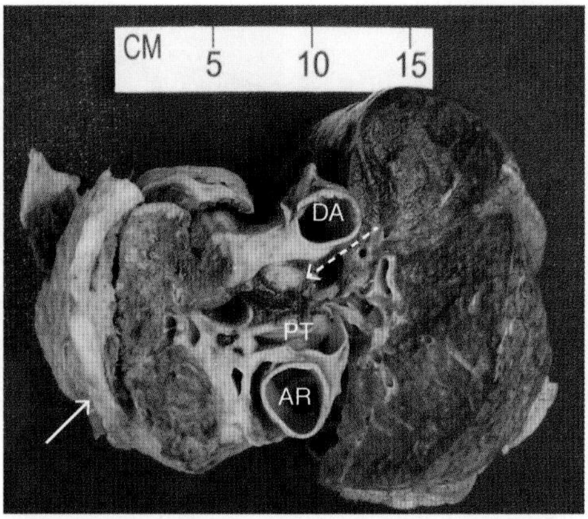

Fig. 32.5 Superior view of transverse section of right and left lung, approximate T5 level. Dense pleural rind of mesothelioma right lung (solid arrow), tumor involving mediastinum (dashed arrow), (AR) aortic root, (PT) pulmonary trunk, and (DA) descending aorta.

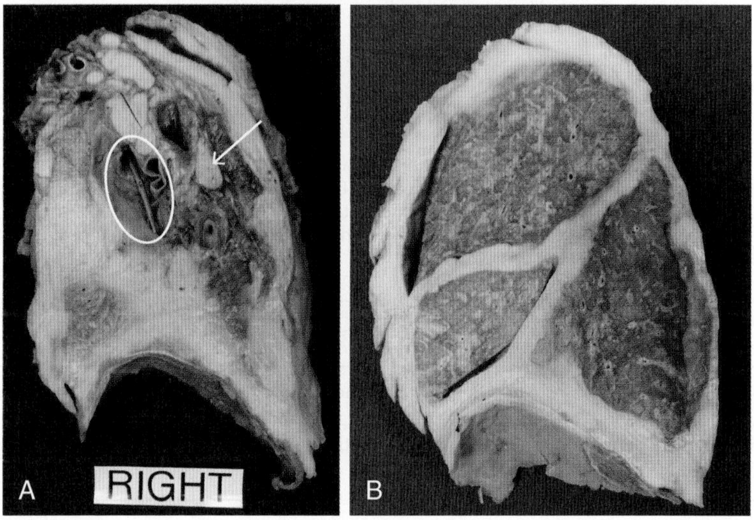

Fig. 32.6 Right lung, epithelioid metastatic mesothelioma. (A) Hilar lymph node involvement (arrow), pleural catheter remnant (circle). (B) Cut surface of the right lung showing complete encasement of parietal pleura mesothelioma. Courtesy of Jillian Brockmann, PA (ASCP)^{CM}.

The main histopathologic subtypes of MM are epithelioid, sarcomatoid, biphasic, and desmoplastic mesothelioma (Fig. 32.7A–C).

CLINICAL PEARL

Histopathologic subtypes of MM
- Epithelioid: tubulopapillary, deciduoid, clear cell and small cell types
- Sarcomatoid: desmoplastic and lymphohistiocytoid types
- Biphasic or mixed
- Desmoplastic

Stromal or fat invasion is helpful for the diagnosis

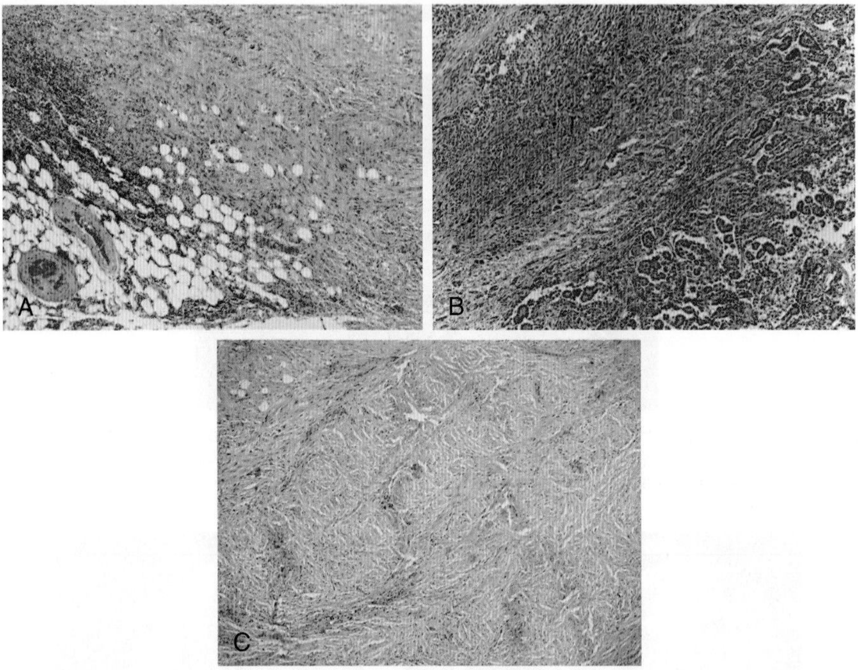

Fig. 32.7 (A) Sarcomatoid mesothelioma composed of spindled mesothelial cells arranged in fascicles showing superficial fat infiltration and fat trapping (H&E stain 100x). (B) Biphasic mesothelioma showing a sarcomatoid (upper left) and epithelioid (lower right) component (H&E stain 100x). (C) Desmoplastic mesothelioma showing a haphazard arrangement of spindled cells with a dense hyalinized fibrous stroma comprising at least 50% of the population (H&E stain 100x).

Case Point 32.7

Histologically, the tumor shows epithelioid mesothelioma with subpleural infiltrative gland-like or acinar proliferation of epithelioid cells mimicking adenocarcinoma (Fig. 32.8). Immunohistochemical staining shows immunoreactivty for mesothelioma markers including calretinin, WT-1, and CK5/6 (Fig. 32.9A–C).

Ferruginous bodies are asbestos fibers coated with calcium and iron and having a distinct microscopic appearance with an iron stain (Fig. 32.10). Ferruginous body formation depends on numerous factors (amphibole fiber type, length, concentration/fiber burden, and quantity of iron in the lung) and may or may not be present, or show a relationship with asbestos fiber count. Light microscopy limits the evaluation of retained asbestos fibers due to the very small size. Amphibole fibers persist; fibers can be counted after lung tissue digestion for quantification; however, this is not routinely performed in most pathology laboratories.

What is the prognosis of mesothelioma?
Mesothelioma has a low cure rate but can be a slow-growing malignancy. Overall prognosis is poor, with epithelioid type having more favorable prognosis, and sarcomatoid and mixed (biphasic) tumors unfavorable. Prognosis depends on the stage of disease when diagnosed and if treatable, the tumor response to therapy. Most patients are diagnosed in the later stages of disease and die within a year of diagnosis.

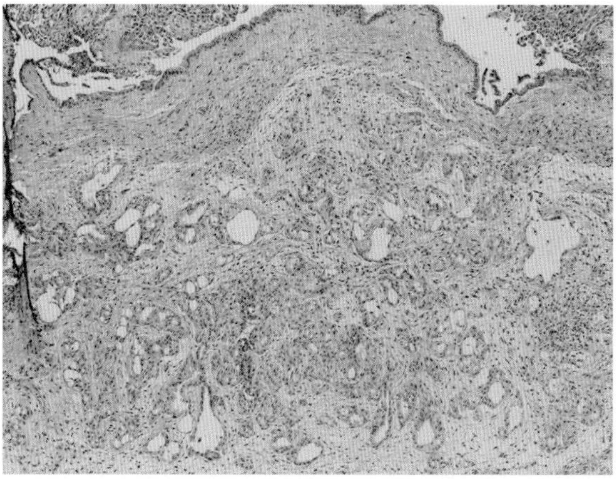

Fig. 32.8 Epithelioid mesothelioma. Subpleural infiltrative gland-like or acinar proliferation of epithelioid cells mimicking adenocarcinoma (H&E stain 100x).

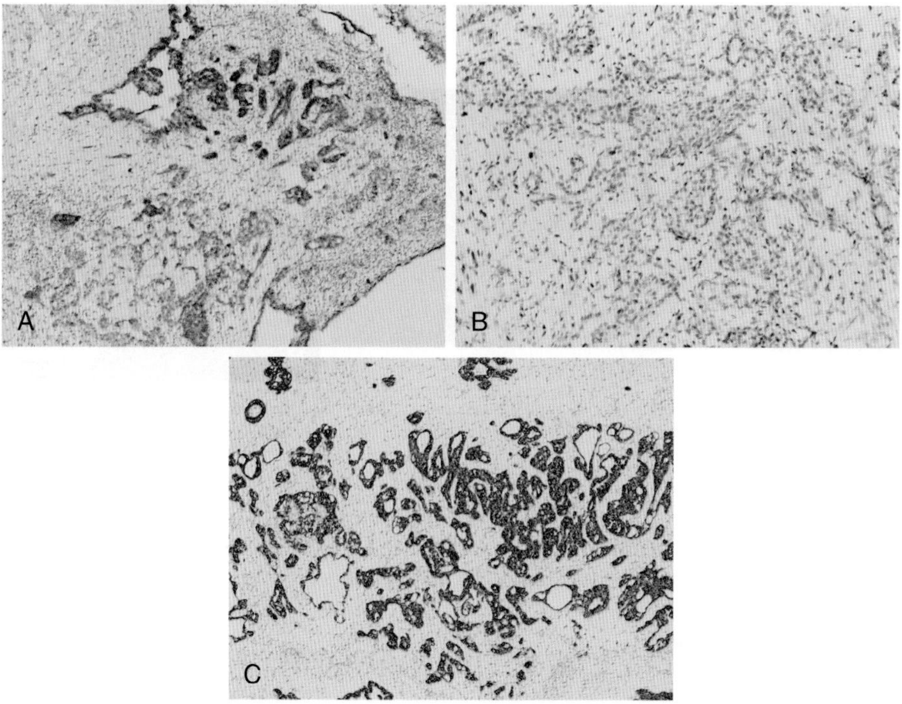

Fig. 32.9 Gland-like or acinar proliferation of epithelioid cells showing immunoreactivty for mesothelioma markers including (A) calretinin stain 100x, (B) WT-1 stain 200x, and (C) CK5/6 stain 100x.

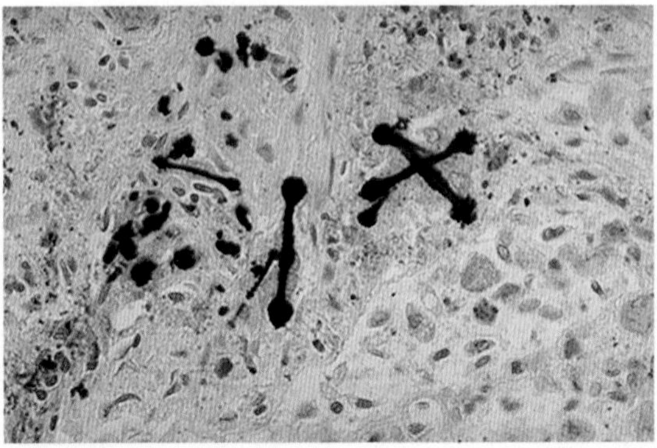

Fig. 32.10 Ferruginous bodies. Asbestos fibers coated with calcium and iron, with characteristic barbell shape, Prussian blue iron stain. From Klatt, EC. Chapter 5 *The Lung in Robbins and Cotran Atlas of Pathology*, Third Edition. Elsevier 2015: 107-158, Fig 5-40.

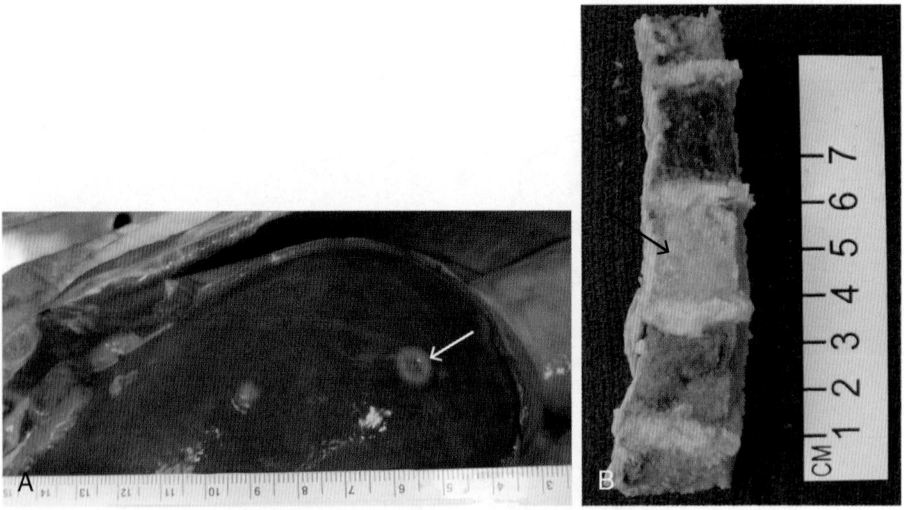

Fig. 32.11 (A) Metastatic mesothelioma, right lobe of liver in situ. Arrow indicates central depression in previously biopsied lesion. (B) Metastatic mesothelioma of thoracic vertebral body (arrow).

Localized spread of the tumor occurs in the mediastinal and regional lymph nodes and diaphragm. Metastases frequently involve the contralateral lung, liver, adrenal gland, and kidney. Rare metastases occur in the bone (Fig. 32.11A and 32.11B).

BEYOND THE PEARLS

- Differential diagnosis in mesothelioma:
  Adenocarcinoma
  Atypical mesothelial hyperplasia
  Fibrous pleurisy
  Synovial sarcoma
- Simian vacuolating 40 virus: Polyomavirus of rhesus macaque, inadvertently discovered in polio vaccines administered between 1955 and 1963; oncogenic and may play a role in

human cancers (mesothelioma, osteosarcoma, pediatric and adult brain tumors, and non-Hodgkin lymphomas)

- Occupation-associated lung diseases (pneumoconiosis)
  Coal worker's pneumoconiosis
  Silicosis
  Berylliosis
- Caplan syndrome: Pneumoconiosis of any type associated with rheumatoid arthritis
- International Mesothelioma Interest Group: developed TNM staging system for primary pleural mesothelioma

References

Dognini DV, Arcangeli S, Melis E, Facciolo F. Malignant pleural mesothelioma: management and role of radiation therapy. *J Nucl Med Radiat Ther*. 2013(suppl 2):011. doi:10.4172/2155-9619.S2-011.

Klatt EC. *Chapter 5 The Lung in Robbins and Cotran Atlas of Pathology*. 3rd ed. Elsevier; 2015:107-158. Available at: https://www.clinicalkey.com//#!/content/book/3-s2.0-B9781455748761000050?scrollTo=%233-s2.0-B9781455748761000050-f05-040-9781455748761.

Mossman BT, Shukla A, Heintz NH, Verschraegen CF, Thomas A, Hassan, R. New insights into understanding the mechanisms, pathogenesis, and management of malignant mesotheliomas. *Am J Pathol*. 2013; 182(4):1065-1077.

Ordóñez NG. Value of claudin-4 immunostaining in the diagnosis of mesothelioma. *Am J Clin Pathol*. 2013;139(5):611-619.

Roggli VL, Gibbs AR, Attanoos R, et al. Pathology of asbestosis—an update of the diagnostic criteria. Report of the asbestosis committee of the college of American pathologists and pulmonary pathology society. *Arch Pathol Lab Med*. 2010;134:462-480.

CASE 33

A 33-Year-Old Female Presenting with Shortness of Breath and Cough

Anish R. Patel ■ Sahar Rabiei-Samani ■ Raj Dasgupta

A 33-year-old woman who recently moved to the United States from Nigeria presents to the urgent care seeking medical evaluation for cough and shortness of breath that has progressed over the past 6 months. Her past medical history is significant for asthma and diabetes mellitus. Medications include albuterol and metformin. She is diagnosed with bronchitis and is prescribed a short course of oral antibiotics. After 2 weeks, she presents to the emergency department with persistent cough, shortness of breath, and wheezing. Upon further questioning, she notes a 15-lb weight loss over the past 3 months. She has been experiencing fatigue and excessive sweating at night to the extent that her bedclothes and bedsheets are soaked in the morning. She is nebulized twice, with mild relief of symptoms.

What are the risk factors of sarcoidosis?

Sarcoidosis affects adults aged 20–50 years, with a slight predominance in females. It is more prevalent among Blacks and Northern Europeans. Certain occupational exposures have been related to development of sarcoidosis, including agriculture, the water industry/high-humidity environments, metal machining, construction, and radiation exposure. *Mycobacteria* and *Propionibacteria* are two major infectious risk factors. They have lipid-rich cell walls, which makes them amenable to macrophages. Fungi cell wall (β-glucan) can also stimulate a hypersensitivity reaction that leads to granuloma formation.

How else should her dyspnea be evaluated?

Wheezing is frequently reported as a respiratory symptom in sarcoidosis and can be mistaken for asthma. More frequent presenting symptoms include cough and shortness of breath. To evaluate the dyspnea or the severity of sarcoidosis further, pulmonary function test (PFT) needs to be performed. It may be normal in the earlier stages but may demonstrate a restrictive pattern and reduce the diffusing capacity for carbon monoxide as the severity increases.

Case Point 33.1

Upon physical examination at the time of triage, the patient is febrile with an oral temperature of 38.6°C (101.4°F), blood pressure of 110/63 mm Hg, pulse rate of 117 beats per minute (tachycardic), respiratory rate of 32 breaths per minute (tachypneic), and she is hypoxic. The patient is in moderate distress and diaphoretic. Erythematous plaques are present on the eyelids, central face, neck, and hairline (Fig. 33.1). Scarring alopecia is noted on the frontal scalp. Multiple tender, erythematous, subcutaneous plaques and nodules of varying sizes, ranging from 0.5 to 6.0 cm, are located on the anterior shins bilaterally. The rash spares the mucous membranes, palms, and soles. There is no chest pain, and troponin levels are within normal limits. Complete blood count is significant for an elevated white cell count of 23.7 Th/mm^3 (reference range: 4.0–10.0 Th/mm^3) and elevated serum calcium level of 11.1 mg/dL (reference range: 8.5–10.5 mg/dl). Remaining blood work is unremarkable; platelet count, mean corpuscular volume, ferritin level, total iron-binding capacity, and iron saturation are normal.

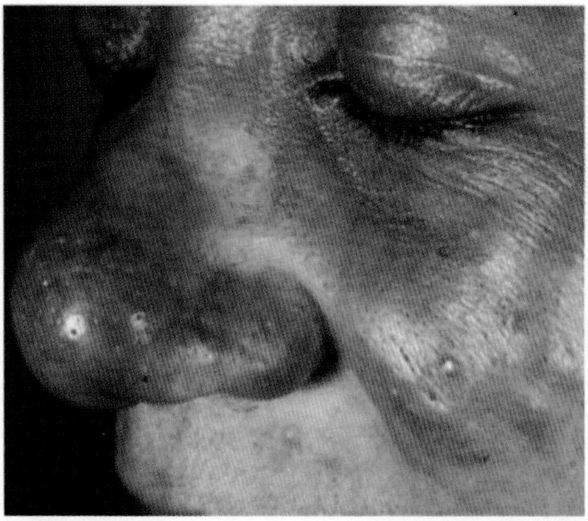

Fig. 33.1 Lupus pernio. A photo of the patient with reddish/purple violaceous, shiny, and indurated places over central face region.

Why is calcium elevated in sarcoidosis?

Hypercalcemia is common in sarcoidosis. The granulomas in sarcoidosis secrete an enzyme called 1-alpha-hydroxylase, responsible for converting 25-hydroxyvitamin D to calcitriol (1,25-dihydroxyvitamin D). Subsequently, calcitriol increases the resorption of calcium from the intestines and kidneys.

Case Point 33.2

Chest radiograph (CXR) shows interstitial fibrosis and reticulonodular infiltrate with bilateral hilar lymphadenopathy (Fig. 33.2). Upon further workup, test results were negative for HIV, syphilis, hepatitis, autoimmune disease, and tuberculosis. Results of antinuclear antibody and rheumatoid factor tests were negative. Results of blood culture, urine culture, and potassium hydroxide preparation were negative for pathogens. The erythrocyte sedimentation rate and C-reactive protein levels were elevated.

CLINICAL PEARL

Different Lung Presentations: Sarcoidosis can present in the thoracic cavity in various ways: (1) moderate to marked perihilar lymph node involvement without pulmonary disease; (2) adenopathy WITH diffuse pulmonary disease; or (3) pulmonary infiltrates only to include pulmonary interstitial fibrosis, localized bronchostenosis with distal bronchiectasis, and atelectasis. Infiltrate and node involvement typically has a predilection for the upper lobes. Progressive lung disease occurs in approximately 25% and disabling organ failure in up to 10%.

CLINICAL PEARL

Grossly, lungs with sarcoidosis may reveal diffuse interstitial fibrosis with honeycomb changes in the worst-affected areas. Small pale, millimeter-sized nodules representing granulomas often may be seen throughout the lungs and on the pleural surfaces.

Hilar lymph nodes may be markedly large, firm, and pale (Fig. 33.3).

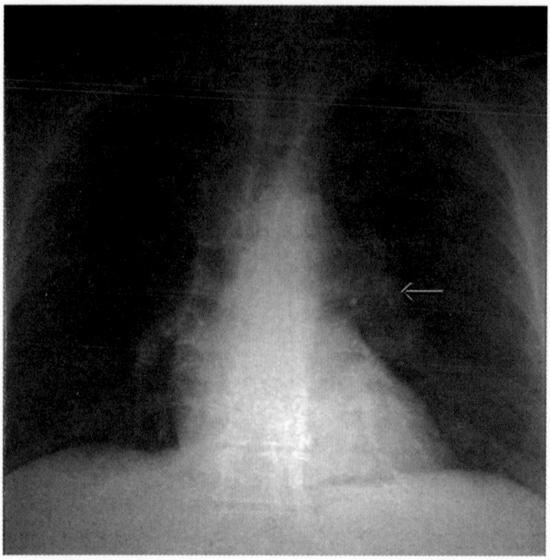

Fig. 33.2 Posteroanterior chest radiograph showing pulmonary interstitial fibrosis and hilar lymphadenopathy (red arrow).

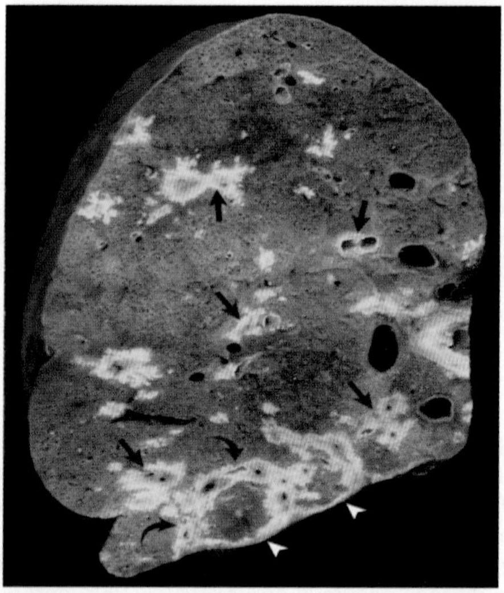

Fig. 33.3 Gross lung specimen from a patient with sarcoidosis demonstrating perilymphatic distribution of sarcoid granulomas. The image shows characteristic perilymphatic distribution of granulomas along the bronchi and vessels (straight arrows), interlobular septa (curved arrows), and interlobar fissure (arrowheads).

What other diagnostic workup should be ordered?

Serum angiotensin-converting enzyme (ACE) is made in the epithelioid cell of the sarcoid granuloma. It is not diagnostic of sarcoidosis due to poor sensitivity and specificity, but when it is elevated to twice the upper limited of the normal, the likelihood of sarcoidosis also increases.

Case Point 33.3

At this point, an ACE test is obtained, revealing a level of 234 U/L, more than three times the normal range. High-resolution computed tomography (CT) scan of the chest demonstrates thickened bronchi, diffuse ground-glass opacities, and fine nodularity (Fig. 33.4). Incidental multiple spleen lesions are noted. Skin biopsy results of the lower back and posterior neck demonstrate granulomatous dermatitis with scattered multinucleated giant cells (Fig. 33.5). Fungal and acid-fast bacilli stains are negative.

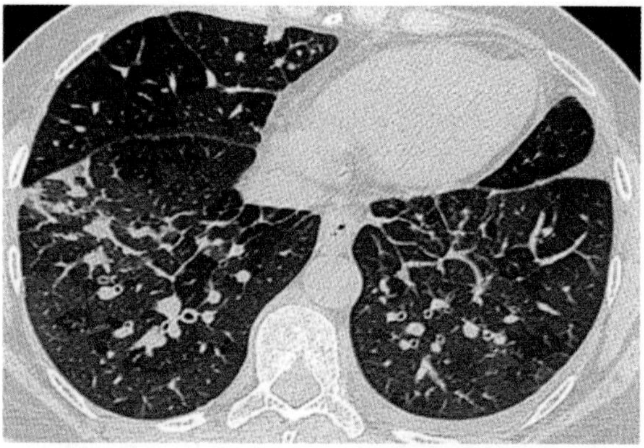

Fig. 33.4 High-resolution computed tomography scan in a patient with sarcoidosis shows extensive bilateral ground-glass opacities and fine nodularity resulting in a granular appearance. Thickening of bronchi, interlobular septa, and interlobar fissures also are noted.

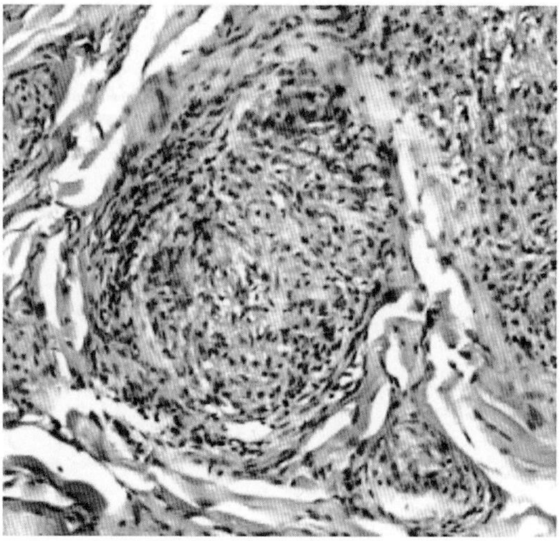

Fig. 33.5 Skin biopsy demonstrating noncaseating granuloma mainly composed of epithelioid cells, with a few lymphocytes and giant cells but no necrosis, located in the deep dermis next to a small venule (H&E stain, original magnification ×250).

What is a granuloma?

Granuloma is a local, chronic inflammatory reaction formed by collection of epithelioid cells (derived from macrophages and secrete ACE) with pale staining nuclei and multinucleated giant cells (a collection of epithelioid cells sharing the same cytoplasm and have multiple nuclei) at the core, surrounded with a rim of lymphocytes mainly made up of helper T cells.

Granulomas are divided into two subtypes, caseating and noncaseating. Caseating granulomas are formed as a result of cell destruction (necrosis), which converts into amorphous debris in the center of the granuloma. It resembles a clumped friable cheese. It is most commonly found in mycobacterial and fungal infections. Noncaseating granulomas characteristically lack central necrosis. They are commonly found in sarcoidosis, Crohn's disease, leprosy, cat-scratch disease, and beryllium exposure (Fig. 33.6).

CLINICAL PEARL

Pathogenesis of a granuloma: When an antigen is presented, monocytes differentiate into antigen-presenting cells (APCs)—macrophages and dendritic cells. The APC presents the antigen to CD4+ Th1 cells, which release interleukin-2, interferon gamma, and TNF-α. This promotes macrophage accumulation, activation, and aggregation, which in turn leads to granulomatous formation. The center of a mature granuloma comprises macrophages, epithelioid cells, and multinucleated cells.

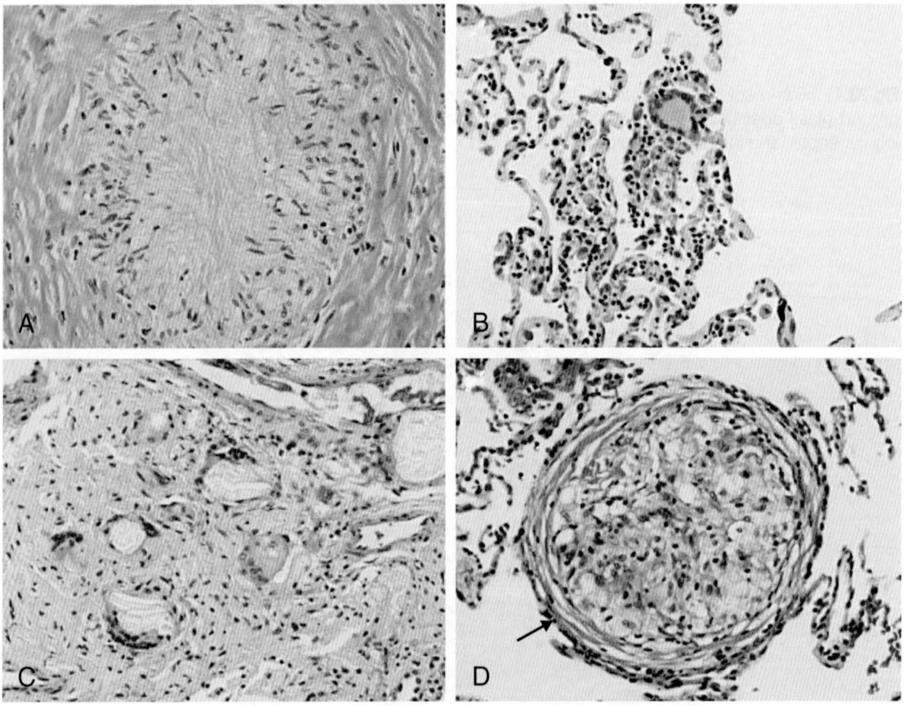

Fig. 33.6 A comparison of caseating and noncaseating granulomas in diffuse lung diseases. (A) Infectious granulomas are necrotizing and tightly formed. (B) In hypersensitivity pneumonitis, the granuloma is non-necrotizing and loosely formed. (C) Foreign body reactions, as seen in this slide of a patient who injected talc intravenously, can resemble granulomas. (D) In sarcoidosis, the granulomas are non-necrotizing and tightly formed. In this case, the granuloma probably is resolving, as indicated by the concentric layer of fibrotic connective tissue (H&E stain, original magnification ×40).

CLINICAL PEARL

The granulomas often surround bronchioles (but not large bronchi). The location of granulomas in and around airways allows for high degree of diagnostic accuracy by transbronchial biopsy with up to 90% sensitivity. Granulomas are also frequently present around and within blood vessel walls, including predominantly pulmonary veins, and may contribute to pulmonary hypertension. Vascular necrosis, however, is not a feature.

How to diagnose pulmonary sarcoidosis?

No pathognomonic diagnostic test exists for sarcoidosis, so the diagnosis remains one of exclusion. Workup is aimed at excluding critical organ involvement, determining extent and severity of disease, and excluding other disease. The presence of noncaseating granulomas does not establish the diagnosis, because conditions such as tuberculosis and malignancies, among others, can cause granulomas. A complete neurologic and ophthalmologic examination is mandatory. A complete occupational and environmental exposure history is recommended. A compatible clinical and radiologic presentation, histologic evidence of noncaseating granulomatous inflammation, and evidence of at least two separate organs involved with the disease are sufficient to diagnose sarcoidosis. Biopsy is done on the most accessible and safest lesion. Biopsy of a second site is not always needed.

CLINICAL PEARL

Differential diagnosis of granuloma in the lungs:

- Tuberculosis
- Atypical mycobacteriosis
- Mycoplasma infections
- Fungal granuloma (aspergillosis, histoplasmosis, cryptococcosis, coccidioidomycosis, blastomycosis)
- Drug reactions
- Aspiration of foreign material
- Hypersensitivity pneumonitis
- Pneumoconiosis (beryllium, aluminum, titanium)
- Lymphocytic interstitial pneumonia
- Necrotizing sarcoid granulomatosis
- Pneumocystis carinii
- Wegener's granulomatosis

CLINICAL PEARL

Differential diagnosis of granuloma in the lymph nodes:

- Brucellosis
- Toxoplasmosis
- Cat-scratch disease
- Sarcoid-like reactions in regional lymph nodes to carcinoma
- Hodgkin's disease
- Non-Hodgkin's lymphoma
- Granulomatous histiocytic lymphadenitis
- (Kikuchi's disease)
- Granulomatous lesions of unknown significance—the GLUS syndrome

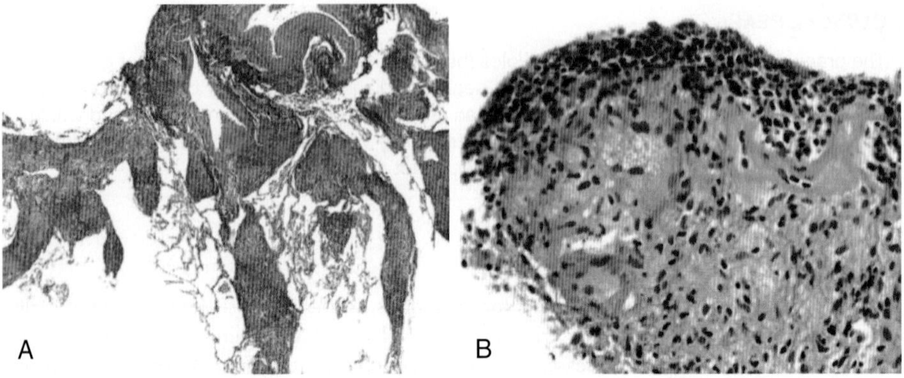

Fig. 33.7 Histopathologic images of bronchial biopsies of patient with sarcoidosis. (A) In bronchoscopic or transbronchial biopsies, granulomas may be quite dramatic in appearance, but sometimes the histopathologic pattern is more subtle. (B) In bronchial mucosal biopsies, lesions are typically present in the immediate subepithelial region of the airway.

Case Point 33.4

Transbronchial biopsy was performed with lymph node sampling and left upper lobe biopsies. Epithelioid granulomas are found on histology to confirm the diagnosis of sarcoidosis (Fig. 33.7).

CLINICAL PEARL

When observing a granuloma, infectious causes need to be ruled out using the following special stains:

- Ziehl–Neelsen:
  - Acid-fast organisms such as Mycobacteria
- Gomori methenamine silver:
  - Fungal infections and *P. carinii*
- Periodic acid–Schiff:
  - Detects lymphocytes and mucopolysaccharide
- Helpful in diagnosis of glycogen storage disease, macrophages in Whipple's disease, adenocarcinoma that secrete mucin and fungal infection (cell wall stains magenta).

CLINICAL PEARL

Histologically, the cardinal feature of sarcoidosis is the presence of numerous non-necrotizing granulomas that are well formed and consist of clusters of multinucleated giant cells with admixed epithelioid histiocytes. Giant cells may contain asteroid bodies, Schaumann bodies, calcium oxalate, or carbonate crystals and Hamazaki-Wesenberg bodies. These compact, well-formed granulomas are confined to the interstitium where they tend to be distributed along the lymphatic pathways and may coalesce to form macroscopic nodules (nodular sarcoidosis).

- Asteroid bodies: stellate arrangement of needle-shaped eosinophilic structures within the cytoplasm of a multinucleated giant cell (Fig. 33.8A)
- Schaumann bodies: fragmented, irregular, calcified, basophilic refractile structure in the cytoplasm of a multinucleated giant cell (Fig. 33.8B)
- Birefringent crystalline particles: oxalate crystal in the cytoplasm of a multinucleated giant cell in a sarcoid granuloma is highly birefringent under polarized light.

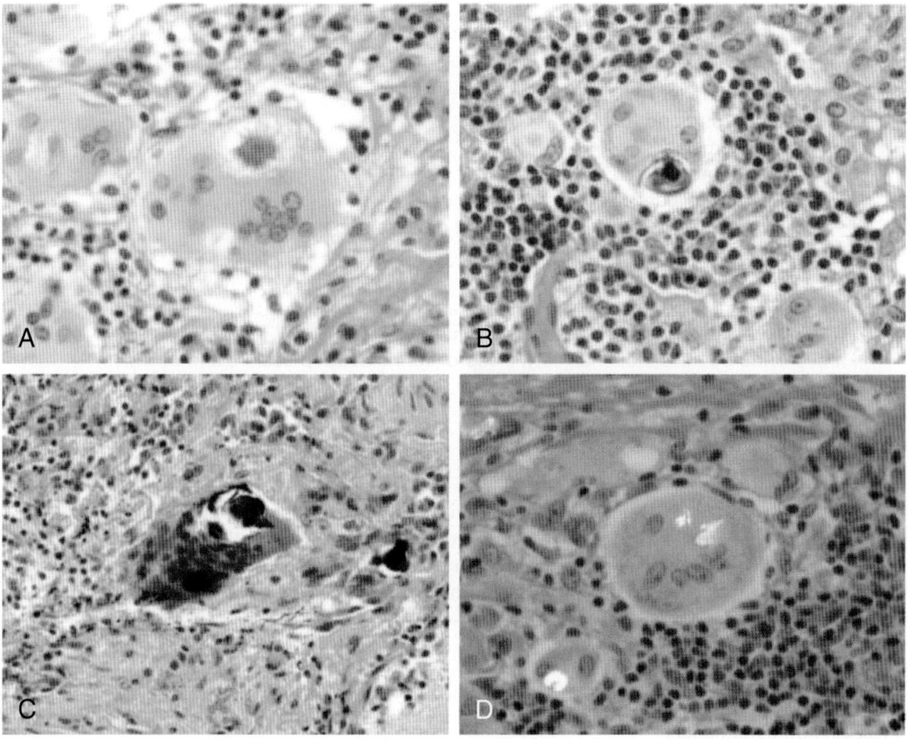

Fig. 33.8 Histologic sections showing multinucleate giant cells with a variety of distinctive (but not specific) cytoplasmic inclusions. (A) Asteroid body. (B) Schaumann body. (C) Schaumann (conchoidal) bodies. (D) Schaumann body in polarized light.

How to treat pulmonary sarcoidosis?

Many patients with sarcoidosis will not require any treatment. In general, treatment should be instituted when organ function is threatened. The goal is to target the initial inflammatory pathway that leads to formation of a granuloma. General targets include CD4+ lymphocytes, macrophages, and tumor necrosis factor (TNF). Glucocorticoids are the mainstay of treatment to inhibit both macrophages and lymphocyte activation (e.g., prednisone 40 mg daily for 8–12 weeks with gradual tapering of the dose to 10 mg daily over 8–12 months). Glucocorticoids should be considered in patients with severe symptoms (e.g., dyspnea, chest pain); hypercalcemia; ocular, central nervous system, or cardiac involvement; or progressive pulmonary disease. Patients with interstitial lung disease benefit from oral glucocorticoid therapy for 6–24 months. It should be noted that it has significant side effects and is not shown to improve mortality but rather alleviate symptoms.

Other agents include methotrexate and leflunomide, which inhibit the inflammatory response of macrophages. Azathioprine and mycophenolate inhibit inflammation by inhibiting macrophages and lymphocyte function. Thalidomide and pentoxifylline (a phosphodiesterase-4 inhibitor) work to specifically reduce TNF release by macrophages. Hydroxychloroquine also inhibits the inflammatory response of the activated macrophage.

Monoclonal anti-TNF antibodies have proven to be effective in patients with refractory disease despite glucocorticoids and other treatments.

CLINICAL PEARL

Side effect of glucocorticoid therapy:

- Weight gain and fat redistribution
  - Osteoporosis and fracture
  - Osteonecrosis
  - Ocular complications: cataract
  - Hyperglycemia and diabetes
  - Cardiovascular effects: ischemic heart disease and heart failure
  - Infection
  - Peptic ulcer disease
  - Steroid-induced myopathy
  - Hypothalamic–pituitary–adrenal axis suppression
- Psychiatric complications: anxiety, sleep disturbance, depression, and delirium.

Case Point 33.5

The patient was started on prednisone 40 mg daily. Outpatient follow-up with rheumatology and ophthalmology specialists was arranged. On further outpatient workup, the patient was found to have ocular involvement, manifesting as uveitis and eyelid granulomas (Fig. 33.9). Her respiratory symptoms and rash had improved after 1 month of treatment with systemic prednisone.

CLINICAL PEARL

Associated conditions:

- Neurosarcoidosis
- Dilated and restrictive/infiltrative cardiomyopathy
- Myocarditis
- Hypercalcemia
- Erythema nodosum
- Uveitis
- Acute interstitial nephritis
- Lupus pernio
- Restrictive lung disease
- Rheumatoid arthropathy

CLINICAL PEARL

Factors associated with a poor prognosis:

- Age of onset > 40 years old
- Cardiac involvement
- Pulmonary hypertension
- Neurosarcoidosis
- Progressive pulmonary fibrosis
- Chronic hypercalcemia or nephrocalcinosis
- Chronic uveitis
- Splenic involvement
- Involvement of nasal mucosa
- Presence of cystic bone lesions
- Lupus pernio

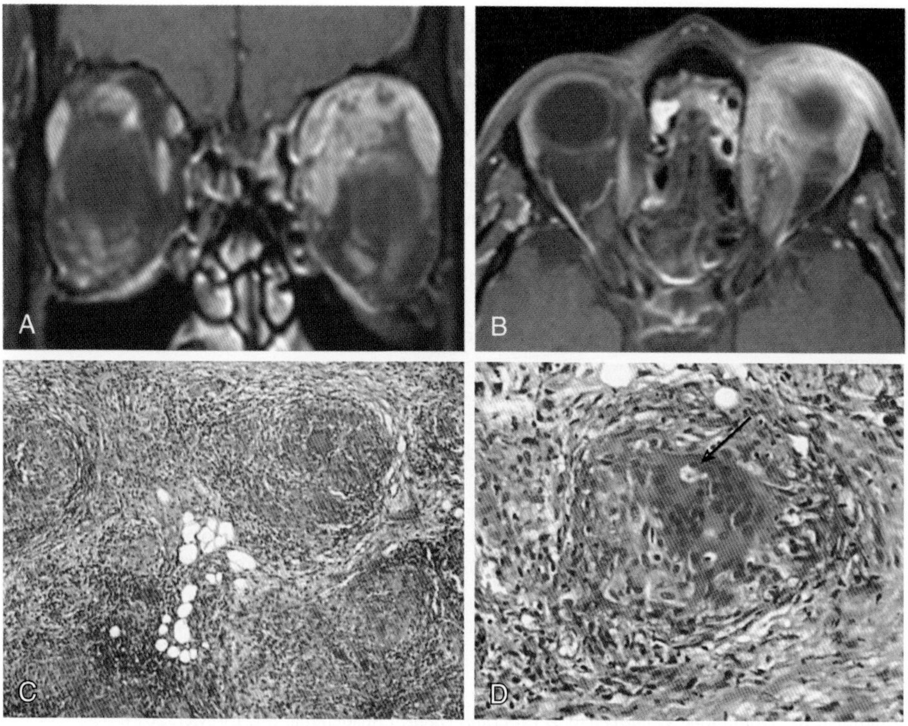

Fig. 33.9 (A and B) Magnetic resonance imaging of the brain showing a diffuse soft tissue mass with irregular borders involving the superior orbital quadrant and enveloping the medial rectus muscle, with an enlarged lacrimal gland. (C) Histology of the orbital specimen showed the typical features of sarcoidosis, consisting of non-necrotizing granulomas with histiocytes and multinucleated giant cells, some of which contained asteroid bodies. Naked granulomas as well as granulomas discretely surrounded by small lymphocytes were present. Special stains for fungal and tuberculous infection were negative (H&E, original magnification ×100). (D) Asteroid body (arrow) in the cytoplasm of a multinucleated giant cell (H&E, original magnification ×200).

BEYOND THE PEARLS

Pulmonary radiograph changes are staged as follows:

Stage 0: normal
Stage I: bilateral hilar and/or paratracheal adenopathy
Stage II: adenopathy with pulmonary infiltrates
Stage III: pulmonary infiltrates only
Stage IV: pulmonary fibrosis (honeycombing)

Organ system involvement in sarcoidosis:

- Dermatology: erythema nodosum, lupus pernio, maculopapular rash, scars, keloids, nodules
- Cardiology: dyspnea, cardiac failure, heart block, arrhythmias, abnormal electrocardiogram, sudden death
- Pulmonology: dyspnea, cough, wheezing abnormal CXR/CT, cor pulmonale, lung function impairment
- Rheumatology: arthritis, bone cysts
- Nephrology: renal failure, hypercalciuria
- Ophthalmology: iritis, choroiditis, keratoconjunctivitis, glaucoma, cataracts, enlarged lacrimal glands, dry eyes

- Neurology: cranial nerve palsies, papilledema, meningitis, myopathy, peripheral neuropathy, space-occupying lesions.
- Endocrinology: diabetes insipidus, hypercalcemia, hyperthyroidism
- Hepatology: liver granuloma, portal hypertension
- Hematology: anemia, leukopenia, thrombocytopenia, hypersplenism
- Otorlaryngology: parotid enlargement, hoarseness, nasal stuffiness

***This list does not include all of the manifestations of sarcoidosis.

*All patients with cutaneous sarcoidosis, even without any respiratory symptoms, should be evaluated with CXR and PFTs annually.

*Löfgren syndrome: acute presentation of fever, bilateral hilar adenopathy, arthralgia, and erythema nodosum

*Heerfordt syndrome: chronic fever, parotid gland enlargement, facial palsy, and anterior uveitis.

*Sarcoidosis is currently a biopsy-proven diagnosis, especially if you are committing a patient to immunosuppressive therapy.

*DO NOT perform biopsy on erythema nodosum lesions; it will show panniculitis and not a granuloma.

*Respiratory corticotropin injection (Acthar) is an adrenocorticotropic hormone that has steroid- and nonsteroid-dependent pathways through the activation of melanocortin receptors located on the adrenal gland and in the immune system. It is approved for symptomatic refractory sarcoidosis.

References

Baughman RP, Dominique V. *Sarcoidosis: A Clinicians Guide*. Philadelphia, PA: Elsevier; 2019.

Fontenot A, King TE. Pathology and pathogenesis of sarcoidosis. In: Hollingsworth H, ed. *UpToDate*. 2018. Available at: https://www.uptodate.com/contents/pathology-and-pathogenesis-of-sarcoidosis.

Gensler LS. Glucocorticoids: complications to anticipate and prevent. *Neurohospitalist*. 2013;3(2):92-97. doi:10.1177/1941874412458678.

Judson MA. *Pulmonary Sarcoidosis a Guide for the Practicing Clinician*. Humana Press; 2014. Available at: https://doi-org.libproxy2.usc.edu/10.1007/978-1-4614-8927-6.

McCormack FX, Trapnell BC, Panos RJ. *Molecular Basis of Pulmonary Disease: Insights From Rare Lung Disorders*. Springer; 2010. Available at: https://doi-org.libproxy2.usc.edu/10.1007/978-1-59745-384-4.

Mihailovic-Vucinic V. *Atlas of Sarcoidosis: Pathogenesis, Diagnosis and Clinical Features*. Springer; 2010. Available at: https://doi-org.libproxy2.usc.edu/10.1007/b138736.

Musculoskeletal System

CASE 34

A 12-Year-Old Male with Right Leg Pain

Phoenix D. Bell ■ Aaron R. Huber

A 12-year-old male with no significant past medical history presents to the emergency department with difficulty weight bearing on his right leg, which started when he was playing soccer with his sister the day before. He also reports a 1-month history of right thigh pain just above his right knee. On physical examination, his blood pressure is 141/80 mm Hg, pulse rate is 106 beats per minute, respiratory rate is 18 breaths per minute, and temperature is 37°C (98.6°F). Palpation of the medial and lateral aspects of his right knee elicits tenderness, and there is no evidence of laxity or joint effusion. A plain film radiograph of the right knee demonstrates a predominantly lucent lesion in the distal femur diaphysis with an ill-defined border. There is cortical erosion medially and an associated irregular periosteal reaction (Fig. 34.1).

What radiographic features are concerning for an aggressive tumor in this case?

It is imperative to correlate radiologic and pathologic findings when evaluating bone lesions. The radiologic hallmark of a benign bone lesion is pushing borders with containment of the involved area by a rim of reactive host bone. In a slow-growing benign tumor, the rim of reactive bone often becomes thicker or sclerotic and appears as a radiodense border on plain film. In contrast,

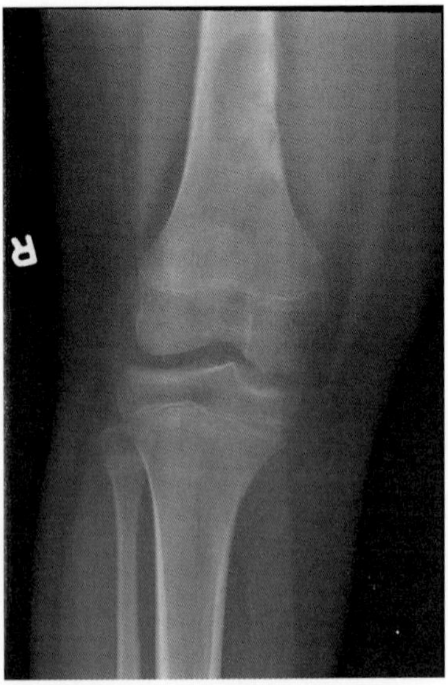

Fig. 34.1 Plain film radiograph of the knee demonstrating a radiolucent lesion involving diaphysis of the distal femur with an associated irregular periosteal reaction.

malignant lesions with potential for local recurrence and metastatic dissemination typically infiltrate surrounding host bone with permeative, ill-defined borders on radiologic imaging.

Several radiographic features to consider when determining whether a bone tumor is benign or malignant include tumor margins, the presence of a periosteal reaction, the presence of extension of the lesion into the soft tissue, and evidence of matrix production calcification. Tumors with sharply demarcated borders contained by a rim of surrounding host bone are generally a feature of benign slow-growing tumors, while poorly defined or indistinct, permeative margins suggest malignancy. In addition, rapid erosion and significant weakening of the cortical bone induces mesenchymal progenitor cells within the periosteum to proliferate and form reactive new bone in an attempt to support the weakened cortex. On plain films, this periosteal reactive process appears as a complex pattern of either layering parallel to the cortical surface ("onion skin"), or spiculation perpendicular to the cortical surface ("sunburst" or "hair on end") on imaging. The presence of a periosteal reaction is indicative of an aggressive process with rapid cortical compromise and favors malignancy. Additionally, the periosteum may be lifted off of the cortex, known as Codman triangle, which is also suggestive of malignancy. Furthermore, the presence of an associated soft tissue mass is more commonly seen in malignant tumors. Cartilaginous tumors produce a chondroid matrix, which, when calcified, can be seen on imaging (described as "rings-and-arcs"), whereas bone-forming tumors produce an osteoid matrix, which can give rise to imaging findings described as "ground glass" and "cloud-like." The majority of bone tumors in pediatric patients are benign, including nonossifying fibroma, unicameral bone cyst, aneurysmal bone cyst, and osteoid osteoma. The most common malignant pediatric bone tumors include osteosarcoma (OSA) and Ewing sarcoma.

CLINICAL PEARL

Aneurysmal bone cysts have a t (16;17)(q22;p13) translocation involving the CDH11 and USP6 genes. The pathogenesis is not fully understood, but this translocation may inhibit osteoblast maturation. This diagnosis is made by fluorescent in situ hybridization.

CLINICAL PEARL

Ewing sarcoma is a small, round, blue cell tumor that affects the diaphysis of long bones, most commonly in males aged <15 years. The most common translocation associated with Ewing is t (11;22)(q24;q12) EWSR1-FLI1.

A biopsy of the femoral lesion is performed. What is your diagnosis based on the histologic findings? The biopsy shows high-grade pleomorphic malignant cells admixed with dense eosinophilic extracellular osteoid matrix production, which is diagnostic of conventional OSA (Fig. 34.2). OSA is a high-grade aggressive neoplasm and is the most common primary malignant bone tumor in both pediatric and adult populations. OSA has a bimodal age distribution with a first peak in adolescence and a later peak in elderly patients. OSA can be primary (typically seen in adolescents) or arise secondary to conditions such as prior radiation, Paget's disease of bone, and bone infarction (most commonly seen in older adults).

CLINICAL PEARL

Patients with Paget's disease of the bone have disordered bone remodeling due to increased osteoblastic and osteoclastic activity. Patients may present with increasing hat size or hearing loss. On laboratory examination, their calcium, phosphorus, and parathyroid hormone levels are within normal ranges; however, their alkaline phosphatase level is increased. Histologically, there is a mosaic pattern of woven and lamellar bone.

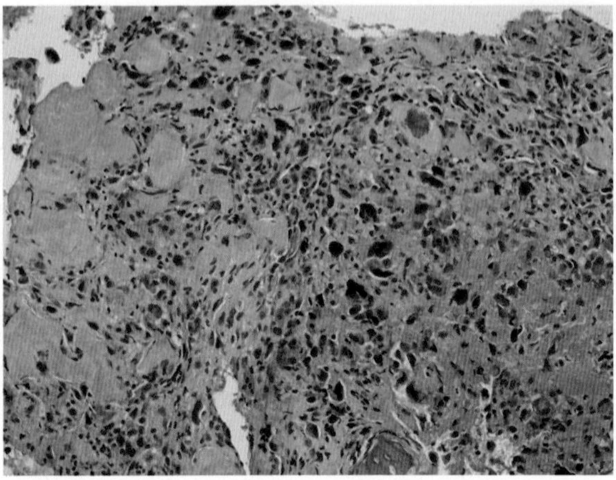

Fig. 34.2 Biopsy of the distal femur lesion demonstrating a tumor with pleomorphic nuclei intimately associated with eosinophilic osteoid matrix, diagnostic of osteosarcoma (H&E, original magnification 200x).

Genetic syndromes that have been associated with OSA include Li-Fraumeni, hereditary retinoblastoma, and Rothmund-Thomson.

CLINICAL PEARL

Li-Fraumeni syndrome occurs due to mutations in the tumor suppressor gene, TP53, leading to uncontrolled cell division. In addition to OSA, patients with this syndrome are at increased risk of breast cancer, soft tissue sarcoma, and leukemia.

Primary OSA may arise in any bone, but are most common in the long bones of the extremities, particularly the metaphyseal region of the distal femur, followed by the proximal tibia and proximal humerus. Patients with OSA often present with a week- to month-long history of deep-seated pain at the tumor site. On physical examination, there may be a palpable mass, but this is not always seen. Although the radiographic appearance may be variable, OSA often demonstrates a destructive, blastic, lytic, or mixed, mass lesion with soft tissue extension and a periosteal reaction. Macroscopically, OSA is typically a destructive intramedullary mass with tan-white or tan-gray cut surfaces that range in consistency from gritty to gelatinous or hemorrhagic, depending upon the predominant matrix component. Histologically, OSA is composed of spindled, epithelioid, or plasmacytoid neoplastic cells within the medullary space, which infiltrate into and destroy the preexisting host bone. The presence of extracellular osteoid matrix production by the neoplastic cells, in any quantity, is required for the diagnosis of OSA. Most often, this neoplastic bone is laid down in a disorganized, haphazard "lace-like pattern" adjacent to and surrounding tumor cells. There are three primary histologic subtypes of conventional OSA based upon the dominant type of matrix production by the tumor, including osteoblastic, chondroblastic, and fibroblastic (Fig. 34.3). These histologic subtypes have no clinical significance and are not related to prognosis. The immunoprofile of OSA is not very specific; thus, immunohistochemical stains are typically not necessary for diagnosis. However, OSA may express osteocalcin, osteonectin, S-100 protein, smooth muscle actin, neuron specific enolase, and CD99. Beware that OSA may express markers of epithelial differentiation, including cytokeratin and epithelial membrane antigen in some cases. Recently, SATB2 has emerged as a reliable marker of osteoblastic differentiation in both benign and malignant tumors. Again, SATB2 is not entirely specific for OSA, as it is also expressed in a

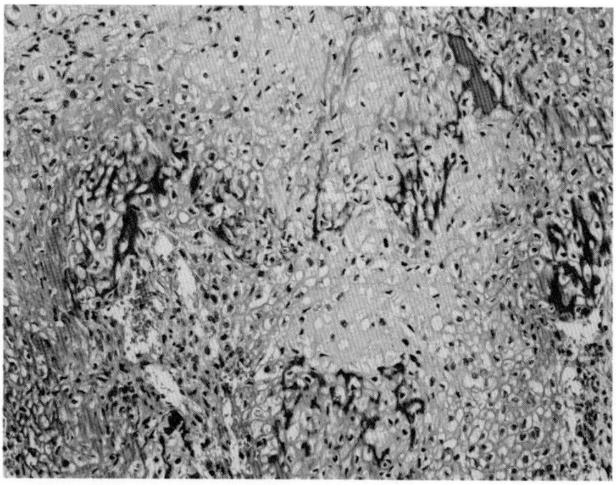

Fig. 34.3 Example of a chondroblastic osteosarcoma with malignant cartilaginous differentiation and lace-like osteoid matrix (H&E, original magnification 200x).

majority of colorectal adenocarcinomas; however, it may be useful in certain situations, such as small biopsies where little woven bone present.

Case Point 34.1

The patient is treated with preoperative chemotherapy and subsequently undergoes a definitive resection that reveals a necrotic tan-white tumor within the medullary space (Fig. 34.4). The tumor is extensively sampled and shows near-complete necrosis histologically (over 90%).

How is OSA treated? What is the role of the pathologist in evaluating the resection specimen?

Currently, high-grade conventional OSA is treated with neoadjuvant chemotherapy, followed by complete surgical resection, which has drastically improved 5-year survival in patients with this disease. Unfortunately, the overall prognosis remains poor in patients with metastatic or unresectable disease. Prior to the use of neoadjuvant chemotherapy, patients were treated with surgery alone and approximately 80% of patients succumbed to the disease; however, with current multimodality treatment, the survival rate is around 60%–70%. According to the World Health

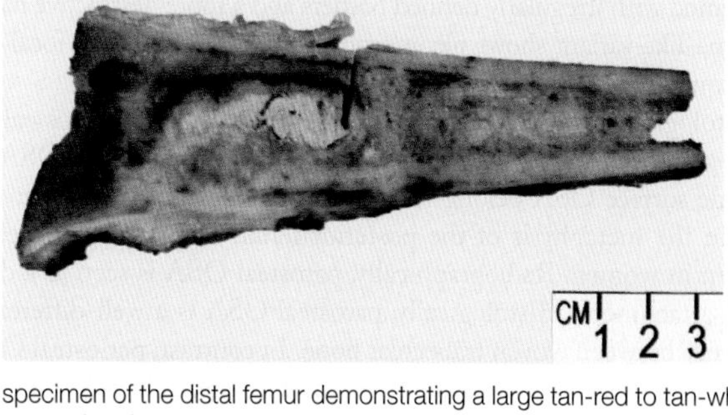

Fig. 34.4 Resection specimen of the distal femur demonstrating a large tan-red to tan-white tumor within the medullary cavity with extension through the cortex into the soft tissue.

Organization (WHO), good prognostic factors include localized disease involving distal sites, greater than 90% tumor necrosis after neoadjuvant chemotherapy, and complete resection with clear margins. Poor prognostic factors include proximal location of disease, large tumor size, metastasis present at diagnosis, and poor response to neoadjuvant chemotherapy. Therefore, the pathologist's examination of a resection specimen for the treatment response (extent of necrosis) and margin status is critical for the patient's clinical outcome.

Case Point 34.2

After 4 years, the patient develops a mass in the left humerus, which is detected on follow-up imaging. The biopsy exhibits metastatic OSA that is morphologically compatible with the original biopsy.

What are the common sites of metastasis for conventional OSA?

OSA has a tendency for hematogenous dissemination, and the most frequent sites of metastasis are the lungs and bone. Patients with metastasis have a survival rate of approximately 20%. Specifically, patients with lung metastasis have a 30% survival rate. In contrast, patients without metastasis have a much higher survival rate, around 65%–70%.

What other histologic subtypes of OSA are there?

The WHO categorizes OSA into several histologic subtypes including giant cell-rich, osteoblastoma-like, epithelioid, and chondroblastoma-like. The giant cell-rich variant occurs in a wide age range (6–67 years), and most patients present with a week- to month-long history of pain, usually in the knee or femur. Radiographically, giant cell-rich OSA are lytic lesions, and a periosteal reaction may be seen. On histology, there are numerous osteoclast-type giant cells admixed with neoplastic spindle cells in a fibrovascular stroma. Minimal osteoid production may be present. Epithelioid OSA occurs in patients from their second to seventh decades in the long bones, ileum, or vertebral column. Radiographically, epithelioid OSA appears as a lytic lesion, which may be associated with mineralization and periosteal reaction. Histologically, epithelioid cells with abundant eosinophilic cytoplasm are seen in various morphologic patterns from cords and trabeculae to nests and glands, and even rosettes. Patients with osteoblastoma-like OSA present at around 25 years of age with pain at various anatomic sites including the tibia, vertebrae, hands, feet, and femur. Radiographically, lesions may mirror those seen in patients with osteoblastoma or OSA. Microscopically, the osteoblastoma-like variant shows neoplastic cells with osteoblastic rimming, similar to that seen in osteoblastoma but with cytologic atypia and an infiltrative growth pattern. The chondroblastoma-like variant is extremely rare, with most cases documented in the metatarsals of young adults in their third decade. The radiologic presentation is variable with reported cases of mixed sclerotic and lytic lesions surrounded by thin to absent cortices and others documented with irregularly defined borders and a more destructive nature. Histologically, the chondroblastoma-like variant shows pleomorphic neoplastic cells, with focal osteoid production, infiltrating the surrounding soft tissue.

Additional histologic variants of OSA include parosteal OSA, periosteal OSA, high-grade surface OSA, low-grade central OSA, telangiectatic OSA, and small cell OSA. Parosteal, periosteal, and high-grade surface OSA belong to the group of "surface OSA". Parosteal OSA is most frequently found in the metaphysis of the posterior femur of patients in their third and fourth decades, more often in women. Radiographically, parosteal OSA is seen as a densely mineralized mass with cortical attachment. Histologically, parosteal OSA is a well-differentiated tumor consisting of spindle cells between woven trabecular bone. In contrast, periosteal OSA presents in late childhood to young adulthood, more frequently in males. Patients have lesions in the metadiaphyseal region of their tibia or femur, and this creates periosteal elevation on radiology. Histologically, there are small nests of malignant cartilage adjacent to atypical spindle cells, and there is no evidence of trabecular bone. Last of the surface OSA, high-grade surface OSA, is an aggressive lesion of the mid femur that is more common in males in their 20s. Radiographically, high-grade OSA is mineralized and is more pronounced near the attachment to the bone. Histologically, neoplastic cells are spindled to pleomorphic. High-grade surface OSA is associated with a poor prognosis, similar to that of conventional OSA.

Low-grade central OSA is rare. It occurs most often in the metaphysis of long bones, especially the distal femur and proximal tibia, of female patients in their 30s. Patients often experience pain for months to years prior to consulting their physician, as there is usually no associated mass or fracture. On radiology, the lesion has variable presentation, often with an intramedullary mass and no soft tissue extension, which favors a more benign lesion. Histologically, this variant is primarily composed of a low-grade fibroblastic proliferation with variable amounts of woven neoplastic bone production, which makes it difficult to distinguish these lesions from fibrous dysplasia. The most helpful histologic features to distinguish low-grade central OSA from other benign tumors include subtle cytologic atypia and an infiltrative growth pattern with permeation of preexisting bony trabeculae. Additionally, low-grade central OSA expresses MDM2 and CDK4, which are not seen in its benign mimics. The prognosis for low-grade central OSA is better than conventional OSA, with an overall 5-year survival rate of 90% following complete surgical resection.

Telangiectatic OSA is another rare variant of OSA that affects a similar demographic as conventional OSA, most commonly occurring in males 15–20 years old. Telangiectatic OSA occurs in the metaphyseal region of long bones, with predilection for the distal femur and proximal tibia. These neoplasms appear as destructive, purely lytic lesions in the metaphysis on radiologic studies. Histologically, this variant can closely mimic an aneurysmal bone cyst (both clinically and morphologically), characterized by variable-sized septae separating cystic spaces filled with blood. The neoplastic cells within the septae are cytologically malignant with atypical mitoses and are admixed with reactive stromal cells. They may also be seen within the cystic spaces. In some cases, there may only be scant, focal, delicate neoplastic woven bone production. Ocasionally, numerous osteoclast-type giant cells are present in the intervening septae, which may be confused with a giant cell tumor of bone (Fig. 34.5). The overall prognosis for telangiectatic OSA is similar to that of conventional OSA.

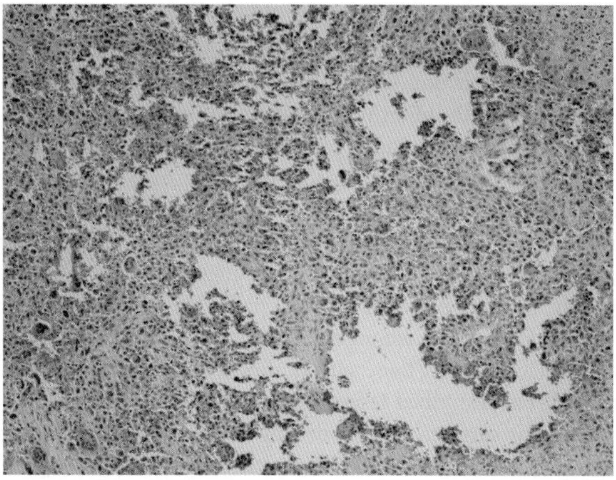

Fig. 34.5 Example of telangiectatic osteosarcoma with cystic spaces filled with blood and surrounded by numerous giant cells; malignant osteoid was seen elsewhere in the tumor (H&E, original magnifications 100x).

CLINICAL PEARL

The most common bone neoplasms that occur within the metaphysis are OSA and osteoblastoma. Ewing sarcoma and osteoid osteoma most commonly arise in the diaphysis. Giant cell tumors and aneurysmal bone cysts occur within the epiphysis.

CLINICAL PEARL

Denosumab, a monoclonal antibody against the RANK ligand (RANKL), may be used to treat patients with giant cell tumor of the bone who are not surgical candidates. RANKL is secreted by stromal cells and binds to the RANK receptor on osteoclasts, stimulating osteoclast differentiation. Denosumab inhibits the binding of RANKL to RANK, thus decreasing osteoclast activity and tumor formation.

Small cell OSA affects a wide age range, yet most patients present in their 20s with associated pain. Many involve the metaphyseal region of the distal femur and proximal tibia. On radiographs, there are both lytic and blastic features, as well as soft tissue extension. Histologically, small, uniform, round to ovoid cells with scant cytoplasm, resembling those in Ewing sarcoma, are present with woven neoplastic osteoid production by the tumor. The lack of osteoid and presence of CD99-positive cells help to distinguish small cell OSA from Ewing sarcoma. This variant has a slightly worse prognosis than conventional OSA.

What are the other benign and malignant bone-forming tumors that may enter the histologic differential diagnosis (Table 34.1)?

Osteoma is a benign tumor that tends to affect the craniofacial bones. Osteomas arise from the endosteal or periosteal surfaces and may occur singly; however, multiple osteomas suggest underlying Gardner's syndrome.

CLINICAL PEARL

Gardner's syndrome is an autosomal dominant condition and is a variant of familial adenomatous polyposis syndrome, in which patients may also develop supernumerary teeth and tumors of the skin and soft tissue (i.e., desmoid tumor or fibromatosis).

When an osteoma involves the medullary space, it is known as an enostosis or bone island. These tumors are typically asymptomatic and thus discovered incidentally. Radiographically, an osteoma appears as a radiopaque mass with uniform ossification and well-demarcated borders. Grossly, an osteoma is a well-circumscribed tumor with a broad-based attachment to the affected bone. Histologically, osteomas are composed of mature lamellar bone that may be lined by osteoblasts, set in a fibrovascular stroma. Osteomas are treated with surgical resection if patients are symptomatic.

Osteoid osteoma is a benign tumor that mainly affects young males. Osteoid osteoma may occur in any bone but most commonly involves the metaphysis or diaphysis of the proximal femur. Characteristically, patients present with dull pain that is relieved by nonsteroidal antiinflammatory drugs (NSAIDs). The radiographic findings are characteristic, revealing a cortical-based lesion with dense sclerotic host bone surrounding a central nidus. Grossly, osteoid osteoma is a cortically-based, well-circumscribed lesion that is usually <2 cm in greatest dimension with red or granular to gritty cut surfaces, surrounded by dense cortical sclerosis. Histologically, the cardinal feature is the presence of a central nidus with osteoblastic activity, surrounded by thick cortical bone. Delicate capillaries are distributed between fairly orderly and organized trabeculae of woven bone with an intervening fibrovascular stroma, and there is no cytologic atypia or mitotic

TABLE 34.1 ■ **Summary of Bone-Forming Tumors**

Tumor	Salient Clinical Features	Radiographic Findings	Pathology Findings	Outcome and Treatment
Osteoma	Craniofacial bones; may be associated with Gardner's syndrome (FAP variant)	Well demarcated, uniform ossification	Trabeculae of lamellar bone, osteoblasts, fibrovascular stroma	Benign, no treatment if asymptomatic
Osteoid osteoma	Young males, proximal femur, pain that responds to NSAIDs	Characteristic: cortical lesion with central nidus and dense sclerosis, <2 cm	<2 cm, central nidus composed of woven bone with osteoblasts, dense cortical bone at the periphery	Benign, may spontaneously resolve, radiofrequency ablation
Osteoblastoma	Young males, posterior spinal elements, pain does not respond to NSAIDs	Well demarcated, round to oval lytic lesion	>2 cm, same as osteoid osteoma	Benign, curettage if small, resection if large
Conventional OSA	Most common primary malignant tumor of bone, painful mass, bimodal age distribution, primary and secondary categories, usually distal femur or proximal tibia, associated with Li-Fraumeni and retinoblastoma, prior radiation, Paget's disease	Poorly demarcated, blastic or lytic mass, soft tissue extension	Permeative pattern of woven bone created by malignant cells: three primary variants include fibroblastic, chondroblastic, and osteoblastic, evaluation of the post-treatment resection specimen for percentage of tumor necrosis is the key	Malignant; with multidrug chemotherapy, prognosis has improved with ~70% long-term survival
Parosteal OSA	Most common type on surface of the bone, women, 30 years old, Distal posterior femur (popliteal fossa)	Mineralized mass attached to the surface of the bone	Spindle cells with parallel trabeculae of woven bone, 50% cartilaginous differentiation	Malignant, low grade, excellent prognosis
Periosteal OSA	Less common than parosteal osteosarcoma, 20–30 years old, men, distal femur and proximal tibia	Soft tissue mass with mineralization on the surface of the bone with cortical scalloping	Predominantly atypical cartilaginous differentiation with woven bone	Malignant, relatively good prognosis
High-grade surface OSA	Men, 20 years old, femur most common, pain and mass	Partially mineralized soft tissue mass on the surface of the bone	High grade with same histologic features and types as conventional OSA	Malignant, high grade, similar prognosis to conventional OSA

Continued on following page

TABLE 34.1 ■ **Summary of Bone-Forming Tumors** (Continued)

Tumor	Salient Clinical Features	Radiographic Findings	Pathology Findings	Outcome and Treatment
Telangiectatic OSA	Rare subtype, 20 years old, men, metaphysis of distal femur	Purely lytic, soft tissue mass, bony destruction	Blood-filled and cystic spaces, septae with pleomorphic tumor cells and woven bone (may be focal)	Malignant, high grade, similar prognosis to conventional OSA
Small cell OSA	Women, 20 years old, metaphysis of long bones	Similar to conventional OSA	Small cells with scant cytoplasm, associated with woven bone, may have spindled cells	Slightly worse prognosis than conventional OSA

FAP, familial adenomatous polyposis; *NSAID*, nonsteroidal antiinflammatory drug; *OSA*, osteosarcoma.

activity. Osteoid osteoma is entirely benign and usually does not recur. In fact, when the lesion is confidently felt to be an osteoid osteoma clinically and radiographically, it can be treated by radiofrequency ablation, and some actually spontaneously resolve.

Osteoblastoma is a rare benign bone tumor that primarily affects the axial skeleton of men in their second to third decade. Patients present with back pain or pain associated with the involved bone of the axial skeleton, which does not respond to NSAID. Radiographically, osteoblastoma demonstrates a large, well-demarcated, round to oval lytic lesion, which can range in size from 2 to 15 cm. Grossly, osteoblastoma is a round to oval lesion that appears red or reddish-brown due to the extremely vascular nature of the tumor. Histologically, osteoblastoma is identical to osteoid osteoma, with anastomosing trabeculae of woven bone with osteoblastic rimming in a fibrovascular stroma (Figs. 34.6 and 34.7). Although osteoblasts do not show cytologic atypia, mitotic figures may be identified. Additionally, there may be osteoclast-type giant cells scattered within the tumor. Osteoblastoma rarely recurs, and smaller lesions may be treated adequately with curettage.

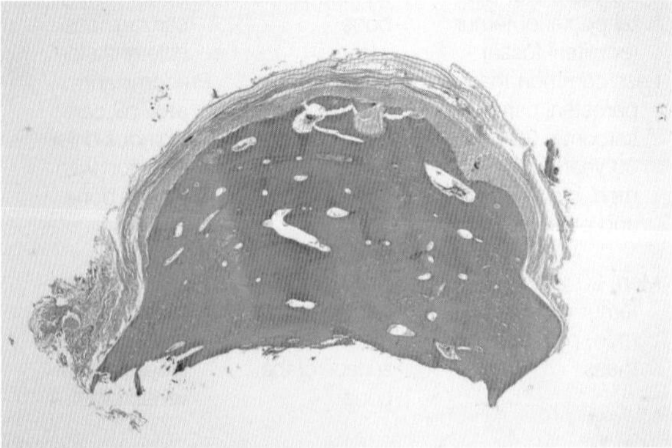

Fig. 34.6 Osteoma composed of mature lamellar bone with a broad base (H&E, original magnification 20x).

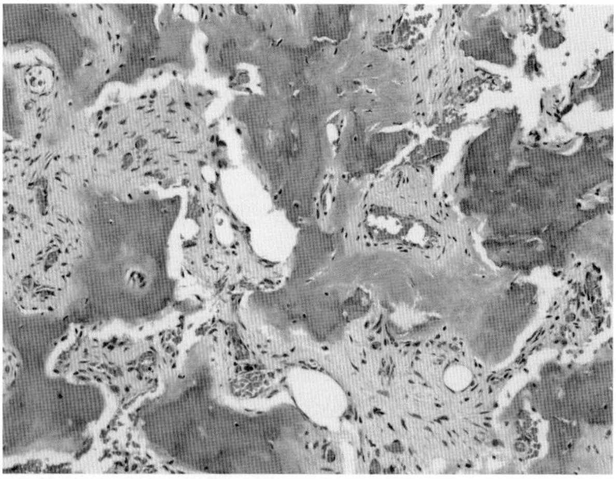

Fig. 34.7 Osteoblastoma demonstrating woven bone with benign osteoblasts in a fibrovascular stroma (H&E, original magnification 200x).

BEYOND THE PEARLS

- Bone is formed via endochondral or intramembranous ossification. Endochondral ossification lays down bone on preexisting cartilage and results in the development of long bones (e.g., femur). Intramembranous ossification results from the development of osteoblasts from mesenchymal stem cells. The osteoblasts produce osteoid, which eventually forms trabeculae and results in flat bones (e.g., skull).
- Metastatic malignant neoplasms to the bone are more common than primary bone tumors.
- Common metastases to the bone resulting in lytic lesions include multiple myeloma, renal cell carcinoma, melanoma, non–small cell lung carcinoma, and thyroid cancer. The common metastases causing blastic (sclerotic) lesions include prostate, small cell lung carcinoma, and medulloblastoma.
- Rothmund-Thompson syndrome is an autosomal recessive condition often associated with RECQL4 mutations. It often presents in infants as an enlarging skin rash, followed by telangiectasia, loss of hair from the eyelashes and eyebrows, dental abnormalities, short stature, and skeletal defects.
- Brown tumor is considered in the radiographic differential for giant cell tumor of the bone. These tumors are found in patients with hyperparathyroidism and most commonly present in the maxilla or the mandible. Histologically, it is composed of woven bone surrounded by fibroblasts, osteoclast-type giant cells, and hemosiderin-laden macrophages.

References

Andresen KJ, Sundaram M, Unni KK, Sim FH. Imaging features of low-grade central osteosarcoma of the long bones and pelvis. *Skeletal Radiol.* 2004;33(7):373-379.

Aycan OE, Vanel D, Righi A, Arikan Y, Manfrini M. Chondroblastoma-like osteosarcoma: a case report and review. *Skeletal Radiol.* 2015;44(6):869-873.

Bertoni F, Bacchini P, Donati D, Martini A, Picci P, Campanacci M. Osteoblastoma-like osteosarcoma. The Rizzoli Institute experience. *Mod Pathol.* 1993;6(6):707-716.

Bishop JA, Shum CH, Sheth S, Wakely PE, Ali SZ. Small cell osteosarcoma cytopathologic characteristics and differential diagnosis. *Am J Clin Pathol.* 2010;133(5):756-761.

Choong PF, Pritchard DJ, Rock MG, Sim FH, McLeod RA, Unni KK. Low grade central osteogenic sarcoma. A long-term followup of 20 patients. *Clin Orthop Relat Res.* 1996;(322):198-206.

Chow LT. Giant cell rich osteosarcoma revisited-diagnostic criteria and histopathologic patterns, Ki67, CDK4, and MDM2 expression, changes in response to bisphosphonate and denosumab treatment. *Virchows Arch.* 2016;468(6):741-755.

Discepola F, Powell TI, Nahal A. Telangiectatic osteosarcoma: radiologic and pathologic findings. *Radiographics.* 2009;29(2):380-383.

Enneking WF, Spanier SS, Goodman MA. A system for the surgical staging of musculoskeletal sarcoma. 1980. *Clin Orthop Relat Res.* 2003;(415):4-18.

Fletcher CDM, World Health Organization, International Agency for Research on Cancer. *WHO Classification of Tumours of Soft Tissue and Bone.* 4th ed. Lyon: IARC Press; 2013:468.

Gambarotti M, Dei Tos AP, Vanel D, et al. Osteoblastoma-like osteosarcoma: high-grade or low-grade osteosarcoma? *Histopathology.* 2019;74(3):494-503.

Gill J, Ahluwalia MK, Geller D, Gorlick R. New targets and approaches in osteosarcoma. *Pharmacol Ther.* 2013;137(1):89-99.

Green JT, Mills AM. Osteogenic tumors of bone. *Semin Diagn Pathol.* 2014;31(1):21-29.

Hakim DN, Pelly T, Kulendran M, Caris JA. Benign tumours of the bone: a review. *J Bone Oncol.* 2015;4(2):37-41.

Hang JF, Chen PC. Parosteal osteosarcoma. *Arch Pathol Lab Med.* 2014;138(5):694-699.

Klein MJ, Siegal GP. Osteosarcoma: anatomic and histologic variants. *Am J Clin Pathol.* 2006;125(4): 555-581.

Kramer K, Hicks DG, Palis J, et al. Epithelioid osteosarcoma of bone. Immunocytochemical evidence suggesting divergent epithelial and mesenchymal differentiation in a primary osseous neoplasm. *Cancer.* 1993;71(10):2977-2982.

Kumar VS, Barwar N, Khan SA. Surface osteosarcomas: diagnosis, treatment and outcome. *Indian J Orthop.* 2014;48(3):255-261.

Larizza L, Roversi G, Volpi L. Rothmund-Thomson syndrome. *Orphanet J Rare Dis.* 2010;5:2.

Macedo F, Ladeira K, Pinho F, et al. Bone metastases: an overview. *Oncol Rev.* 2017;11(1):321.

Malhas AM, Sumathi VP, James SL, et al. Low-grade central osteosarcoma: a difficult condition to diagnose. *Sarcoma.* 2012;2012:764796.

McClure J, Mangham DC, Freemont T. Surface tumours of bone. *Diagn Histopathol.* 2017;23(5):189-199.

Mirabello L, Troisi RJ, Savage SA. Osteosarcoma incidence and survival rates from 1973 to 2004: data from the Surveillance, Epidemiology, and End Results Program. *Cancer.* 2009;115(7):1531-1543.

Miwa S, Shirai T, Yamamoto N, et al. Current and emerging targets in immunotherapy for osteosarcoma. *J Oncol.* 2019;2019:7035045.

Okada K, Hasegawa T, Yokoyama R. Rosette-forming epithelioid osteosarcoma: a histologic subtype with highly aggressive clinical behavior. *Hum Pathol.* 2001;32(7):726-733.

Ordóñez NG. SATB2 is a novel marker of osteoblastic differentiation and colorectal adenocarcinoma. *Adv Anat Pathol.* 2014;21(1):63-67.

Ozger H, Alpan B, Söylemez MS, et al. Clinical management of a challenging malignancy, osteoblastoma-like osteosarcoma: a report of four cases and a review of the literature. *Ther Clin Risk Manag.* 2016;12: 1261-1270.

Sangle NA, Layfield LJ. Telangiectatic osteosarcoma. *Arch Pathol Lab Med.* 2012;136(5):572-576.

Wang CS, Yin QH, Liao JS, Lou JH, Ding XY, Zhu YB. Giant cell-rich osteosarcoma in long bones: clinical, radiological and pathological features. *Radiol Med.* 2013;118(8):1324-1334.

A 50-Year-Old Male with Right Shoulder Mass and Pain

Rana Ajabnoor

A 50-year-old male presents to the orthopedic clinic with history of right shoulder swelling that started 1.5 years ago together with shoulder stiffness and progressively worsening pain. He has a history of trauma 5 years ago, in which he broke his right forearm. Besides this, no significant medical or surgical history is noted. On physical examination, his vital signs are within normal range. There is a hard, diffuse mass measuring 11 cm over the right shoulder with restricted range of motion. No overlying skin changes are identified. The patient's magnetic resonance imaging (MRI) shows a large, lobulated, destructive, heterogenous mass with evidence of chondroid matrix formation and peripheral enhancement, measuring 14 cm and occupying most of the right humeral head and proximal shaft with extension beyond the cortex of the bone into the surrounding soft tissue (Fig. 35.1A and B).

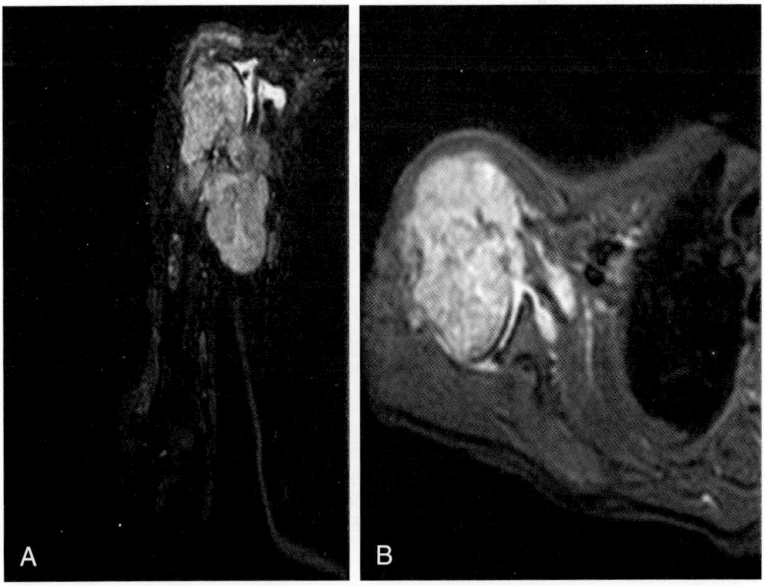

Fig. 35.1 (A) Coronal and (B) Axial magnetic resonance imaging of the right shoulder demonstrating an aggressive T2 hyperintense mass with peripheral lobulated contrast enhancement. Large soft tissue components present.

TABLE 35.1 ■ **Common Types of Cartilaginous Neoplasms**

	Cartilaginous Neoplasm			
Benign	Osteochondroma	Enchondroma	Bizarre parosteal osteochondromatous proliferation	Synovial chondromatosis
Intermediate (locally aggressive)	Chondromyxoid Fibroma	Atypical cartilaginous tumor/grade I chondrosarcoma	Nora's lesion	
Intermediate (minimal risk of metastasis)	Chondroblastoma			
Malignant	Grade II and III chondrosarcoma,	Dedifferentiated chondrosarcoma	Mesenchymal chondrosarcoma	Clear cell chondrosarcoma

CLINICAL PEARL

Computed tomography (CT) and MRI are the gold standard in evaluating bone mass. CT scan visualizes the anatomical site of the tumor with different planes. MRI is excellent in assessing the tumor size, extent and relation to the surrounding soft tissue, and is helpful for planning surgical resection.

What are the types of cartilaginous neoplasm of the bone?

There are many types of cartilaginous neoplasms—benign, intermediate, and malignant tumors (Table 35.1). Benign cartilaginous tumors have no risk for recurrence, whereas intermediate lesions can be locally aggressive with high risk of recurrence and a minimal risk of metastasis. In contrast, malignant cartilaginous tumors have a high risk for distant metastasis.

What is your differential diagnosis for this patient's lesion based on imaging findings?

Based on the history and radiological findings of a large destructive cartilaginous mass in the bone (indicative of malignant behavior), the top differential would include a chondrosarcoma or dedifferentiated chondrosarcoma. Chondroblastic osteosarcoma is also a possibility, especially if there is history of Paget's disease of bone or prior radiotherapy.

Case Point 35.1

The patient undergoes surgical resection of the proximal humerus with surrounding soft tissue and clean surgical resection margin. Grossly, there is large, hard, destructive, lobulated, ill-defined, gray cartilaginous mass measuring 13 × 13 × 10.5 cm within the marrow cavity that invades through the articular cartilage of the humeral head and cortex of the shaft and into the surrounding soft tissue (Fig. 35.2). The microscopic pathology demonstrates irregular lobules of blue-gray myxoid cartilaginous matrix permeating and destructing the host lamellar bone trabecular and cortex extending to the soft tissue (Figs. 35.3 and 35.4). These lobules are hypercellular and show atypical, hyperchromatic neoplastic chondrocytes with size variability (Fig. 35.5). Moreover, myxoid changes to the cartilaginous matrix with cystic formation were readily apparent (Fig. 35.6). The final diagnosis rendered is grade II chondrosarcoma based on the infiltrative growth pattern, the production of an extracellular carilagenous matrix, and the cellularity and cytology of the tumor.

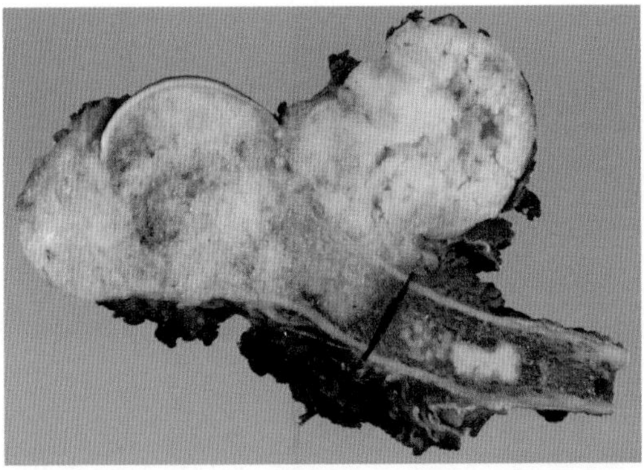

Fig. 35.2 Grossly, large destructive cartilaginous mass within the marrow of proximal humerus infiltrating the humeral head articular cartilage and cortical shaft extending to the soft tissue. Focal cystic areas present.

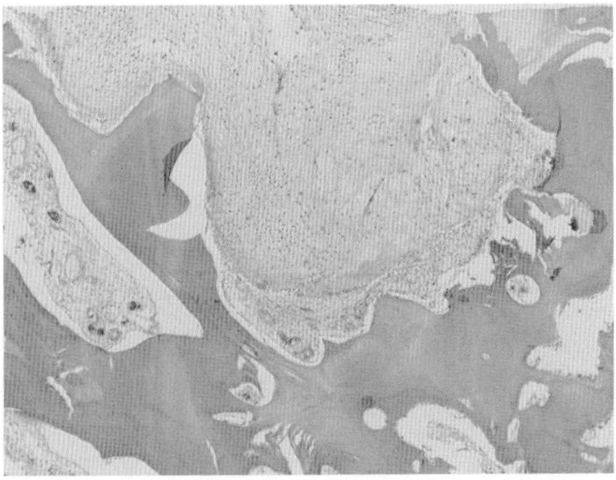

Fig. 35.3 Grade II chondrosarcoma. Irregular hypercellular lobules of blue-gray cartilage with myxoid matrix permeating the host bone (H&E, 40x).

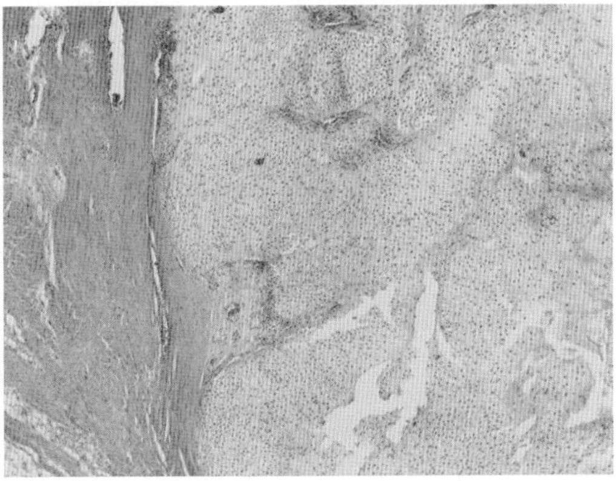

Fig. 35.4 Grade II chondrosarcoma. Neoplastic cellular lobules of myxoid cartilage invading the surrounding soft tissue (H&E, 40x).

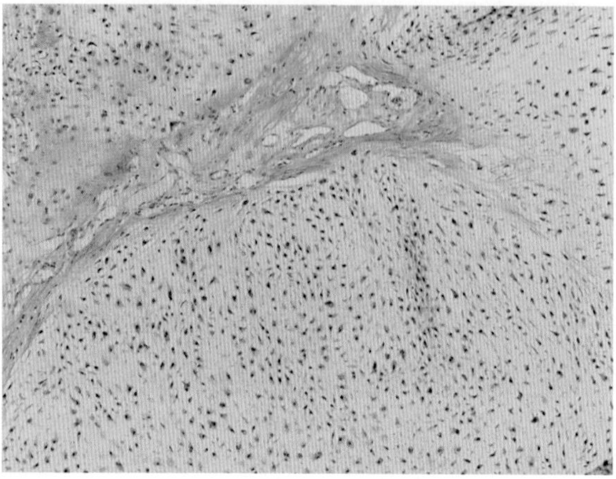

Fig. 35.5 Grade II chondrosarcoma. Hypercellular lobules of cartilage with variable size and shape of atypical hyperchromatic cells (H&E, 100x).

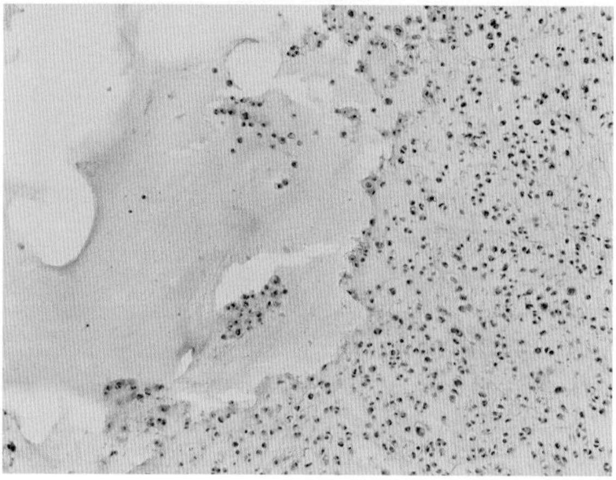

Fig. 35.6 Grade II chondrosarcoma. Foci of myxoid material (H&E, 100x).

What is the natural history of chondrosarcoma?

Chondrosarcomas usually occur in patients older than 40 years and are exceedingly rare in those younger than 20 years. Typically, there is a history of pain (rest pain or night pain), which may be prolonged. Chondrosarcomas may be primary or secondary in a previously benign lesion such as an enchondroma or osteochondroma. Patients with syndromes that include multiple endochondromatosis or multiple osteochondromatosis are at increased risk for developing secondary chondrosarcomas.

Cartilaginous tumors of the skeleton can be diagnostically challenging in histologic specimens. This is partly due to the significant overlap in the morphologic appearance found in the different cartilaginous lesions, especially the low-grade lesions such as enchondrama versus atypical cartilagenous neoplasm / grade 1 chondrosarcoma. Fortunately, differentiating low-grade cartilaginous lesions with minimal or no risk of metastases (i.e., enchondromas and atypical cartilaginous tumor / grade I chondrosarcoma) from higher-grade cartilaginous tumors with a significant risk of metastases (i.e., grade II or grade III chondrosarcomas) is usually not challenging and is the most relevant distinction clinically. Histologic grading is the single most important factor in determining the prognosis for patients diagnosed with chondrosarcoma.

Grade I chondrosarcomas typically behave in a locally aggressive manner and can recur locally; however, metastases are exceedingly rare. In contrast, grade II and III chondrosarcomas have metastatic potential and a much worse prognosis with a 5-year survival rate of approximately 50%. Recurrent tumors may show a higher histologic grade at the time of recurrence and a corresponding worse prognosis.

Why is it important to have clinical and imaging information when evaluating a biopsy from a cartilaginous lesion of bone?

When evaluating a cartilage lesion, it is critical to include relevant clinical data, especially the history of pain as well as all pertinent radiographic findings. Plain films provide important information regarding the location of the lesion within the skeleton, the size of the lesion, as well as the pattern of growth, all of which are important determinants of benign versus malignant behavior. Tumors of the axial skeleton, pelvis, and proximal ends of long bones are more likely to be malignant compared with lesions of the distal extremities and tubular bones of the feet and hands. Likewise, lesions with ill-defined borders with permeative growth are more likely to behave in a malignant fashion than smaller, circumscribed lesions with well-defined pushing borders. Low-grade tumors typically have significant area of matrix mineralization seen radiographically and can produce bone expansion with endosteal scalloping, whereas high-grade tumors have large, radiolucent areas with cortical destruction and may also show extension through the cortex with formation of a soft tissue mass.

What is the most appropriate treatment for a patient diagnosed with chondrosarcoma?

The treatment of chondrosarcoma is heavily dependent on the anatomic location, the histologic grade, and the metastatic potential of the tumor. Low-grade (grade I) chondrosarcomas are often adequately treated with aggressive curettage, particularly if the tumor is located in the appendicular skeleton, with clinical follow-up for possible local recurrence. One exception would be a low-grade chondrosarcoma arising in the pelvis, which would be treated with resection due to the fact that a local recurrence in this anatomic location would be difficult to treat. Grade II or grade III chondrosarcomas are typically treated with wide surgical resection for clear margins if possible. For unresectable tumors, radiation therapy may be offered and is frequently used for chondrosarcoma arising in the spine or skull base.

CLINICAL PEARL

Primary chondrosarcomas are tumors that arise de novo in the bone without evidence of preexisting precursor lesion.

Secondary chondrosarcomas are tumors that arise on preexisting benign bone tumor such as enchondroma or osteochondroma, associated with syndromes such as Maffucci, and might occur in patients with history of radiation or Paget's disease.

What are the clinicopathological differences between enchondroma and atypical cartilaginous tumor/grade I chondrosarcoma?

Enchondroma usually occurs in younger age group in second to fifth decade and tends to arise in short tubular bones of the hand as well as long bones. The majority of these lesions are asymptomatic and detected as an incidental finding during investigation of some other condition. They may

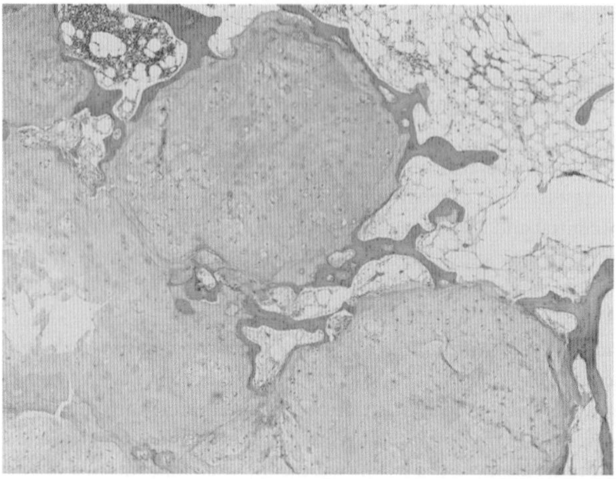

Fig. 35.7 Enchondroma. Regular lobules of hypocellular cartilaginous neoplasm with the surrounding reactive bone (H&E, 40x).

present as swelling with or without pain, particularly in lesions arising in phalanges. Radiologically, enchondromas are usually less than 5 cm, well-circumscribed, sharply demarcated lucent mass within the medullary cavity, without cortical destruction. Microscopically, the typical enchondroma shows well-circumscribed hypocellular lobules of mature hyaline cartilage (Fig. 35.7), without permeation or extension into the surrounding host cancellous bone. The matrix is usually hyaline-type and frequently calcified, with myxoid changes either being absent or very focal. Prominent myxoid changes should raise suspicion for a chondrosarcoma. The hyaline matrix contains chondrocytes that have uniform, small, round hyperchromatic cells that lack atypia. Enchondroma of the hand tend to be more cellular.

Atypical cartilaginous tumor/chondrosarcoma grade I occur in older age group in the fifth to seventh decade, usually arise in the axial and appendicular skeleton, and commonly present with an enlarging mass and pain and sometime pathological fracture. Radiologically, these tumors are usually larger than 5 cm; radiolucent fusiform intramedullary masses with extensive endosteal scalloping and cortical destruction may also show soft tissue extension. Microscopic examination reveals moderately cellular infiltrating lobules of cartilage with more myxoid matrix permeating into the surrounding host bone. The atypia seen in these tumors is mild, with true host bone trabeculae permeation present; however, this might be difficult to discern from limited biopsy material or curetted specimens (Table 35.2).

Given the important clinical significance, what is the best way to differentiate between chondrosarcoma grades I, II, and III histologically?

The degree of cellularity, atypia, presence of mitotic figures, architecture, and myxoid matrix are the histologic findings that are most useful for grading chondrosarcoma, as these features tend to progressively increase from grade I to grade III chondrosarcoma. Grade I chondrosarcoma tends to show hypocellular chondroid matrix with small hyperchromatic nuclei and minimal atypia (Fig. 35.8A). Grade II chondrosarcoma becomes more cellular with medium-sized, regular nuclei and more opened chromatin (Fig. 35.8B). Grade III chondrosarcoma is hypercellular and shows enlarged nuclei, with marked pleomorphism and frequent mitotic figures (Fig. 35.8C).

TABLE 35.2 ■ **Differences Between Enchondroma and Atypical Cartilaginous Tumor/Grade I Chondrosarcoma**

Features	Enchondroma	Atypical Cartilaginous Tumor/ Grade I Chondrosarcoma
Age	2nd to 5th decades	5th to 7th decades
Site	Short tubular bone of the hand, proximal humerus, distal tibia, and proximal and distal femur	Pelvis, proximal and distal femur, proximal humerus, and rib
Clinical	Found incidentally, may cause swelling with or without pain	Swelling and pain for long duration. May present with pathological fractures
Radiological	Well-circumscribed, sharply demarcated lucent mass within the medullary cavity. Highly mineralized with ring or arch pattern of calcification. Endosteal scalloping, cortical erosion, and cortical thinning are common findings.	Radiolucent fusiform intramedullary mass with less mineralization with popcorn-like and punctate calcification. Extensive endosteal scalloping, cortical thickening, and destruction with soft tissue extension are common findings.
Size	Usually <5 cm	>5 cm
Grossly	No cortical destruction No myxoid material	Cortical destruction Myxoid material
Microscopically	Well-circumscribed, less cellular lobules of mature hyaline cartilage with surrounding reactive bone (Fig. 35.7). Granular calcification present. No true host bone permeation. No myxoid matrix. No atypia. Enchondroma of the hand tends to be more cellular.	Moderately cellular infiltrating lobules of cartilage with more myxoid matrix. The atypia are mild. True host bone trabeculae permeation present.
Treatment	Curettage	Curettage with local adjuvant
Risk of recurrence	Uncommon	10% has risk of recurrence
Risk of metastasis	–	Very rare

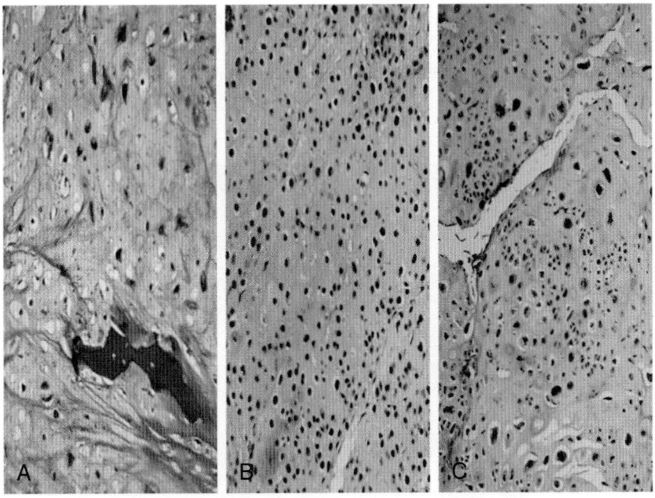

Fig. 35.8 Grading of chondrosarcoma. (A) Grade I: hypocellular chondroid matrix with small hyperchromatic nuclei and minimal atypia. (B) Grade II: more cellular and medium-sized, regular nuclei with loose chromatin structure. (C) Grade III: hypercellular, enlarged nuclei with marked pleomorphism and frequent mitosis (H&E, 200x).

CLINICAL PEARL

Low-grade chondrosarcoma may recur and undergo dedifferentiation into high-grade nonchondrogenic sarcomatous tumor and will be diagnosed as dedifferentiated chondrosarcoma. Dedifferentiated chondrosarcoma is a highly malignant tumor composed histologically of low-grade chondrogenic neoplasm with abrupt transition to high-grade nonchondrogenic sarcoma, such as fibrosarcoma (Fig. 35.9).

What are the molecular genetic findings that have been reported for chondrosarcomas?

Many chondrosarcomas have a specific genetic mutation in the isocitrate dehydrogenase genes IDH1 and IDH2, which can be seen in 40%–70% of primary tumors and in >80% of secondary tumors. Occasionally, mutation analysis can be useful to help distinguish chondrosarcoma from a chondroblastic osteosarcoma in a limited biopsy sample.

CLINICAL PEARL

Isocitrate dehydrogenase IDH1 or IDH2 gene mutations occur in 38%–70% chondrosarcoma.

What are the syndromes associated with increased risk of developing chondrosarcoma?

There are three syndromes associated with chondrosarcoma: Maffucci syndrome, Ollier disease, and hereditary multiple exostoses.

CLINICAL PEARL

Maffucci syndrome is extremely rare, affects bone and skin, and manifests as early as 5 years of age. It present with multiple enchondromas especially in the hand, feet, and limbs. Also, patients develop multiple skin hemangiomas. Patients have a 53% risk of developing secondary chondrosarcoma. This syndrome is caused by mutation on IDH1 or IDH2 gene.

CLINICAL PEARL

Ollier disease is extremely rare, related to Maffucci syndrome, and presents with multiple enchondromas of the long bones and hand. Lesions start to develop just after birth. Patients have a 40% risk for developing secondary chondrosarcoma. This disease is caused by mutation on IDH1 or IDH2 gene.

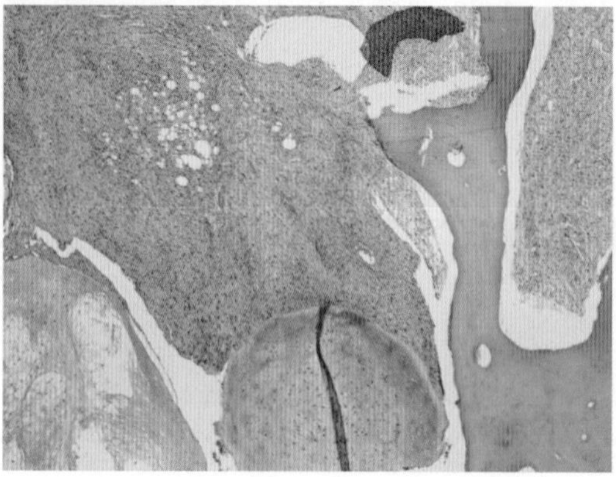

Fig. 35.9 Dedifferentiated chondrosarcoma. Abrupt transition of grade II chondrosarcoma to high-grade nonchondrogenic sarcoma (fibrosarcoma) (H&E, 40x).

CLINICAL PEARL

Hereditary multiple exostosis is a disease of developing multiple benign osteochondromas starting from 12 years of age and causes significant growth deformities. It is caused by EXT1 or EXT2 mutation.

What are the clinicopathological features of other common benign cartilaginous neoplasms?

Osteochondroma: It usually occurs in the second decade of life and involves the bone formed by endochondral ossifications, commonly metaphysis of long bone such as femur, proximal tibia, and upper humerus. Also, it might involve flat bones like scapula and ilium. Radiologically, osteochondroma is a surface bone neoplasm with cartilaginous cap and stalk. The bone cortex and medullary space are in continuity with lesion stalk and medullary cavity, which can be seen radiographically. Grossly, the lesion may be sessile or pedunculated, measuring 3–6 cm, and is covered by a cartilaginous cap with variable thickness of 1–2 cm. In addition, there is direct continuity of the medullary cavity of the lesion with the underlying bone. Microscopically, hyaline cartilaginous cap resembles disorganized growth plate–like cartilage, covered with fibrous perichondrium, and undergoes enchondral ossifications. Beneath the cartilage cap, bony trabeculae and hematopoietic marrow can be observed (Fig. 35.10). The cartilaginous cap displays high cellularity more toward the deeper layer (particularly in younger patients), with columnar arrangement of the chondrocytes, and may exhibit some cellular atypia. Surgical resection with removal of the fibrous perichondrium is curative for osteochondroma. Risk of recurrence is very rare.

CLINICAL PEARL

Less than 1% of osteochondroma might undergo malignant transformation to chondrosarcoma and always arise from the cartilaginous cap.

Bizarre parosteal osteochondromatous proliferation (Nora's lesion): This is a rare lesion commonly occurring in the third and fourth decade and usually involving small bones of hand and feet. Frequently, there is a history of prior trauma with rapid growth of the lesion. Radiologically, it is a heavily calcified, well-circumscribed, radiolucent nodule on the surface of small long bone with cartilaginous cap. The medullary cavity of the lesion is not in continuity with the underlying bone trabeculae. Grossly, it is approximately 1 cm, nodular lesion with lobulated

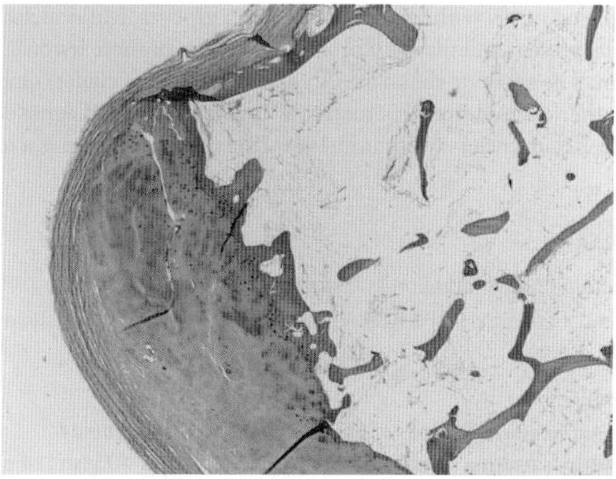

Fig. 35.10 Osteochondroma displaying the three layers of fibrous perichondrium, cartilaginous cap, and bone trabeculae. The center of the neoplasm is in continuity with underlying bone medullary cavity (H&E, 20x).

cartilaginous cap and bony stalk. Microscopically, it comprises three components: fibrous tissue, cartilage, and bone arranged in disorganized manner. The fibrous tissue is spindle and cellular. The cartilage is hypercellular with enlarged chondrocytes and undergoes enchondral ossifications with the formation of blue mineralized woven bone trabeculae. The center of the lesion is not in continuity with the underlying originating bone. Surgical resection is the treatment of choice.

Synovial chondromatosis: Commonly occurs in third and fifth decades, and two-thirds of the cases occur in the knee. Radiologically, it is multiple, small, round calcified nodules in the joint. Microscopically, it shows nodules of hypercellular hyaline cartilage and is often surrounded by synovial tissue. Malignant transformation is very rare, but recurrence may occur after resection.

What are the clinicopathological features of cartilaginous neoplasms with a potential for local recurrence?

Chondromyxoid fibroma: Very rare and commonly occurs under age of 40 years. It usually involves the medullary cavity of the metaphysis of long bone around the knee. Radiologically, it is an eccentric, metaphyseal, radiolucent lesion with sharply circumscribed, sclerotic margins. The borders typically have a scalloped appearance. Cortical thinning is typical and may be marked. If present, cortical expansion is usually minimal. Periosteal reaction is absent. Grossly, it is multilobulated, well-circumscribed mass with bluish-grey or white cut surface. Microscopic features include a lobular appearance, in which the lobules are densely cellular peripherally and hypocellular centrally. The central portions of the lobules are composed of watery, chondromyxoid ground substance in which the stellate or spindled cells appear to float. The cells have round, oval, stellate, or triangular nuclei in which chromatin varies from finely clumped and pale to dense and darkly staining. The nuclei are minimally atypical, and occasional binucleated, multinucleated, or even "bizarre" forms may be seen. At the periphery of the lobules are dense condensations of round or ovoid cells with little intervening matrix. These cells have relatively uniform, round nuclei with finely clumped chromatin. Surgical resection is the mainstay of treatment; the risk of recurrence is 15%–20%, predominantly in patients treated by curettage. Multiple recurrences are distinctly uncommon and should raise a suspicion of chondrosarcoma.

Chondroblastoma: Is a rare lesion, commonly occurring between 10 and 25 years of age. These lesions usually involve epiphysis of long bone, such as femur, humerus, and tibia. Radiologically, chondroblastomas are small lesions (usually <5 cm) showing lytic defects with sharply circumscribed, sclerotic borders. Speckled calcifications may be present. Histologic sections demonstrate sheets of uniform, polygonal cells with sharply demarcated cell borders, eosinophilic cytoplasm, and indented nuclei with longitudinal nuclear grooves. Multinucleated osteoclast-like giant cells are usually present and may be a prominent feature of these lesions. Discrete islands of chondroid matrix may be scant or abundant. A characteristic pericellular "chicken-wire" pattern of calcifications is often seen within this matrix, which is a helpful diagnostic feature. Surgical curetting is curative. Recurrence may occur in 14%–18% cases, and there is a less than 1% risk of metastasis.

CLINICAL PEARL

Most chondroblastoma show mutation in histone gene H3F3A.

Immunohistochemical stain for H3F3 K36M mutant protein is highly sensitive and specific for chondroblastoma.

What are the clinicopathological features of mesenchymal chondrosarcoma?

Mesenchymal chondrosarcoma usually occurs between 10 and 40 years of age and commonly involves the craniofacial bone, jaw, pelvis, vertebra, ribs, and long bones. Radiologically, it is an ill-defined, highly destructive lytic tumor with poorly defined margins and may show stippled calcifications. Grossly, these lesions are usually more than 5 cm, solid, gritty, fleshy, destructive tumors. Microscopically, one sees sheets of small, hyperchromatic, malignant small round blue cells with scattered interspersed islands of malignant cellular hyaline cartilage matrix. The transition between the two histologic components is characteristically abrupt. A hemangiopericytomatous-like vascular pattern commonly occurs and is a helpful diagnostic feature. Mesenchymal chondrosarcoma is an aggressive, high-grade malignant tumor; surgical resection with adjuvant radiotherapy and chemotherapy is the treatment of choice. The clinical course is aggressive with frequent metastasis.

CLINICAL PEARL

Mesenchymal chondrosarcomas are associated with recurrent fusion mutation of HEY1-NCOA2.

BEYOND THE PEARLS

- Primary chondrosarcoma is the second most common malignant bone tumor after osteosarcoma.
- Histologic grade is the most prognostic predictor for local recurrence and metastasis in chondrosarcoma.
- The standard-of-care for treatment of chondrosarcoma is surgical resection because it is resistant to chemotherapy and radiotherapy.
- Diagnosing atypical cartilaginous tumor/grade I chondrosarcoma on needle biopsy is challenging and needs radiological correlation to differentiate it from enchondroma.
- Conventional chondrosarcoma in children and teens is rare and always exclude chondroblastic osteosarcoma.

Case Point 35.2

The patient recovered uneventfully from the surgery of the radical resection of the chondrosarcoma of the proximal humerus with endoprosthetic reconstruction. The surgical resection margins were clear, and his pathological stage is pT2 pN0. The patient was followed up for 3 years with no history of recurrence.

References

Cho HS, Han I, Kim HS. Secondary chondrosarcoma from an osteochondroma of the proximal tibia involving the fibula. *Clin Orthop Surg*. 2017;9(2):249-254.

Deyrup AT, Siegal GP. *Practical Orthopedic Pathology: A Diagnostic Approach: A Volume in the Pattern Recognition Series*. Philadelphia, PA: Elsevier Health Sciences; 2015:127-148.

Fletcher CDM, Bridge JA, Hogendoorn, PCW, Mertens F. *WHO Classification of Tumours of Soft Tissue and Bone*. 4th ed. vol 5. Pathology. 2013.

Kim MJ, Cho KJ, Ayala AG, Ro JY. Chondrosarcoma: with updates on molecular genetics. *Sarcoma*. 2011;2011:405-437.

Nielsen GP, Rosenberg AE. *Diagnostic Pathology: Bone*. 2nd ed. Philadelphia, PA: Elsevier Health Sciences; 2017:84-162.

CASE 36

A 30-Year-Old Female with Right Foot Mass

Rana Ajabnoor

A 30-year-old female presents to the primary health care physician with a slow-growing right foot mass over 1 year. She started to feel intermittent pain over the mass 6 months earlier and could not fit her foot in a closed shoe due to the bulkiness of the mass over the dorsum surface. She does not have any walking limitation. She is an administrative secretary and did recall a history of fall 2 months ago before she noticed the mass while walking downstairs. Otherwise her past medical history is not significant. Physical examination of the right foot shows a mass, measuring approximately 4 cm, on the dorsal aspect of her foot overlying the first and second metatarsals bones. It is largely firm to palpation with some soft areas. It is not mobile. Motor function is preserved together with flexion and extension of the toes. Numbness is identified over the mass. Magnetic resonance imaging shows a soft tissue mass on the dorsum of the foot with diffuse enhancement of the surrounding soft tissue and cortical bone destruction of the first metatarsal bone (Fig. 36.1).

What are the causes of a soft tissue mass in the foot of an adult patient?
The causes are variable ranging from reactive process, such as nodular fasciitis (NF) or proliferative fasciitis (PF), to neoplastic that could be benign, such as superficial fibromatosis, fibroma of tendon sheath, and localized or diffuse tenosynovial giant cell tumor, or malignant, such as epithelioid sarcoma (ES), clear cell sarcoma (CCS) of soft tissue, and metastasis (Table 36.1).

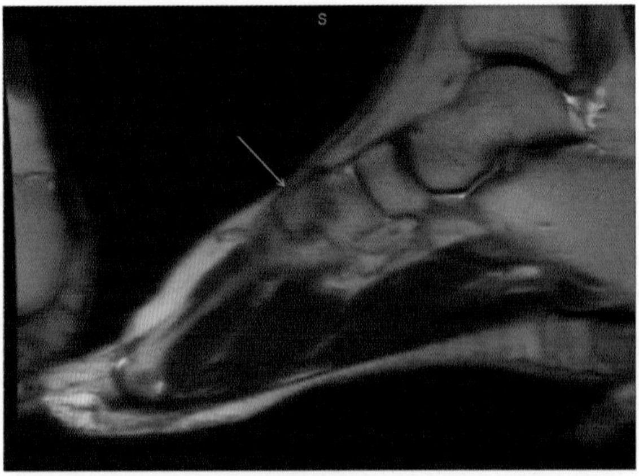

Fig. 36.1 Magnetic resonance imaging shows a soft tissue mass on the dorsum of the foot with diffuse enhancement of the surrounding soft tissue and cortical bone destruction of the first metatarsal bone (arrow).

TABLE 36.1 ■ **Common Soft Tissue Masses in the Foot of an Adult**

Cell of Origin	Benign	Intermediate Malignancy	Malignant
Fibroblastic	Nodular fasciitis Proliferative fasciitis Fibroma of tendon sheath	Superficial fibromatosis	
Fibrohistiocytic Tumors	Tenosynovial giant cell tumor: localized and diffuse type		Malignant tenosynovial giant cell tumor
Uncertain Differentiation	Acral fibromyxoma	Hemosiderotic fibrolipomatous tumor	Epithelioid sarcoma Clear cell sarcoma of soft tissue

What is your differential diagnosis?

Based on the patient's age and the clinical presentation of the lesion, which is locally aggressive, this is suggestive of a malignant process such as CCS of soft tissue or ES; however, diffuse-type tenosynovial giant cell tumor should be included, as it could infiltrate the surrounding soft tissue with destruction of the underlying cortical bone.

Case Point 36.1

The patient undergoes an open biopsy, which shows infiltrating neoplastic growth with alternating cellularity composed of abundant mononuclear cells, small spindle histiocyte-like and epithelioid cells, osteoclast-like giant cells, and chronic inflammatory cells (Fig. 36.2A–E). These cells invade the underlying tendon and surrounding soft tissue. No atypia or mitosis is present. The stroma is focally myxoid and collagenous.

What are the clinicopathologic features of proliferative fasciitis (PF)?

It is a pseudosarcomatous myofibroblastic lesion in the same spectrum of NF but less common. PF occurs in an older age than NF, usually in middle-aged adults, and could occur subcutaneously in any site but more commonly in the upper extremity. It presents as a rapidly growing mass within 2 months. Grossly, it is an ill-defined mass, extending horizontally along the fascia and most often less than 3 cm. Histologically, it is an infiltrative lesion composed of plump fibroblastic and myofibroblast spindle cells arranged in a similar fashion as in NF; however, it contains a large epithelioid or ganglion-like cells with eccentrically placed rounded nuclei, prominent nucleoli, and amphophilic cytoplasm (Fig. 36.3A and B). These cells do not exhibit atypia or mitosis and are admixed with lymphocytes. The stroma shows variable myxoid and fibrous background. Immunohistochemical analysis demonstrates spindle cells stained by smooth muscle actin (SMA) and muscle-specific actin (MSA). Also, the ganglion-like cells are focally positive for SMA. Cytokeratin, desmin, and S100 are negative. These lesions are usually managed conservatively, but may be excised occasionally and have no risk of recurrence.

CLINICAL PEARL

PF is associated with history of trauma in one-third of the cases.

The characteristic ganglion cells of PF are actually fibroblasts.

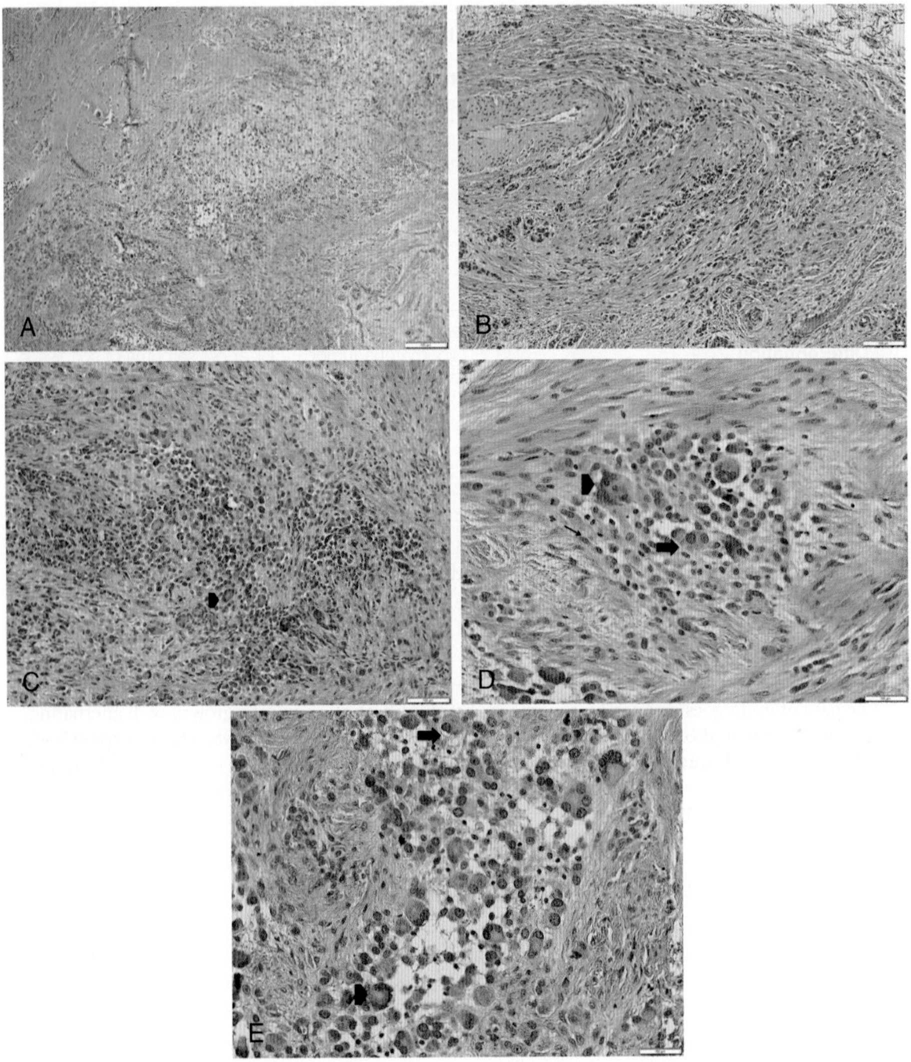

Fig. 36.2 Diffuse-type tenosynovial giant cell tumor: (A) Microscopically, low power shows an infiltrative neoplastic growth composed of sheets with alternating and variable cellularity (H&E 40x). (B) It is seen infiltrating the underlying soft tissue (H&E 100x). (C, D, and E) At high power, it is composed of polymorphous cellularity of osteoclast-like giant cells (arrowhead), mononuclear cells that consist of small spindle histiocyte-like cells (thin arrow), and large epithelioid-like cells (arrow) admixed with inflammatory cells (H&E 100x & 200x).

What are the clinicopathologic features of the other fibroblastic neoplasms that might occur in the foot of an adult?

Fibroma of tendon sheath: Slow-growing neoplasm commonly occurs in patients aged 20–50 years. Upper extremities are the common sites of occurrence, with predilection to fingers and hands; it could also occur in the foot. Grossly, it is a well-circumscribed nodule with tendon attachment. Histologically, it shows well-demarcated, multilobulated neoplasm with elongated cleft-like spaces mainly at the periphery and lined by flattened cells. The lobules are usually

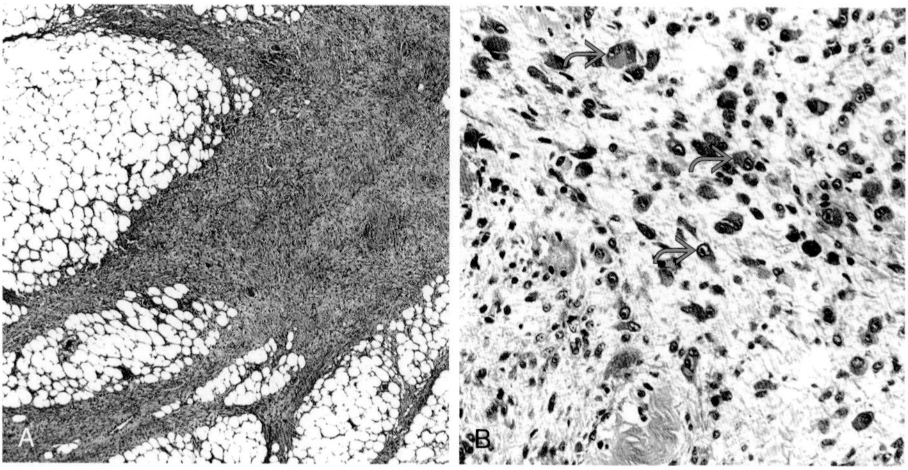

Fig. 36.3 Proliferative fasciitis: Histologically, low power shows (A) subcutaneous spindle cell neoplasm infiltrating the fat. (B) Enlarged epithelioid, ganglion-like cells (arrow) are characteristic of proliferative fasciitis. (From *ExpertPath*. Copyright Elsevier)

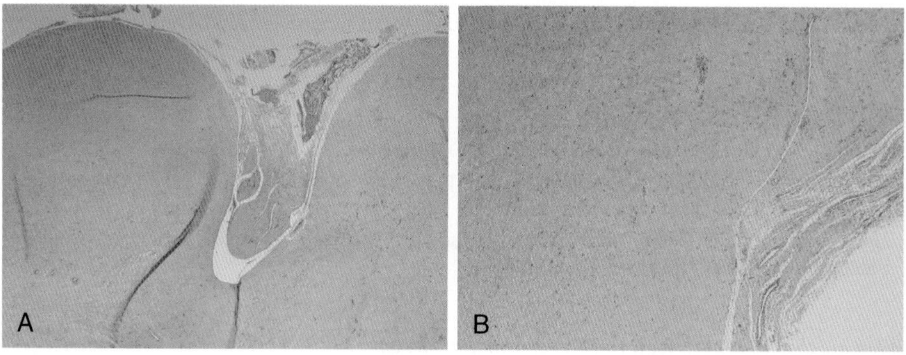

Fig. 36.4 Fibroma of tendon sheath: (A) Histologically, a well-demarcated, multilobulated hypocellular fibrous neoplasm is seen (H&E x20). (B) Elongated slit-like vascular spaces at the periphery of the lobules (H&E 40x).

hypocellular with collagenous background formed by proliferating bland-looking fibroblasts with oval nuclei exhibiting fine, open chromatin and small nucleoli, with no atypia (Fig. 36.4A and B). This neoplasm commonly tends to show a cellular phase resembling NF-like features. Immunohistochemical analysis shows MSA and SMA positivity. Tendency for recurrence has been documented, especially in the incompletely excised lesions. Surgical excision is the treatment of choice.

Plantar fibromatosis (superficial fibromatosis): According to the World Health Organization, it is classified as an intermediate malignant neoplasm due to its local aggressiveness. It commonly occurs in adults aged approximately 30 years, and the incidence increases with advanced age. It usually arises within the plantar aponeurosis in nonweight-bearing areas and presents as a subcutaneous nodule that might be associated with pain and, rarely, toe contraction. Grossly, it is composed of ill-defined, multinodular growth with attachment to tendon or aponeurosis. Microscopically, it shows hypercellular, multinodular growth composed of proliferating uniform bland spindle fibroblastic cells, with pinpoint nucleoli. No mitosis or

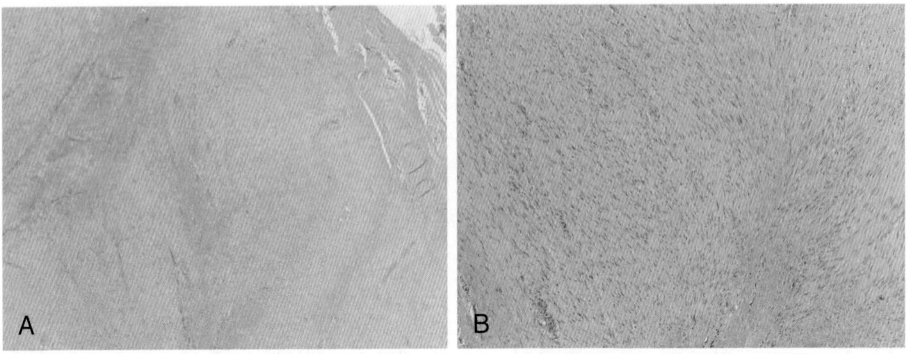

Fig. 36.5 Plantar fibromatosis (superficial fibromatosis): (A) Microscopically, low power shows cellular, multinodular, infiltrating spindle cell neoplasm (H&E, 40x). (B) It is composed of bland spindle cells with background of collagenous stroma (H&E, 100x).

atypia is present. The stroma is collagenous (Fig. 36.5A and B), and scattered osteoclast-like giant cells are present. Immunohistochemistry usually shows positivity for SMA and MSA, approximately 50% of the cases might have nuclear positivity for beta-catenin. The risk of recurrence is closely related with the extent and adequacy of surgical excision. Dermatofasciectomy is the treatment of choice.

CLINICAL PEARL

Plantar fibromatosis is also known as Ledderhose disease.

Plantar fibromatosis etiology is multifactorial that might occur in patients with diabetes, epilepsy, and alcoholism with liver disease.

Usually recurrence occurs within the 1st year after the excision, and risk increases in patients with multiple nodules and bilaterality.

What are the clinicopathologic features of acral fibromyxoma?

It is a benign neoplasm of uncertain lineage, commonly affecting adults in the fifth decade. It commonly arises in ungual or periungual location in the hand palm or foot sole, with big toe being the most common site of involvement. It presents as a single, superficial, slow-growing mass. Grossly, it is a soft to firm, well-circumscribed, polypoid lesion with a median size of 1.5 cm. Histologically, it is a dermal-based, moderately cellular neoplasm composed of proliferating bland spindle or stellate cells arranged in a loose fascicular or storiform growth pattern in a background of myxoid or collagenous stroma (Fig. 36.6A and B). No nuclear atypia or increased mitosis is present. Mild increased vascularity and mast cells are seen. The overlying epidermis may show verrucoid changes. Immunohistochemical analysis shows diffuse positivity for CD34 and rare focal positivity for epithelial membrane antigen (EMA) and SMA. S100, desmin, and keratin are negative. Surgical excision is the treatment of choice, and the risk of recurrence is 15% to 20%.

What are the clinicopathologic features of hemosiderotic fibrolipomatous tumor (HFLT)?

It is a locally aggressive, intermediate malignant neoplasm that commonly arises in the dorsum of the foot at the ankle region and affects more women in the fifth or sixth decade. It presents as a slow-growing, painful, subcutaneous mass. Grossly, it is an ill-defined lesion with a median size of

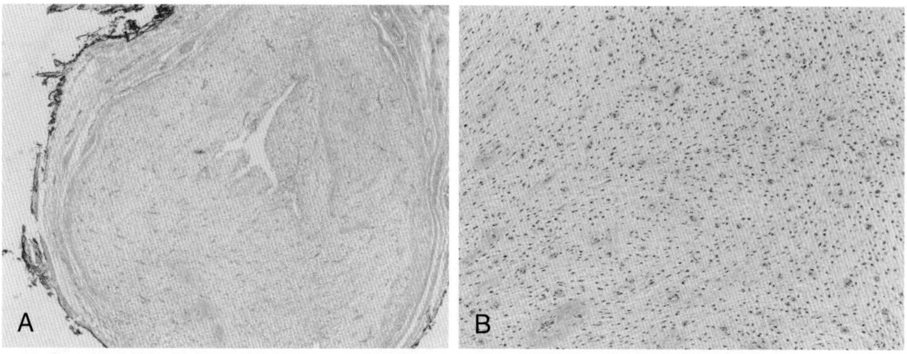

Fig. 36.6 Acral fibromyxoma: Microscopically, (A) a well-circumscribed, dermal-based neoplasm (H&E 40x) is seen composed of (B) bland spindle and stellate cells arranged in myxoid stroma with increased vascularity (H&E 100x).

7.7 cm and has yellow cut surface with foci of hemorrhage. Microscopically, it is a fibrolipomatous neoplasm resembling a reactive process that is composed of fascicles of bland fibroblastic spindle cells and hemosiderin pigment deposition admixed with mature adipocytes, hemosiderin-laden macrophages, and osteoclast-like giant cells (Fig. 36.7A and B). The spindle cells are arranged in periadipocytic, septal, and perilobular fashion. Large cells with atypical nuclei are occasionally seen (Fig. 36.7C). No necrosis or mitosis is identified. There is no specific immnohistochemical stains for HFLT, as it usually stains positive for CD34 and negative for S100, desmin, and SMA. HFLT has 30% to 50% risk of local recurrence if not completely excised, and no risk of metastasis. Surgical excision is the mainstay of treatment.

CLINICAL PEARL

HFLT shares morphological and cytogenetical features with myxoinflammatory fibroblastic sarcoma.

What are the clinicopathologic features of epitheliod sarcoma (ES)?

It is a malignant mesenchymal neoplasm of unknown lineage. It has two subtypes, classic and proximal. Classic ES usually occurs distally in the extremities, especially in the volar surface of the hand and foot with predilection to upper extremity. Classic ES commonly affects young adults aged 10–40 years, whereas proximal ES affects older population aged 20–65 years. Proximal ES tends to arise from the deep soft tissue of the trunk, pelvoperineal, inguinal, and genital areas. Classic ES usually presents as superficial, painless, slow-growing, firm nodule with skin ulceration ranging in size from few millimeters to 5 cm, whereas proximal ES presents as a large infiltrative mass measuring up to 15 cm. Grossly, classic ES shows ill-defined, dermal or subcutaneous nodule that has white to yellow cut surface with necrotic center and may also involve the underlying tendon and fascia. Microscopically, classic ES consists of multiple proliferating malignant nodules with central necrosis, simulating granulomatous formation (Fig. 36.8A–C). These nodules are composed of large polygonal epithelioid and spindled plump cells with eosinophilic cytoplasm, mild nuclear atypia, vesicular chromatin, and prominent small nucleoli (Fig. 36.8D and E). Mitosis is usually low (<5/10 HPF). The stroma is collagenous, with occasional dystrophic calcifications and metaplastic osteoid formation. Proximal ES is composed of sheets and multinodular growth pattern that consists of large,

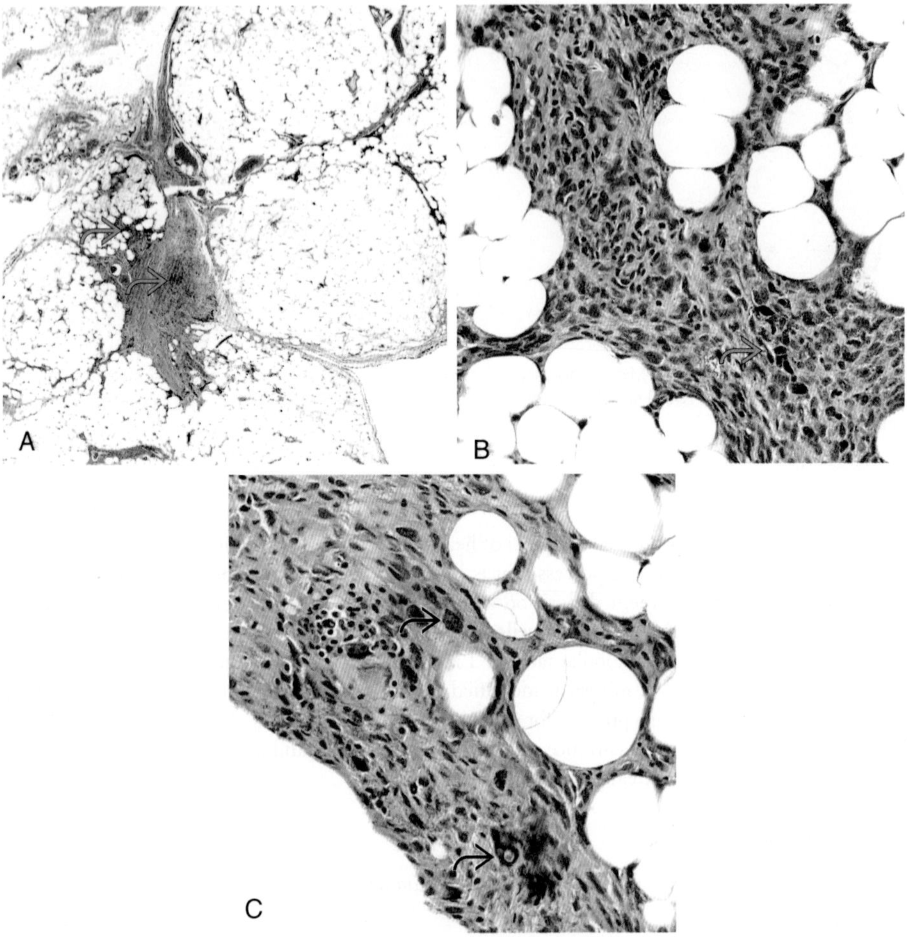

Fig. 36.7 Hemosiderotic fibrolipomatous tumor: Microscopically, (A and B) lobules of mature adipose tissue are seen with bland spindle cells arranged in perilobular and septal fashion admixed with hemosiderin deposition (arrow). (C) Focal nuclear pleomorphism and intranuclear pseudoinclusion (arrow) are occasionally present in some cases. (From *ExpertPath*. Copyright Elsevier).

pleomorphic epithelioid cells with deeply eosinophilic cytoplasm, marked nuclear atypia, vesicular nuclei, and prominent nucleoli. Foci of necrosis are present but without pseudogranulomatous pattern (Table 36.2). Collection of cells with rhabdoid features is more frequently seen in proximal ES exhibiting glassy intracytoplasmic hyaline inclusion and eccentrically placed vesicular nuclei. Immunohistochemistry for both subtypes demonstrates positive staining for epithelial markers, specifically high- and low-molecular-weight cytokeratin and EMA. Also, it shows positive nonspecific staining for vimentin and CD34 in >50% cases. It is negative for S100, CD31, and desmin. Approximately 90%–95% cases show loss of expression of INI1. Radical surgical excision with wide resection margin is the mainstay of treatment with adjuvant radiotherapy. Risk of recurrence ranges from 30% to 85% and depends on the margin status of the excision. Metastasis rate increases up to 40%–60% in the patients after they develop recurrence. Usually ES tends to metastasize to the lung and regional lymph nodes.

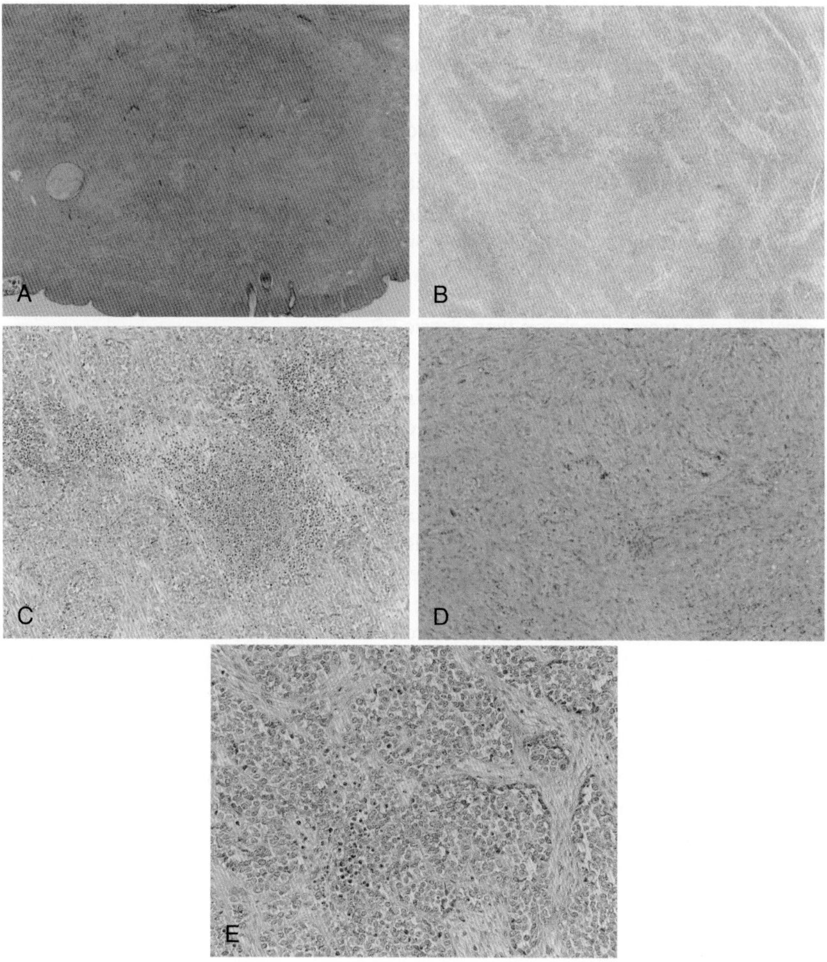

Fig. 36.8 Epithelioid sarcoma: Microscopically, (A–C) dermal-based, multinodular, malignant neoplasm is seen with central necrosis, simulating granulomatous formation (H&E x20, 40x, 100x). (D and E) The nodule is composed of large epithelioid cells with moderate atypia, vesicular chromatin, and prominent small nucleoli admixed with plump spindle-shaped cells with atypical nuclei (H&E 200x).

TABLE 36.2 ■ **Differences Between Distal and Proximal Type of Epithelioid Sarcoma**

Parameters	Distal (Classic) Type	Proximal Type
Age	Younger age: 10–40 years	Older age: 20–65 years
Site	Upper extremities; hand and fingers	Pelvoperineal, genital, and inguinal
Size	Mean 5 cm	Up to 15 cm
Gross features	Superficial dermal-based or subcutaneous nodule	Deep-seated infiltrative multinodular mass
Histologic features	- Pseudogranulomatous pattern present - Mild nuclear atypia - Rare rhabdoid cells	- No pseudogranulomatous pattern - Marked nuclear atypia - Frequent rhabdoid cells
Prognosis	Protracted clinical course	More aggressive clinical course

CLINICAL PEARL

ES is one of the few sarcomas that always metastasizes to the lymph node.

Rheumatoid nodule and granuloma annulare are great mimickers for classic ES.

SMARCB1 (INI1) is a tumor suppressor gene located on chromosome 22q that undergoes genetic alteration, resulting in inactivation of the gene in both types of ES; this is demonstrated by the loss of INI1 immunohistochemical stain.

High-risk factors for aggressive course include male patient, age >75 years, tumor size >5 cm, deep-seated and proximal sites, extensive necrosis, nuclear pleomorphism, vascular and nerve invasion, presence of rhabdoid cells, regional lymph node metastasis, and inadequate excision.

Proximal ES has a worse prognosis than classic ES.

What are the clinicopathologic features of CCS of soft tissue?

It is a rare malignant tumor with melanocytic differentiation that mainly affects young adults aged 10–40 years. Approximately 40% of the cases occur in the ankle and foot region associated with tendon and aponeuroses, followed by knee, wrists, and hands. It usually presents as a slow-growing, deeply seated mass, possibly present for several years before the patient seeks medical attention. Grossly, it is a multilobular, firm mass (2–5 cm) with infiltrative boarder and gray-white cut surface and occasional pigmented areas. Histologically, it is composed of malignant epithelioid to spindle cells arranged in a nesting or fascicular pattern that are separated by fibrocollagenous bands (Fig. 36.9A and B). These cells exhibit pale eosinophilic to clear cytoplasm with intracellular glycogen, vesicular nuclei, and prominent macronucleoli resembling melanoma (Fig. 36.9C and D). Mitosis and pleomorphism are minimal. Wreath-like multinucleated giant cells are often present and good diagnostic clue. Immunohistochemical analysis consistently shows strong and diffuse positivity for melanocytic markers, including S100, SOX10, HMB-45, melan A, and microphthalmia transcription factor. The molecular genetic signature of CCS is a reciprocal translocation t(12;22)(q13;q12) that results in the *EWSR1-ATF1* fusion oncogene. The treatment of choice is surgical excision with wide margins; however, it is associated with high rate of local recurrence and late metastasis. The common sites of metastasis are lymph nodes, followed by lung and bone.

CLINICAL PEARL

CCS of soft tissue shows low nuclear pleomorphism and mitosis compared with malignant melanoma.

Lymph node metastasis occurs in 50% of the cases.

What are the types and clinicopathologic features of tenosynovial giant cell tumors?

Localized-type tenosynovial giant cell tumor (giant cell tumor of tendon sheath): It usually occurs in adults aged 30–50 years, and approximately 85% cases arise in the fingers but could also occur in the foot, wrist, and ankles. Commonly, this lesion develops in the vicinity of the synovium of the tendon and presents as a slow-growing mass; some patients report history of trauma. Grossly, it is typically a well-circumscribed, lobulated white to grey mass measuring 0.5–4 cm. Histologically, it is well-demarcated, lobulated neoplasm focally covered by fibrous pseudocapsule and composed of mononuclear cells, multinucleated osteoclast-like giant cells, and foamy macrophages with variable proportions (Fig. 36.10A and B). Mononuclear cells are either small histiocytoid spindle cells with nuclear groove or more abundant large epithelioid cells with eosinophilic cytoplasm, eccentric nuclei, and prominent nucleoli. Hemosiderin granules are commonly present in the large epithelioid mononuclear cells (Fig. 36.10C). Mitoses are frequent up to 5/10 HPF.

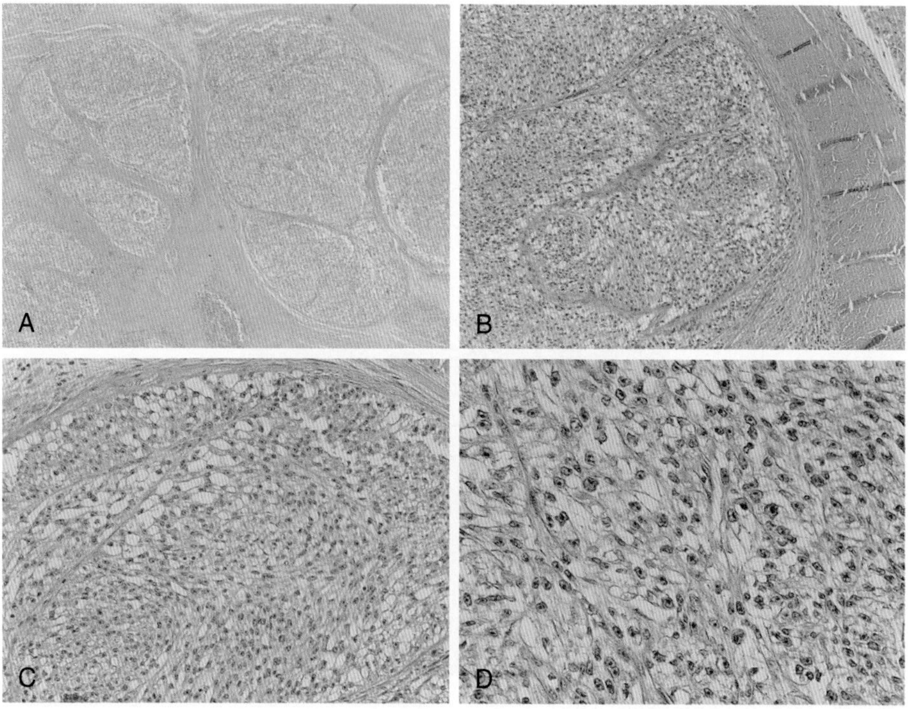

Fig. 36.9 Clear cell sarcoma of soft tissue: Microscopically, low power shows (A) multilobular, nesting neoplasm separated by collagenous band and (B) infiltrating along the tendon (H&E 40x, 100x). (C and D) These nests are composed of alternating spindle and epithelioid cells that display clear to pale eosinophilic cytoplasm with intracellular glycogen, vesicular nuclei, and prominent nucleoli (H&E 200x, 400x).

The stroma is collagenized and variably hyalinized; this type shows less cleft-like spaces than the diffuse type. Immunohistochemistry has no pivotal role in the diagnosis of tenosynovial giant cell tumor. The osteoclast-like giant cells and small histiocytoid cells are positive for CD68 and CD163 due to their histiocytic nature. The large epithelioid mononuclear cells are occasionally positive for desmin. Surgical excision is the treatment of choice with low risk of recurrence.

Diffuse-type tenosynovial giant cell tumor (pigmented villonodular synovitis): usually affects younger patients aged <40 years, more than the localized type. It has two subtypes: intra-articular, which occurs commonly in the knees (about 70% cases); and extra-articular, which occurs in the soft tissue surrounding the joint, such as knee, hip, or foot. Patients present with long duration of pain, tenderness, limitation of motion, and slow-growing swelling. Radiologically, it shows ill-defined masses near the joint with degenerative joint disease and occasional cortical erosion of adjacent bones. Grossly, the intra-articular subtype is commonly >5 cm and has villous growth pattern with pigmentation, thus named *pigmented villonodular synovitis*. The extra-articular subtype does not have the villonodular pattern; instead, it is firm, spongy, and has multinodular whitish cut surface with areas of brown pigmentation. Histologically, it is infiltrative neoplasm with diffuse sheets with variable cellularity displaying cleft-like spaces reminiscent of pseudoglandular spaces (Fig. 36.11A). The cellular composition is similar to the localized variant, but with fewer osteoclast-like giant cells. The predominant cell is the large mononuclear epithelioid cell with eosinophilic cytoplasm and exuberant hemosiderin pigment deposition. Histiocytoid spindle cells, foamy macrophages, and chronic inflammatory cells are present. (Fig. 36.11B). Mitosis is usually

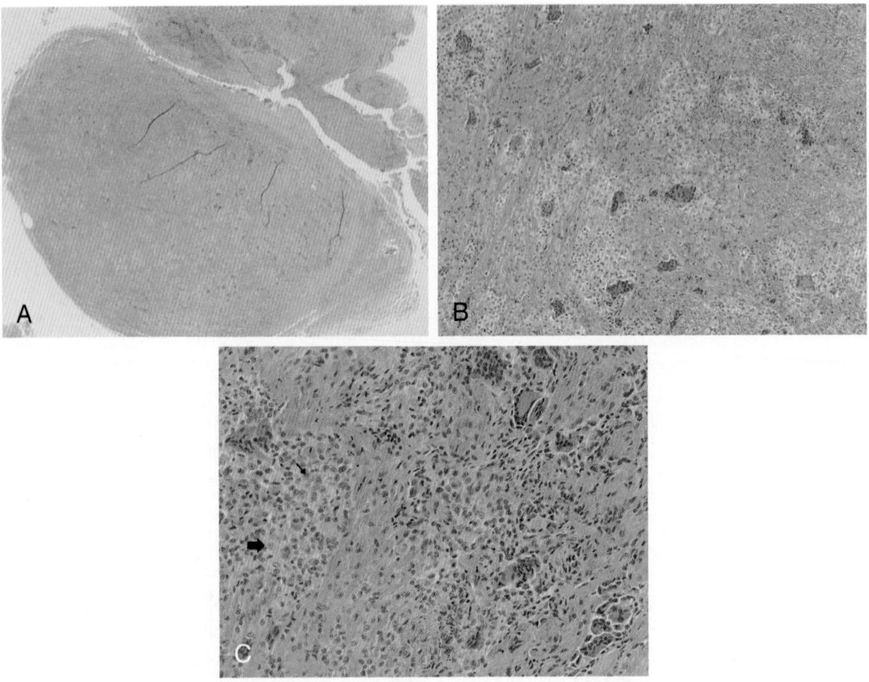

Fig. 36.10 Localized-type tenosynovial giant cell tumor: Microscopically, (A and B) well-circumscribed, lobulated neoplasm is seen surrounded focally by fibrous pseudocapsule and composed of mononuclear cells, multinucleated osteoclast-like giant cells, and foamy macrophages (H&E 40x, 100x). (C) Mononuclear cells consist of small histiocytoid spindle cells with nuclear groove (thin arrow) and large epithelioid cells with eosinophilic cytoplasm, eccentric nuclei, and prominent nucleoli (thick arrow), and some have hemosiderin deposition (H&E 200x).

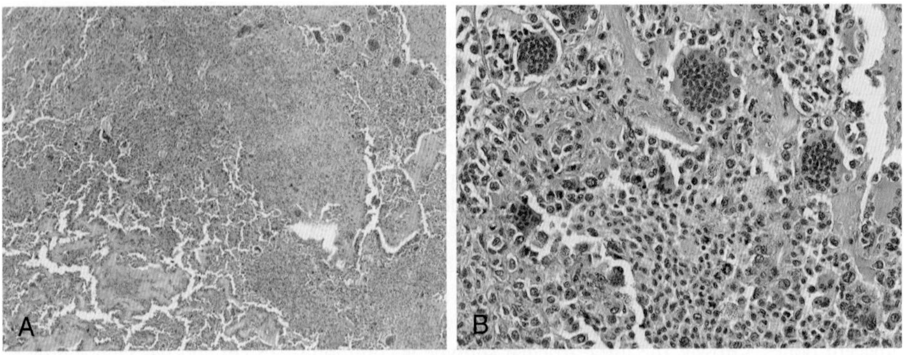

Fig. 36.11 Diffuse-type tenosynovial giant cell tumor: Histologically, (A) at low power, pseudoglandular or pseudoalveolar pattern is seen (H&E 40x). (B) It is composed of mononuclear epithelioid and histiocytoid cells with hemosiderin deposition, osteoclast-like giant cells, and foamy macrophages (H&E 200x).

frequent, >5/10 HPF. Features that are associated with malignancy include high mitotic count >20/10 HPF, extensive necrosis, spindling of multinucleated giant cells, abundant eosinophilic cytoplasm, marked nuclear pleomorphism with enlarged nuclei and nucleoli, and myxoid stoma (Fig. 36.12). Immunophenotypically, it is similar to the localized variant. Recurrence is common in both intra-articular (20%–50%) and extra-articular (30%–60%) subtypes, resulting in limitation

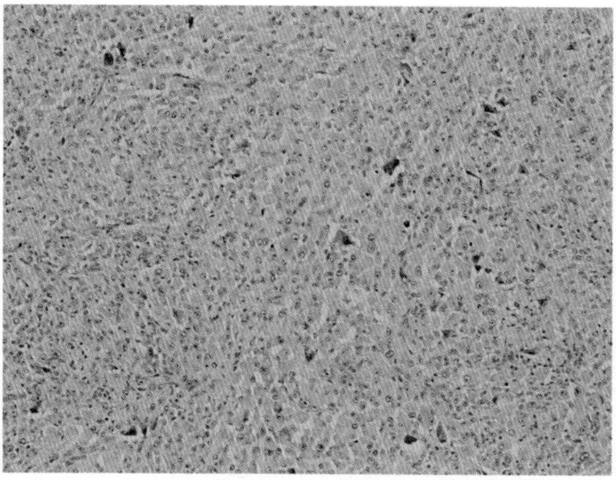

Fig. 36.12 Malignant diffuse-type tenosynovial giant cell tumor: Microscopically, sheets of highly malignant epithelioid cells are seen with abundant eosinophilic cytoplasm and pleomorphic nuclei with prominent nucleoli (H&E, 100x).

of joint function. Total synovectomy and complete surgical excision with wide margin is the treatment of choice for intra-articular and extra-articular subtypes, respectively.

CLINICAL PEARL

The risk of recurrence for the diffuse-type tenosynovial giant cell tumor depends on adequate surgical excision.

Malignant diffuse-type tenosynovial giant cell tumor is exceedingly rare.

The criteria to diagnose malignant diffuse-type tenosynovial giant cell tumor are 1) the presence of component of conventional diffuse-type giant cell tumor admixed with malignant sarcomatous areas and 2) conventional diffuse-type giant cell tumor recur as malignant sarcoma.

Case Point 36.2

Immunohistochemistry on the patient biopsy shows strong positivity for CD68, CD163 (Fig. 36.13A and B), and CD45 in most of the histiocytic-like cells and osteoclast-like giant cells and negative for CD34, EMA, pancytokeratin, and HMB45. INI1 is preserved. Based on the histologic and immunohistochemical findings, the patient is diagnosed to have extra-articular diffuse-type tenosynovial giant cell tumor (pigmented villonodular synovitis). The patient underwent a complete surgical excision with wide clear margins and extended curettage of the first metatarsal bone. Although she still complains of numbness and tingling sensation on her right great toe, the patient recovered in good condition and was followed up without evidence of recurrence.

BEYOND THE PEARLS

ES may show overlapping features of both classic and proximal subtypes.

Reverse transcription–polymerase chain reaction (RT-PCR) or fluorescence in situ hybridization (FISH) for EWSR1 gene translocation helps to aid in the diagnosis of CCS and to differentiate it from malignant melanoma.

CCS of Soft tissue usually follows a dismal clinical course.

Diffuse-type tenosynovial giant cell tumor occasionally can be diagnostically challenging because it radiologically presents as an ill-defined, destructive mass along with marked cellularity of epithelioid cells histologically.

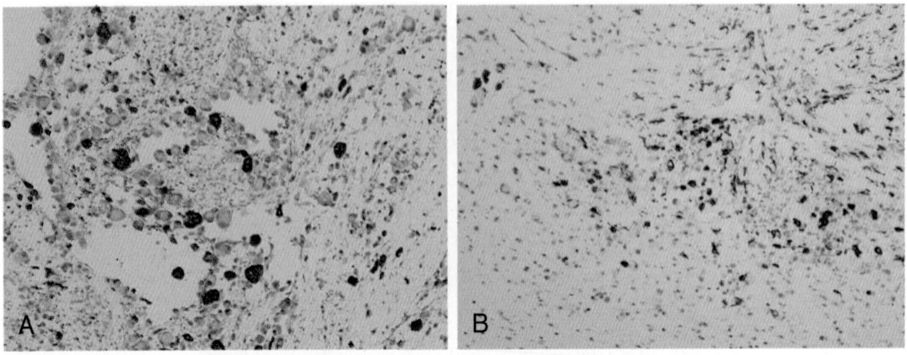

Fig. 36.13 Diffuse-type tenosynovial giant cell tumor: (A) CD68 and (B) CD163 show strong positivity in histiocytoid-like cells and osteoclast-like giant cells (H&E, 100x).

References

Clay MR, Martinez AP, Weiss SW, Edgar MA. MDM2 amplification in problematic lipomatous tumors: analysis of FISH testing criteria. *Am J Surg Pathol.* 2015;39(10):1433-1439. doi:10.1097/PAS.000000 0000000468.

Fletcher CDM, Unni KK, Mertens F, eds. WHO classification of tumours of soft tissue. *Pathology.* 2014;5:250-272.

Mariani O, Brennetot C, Coindre JM, et al. JUN oncogene amplification and overexpression block adipocytic differentiation in highly aggressive sarcoma. *Cancer Cell.* 2007;11(4):361-374.

Shimada S, Ishizawa T, Ishizawa K, Matsumura T, Hasegawa T, Hirose T. The value of MDM2 and CDK4 amplification levels using real-time polymerase chain reaction for the differential diagnosis of liposarcomas and their histologic mimickers. *Hum Pathol.* 2006;37(9):1123-1129.

CASE 37

A 68-Year-Old Woman with Right Thigh Mass

Rana Ajabnoor

A 68-year-old female presents to the primary health care physician with slow-growing, painless right thigh mass over a period of 18 months. She is a housewife and does not recall any history of trauma. Her past medical history is significant for controlled diabetes, for which she takes metformin daily. On physical examination, her vital signs are within normal range. There is large, mobile, oval firm mass in her thigh measuring 15 × 10 cm, with unremarkable overlying skin and normal range of motion.

What are the causes of a thigh soft tissue mass in the elderly?
There are various causes for soft tissue mass in the thigh of an elderly patient ranging from non-neoplastic process to neoplastic tumors (Table 37.1). Abscess usually presents with a very painful mass, skin redness and hotness due to inflammation caused by bacterial infection, and the patient might experience high fever. Myositis ossificans is a pseudotumor and non-neoplastic lesion commonly occurring in young adults and associated with a history of trauma. Neoplastic tumor includes benign and malignant mesenchymal tumor and metastatic carcinoma, with lipoma and liposarcoma being the most common benign and malignant mesenchymal tumor in humans, respectively.

What is your differential diagnosis?
The patient is an elderly lady with a slow-growing, painless right thigh mass. It is most likely neoplastic process. The patient's physical examination shows a slow-growing, freely mobile, large soft tissue lesion without fixation to the skin, rendering a lipomatous neoplasm very high on the differential diagnoses. The diagnostic distinction as to whether this is a benign lipoma or atypical

TABLE 37.1 ■ **Differential Diagnosis of Soft Tissue Thigh Mass**

Non-neoplastic		
• Abscess • Myositis ossificans		
Neoplastic		
Benign	**Intermediate Malignancy**	**Malignant**
• Lipoma • Myxoma • Neurofibroma • Deep benign fibrous histiocytoma	• Solitary fibrous tumor	• Liposarcoma • Leiomyosarcoma • Malignant peripheral nerve sheath tumor • Low-grade fibromyxoid sarcoma • Myxofibrosarcoma • Undifferentiated pleomorphic sarcoma • Metastasis

BOX 37.1 ■ Features Suspicious of Malignancy in a Lipomatous Tumor

- Size >5 cm.
- Infiltration into surrounding tissue
- Deep-seated tumor, near spermatic cord or retroperitoneal
- History of recurrence
- Unusual gross appearance (necrosis, fibrous bands, and gelatinous areas)

lipomatous tumor (ALT)/well-differentiated liposarcoma (WLDS) depends on histopathological examination of the mass after biopsy or surgical excision. Also, this patient has some features that are worrisome for malignancy such as large size of the lesion and its location in deep soft tissues (Box 37.1). Another consideration in the differential diagnosis is leiomyosarcoma, which is common in this age group and presents with firm soft tissue mass. Other differential diagnostic considerations would include solitary fibrous tumor, malignant peripheral nerve sheath tumor (commonly associated with neurofibromatosis), and synovial sarcoma (which would be more likely in a young adult). Metastatic carcinoma and melanoma should also be considered as well.

How should this patient be investigated?

Imaging studies should be the first diagnostic modality to be pursued in the evaluation of this patient. Magnetic resonance image (MRI) and computerized tomography (CT) scan are the mainstay for evaluation of the soft tissue tumor and its relationship with surrounding structures, followed by imaging-directed core needle tissue biopsy or open surgical incisional biopsy to be evaluated histologically and cytogenetically.

CLINICAL PEARL

MRI is the gold standard imaging modality to evaluate the soft tissue tumor and its relation with surrounding structures.

CT scan is helpful for staging and evaluating bone involvement.

Case Point 37.1

The patient's MRI shows large heterogeneous, hyperintense, intramuscular mass measuring 30 × 16 × 13 cm with fatty component and multiple septation. No cortical bone destruction was identified (Fig. 37.1). Imaging studies were followed by a CT-guided core needle biopsy where cylindrical cores of soft tissue from the mass were taken for histopathological examination. On microscopic examination, the biopsy showed a fatty tumor with variable sized adipocytes with focal atypia in both adipocytes and stromal cells in a fibrillary collagenous background arranged in septae throughout the lesion (Fig. 37.2). These features are quite suggestive of ALT/WDLS.

What confirmatory tests are helpful in making a diagnosis of ALT/WDLS?

A characteristic cytogenetic finding in ALT/WDLS on karyotype analysis is the presence of supernumerary ring and giant marker chromosome containing amplified sequences originating from the 12q14-15 region on chromosome 12. Fluorescence in situ hybridization (FISH) and real-time polymerase chain reaction (PCR) testing for MDM2 gene amplification on chromosome 12 is a consistent finding in ALS/WDLS and is present in >95% of these tumors. Furthermore, the genes CDK4, CPM, HMGA2, and FRS2 are frequently co-amplified (Table 37.2). Nuclear expression of MDM2 and CDK4 can also be detected by immunohistochemistry (IHC), which may also be helpful diagnostically.

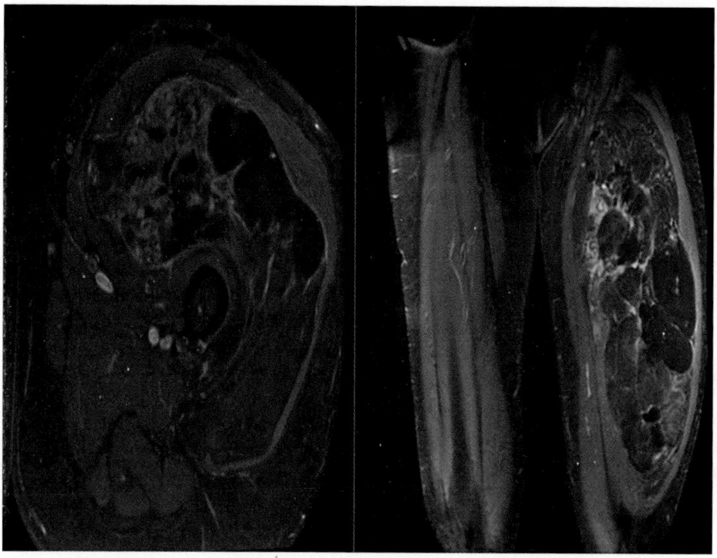

Fig. 37.1 Axial and coronal post-contrast T1-magnetic resonance imaging images demonstrating large, heterogenous intramuscular mass with soft tissue nodularity, fatty component, and septations.

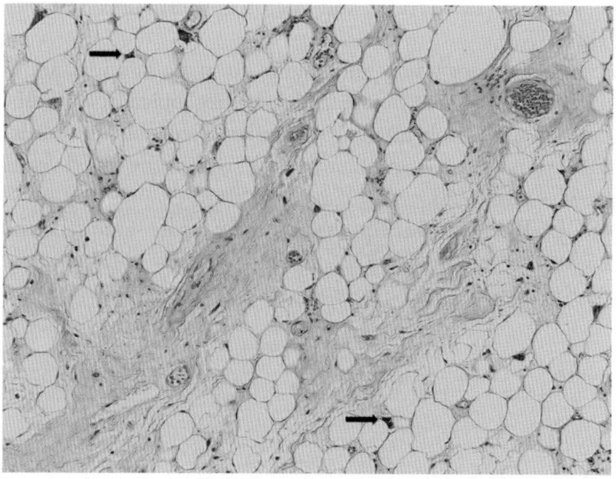

Fig. 37.2 Atypical lipomatous tumor / well-differentiated liposarcoma on core needle biopsy shows variable sized adipocytes with focal atypia (arrow; H&E, 100x).

TABLE 37.2 ■ **Molecular Genetic Signature of Certain Lipomatous Tumor**

Tumor	Molecular Genetic
Spindle cell lipoma / pleomorphic lipoma	Deletion of 13q and 16q
Atypical lipomatous tumor / well-differentiated liposarcoma	Ring chromosome (12q13 and MDM2 amplification)
Dedifferentiated liposarcoma	Ring chromosome (12q13 and MDM2 amplification)
Myxoid liposarcoma	t(12;16)(q13;p11) DDIT3–FUS

Case Point 37.2

The patient's tissue biopsy is tested for MDM2 gene amplification on chromosome 12 cytogenetically by FISH and is positive. The diagnosis of ALT/WDLS is rendered.

CLINICAL PEARL

MDM2 amplification is almost always present in ALT/WDLS and dedifferentiated liposarcoma. **Dedifferentiated liposarcoma** has more complex karyotype changes and mutations in addition to MDM2 gene amplification.

CLINICAL PEARL

It is recommended to use FISH for MDM2 amplification in lipomatous neoplasm that has: history of recurrence; deep-seated mass in the extremity; measuring >10 cm in patients; in cases with equivocal atypia; also, in masses occurring in the retroperitoneum, pelvis, or abdomen, and in situation were clinically suspicious.

What are the common types of lipomas and their clinicopathological features?

- **Lipoma**: Usually affects adults in their fourth and fifth decades. It may occur at any anatomical site, either superficial or deep, and may be seen in an intramuscular location. Grossly, lipomas are well demarcated and microscopically show uniform mature adipocytes of equal size (Fig. 37.3).
- **Angiolipoma**: Affects young adults and tend to be small, multiple, and painful. Commonly arise in the subcutaneous tissue of the limbs. Microscopically, angiolipoma shows mature adipocytes admixed with proliferation of capillary sized blood vessels, commonly at the periphery of the lesion. Also, fibrin microthrombi within the blood vessels are characteristic features (Figs. 37.4 and 37.5).
- **Spindle cell (SCL)/Pleomorphic lipoma**: Both are in the same spectrum of benign adipocyte tumors with variable admixture of spindle cells, ropy collagen, mature fat, and multinucleated tumor giant cells in the case of pleomorphic lipoma. These lesions commonly

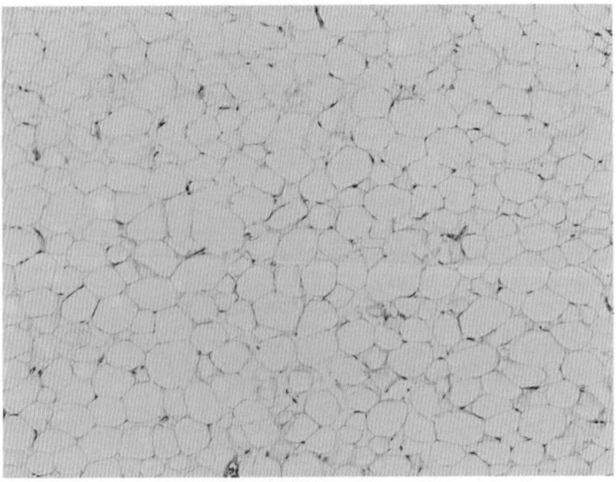

Fig. 37.3 Lipoma shows uniform mature adipocytes (H&E, 40x).

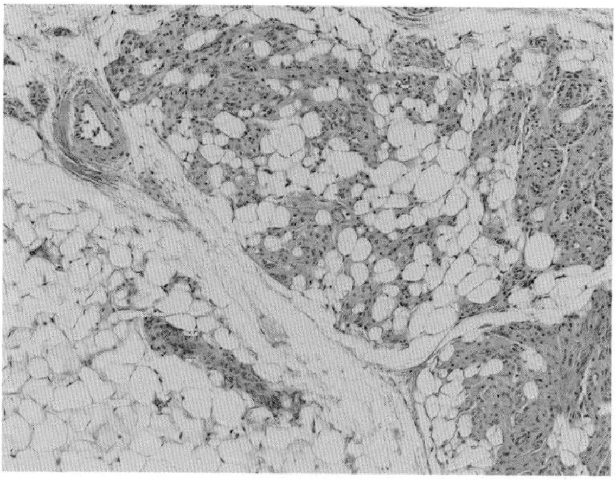

Fig. 37.4 Angiolipoma shows benign adipocytes admixed with capillary sized blood vessels (H&E, 100x).

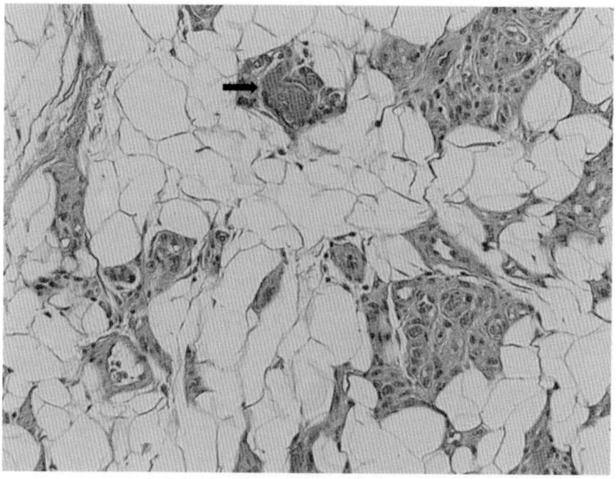

Fig. 37.5 Angiolipoma shows fibrin microthrombi in capillary-sized blood vessels (arrow) (H&E, 200x).

affect middle-aged men, arising most commonly in the upper back, neck, and shoulder. Grossly, they are often <5 mm. Microscopically, SCL shows mature adipocytes admixed with bland elongated and tapered-end spindle cells that are haphazardly arranged in myxoid background with ropy collagen bundles (Fig. 37.6). Mitoses are rare. Pleomorphic lipoma shares the same morphological features with SCL in addition to the presence of multinucleated floret giant cells in which hyperchromatic nuclei are arranged in concentric fashion (Fig. 37.7). On the molecular level, SCL/pleomorphic lipoma shows usually the combination loss of long arm of chromosome 13q and 16q (Table 37.2).

What is the treatment of liposarcoma?

The treatment of liposarcoma mainly depends on the grade and location of the tumor. For ALT/WDLS that occur in the limbs, the mainstay of treatment is surgical resection with clean margins. High-grade dedifferentiated liposarcoma and pleomorphic liposarcoma usually receive neoadjuvant radiotherapy to downsize the tumor, followed by surgical resection with clear margin.

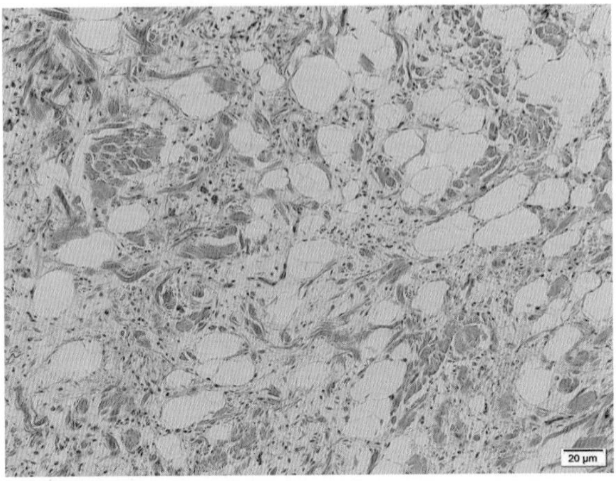

Fig. 37.6 Spindle cell lipoma shows mature adipocytes admixed with spindle cells and ropy collagen bundles in myxoid background (H&E, 100x).

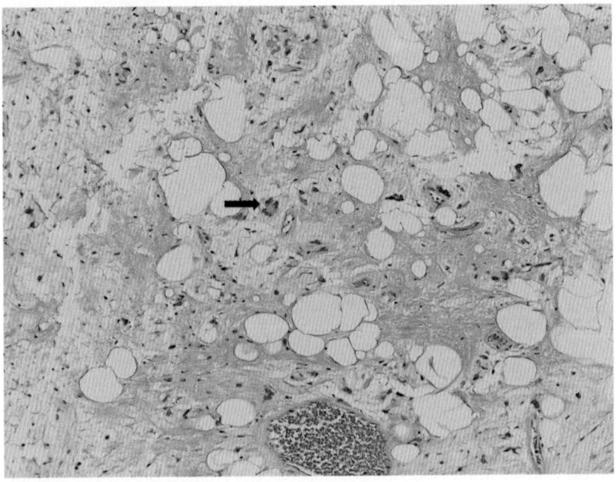

Fig. 37.7 Pleomorphic lipoma shows mature adipocytes with spindle cells and associated floret giant cells in myxoid background (arrow, H&E, 100x).

CLINICAL PEARL

Liposarcoma that arises retroperitoneally has dismal prognosis because it is difficult to surgically resect it completely with clear margins. Therefore, the risk of recurrence is high.

Case Point 37.3

This patient undergoes surgical resection of the tumor. Grossly, there is a large, deep-seated, multilobulated adipocytic mass measuring 28 × 25 × 10 cm. The cut surface shows bands of fibrosis areas of gelatinous material, necrosis, and hemorrhage (Fig. 37.8).

The histology of the resection specimen exhibits the same morphology as seen in the core needle biopsy.

TABLE 37.3 ■ **Liposarcoma Classification**

Type of Liposarcoma	WHO Category	Prognosis
Atypical lipomatous tumor/ well-differentiated liposarcoma	Intermediate malignancy	Locally aggressive due to high recurrence rate up to 50%. Extremely low risk of metastasis
Dedifferentiated liposarcoma	Malignant	High risk of metastasis up to 20%. Prognosis better than pleomorphic sarcoma
Myxoid liposarcoma	Malignant	Low-grade myxoid liposarcoma has very low risk of metastasis. High-grade (round cell) liposarcoma is associated with unfavorable prognosis
Pleomorphic liposarcoma	Malignant	Very aggressive with up to 50% risk of metastasis

WHO = World Health Organization.

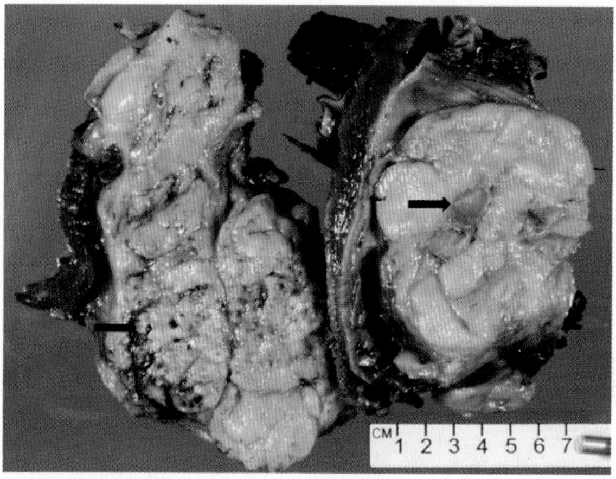

Fig. 37.8 Gross image of atypical lipomatous tumor / well-differentiated liposarcoma shows deep-seated, multilobulated, adipocytic tumor with focal gelatinous area (arrow) and focal necrosis (arrow).

What are the types of liposarcoma and their clinicopathological features? (Table 37.3)

- **ALT/WDLS:** This is the most common type of liposarcoma and commonly occurs in middle-age adults in the sixth decade, in the deep soft tissues of the limbs, retroperitoneum, and rarely around the spermatic cord and head and neck area. Grossly, these lesions usually show a large, multilobulated adipocytic mass, with fibrosis and a fatty to gray-tan cut surface. Foci of necrosis and hemorrhage may be seen in larger tumors (Fig. 37.8). Microscopically, ALT/WDLS shows variabley sized adipocytes with focal atypia in the adipocytes and stromal cells. Variably prominent, thickened, irregular fibrous septae are typically present. The hyperchromatic atypical stromal cells tend to be present in the fibrotic areas and around blood vessels. A background of fibrillary collagenous or myxoid stroma might be seen (Figs. 37.9 and 37.10). Also, lipoblasts are rarely seen and is not required for diagnosis. The vast majority of the cases of ALT/WDLS show high levels of MDM2 gene amplification; this molecular genetic finding is extremely helpful for confirming the diagnosis. There are four morphologic types of WDLS: 1) lipomatous-like, 2) inflammatory, 3) sclerosing, and 4) spindle cell. There

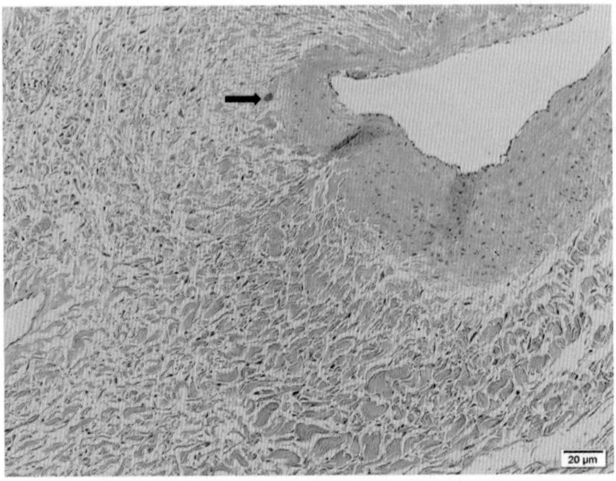

Fig. 37.9 Atypical lipomatous tumor / well-differentiated liposarcoma shows atypical spindle cells around the blood vessel wall (arrow; H&E, 100x).

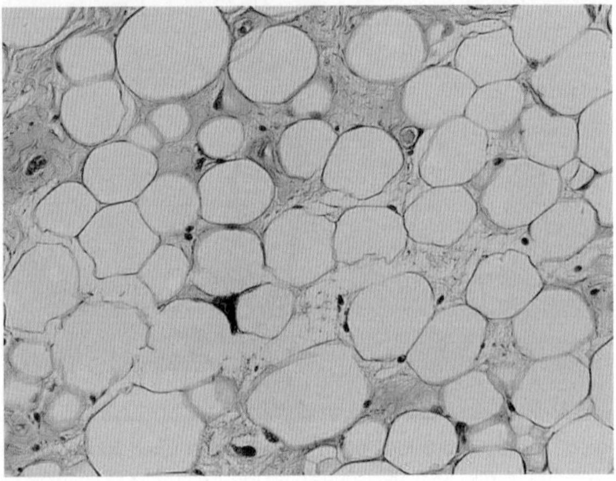

Fig. 37.10 Atypical lipomatous tumor / well-differentiated liposarcoma shows lipoblast with indented hyperchromatic nuclei (H&E, 100x).

is no clinical significance regarding these morphologic types. Atypical spindle cell tumor / spindle cell liposarcoma is in the differential diagnosis for ALT/WDLS, and the distinction can be challenging at times. These tumors contain bland spindle cells with myxoid to fibrous stroma and variable adipocytic differentiation and can show significant morphologic overlap with ALT/WDLS. Unlike ALT/WDLS, these lesions do not show MDM2 gene amplification and are negative for MDM2 and CDK4 expression by IHC, which can be helpful diagnostically.

- **Dedifferentiated liposarcoma:** Dedifferentiated liposarcoma is a more cellular neoplasm, which usually contains a nonlipogenic sarcomatous component and can show a wide morphologic spectrum of findings. Many lesions also contain a component of ALT/WDLS, and these tumors are thought to represent a progression of ALT/WDLS to nonlipogenic dedifferentiation. Similarly, at the molecular level, dedifferentiated liposarcoma shows

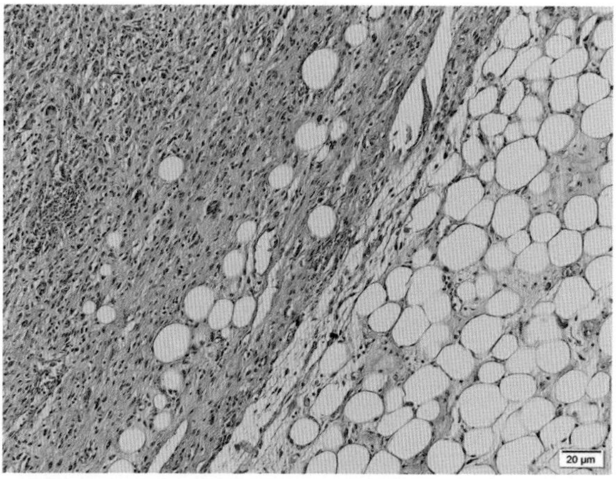

Fig. 37.11 Dedifferentiated liposarcoma shows abrupt transition between high-grade nonlipogenic sarcoma (upper left) and atypical lipomatous tumor / well-differentiated liposarcoma (lower right) (H&E, 40x).

MDM2 amplification, expression of MDM2 and CDK4 by IHC, and commonly occurs in the retroperitoneum, deep soft tissue, mediastinum, and head and neck. Patients are most commonly adults in the sixth and seventh decades. Grossly, the tumors are large and multinodular, with a yellow cut surface depending on the amount of fatty component of the tumor, and these areas are admixed with nodules of more dense, firm gray tissue corresponding to areas showing dedifferentiation. Microscopically, one sees areas of typical ALT/WDLS that display either abrupt or gradual transition to nonlipogenic high-grade pleomorphic sarcoma (Fig. 37.11). The dedifferentiated component of the tumor might contain leimyosarcomatous, rhabdomyosarcomatous, osteosarcomatous, myxofibrosarcomatous differentiation, and solitary fibrous tumor morphology as well. Dedifferentiated liposarcoma share the same molecular signature of MDM2 amplification as does ALT/WDLS, providing a molecular genetic link between these two entities (Table 37.2).

CLINICAL PEARL

Dedifferentiated liposarcoma is the most common sarcoma that arises in the retroperitoneum and account for up to 75%.

- **Myxoid liposarcoma**: Myxoid liposarcoma is a malignant mesenchymal neoplasm composed of nonlipogenic cells, variable numbers of lipoblasts, with a characteristic prominent myxoid stromal background containing a delicate capillary vasculature. These tumors commonly occur in younger adults in the fourth and fifth decades and usually arise within the deep muscles of the limbs, with predilection for thigh muscles. Grossly, one sees an intramuscular, circumscribed, multinodular tumor with a gelatinous cut surface. High-grade lesions can appear tan-white and firm or fleshy. Microscopically, these tumors show a lobulated myxoid neoplastic growth with chicken wire vasculature and bland spindle cells more pronounced at the periphery of the lobules. The abundant myxoid stroma may show pools of myxoid material imparting a pulmonary edema-like pattern (Fig. 37.12). The small spindled, stellate, and ovoid nonlipogenic tumor cells exhibit minimal atypia and are admixed with variable numbers of lipoblasts with different morphology including signet ring features (Fig. 37.13). Mitotic count is usually very low. Myxoid liposarcoma can undergo

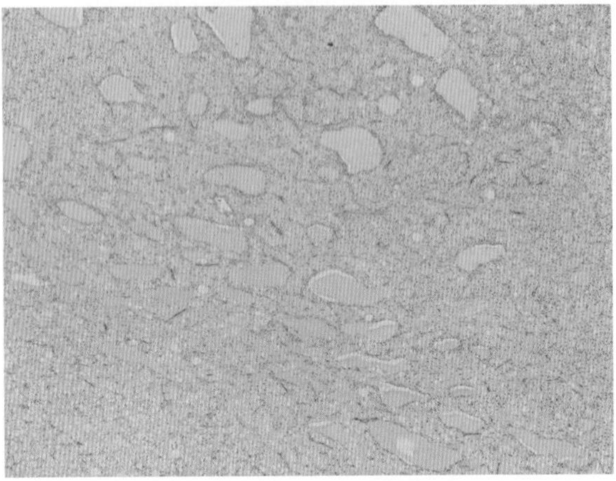

Fig. 37.12 Myxoid liposarcoma shows pools of myxoid material with chicken wire blood vessels that resemble pulmonary edema (H&E, 40x).

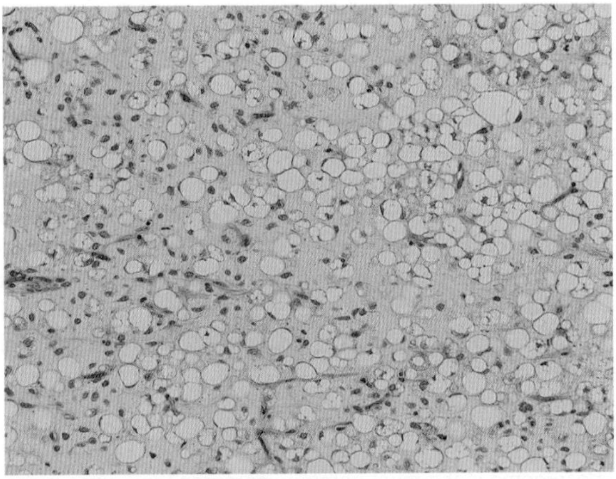

Fig. 37.13 Myxoid liposarcoma shows bland oval spindle cells admixed with lipoblasts and chicken wire blood vessels present in myxoid background (H&E, 20x).

dedifferentiation to high-grade round cell sarcoma with increased mitotic activity, which is associated with much worse prognosis. Molecularly, myxoid liposarcoma shows a characteristic specific translocation of t (12;16) (q13;p11) that is a fusion of DDIT3 gene on12q13 with FUS gene on 16p11 (Table 37.2). TP53 mutations can be found in up to one-third cases, which is independent of the histologic grade.

- **Pleomorphic liposarcoma**: Pleomorphic liposarcoma is a high-grade malignant mesenchymal neoplasm showing evidence of lipoblastic differentiation without a component of WDLS or other lines of differentiation. These tumors most commonly affect older adults in their sixth decade and usually arise in the deep soft tissues of the extremities. Grossly, one sees a well-defined or irregular lesion with infiltrating borders, extensive necrosis, and hemorrhage. The histologic features are variable and include high-grade pleomorphic lipoblasts (a requisite finding) with large, hyperchromatic, and bizarre nuclei that are scalloped

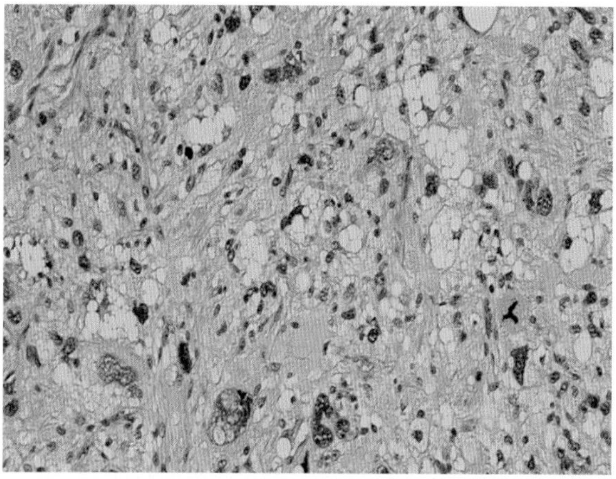

Fig. 37.14 Pleomorphic liposarcoma shows proliferation of high-grade pleomorphic multivaculated lipoblasts (H&E, 20x).

by cytoplasmic vacuoles. Mitoses are extremely high with extensive necrosis (Fig. 37.14). Multiple morphologic patterns can be seen, with cellular pleomorphic sarcoma being the most common. Molecularly, it has a complex karyotype with multiple nonspecific chromosomal abnormalities.

Case Point 37.4

The patient recovered from surgery without any complications. The surgical resection margins were clear, and her pathologic stage is pT4, pN0. The patient is being followed-up without any history of recurrence or metastasis.

BEYOND THE PEARLS

- The term ALT tends to be used for tumor arising in the limbs, whereas WDLS is used to for tumor in the retroperitoneum and intra-abdominal regions.
- Giant ring chromosome in ALT/WDLS and dedifferentiated liposarcoma can be tested cytogenetically by karyotype analysis of the fresh tissue from the tumor.
- MDM2 amplification with protein overexpression can be tested by IHC and cytogenetically by FISH and real-time PCR.
- Extensive sampling of ALT/WDLS is important for not to overlook as areas of dedifferentiation.
- Lipoblast is not required for the diagnosis of liposarcoma, as it could be seen in other benign mimickers such as lipoma with fat necrosis.

References

Clay MR, Martinez AP, Weiss SW, Edgar MA. MDM2 amplification in problematic lipomatous tumors: analysis of FISH testing criteria. *Am J Surg Pathol.* 2015;39(10):1433-1439.

Fletcher CDM, Bridge JA, Hogendoorn PCW, Mertens F. WHO classification of tumours of soft tissue and bone, vol. 5. 4th ed. *Pathology.* 2013.

Goldblum JR, Folpe AL, Weiss SW. *Enzinger and Weiss's Soft Tissue Tumors.* 6th ed. Philadelphia, PA: Elsevier; 2014.

Hornik JL. *Practical Soft Tissue Pathology: A Diagnostic Approach.* 2nd ed. Philadelphia, PA: Elsevier; 2019.
Mariani O, Brennetot C, Coindre JM, et al. JUN oncogene amplification and overexpression block adipocytic differentiation in highly aggressive sarcomas. *Cancer Cells.* 2007;11(4):361-374.
Shimada S, Ishizawa T, Ishizawa K, Matsumura T, Hasegawa T, Hirose T. The value of MDM2 and CDK4 amplification levels using real-time polymerase chain reaction for the differential diagnosis of liposarcomas and their histologic mimickers. *Hum Pathol.* 2006;37(9):1123-1129.

An 18-Year-Old Male with Left Knee Pain and Mass

Rana Ajabnoor

An 18-year-old male high-school student presents to the orthopedic clinic with a history of left knee pain that began 1 year ago, gradually and progressively worsening over time. The pain intensity is in the range of 8/10 points scale, increases with activity, and stops him from running or doing any strenuous activity. After 7 months, he noticed swelling on the lateral side of his left knee that was slowly increasing in size. He has no neurological symptoms or history of trauma; he has no significant medical history. He went to a physical therapy session, but there was no improvement. On physical examination, his vital signs are within normal range. There is deep, firm mass in the lateral aspect of the left knee that measures around 2 cm. There is mild tenderness over the mass, and it is not freely mobile on clinical examination. He has a full range of motion of the left knee and no overlying skin changes.

What is your differential diagnosis?

The patient is a young adult with a slow-growing, painful left knee mass for a long time. It is most likely a neoplastic process. It is unlikely to be a reactive process such as nodular fasciitis, proliferative fasciitis, and myositis ossificans, which are pseudotumor or non-neoplastic lesions, commonly occurring in young adults, associated with history of trauma, and usually located subcutaneously. These reactive lesions are self-limited and may subside spontaneously. Given the patient's physical examination that shows firm, deep soft tissue mass near the knee, fibrous, neural, and muscular tumors (benign or malignant) must be considered in the differential diagnosis. These considerations would include deep benign fibrous histiocytoma (DBFH), fibromatosis, solitary fibrous tumor (SFT), schwannoma, neurofibroma, rhabdomyosarcoma (RMS), dermatofibrosarcoma protuberans (DFSP), leiomyosarcoma (LMS), and malignant peripheral nerve sheath tumor (PNST). Absence of history of neurofibromatosis would put malignant PNST lower on the list, and LMS occurs mostly in an older patients. Also, one would have to consider other neoplastic tumors of unclear origin that occur in young adults, such as myxoma, angiomatoid fibrous histiocytoma, synovial sarcoma (SS), and Ewing sarcoma. Metastatic carcinoma and melanoma are unlikely to occur in this age group.

What is the most appropriate initial workup for this patient?

Imaging of the area either by computed tomography (CT) scan or magnetic resonance imaging (MRI) should be considered. Primary excision would be an option for this patient, but a biopsy to establish the diagnosis before surgery was also considered. This would also provide an option for preoperative radiation and/or chemotherapy, which might shrink the tumor to make surgical removal easier.

Case Point 38.1

The patient undergoes an MRI, which shows a large, lobulated, well-circumscribed soft tissue mass in the lateral aspect of the knee adjacent to the lateral menisci and has intermediate signal. All the adjacent ligaments and menisci are intact, and there is no cortical bone destruction. The radiological features support a neoplastic process (Fig. 38.1).The patient undergoes a complete excision of the mass with a wide-margin resection. The gross specimen shows a well-circumscribed, lobulated, firm, deep soft tissue mass with a yellow-tan cut surface and focal areas of hemorrhage (Fig. 38.2A). Microscopically, the tumor shows a highly cellular proliferation of sheets of monotonous neoplastic spindle cells with areas of ectatic dilated branching blood vessels exhibiting a hemangiopericytomatous (HPC) pattern (Fig. 38.2B and C). The malignant spindle cells are overlapped and show high nuclear-to-cytoplasmic ratio with hyperchromatic nuclei. Mitotic figures are infrequent (Fig. 38.3). Based on the clinical and histologic features, the diagnosis of monophasic SS is the top differential.

What is the differential diagnosis of spindle cell lesions in adolescents and young adults?

This differential diagnosis is broad, including reactive fibroblastic lesions and neoplastic entities that range from benign to intermediate malignancy (due to local recurrence or low risk of metastasis) to malignant neoplasms with significant metastatic potential. The cell of origin for spindle cell neoplasms could be fibroblastic, neural, smooth muscle, skeletal muscles, as well as tumors of uncertain histologic origin. Spindle cell carcinoma and melanoma are in the differential as well but unlikely to occur in young adults (Table 38.1).

What are the clinicopathological features of the reactive fibroblastic lesions?

Nodular fasciitis: Occurs in any age group, but most commonly during the age of 20–40 years. These lesions can arise at any site, with predilection for the volar aspect of the upper extremity and head and neck area, typically within subcutaneous tissues. A history of trauma and injury might be associated with the development of these lesions, which are reported to have a rapid growth phase usually 1 month or less. Grossly, nodular fasciitis is usually 2–3 cm or less in greatest dimension, well circumscribed, nonencapsulated, in the subcutaneous tissue, and has variable fibrous to myxoid and gelatinous cut surface. Microscopically, these lesions are composed of short intersecting fascicles of plump reactive fibroblasts and myofibroblasts with oval-shaped nuclei, open pale chromatin, and prominent nuclei. Frequent mitotic figures are commonly seen and may be numerous, but no

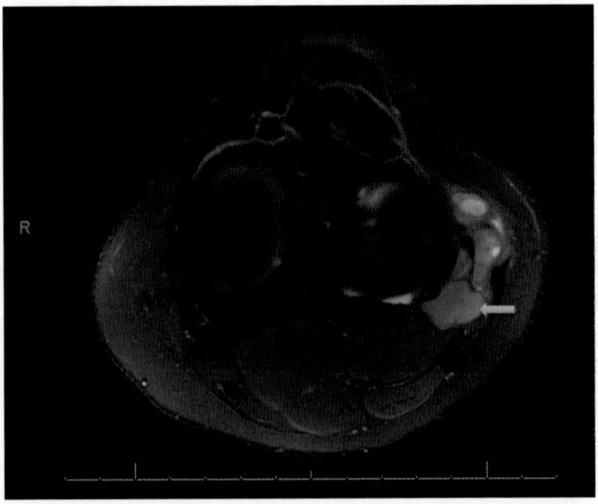

Fig. 38.1 Cross-sectional magnetic resonance imaging showing lobulated, well-circumscribed soft tissue mass in the lateral aspect of the knee with intermediate signal.

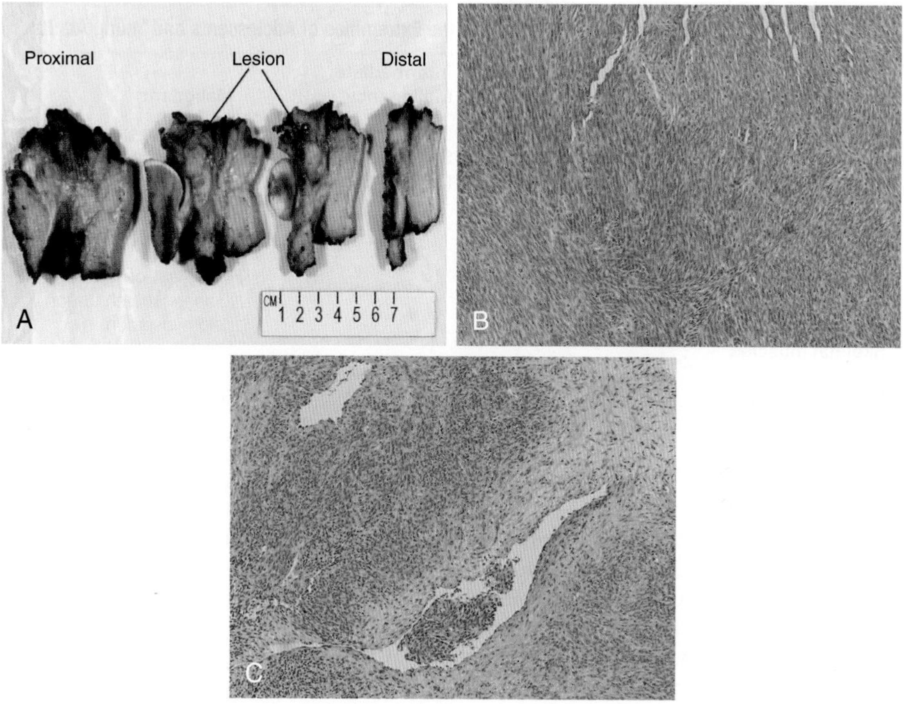

Fig. 38.2 (A) Grossly, synovial sarcoma shows well-circumscribed, lobulated soft tissue mass with hemorrhagic foci in the cut surface. Monophasic synovial sarcoma (B) shows highly cellular compact sheets of malignant spindle cells with herringbone pattern and (C) areas of hemangiopericytomatous pattern (H&E 100x).

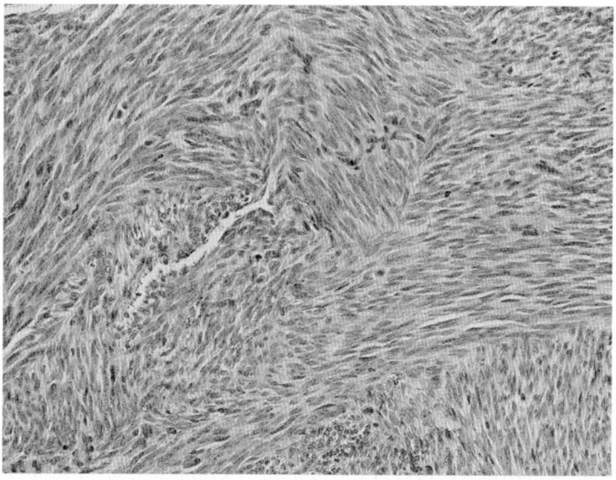

Fig. 38.3 Monophasic synovial sarcoma shows overlapped malignant monotonous spindle cells with high nuclear-to-cytoplasmic ratio and hyperchromatic nuclei (H&E 100x).

TABLE 38.1 ■ **Common Spindle Cell Lesions in the Extremities of Adolescents and Young Adults**

Cell of Origin	Benign	Intermediate Malignancy	Malignant
Fibroblastic	Nodular fasciitis Myositis ossificans	Deep fibromatosis Solitary fibrous tumor Dermatofibrosarcoma protuberans	Low-grade fibrosarcoma Myxofibrosarcoma
Fibrohistiocytic tumors	Deep benign fibrous histiocytoma		
Neural	Schwannoma Neurofibroma		Malignant peripheral nerve sheath tumor
Smooth muscle			Leiomyosarcoma
Skeletal muscles			Spindle cell/sclerosing rhabdomyosarcoma
Uncertain origin	Myxoma		Synovial sarcoma

atypical mitotic forms should be present. The spindle cells are intermingled with lymphocytes, extravasated red blood cells, and infrequently giant cells. Areas of loose myxoid changes are usually present (Fig. 38.4A and B). On immunohistochemistry (IHC), nodular fasciitis is positive for smooth muscle actin (SMA) (tram-track pattern, Fig. 38.4C) and muscle-specific actin (MSA) and negative for desmin, h-caldesmon, S100, CD34, beta-catenin, and cytokeratin. Although spontaneous regression is well documented, and risk of recurrence is very low, this lesion is usually treated by surgical excision. Nodular fasciitis does not metastasize or show malignant transformation.

CLINICAL PEARL

Nodular fasciitis is the most common reactive mesenchymal lesion that is overdiagnosed as sarcoma.

Most nodular fasciitis show MYH9–USP6 gene fusion.

Myositis ossificans: It is a reactive, non-neoplastic soft tissue lesion that commonly occurs in active adolescents and young adults, with predilection for skeletal muscles of the lower extremity. A history of trauma can be elicitied in 50% cases. Additionally, most of the cases present with a history of pain and rapid growth phase over 4 weeks on average. On imaging, myositis ossificans shows a ring-like lesion with a central lucency and a peripheral rim of ossification. Grossly, it is a well-circumscribed lesion, with soft hemorrhagic center and a firm periphery, with an average size of 5 cm. Histologically, it shows zonal proliferation of fibroblasts and myofibroblasts in the center with features mimicking nodular fasciitis mixed with chronic inflammatory cells, osteoclasts giant cells, and hemorrhage, and may show early immature woven bone formation. The peripheral zone shows more mature lamellar bone (Fig. 38.5A and B). Areas of cystic changes are commonly present. Immunohistochemical stains are not diagnostically helpful. Recurrence rate is extremely rare; it is a self-limited condition, and surgical excision is indicated in certain complicated or symptomatic cases.

What are the clinicopathological features of the common fibroblastic/myofibroblastic neoplasms with intermediate malignancy?

Deep fibromatosis (desmoid-type fibromatosis) has three forms in terms of sites of development, including extra-abdominal, abdominal wall, and intra-abdominal. The extra-abdominal

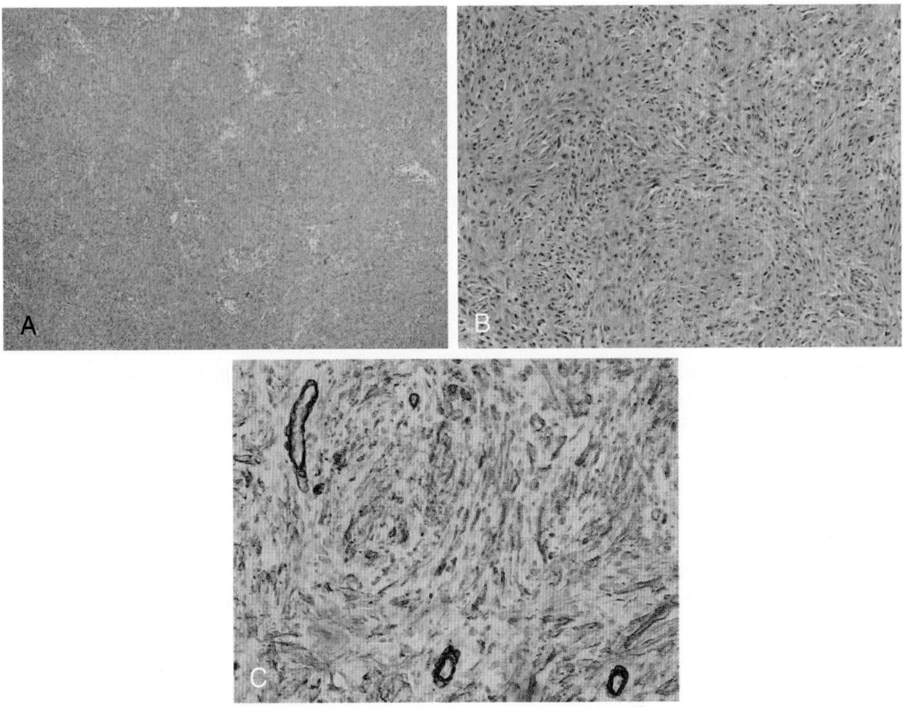

Fig. 38.4 Nodular fasciitis: (A) Microscopically shows short intersecting fascicles of reactive fibroblasts and myofibroblasts intermixed with foci of myxoid changes (H&E 40x). (B) Reactive plump fibroblasts and myofibroblasts with oval nuclei, open chromatin, and prominent nuclei (H&E 100x). (C) Immunohistochemistry shows positive staining of SMA in the fibroblasts with tram-track pattern (H&E 200x).

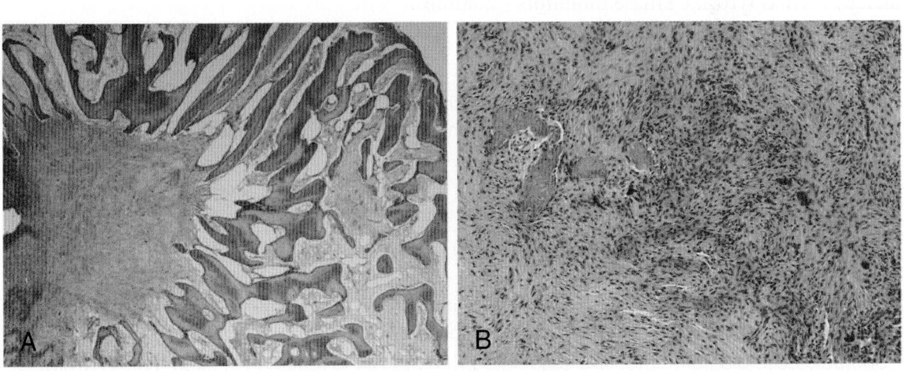

Fig. 38.5 Myositis ossificans: (A) Microscopically, low-power view shows the zonation pattern in which there is a peripheral shell of reactive bone formation (H&E 20x) and (B) central zone of reactive fibroblast formation (H&E 100x).

form is usually a deep-seated, infiltrative neoplasm that arises in the muscle of the shoulder, back, pelvis, thigh, or head and neck region. Grossly, it is a firm mass with ill-defined margin and size ranges from 5 to 10 cm and has white fibrous cut surface with whorl formation. Histologically, the majority of cases of fibromatosis show infiltration of adjacent adipose tissue or skeletal muscle by a proliferation of spindle myofibroblasts arranged in long sweeping fascicles. Usually this

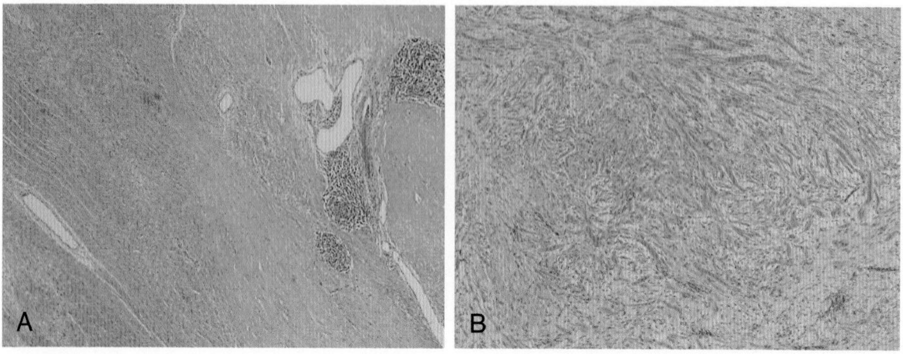

Fig. 38.6 Deep fibromatosis (desmoid): (A) Histologically, low-power view shows long sweeping hypocellular fascicles of bland spindle cells. Aggregates of lymphocytes are present (H&E 20x). (B) Bland spindle cells with keloid like collagen in the stroma (H&E 40x).

neoplasm does not display high cellularity, and the spindle cells do not overlap. These spindle cells are uniform, bland, and have stellate shape with eosinophilic cytoplasm, ill-defined border, and small nucleoli. Mitosis and atypia are rare. The stroma may show keloid-like collagen and extensive hyalinization. Myxoid changes may also be present. Scattered lymphocytes aggregates might present, particularly at the periphery of the lesion (Fig. 38.6A and B). IHC shows frequent expression of SMA and MSA in most cases, with occasional positivity for desmin. S100 and CD34 are usually negative. Beta-catenin nuclear and cytoplasmic positivity are seen in approximately 80% cases. Fibromatosis is a benign lesion that does not metastasize. However, these lesions are prone to local recurrence and therefore classified as a neoplasm with intermediate malignant potential. Aggressive cases might be treated with radiotherapy or adjuvant systemic therapy such as tyrosine kinase inhibitors (imatinib).

CLINICAL PEARL

Abdominal form of desmoid fibromatosis usually arise from the rectus abdominis muscles and aponeuroses of the abdominal wall in young female during pregnancy or after a childbirth, especially after cesarean section.

Intra-abdominal form of desmoid fibromatosis usually arises in the mesentery, pelvis, and retroperitoneal region. Usually occurs in adults aged 20–35 years.

Desmoid fibromatosis could be sporadic (90%) or familial, and both settings are associated with dysregulation of Wnt signaling pathway.

Familial desmoid fibromatosis is associated with Gardner syndrome (familial adenomatous polyposis) in which there is inactivating mutation of APC gene.

Sporadic desmoid fibromatosis is associated with activating mutation in exon 3 of CTNNB1 oncogene, coding for beta-catenin.

Both APC and CTNNB1 gene mutations results in intranuclear accumulation of beta-catenin.

SFT usually arises in the pleura but can occur in any anatomical site. The common extrapleural sites are deep soft tissue of the extremities and head and neck, and the patients are usually middle-aged adults. Grossly, SFT is a firm, well-circumscribed, encapsulated mass with median size of 5–8 cm and has multinodular gray-white cut surface. Occasionally, hemorrhage and myxoid changes might be present. Microscopically, SFT shows a classic “patternless pattern” with alternating

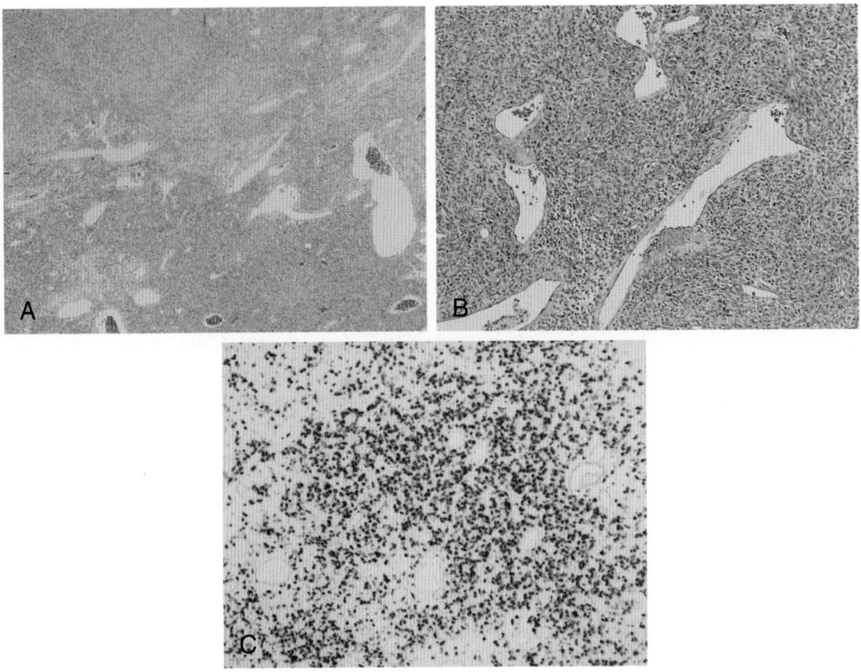

Fig. 38.7 Solitary fibrous tumor: (A) Histologically, low-power view shows hypocellular and hypercellular areas of spindle cells with dilated branched blood vessels (hemangiopericytomatous pattern) (H&E 40x). (B) High-power view shows the bland spindle tumor cells arranged in a patternless manner around the branched blood vessels (H&E, 100x). (C) Immunohistochemistry shows positive nuclear staining of STAT6 (H&E, 100x).

hypo- and hypercellular areas with variable hyalinized and keloid-like collagen deposited in the stroma. The cellular areas are composed of oval to spindle cells with pale cytoplasm and indistinct cell borders, open vesicular chromatin, and inconspicuous nucleoli. The tumor cells are not arranged in distinct pattern and are condensed around dilated, stag-horn-like branched blood vessels displaying HPC architecture. Perivascular hyalinization is a common finding. Mitotic figures are rare, usually <3/10 HPF. Myxoid changes, fat formation, fibrous stroma, and interstitial mast cell are common features (Fig. 38.7A and B). Immunohistochemical stains almost always show diffuse positive staining of CD34 in the tumor cells (up to 95%) and variable expression of CD99, bcl2, SMA, and EMA. More than 95% of SFT cases show strong and diffuse nuclear expression of transcription factor immunostain STAT6 (Fig. 38.7C). Molecular genetics shows that most of the cases of SFT harbor NAB2–STAT2 gene fusion that leads to overexpression of STAT6, which can be detected by IHC. Clinically, the majority of SFT follow a benign course, but it has a 5%–10% risk of metastasis; therefore, it is classified as a tumor with intermediate malignancy. It is usually treated with surgical excision and adjuvant radiotherapy.

CLINICAL PEARL

Criteria of malignancy in SFT are increased cellularity, increased mitosis (>4/10 HPF), necrosis, and nuclear pleomorphism. Moreover, another form of malignancy is dedifferentiation, in which SFT shows abrupt transition from typical histology to anaplastic transformation such as pleomorphic malignant round cell or spindle cell associated with loss or decrease in the expression of CD34 and STAT6 in these areas and strong expression of p53 and p16.

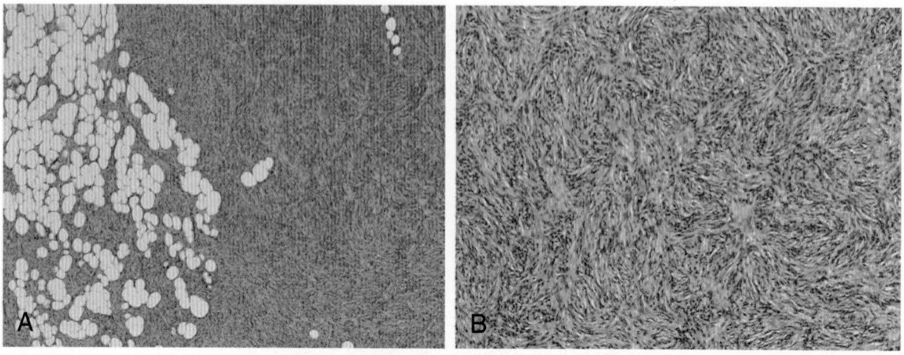

Fig. 38.8 Dermatofibrosarcoma protuberans: (A) Monotonous spindle cells neoplasm infiltrating the fat lobules exhibiting honeycomb appearance (H&E, 40x). (B) Closer view shows monotonous mildly atypical spindle cells arranged in storiform pattern (H&E 100x).

DFSP is a rare neoplasm, which most commonly occurs in young adults in their second and fourth decades with a site predilection for the trunk and extremities. Clinically, it is a slow-growing neoplasm that usually starts as an indurated skin plaque for a long history of up to 10 years before it shows a large, firm nodule with red discoloration in the skin and an average size of 5 cm. Histopathologically, DFSP is a dermal-based, ill-defined infiltrative spindle cell proliferation involving the underlying dermis and subcutaneous tissues. Also, DFSP might involve the overlying epidermis, but these lesions do not show epidermal hyperplasia similar to that occurring in cutaneous benign fibrous histiocytoma (dermatofibroma). DFSP is composed of monotonous, uniform, mildly atypical plumb or elongated spindle cells arranged in tight storiform pattern. The mitoses are low to moderate up to 5/10 HPF. The peripheral edges of the tumor show infiltrating tumor cells between collagen fibers or deep between fat lobules creating honeycomb appearance (Fig. 38.8A and B). IHC mostly shows diffuse positivity of CD34, which is often lost or decreased in areas undergoing fibrosarcomatous transformation. Genetically, most of the cases show fusion translocation of collagen type 1 alpha 1 (COL1A1) on chromosome 17 and platelet-derived growth factor beta (PDGFB) gene on chromosome 22 t (17:22)(q22;q13). This translocation usually presents as supernumerary ring chromosome on karyotype analysis, especially in adults. DFSP is an intermediate malignant neoplasm according to the World Health Organization classifications in 2013, as it is a locally aggressive neoplasm with the risk of recurrence in about half of the cases. DFSP is usually treated surgically with wide-margin excision. Metastasis usually occurs several years after the initial diagnosis, especially in the recurring lesions; therefore, a close follow-up of the patient is recommended.

CLINICAL PEARL

DFSP might undergo fibrosarcomatous transformation, presenting as a rapidly growing nodule. Microscopically, transformation shows an abrupt or gradual transition to fibrosarcomatous component displaying highly cellular spindle cells area with herringbone appearance, increased cytological atypia, and frequent mitosis. CD34 shows low or loss in expression in the fibrosarcomatous areas.

The risk of recurrence in DFSP mainly depends on the margin of excision, with at least 4 cm recommended.

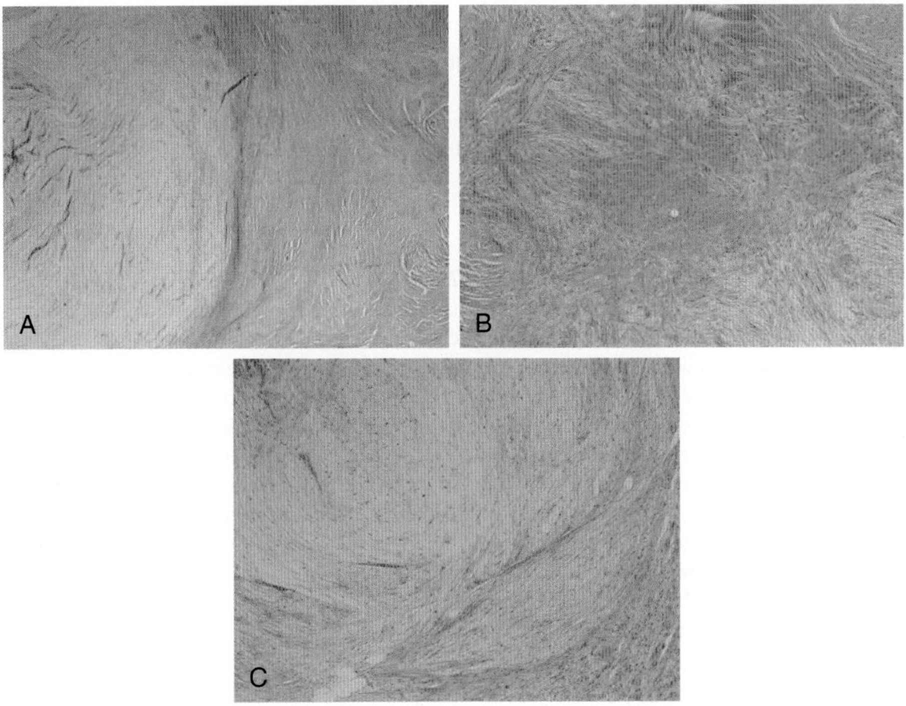

Fig. 38.9 Low-grade fibromyxoid sarcoma: (A) Low-power view shows abrupt transition between the collagenous fibrous area and the myxoid area (H&E 20x). (B) Hypocellular collagenized and hyalinized area (H&E 40x). (C) Myxoid area shows bland spindle cells and arcade of blood vessels (H&E, 40x).

What are the clinicopathologic features of low-grade fibromyxoid sarcoma (LGFMS)?

Low-grade fibromyxoid sarcoma usually presents as a deep, slow-growing soft tissue mass in young adults with a median age of 35 years. The common sites of occurrence are lower extremity, especially the thigh and limb girdle. LGFMS mostly occurs in the subfascial plane and is rarely superficial. Grossly, it is well-circumscribed, firm, fibrous mass with whitish cut surface and a median size of 5 cm. Histologically, LGFMS shows a combination of an alternating hypocellular, fibrous, collagenized areas with cellular, myxoid areas that contain monomorphic, bland-looking spindle cells with open chromatin and ill-defined cell border arranged in a short fascicle and whorling pattern. Scattered hyperchromatic cells might be present, and mitotic figures are rare (Fig. 38.9A–C). The tumor shows arcade of small blood vessels and arteriole-sized vessels with perivascular sclerosis. Necrosis is rare but may be focally present in larger lesions. Around 30% cases comprise of giant collagen rosettes consisting of nodules that are centrally hyalinized and collagenized, surrounded by a cuff of palisaded round to ovoid epithelioid fibroblasts. MUC4 is an immunohistochemical stain for epithelial mucin and is highly sensitive and specific for LGFMS, as nearly all the cases show strong and diffuse expression of MUC4. Genetically, real-time polymerase chain reaction (RT-PCR) detects a specific translocation of t(7:16) resulting in gene fusion of FUS on chromosome 16 with CREB3L2 on chromosome 7 in up to 95% of cases. Surgical resection is the mainstay of treatment. LGFMS has a low rate of recurrence and metastasis in the first few years after the initial surgery, and lung is the common site for metastasis. Higher rates of recurrence and metastatic disease are seen with longer clinical follow-up.

CLINICAL PEARL

LGFMS can infiltrate the surrounding tissue, although it has well-circumscribed growth by gross examination.

Occasionally, LGFMS may show distinctively hypercellular areas with nuclear pleomorphism and high mitosis; the significance of these features is still unclear.

LGFMS originally was named *Evans tumor*.

What are the clinicopathological features of DBFH?

It is a rare benign fibrous histiocytoma of deep soft tissue, usually occurring in young adults and commonly in the extremities and head and neck. It presents as a slow-growing painless mass. Grossly, the lesion is a well-circumscribed, firm mass with pseudocapsule measuring around 4 cm on average. Microscopically, DBFH shows a noninfiltrative neoplasm composed of bland spindle-shaped cells arranged in storiform pattern. These cells have oval vesicular nuclei, inconspicuous nucleoli, and pale eosinophilic cytoplasm (Fig. 38.10). Nuclear pleomorphism, necrosis, or increased mitotic activity should not be present. Scattered lymphocytes, foam cells, and osteoclast giant cells are typically seen in these lesions. DBFH is a diagnosis of exclusion, as there are no specific immunohistochemical stains or genetic mutation that can be used for diagnostic conformation. The most important entities that need to be thoroughly excluded before the diagnosis of DBFH is rendered are SFT and DFSP. Surgical resection is the treatment of choice, and the risk of recurrence or metastasis is exceedingly low.

What are the clinicopathological features of the common PNSTs that occur in young adult?

Schwannoma is one of the common benign PNST that occur in all age groups with peak incidence in middle-aged adults. These lesions usually occur subcutaneously along the peripheral nerves in the skin of the extremities and head and neck areas. Furthermore, it can arise in deep sites such as the retroperitoneum and mediastinum. It is a slow-growing lesion and could be asymptomatic or painful. Grossly, schwannoma is a well-circumscribed, encapsulated globoid lesion, measuring <10 cm, which may show attachment to a peripheral nerve. Microscopically, schwannomas have a thickened capsule that might contain intracapsular lymphoid aggregates.

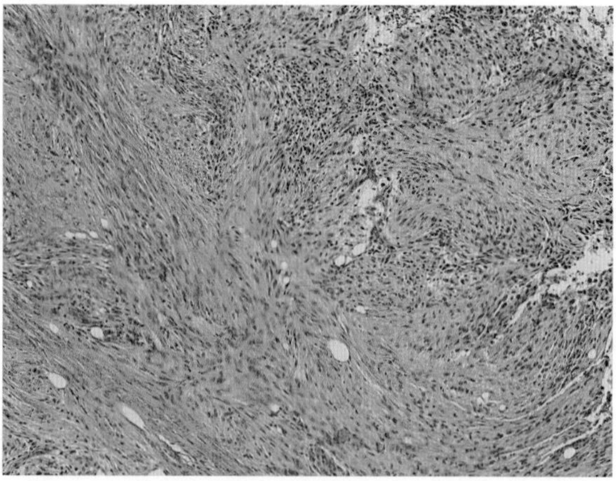

Fig. 38.10 Deep benign fibrous histiocytoma histologically shows benign spindle cells arranged in storiform pattern and short fascicles.

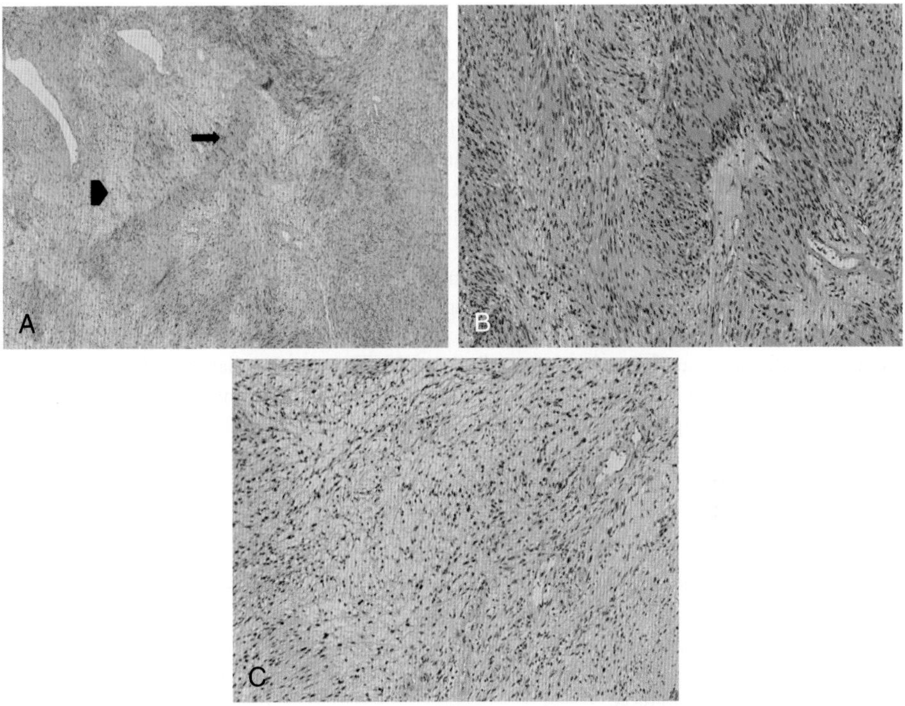

Fig. 38.11 Schwannoma: (A) Histologically shows hyalinized walled blood vessels with alternating areas of hypercellular (Antoni A; arrow) and hypocellular area (Antoni B; arrowhead) (H&E, 40x). (B) Antoni A area shows hypercellularity with nuclear palisading and Verocay bodies (H&E 100x). (C) Antoni B shows loose hypocellular area (H&E 100x).

This neoplasm is biphasic showing compact hypercellular areas (Antoni A) with nuclear palisading (Verocay bodies) alternating with loose hypocellular areas (Antoni B) (Fig. 38.11A). The cells in Antoni A areas are spindle-shaped Schwann cells in short or interconnecting fascicles with elongated, tapered nuclei with eosinophilic cytoplasm and no distinct border (Fig. 38.11B). Antoni B areas commonly show thick hyalinized blood vessels and hemosiderin-laden histiocytes (Fig. 38.11B). Sometimes nuclear pleomorphism might be seen especially with ancient schwannoma as part of degenerative changes; however, such cases will not show increase in the mitotic activity. IHC shows diffuse and strong expression of S100 in the spindle tumor cells. Schwannomas are usually treated by complete surgical excision, and the risk of recurrence is rare.

CLINICAL PEARL

More than 90% of schwannomas are solitary and sporadic. Multiple schwannomas and those that arise bilaterally from intracranial vestibular nerves are a feature of neurofibromatosis type 2.

Variants of schwannoma are ancient, cellular, plexiform, microcystic/reticular, epitheloid, and melanotic schwannoma.

Melanotic schwannoma is associated with Carny's complex a familial, autosomal dominant, multiple neoplasia syndrome.

Neurofibroma is the most common benign PNST that usually occurs solitary and sporadically. It affects all ages and both sexes, but is more common in young adults. There are five macroscopic variants of neurofibroma: localized cutaneous, diffuse cutaneous, localized intraneural, plexiform intraneural, and massive diffuse soft tissue plexiform tumor. Histologically, neurofibroma is composed of admixture of axon cells, fibroblasts, and mast cells. These cells are loosely arranged in a myxoid stroma and diffusely infiltrate the involved nerve. The proportion of the cellular and stromal component is variable. The classic appearance consists of vaguely whorled proliferation of elongated spindle cells with eosinophilic cytoplasmic processes and wavy hyperchromatic nuclei, admixed with a population of short spindle cells with scattered mast cells and occasional nerve fibers. Thick or course collagen fiber bundles often described as having an appearance of shredded carrots are also present (Fig. 38.12A and B). IHC shows S100 and SOX10 positivity in the axonal spindle cells and CD34 highlights the stromal cells (Fig. 38.12C). The criteria of malignant transformation into malignant PNST are a constellation of features including hypercellularity, nuclear atypia defined by hyperchromatic enlarged nuclei, increased mitosis, and loss or decreased expression of S100, SOX10, and CD34 (Fig. 38.13). Localized and diffuse cutaneous neurofibromas are usually benign and do not recur. Plexiform neurofibroma and localized intraneural neurofibroma are a precursor to malignant PNST.

CLINICAL PEARL

Multiple neurofibromas usually occur in patients with neurofibromatosis type 1 (NF1).

Plexiform neurofibroma is a pathognomonic in patients with NF1.

Malignant PNST is very rare tumor with median age of 35, and around 50% of the cases arise in patients with NF1 and 10% are induced on radiation. Other cases might arise sporadically from preexisting neurofibroma.

Patients with NF1 have 10% lifetime risk to develop MPNST.

Soft tissue **perineuroma** is an uncommon tumor composed exclusively of perineural cells. These tumors have a wide age range and arise most commonly in middle-aged adults, with predilection for limbs, and can occur superficially or deep. Grossly, it is a well-circumscribed, nonencapsulated mass with fibrous cut surface. Histologically, the tumor comprises of slender spindle cells with wavy nuclear and bipolar cytoplasmic process arranged in whorled and storiform growth pattern. Nuclear atypia or mitosis should not be present. The stroma is variable, ranging from collagenous to myxoid. On IHC, perineuromas show expression of EMA and focal expression for CD34. Sometimes the positivity of EMA could be weak and focal due to the thin and delicate processes of perineural cells requiring careful examination. It is treated surgically and rarely recurs.

What are the clinicopathological features of LMS?

LMS of the soft tissue in the extremities is very rare and most commonly occurs in middle-aged adults or the elderly. Grossly, LMS is usually well circumscribed, with fleshy white-tan and whorled cut surface. High-grade LMS tends to have necrosis and hemorrhage. Microscopically, LMS is composed of compact intersecting fascicles and bundles of malignant spindle cells. The cells exhibit cigar-shaped nuclei with blunt ends, bright eosinophilic cytoplasm, and distinct cell borders. Nuclear atypia varies from mild, to moderate, to high. Mitosis is common, and atypical forms are frequent in high-grade LMS (Fig. 38.14A and B). Areas of coagulative necrosis are common. IHC shows diffuse strong expression of SMA, HHF35, and desmin (Fig. 38.14C). Also, caldesmon is more specific for smooth muscle differentiation but is less sensitive. LMS has high risk of metastasis, especially to the lung and bone. LMS is usually treated surgically, followed by adjuvant radiotherapy to decrease the recurrence. Patients with metastatic LMS may also be treated with chemotherapy.

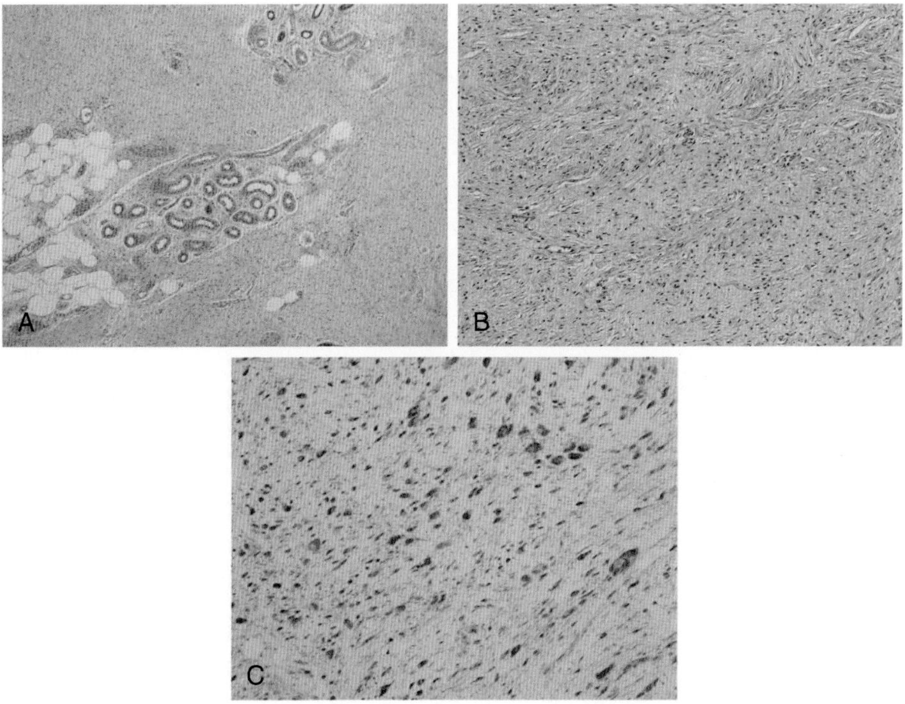

Fig. 38.12 (A) Diffuse cutaneous neurofibroma: (A) Sheets of bland spindle cell with fibrous stroma trapping the skin adnexal structure and infiltrating the fat (H&E 40x). (B) The neural axon cells are short and stubble admixed with fibroblasts and short collagen fibers (Shredded carrots) (H&E 100x). (C) Immunostain of S100 is expressed in the majority of axon neural cells (H&E 100x).

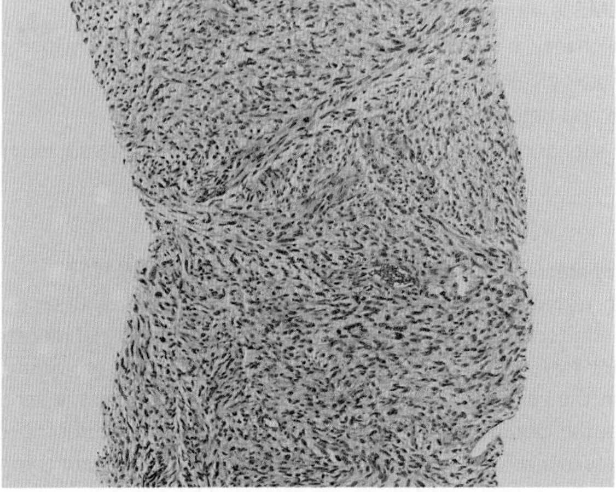

Fig. 38.13 Malignant peripheral nerve sheath tumor shows hypercellular spindle cell neoplasm with nuclear atypia and frequent mitosis (H&E, 100x).

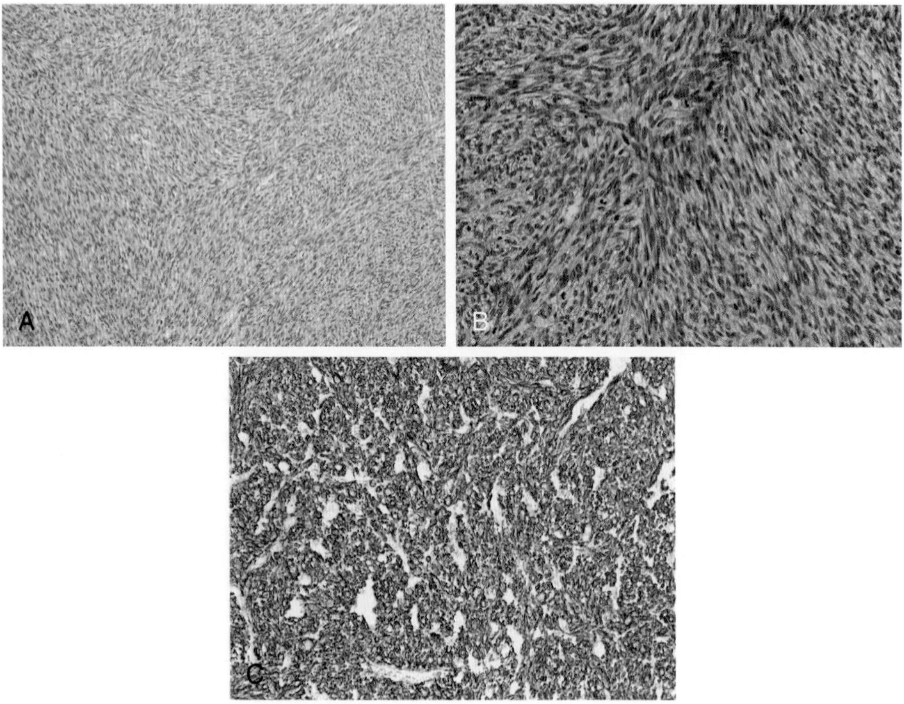

Fig. 38.14 Leiomyosarcoma: (A) Histologically, low-power view shows intersecting fascicles of malignant spindle smooth muscle cells (H&E 40x). (B) The malignant smooth muscle cells show cigar-shaped blunted end nuclei with frequent mitoses (H&E 200x). (C) Immunohistochemistry shows diffuse positivity of SMA in the malignant smooth muscles (H&E 200x).

CLINICAL PEARL

Retroperitoneal LMS is more common in women.

The criteria of malignancy in smooth muscle tumors are nuclear atypia, mitosis, and necrosis.

LMS is graded histologically from mild to moderate to high grade.

LMS has variable and heterogeneous molecular background.

Grade, anatomic site, and depth are the most significant prognostic factors for LMS.

What are the clinicopathological features of spindle cell / sclerosing RMS?

It is an uncommon variant of RMS, which accounts for 5%–10% of all cases of RMS, occurs in both children and adults, and features prominent fascicular spindle cell morphology. Spindle and sclerosing RMS are two entities from the same neoplastic spectrum. Spindle cell RMS more commonly arises in the paratesticular region and head and neck areas, whereas sclerosing RMS commonly arises in the extremities. Grossly, the tumor is a well-circumscribed, nonencapsulated firm mass with a mean size of 4–6 cm. Histologically, these lesions are composed of malignant spindle cells arranged in fascicles and storiform pattern. These spindle cells exhibit cigar-shaped nuclei, vesicular chromatin, inconspicuous nucleoli, and eosinophilic fibrillar cytoplasm with distinct cell borders. Occasional cytoplasmic cross striations are present. Scattered large polygonal rhabdomyoblasts with nuclear atypia and mitosis are commonly present (Fig. 38.15A and B).

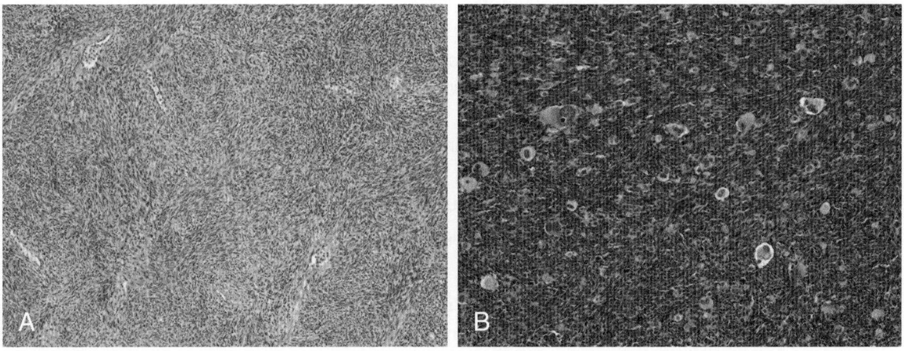

Fig. 38.15 Spindle cell rhabdomyosarcoma: (A) Microscopically shows elongated intersecting fascicles of malignant spindle cells (H&E 40x). (B) Scattered large polygonal malignant rhabdomyoblasts are commonly present (H&E 100x).

Sclerosing RMS shows sclerosed collagenous stroma. IHC in spindle cell RMS shows diffuse expression of desmin and SMA and nuclear staining of myogenin in the rhabdomyoblasts in most of the cases. In contrast, IHC in sclerosing RMS shows strong and diffuse nuclear positivity of MyoD1 and weak and focal positivity for myogenin. Spindle cell RMS in a pediatric age group has more favorable prognosis than other variants of RMS. Spindle/sclerosing RMS in adults is associated with high risk of recurrence and metastasis.

What are the clinicopathological features of myxoma?

There are two forms of myxoma—juxta-articular and intramuscular; both the entities are histologically similar, most commonly occurring in middle aged-adults. Intramuscular myxoma is more common in men, with a predilection to occur in the muscles of the thigh and shoulder. In contrast, juxta-articular myxoma is more common in women and usually arises near joints, especially the knee joint. Grossly, the lesion is well circumscribed, with lobulated and gelatinous cut surface. Microscopically, the tumor is a hypocellular and hypovascular neoplasm that contains uniform benign spindle and stellate-shaped cells embedded in abundant extracellular myxoid matrix (Fig. 38.16). The stroma may show vacuolation and cystic changes. No atypia or increased mitosis is present. Scattered capillary-sized blood vessels are present. IHC shows CD34 positivity in the spindle cells. These lesions harbor no risk of recurrence if treated surgically.

Fig. 38.16 Myxoma, histologically, is hypocellular and hypovascular, consisting of benign spindle cells in abundant myxoid stroma (H&E 40x).

CLINICAL PEARL

Intramuscular myxoma might show areas of increased cellularity, collagen fibers, and blood vessels; such lesions have been termed *cellular myxoma*. Cellular myxoma has minimal risk of local recurrence.

Intramuscular myxoma tends to harbor activating mutation of GNAS gene.

Myxoma can occur sporadically or associated with Mazabraud syndrome, which presents with intramuscular myxomas and skeletal fibrous dysplasia.

Juxta-articular myxoma lacks the GNAS mutation.

What are the clinical and radiological characteristics of SS?

SS could occur at any age but more commonly in the teenage and young adults, and around 70% of the cases arise from the deep soft tissue of the extremities with a predilection to occur near the joints. SS can also occur in the trunk and head and neck areas. The tumor usually presents as a slow-growing, deep-seated, small painful mass that might be associated with minimal limitation of motion. MRI and CT scan usually show septate heterogenous mass with irregular calcifications and might show cystic and hemorrhagic changes. Also, MRI and CT scan will help to identify the extent and anatomical relation of the mass and are helpful in planning for surgical resection.

What are the pathological features of SS?

Grossly, SS is a well-circumscribed, multilobulated mass with pseudocapsule measuring 3–10 cm. The appearance of the cut surface will correlate with the proportion of collagenous stroma that is present in the tumor. Prominent multicystic changes are commonly seen together with calcifications. Poorly differentiated SS tends to be less circumscribed, friable, and shows more necrosis and hemorrhage.

Microscopically, there are three variant of SS including monophasic, biphasic, and poorly differentiated. Monophasic SS is composed of solid compact sheets of uniform, plump, malignant spindle cells with minimal amount of cytoplasm, hyperchromatic nuclei, fine granular chromatin, and inconspicuous nucleoli. The atypia is usually mild, and mitotic figures can be frequent. The malignant spindle cells are arranged in long fascicles or show a herringbone pattern, in which there is nuclear overlapping due to indistinct cell border (Figs. 38.2 and 38.3). Areas of a distinctive HPC vascular pattern, hyalinized or wiry collagenous stromal fibers, and dystrophic calcifications are commonly present. Biphasic SS comprises of spindle cell component, similar to that seen in the monophasic variant together with an epithelial component. The epithelial component will show cords, nests, tubules, and glands of malignant epithelial cells that are tall or cuboidal exhibiting vesicular nuclei and pale eosinophilic cytoplasm. The glandular and tubular structures merge indistinctly with the surrounding spindle cell component, forming cleft-like pattern and containing eosinophilic secretion (Fig. 38.17A and B). Poorly differentiated SS can be monophasic or biphasic SS showing hypercellular areas of round or spindle cells with marked nuclear atypia, high mitotic activity more than 15/10 HPF, and necrosis. These areas may resemble Ewing sarcoma or malignant PNST. On IHC, SS will demonstrate expression of epithelial markers, specifically EMA, pancytokeratin, and cytokeratin 7 in most cases. The patterns of staining of the epithelial markers are frequently focal and require careful examination (Fig. 38.17C). TLE 1 is a nuclear transcription corepressor that demonstrates diffuse strong positivity in 90% of the SS cases.

Case Point 38.2

On IHC, the patient's biopsy demonstrates positivity for cytokeratin 7 and EMA and negativity for S100, CD34, SMA, and desmin. TLE1 shows strong, diffuse nuclear positivity. Based on the histologic and immunophenotypic features, the diagnosis is consistent with monophasic SS.

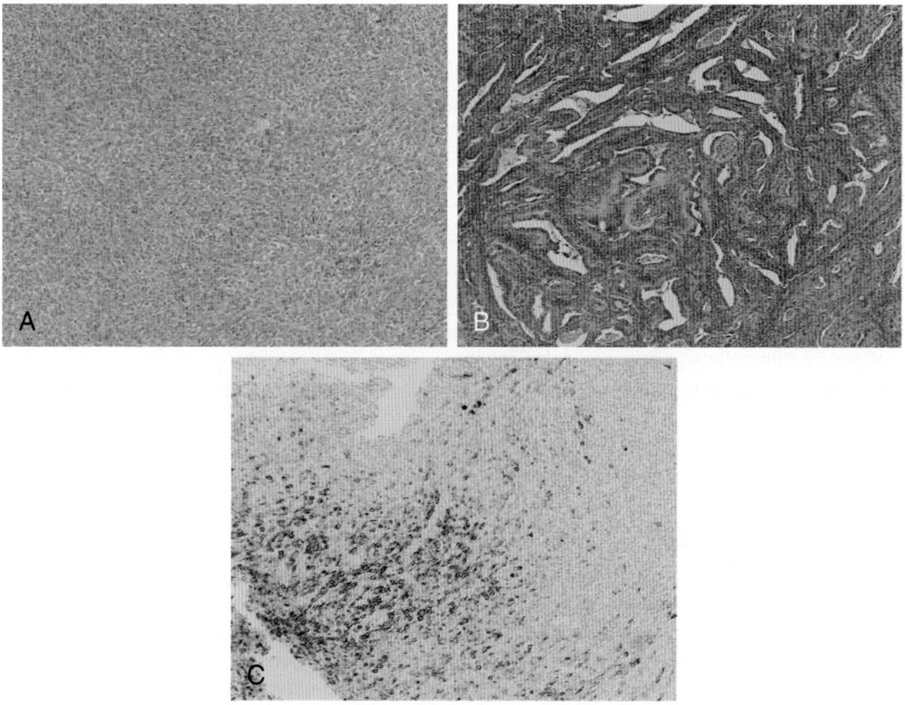

Fig. 38.17 (A) Monophasic synovial sarcoma (SS) shows uniform, monotonous, plump malignant spindle cells with wiry collagen in the stroma (H&E 100x). (B) Biphasic SS shows glandular epithelial component with cleft-like spaces filled with eosinophilic secretion and merges indistinctly with spindle cell component (H&E 100x). (C) EMA immunostain demonstrates focal positivity in SS (H&E 100x).

What is the genetic signature of SS?

Fluorescence in situ hybridization (FISH) or RT-PCR consistently demonstrates t(X;18)(p11;q11) translocation in all cases of SS. The SS18 gene on chromosome 18 fuses to one of the SSX genes on chromosome X. The translocation may involve the SSX1 gene (most common) as well as SSX2 and SSX4.

Case Point 38.3

The patient's biopsy has been tested by FISH, which demonstrates the t(X;18)(p11;q11) translocation, and the diagnosis of monophasic SS is confirmed.

What is the treatment and prognosis of SS?

SS is a highly aggressive tumor, and the mainstay of treatment is complete excision with wide-margin resection, followed by radiotherapy and adjuvant chemotherapy. Neoadjuvant chemotherapy sometimes may be given. Recurrence and metastasis usually occur in the first 2 years after the initial diagnosis; however, late metastases can occur after many years. Metastases occur in 40% of the cases and most commonly to the lungs. Biphasic versus monophasic tumor morphology has no prognostic relevance for disease recurrence or metastatic potential.

Case Point 38.4

After the surgery, the patient recovered uneventfully; he subsequently received adjuvant chemotherapy and radiotherapy and continued to follow up without recurrence or metastasis.

CLINICAL PEARL

Monophasic SS is the most common histological variant.

No clinical significance between monophasic and biphasic SS.

Poorly differentiated SS is associated with more aggressive clinical course.

The most important prognostic factors are tumor stage, size, the patient age, the proportion of poorly differentiated areas and calcifications.

Patients younger than 25 years have a lower risk of metastasis than patient olden than 40 years.

SS is chemosensitive; t(X;18)(p11;q11) is diagnostic for SS.

BEYOND THE PEARLS

- Nodular fasciitis has different growth phases such as a cellular phase, with or without myxoid changes, and a fibrotic phase.
- Neurofibromas are sporadic in about 90% of cases; others are syndromic in association with NF1, which results from a germline mutation in the NF1 gene on chromosome 17q11.2.
- Myxofibrosarcoma is the most common sarcoma in the elderly that occurs superficially in the limb composed of admixture of atypical spindle cell in a myxoid background with fibrous area and has no specific genetic signature (complex karyotype with multiple genomic abnormalities).
- Myxofibrosarcoma could be graded histologically based on the nuclear atypia into low, intermediate, and high grade.
- Leiomyoma of deep soft tissue is extremely rare and should be thoroughly examined for malignant features before giving such a diagnosis.

References

Fletcher CDM, Unni KK, Mertens F. WHO classification of tumors of soft tissue. *Pathology*. 2014;5: 250-272.

Goldblum JR, Folpe AL, Weiss SW. *Enzinger and Weiss's Soft Tissue Tumors*. 6th ed. Philadelphia, PA: Elsevier; 2014.

Hornik JL. *Practical Soft Tissue Pathology: A Diagnostic Approach*. 2nd ed. Philadelphia, PA: Elsevier; 2019.

Skin

CASE 39

A 61-Year-Old Female with a Pruritic Rash

Cynthia Reyes Barron ■ Tatsiana Pukhalskaya

A 61-year-old woman presents to her dermatologist complaining of a multifocal pruritic rash. The rash began on the dorsal aspect of her hands and feet and has spread to her wrists, ankles, lower back, and shoulders. It is not painful, but stings occasionally. She believes the rash worsens when she plays tennis. It has been present for 8 months. The patient denies fever, chills, and weight loss. She has no history of cancer and is a nonsmoker. Other medical history includes hypothyroidism and hypercholesterolemia for which she takes levothyroxine and rosuvastatin. She is allergic to sulfa antibiotics, which give her hives. Her family history is unremarkable other than heart disease in her deceased parents. She is a school teacher and has an active lifestyle.

What is a general differential diagnosis for a pruritic rash?
There are many etiologies of pruritic rashes, such as infections, arthropod bites, cutaneous lymphoma, genetic conditions, and inflammatory diseases including autoimmune and reactive disorders (Table 39.1). Evaluating the clinical history, presentation, physical exam findings, and histologic findings is critical for determining the diagnosis.

TABLE 39.1 ■ **Common Pruritic Skin Disorders**

Diagnosis	Clinical Appearance	Key Histologic Features
Amyloidosis	Variable: often waxy papules or macules in various locations	Variable: subtle deposits or large nodules of amyloid in papillary dermis and perivascular deposits, perivascular lymphoid infiltrate, basal vacuolar change
Arthropod bite	Often excoriated purpuric papules, bullae, nodules, or ulcers	Variable spongiosis, dermal edema, perivascular and interstitial lymphocytic infiltrate, abundant interstitial eosinophils
Atopic dermatitis (eczema)	Papules, plaques, and vesicles acutely progressing to thickened plaques with lichenification	Microvesicles present in acute disease, epidermal edema, superficial perivascular lymphocytic infiltrate, exocytosis of lymphocytes into epidermis, parakeratosis
Contact dermatitis (Fig. 39.1)	May be allergic or irritant type Allergic: usually localized Irritant: confined to exposed area Erythematous lesions with small, fragile vesicles, may have overlying scale	Variable depending on phase with superficial perivascular lymphocytic infiltrate, lymphocyte and eosinophil exocytosis into epidermis, parakeratosis, variable acanthosis, spongiosis
Dermatitis herpetiformis (Fig. 39.2)	Grouped lesions symmetrically involving the elbows, knees, neck, scalp, and sacrum	Early dermal microabscesses with neutrophils; later subepidermal split with possible microabscesses; granular IgA in dermal papillae seen by immunofluorescence

TABLE 39.1 ■ **Common Pruritic Skin Disorders** (continued)

Diagnosis	Clinical Appearance	Key Histologic Features
Dermatophytosis	Scaly, erythematous annular lesions that occur more commonly on extremities and trunk	Foci of parakeratosis, minimal perivascular inflammation with occasional neutrophils and eosinophils, mild spongiosis, PASD stain may help identify hyphae and yeast forms
Drug eruption	Variable: may be fixed, morbilliform, lichenoid (Fig. 39.3), or psoriasiform; associated with many medications	Nonspecific changes that may include perivascular and interstitial dermal infiltrate with lymphocytes and neutrophils, eosinophils often present, pigment incontinence, parakeratosis occasionally
Id (hypersensitivity) reaction	Delayed hypersensitivity reaction at sites distant to previous dermatitis eruption 1–2 weeks after primary occurrence; usually on the forearms, legs, and trunk; papules	Prominent spongiosis, microvesicle formation, lymphocyte exocytosis, superficial perivascular lymphocytic infiltrate with eosinophils; late lesions may show hyperkeratosis, wedge-shaped hypergranulosis, and parakeratosis
Lichen planus	Polygonal, purple papules and plaques with possible overlying Wickham striae	Epidermal hyperplasia, hyperkeratosis without parakeratosis, wedge-shaped hypergranulosis, band-like lymphoid infiltrate that obscures the dermal–epidermal junction, dying keratinocytes (Civatte bodies)
Lichen sclerosus	Tissue paper–like white lesions, often in the genital area	Early: lichenoid and perivascular superficial inflammation, homogeneous eosinophilic material in papillary dermis Late: epidermal atrophy, minimal inflammation, melanophages
Lichen simplex chronicus (Fig. 39.4)	Patches and plaques in areas of persistent rubbing	Hyperkeratosis with occasional parakeratosis, psoriasiform epidermal hyperplasia, epidermis with acral appearance, hypergranulosis, papillary dermal fibrosis, minimal superficial perivascular lymphocytic infiltrate
Prurigo nodularis	Pruritic nodules resulting from skin trauma, dome-shaped lesions with scaly and excoriated surface	Cup-shaped acanthosis, hyperorthokeratosis, hypergranulosis, vascular ectasia and hyperplasia, mild perivascular inflammation
Urticaria (Fig. 39.5)	Transient (24 hours) erythematous patches and plaques, dermal wheals	Slight perivascular edema, sparse infiltrate of lymphocytes, neutrophils, scattered eosinophils and mast cells around superficial vessels, no epidermal changes
Viral exanthem	Erythematous papules and macules with rapid onset and usual rapid resolution	Superficial perivascular lymphohistiocytic infiltrate; rare eosinophils

In particular, the chronicity of the lesions is important. Certain rashes, such as urticaria (Fig. 39.5), are transient, often disappearing within 24 hours. Others may persist for months and years if not treated appropriately. Some conditions, such as dermatitis herpetiformis (Fig. 39.2), are persistent with exacerbations and remissions for life.

What type of rashes commonly present with fever?

Pruritic rashes may be preceded or followed by fever, especially when associated with bacterial and viral etiologies. Many of these are more commonly seen in children, particularly if unvaccinated, including rubeola (measles), varicella, rubella, erythema infectiosum, and roseola infantum.

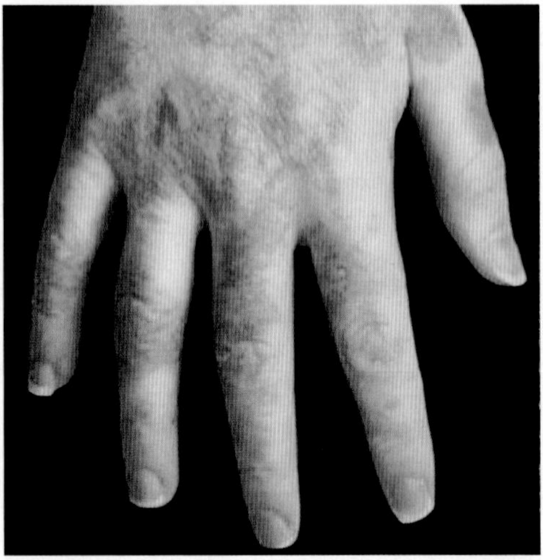

Fig. 39.1 Irritant contact dermatitis with erythematous crusted plaques occurring on the skin that came in contact with a glove. (From *ExpertPath*. Copyright Elsevier.)

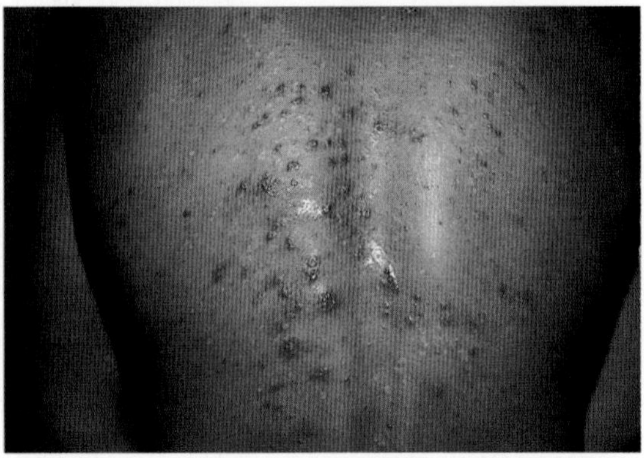

Fig. 39.2 Dermatitis herpetiformis with grouped vesicular lesions on a patient's back (From Goldblum J, Lamps L, McKenney J, Myers J. *Rosai and Ackerman's Surgical Pathology*. 11th ed. Philadelphia, PA: Elsevier; 2018. Figure 2.45)

Scarlet fever and erythema marginatum of acute rheumatic fever are associated with pharyngitis and group A *Streptococcus* infection. Adults are susceptible to herpes zoster (shingles) with a history of a previous varicella infection. Secondary syphilis often presents with fever, malaise, and a maculopapular rash weeks after a primary chancre. Furthermore, rheumatologic diseases such as lupus erythematosus may be accompanied by fever.

CLINICAL PEARL

Secondary syphilis, resulting from the dissemination of bacteria *Treponema pallidum*, may present as a localized or widespread pruritic rash that involves the palms and soles as well as the extremities and trunk. The lesions are typically maculopapular or scaly patches. Syphilis is known as "the great imitator" and may imitate lichen planus histologically. However, the inflammatory infiltrate usually extends deeper into the dermis, and the band-like infiltrate at the DE junction may not obscure the junction. An immunohistochemical stain specific for the spirochete is available.

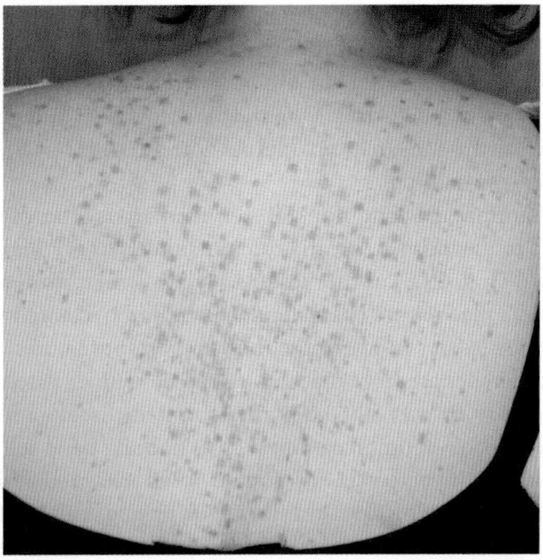

Fig. 39.3 Lichenoid drug eruption with diffuse papules on the patient's back, clinically similar to lichen planus. (From *ExpertPath*. Copyright Elsevier.)

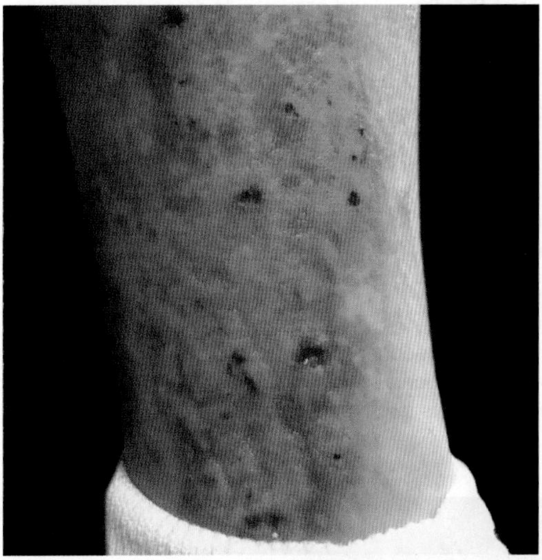

Fig. 39.4 Lichen simplex chronicus with erythematous papules and plaques and signs of excoriation. (From *ExpertPath*. Copyright Elsevier.)

Case Point 39.1

The patient cannot recall any recent febrile illness. Furthermore, she has not had new sexual partners in years.

What features should be noted on physical examination?

The location of the rash is important in narrowing the differential. Some reactive conditions including drug eruptions may be widespread; others occur more commonly on sun-exposed areas, whereas some have characteristic manifestations at particular locations such as the facial malar rash of lupus erythematosus. A focal rash may be caused by contact dermatitis or an arthropod bite, whereas folliculitis is localized to hair follicles.

Not only location but arrangement should also be noted. For example, pityriasis rosea manifests with the appearance of a herald patch, usually on the back, followed by a generalized eruption that is often described as a Christmas tree pattern. Herpes zoster results in a vesicular eruption along a dermatome and rarely crosses midline.

Although most inflammatory conditions are erythematous, the color of the lesions may provide additional clues to diagnosis. Urticaria often manifests as erythematous or white plaques surrounded by a red halo (Fig. 39.5). Other lesions such as lichen planus may have a violaceous color (Fig. 39.6). Psoriasis plaques are characteristically salmon-colored with silvery scales.

The morphology of the lesions is one of the most important features. Macules are discolored lesions that are flat, and patches are large macules. A papule is an elevated lesion measuring 1 cm or less in diameter and may or may not have an associated discoloration. Some papules have characteristic central depression or umbilication, such as nodular basal cell carcinoma, molluscum contagiosum, and sebaceous hyperplasia. A nodule is an elevated lesion measuring greater than 1 cm and may be above or below the skin surface. A plaque is also defined as a lesion greater than 1 cm in diameter and may be either an elevated or thickened circumscribed palpable lesion. Vesicles are small blisters (fluid-containing lesions), while bullae are large blisters greater than 1 cm in diameter. Additional qualities include scaling, which is an increase in the number of dead cells on the skin surface, and ulceration, which is a full-thickness loss of the epidermis with some involvement of the dermis and presence of acute and chronic inflammation.

Case Point 39.2

On physical examination, a full survey of the patient's skin is conducted revealing numerous erythematous and violaceous macules and papules with some scaling (Fig. 39.6). Some of the lesions on her wrists and ankles exhibit the Koebner phenomenon. The lesions are diffusely spread on the lower back, shoulders, wrists, dorsal hands, feet, and ankles.

CLINICAL PEARL

The Koebnerization effect (or Koebner phenomenon) is used to describe a lesion or groups of lesions attributed to trauma, such as scratching or rubbing. The lesion is often linear. It may be observed in other conditions such as psoriasis and vitiligo.

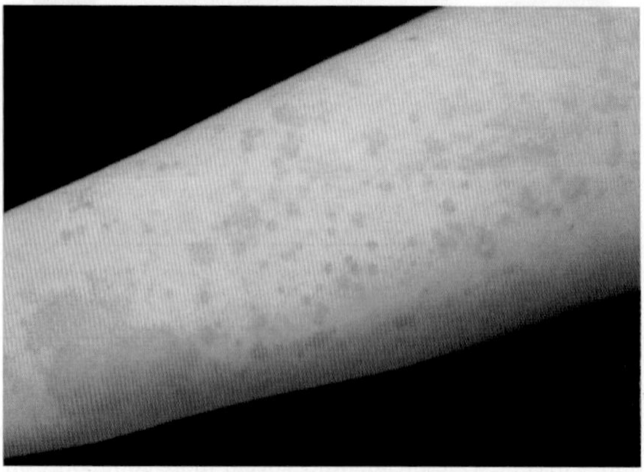

Fig. 39.5 Urticaria with well-demarcated erythematous lesions on the forearm. (From *ExpertPath*. Copyright Elsevier.)

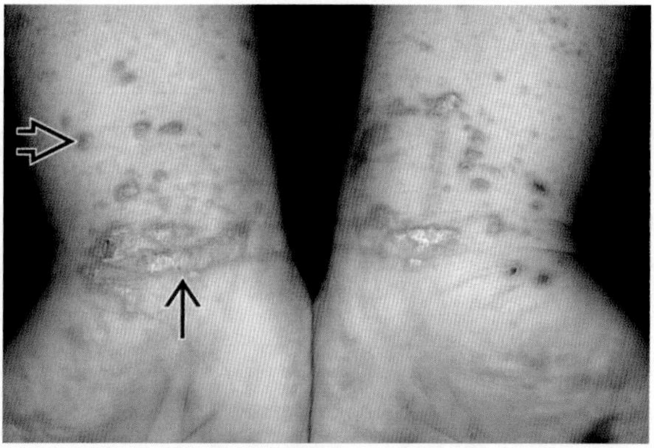

Fig. 39.6 Lichen planus with scattered erythematous polygonal papules and plaques with focal white scaling (black open arrow) and the Koebnerization effect (black solid arrow) on the wrists. (From *ExpertPath*. Copyright Elsevier.)

Case Point 39.3

Shave biopsies of two lesions are taken and sent to pathology for further evaluation.

CLINICAL PEARL

The skin is composed of three principal layers: epidermis, dermis, and subcutis. The epidermis is the most superficial layer and is further subdivided into four layers of squamous epithelium:

1. Stratum basalis: deepest layer composed of proliferating keratinocytes and melanocytes
2. Stratum spinosum: consists of layers of keratinocytes (usually 5–10)
3. Stratum granulosum: flattened cells in one to three layers containing basophilic kertatohyalin granules
4. Stratum corneum: outermost layer composed of anucleate keratinocytes that may intertwine for a basket weave appearance

The DE junction consists of interlocking epidermal ridges (rete ridges) and dermal papillae. Adnexal structures such as hair follicles, eccrine glands, and apocrine glands are rooted in the dermis. The subcutis consists of mature adipose tissue and connective tissue (Fig. 39.7).

What is the difference between a shave biopsy and a punch biopsy?

A shave biopsy is performed with a flat blade or scalpel. A tissue sample is taken by cutting parallel to the skin surface. The epidermis alone may be sampled or a deeper section may be taken to include the dermis depending on the nature of the lesion. Shave biopsies do not require sutures for closure; however, they may result in a depressed scar. Punch biopsies are performed with round circular blades that range in diameter and may be as small as 3 mm. They produce a cone-shaped sample with the base at the epidermis and narrowing into the dermis and subcutis. If a small blade is used, sutures are not required for closure, and minimal scarring occurs. Larger biopsies are sutured to re-approximate the edges of the skin.

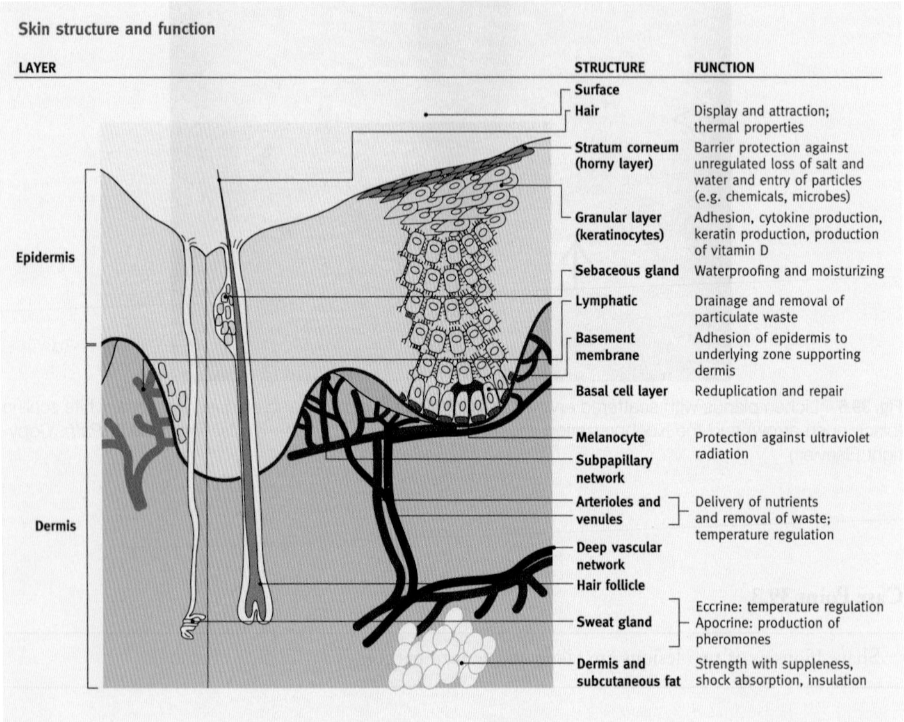

Fig. 39.7 Diagram of skin anatomy and function of structures. (From Venus M, Waterman J, McNab I. Basic Physiology of the skin. *Surgery (Oxford)*. 2011;29(10):471-474. Figure 1. doi:10.1016/j.mpsur.2011.06.010.)

Case Point 39.4

The two biopsies consist of epidermis with a partial thickness portion of dermis and have a similar histologic appearance. There is a band-like infiltrate of lymphocytes focally obscuring the dermal–epidermal (DE) junction (Fig. 39.8). Rare eosinophils are present within the inflammatory infiltrate. There is hypergranulosis and wedge-shaped hyperplasia of the epidermis without parakeratosis (Fig. 39.9). Focal pigment incontinence is present (Fig. 39.10).

CLINICAL PEARL

Pigment (or melanin) incontinence is seen more commonly in dark-skinned patients and in long-standing lesions. As basal cells are damaged, the transfer of melanin from melanocytes to keratinocytes is hampered and the pigment is lost, or it may be released as basal cells die. It is a feature of multiple entities with a damaged basal layer, including lichenoid drug eruptions, which may present with lesions clinically indistinguishable from lichen planus (Fig. 39.3).

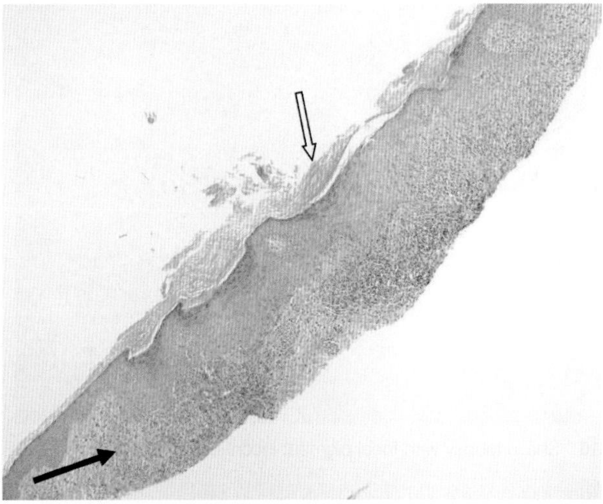

Fig. 39.8 Shave biopsy with a band-like lymphocytic infiltrate at the dermal–epidermal junction (black solid arrow) and hyperkeratosis without parakeratosis (black open arrow) (H&E, 40x).

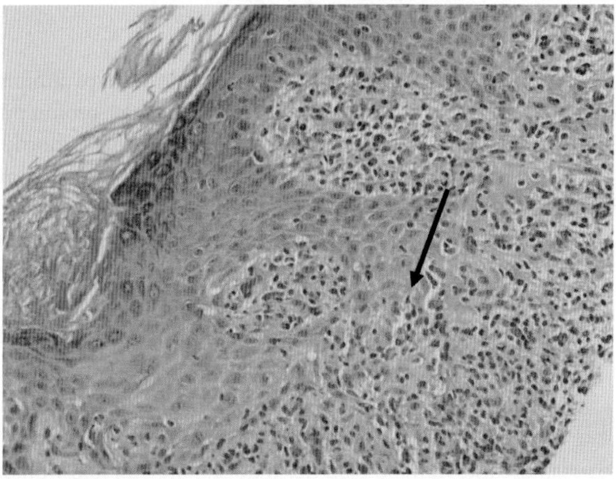

Fig. 39.9 Shave biopsy with focal disruption of the dermal–epidermal junction by the lymphocytic infiltrate (black arrow) (H&E, 200x).

Case Point 39.5

The histologic differential diagnosis includes lichen planus and a lichenoid drug eruption.

CLINICAL PEARL

Lichenoid (lichenoid dermatitis) refers to conditions with a band-like infiltrate of inflammatory cells disrupting the DE junction.

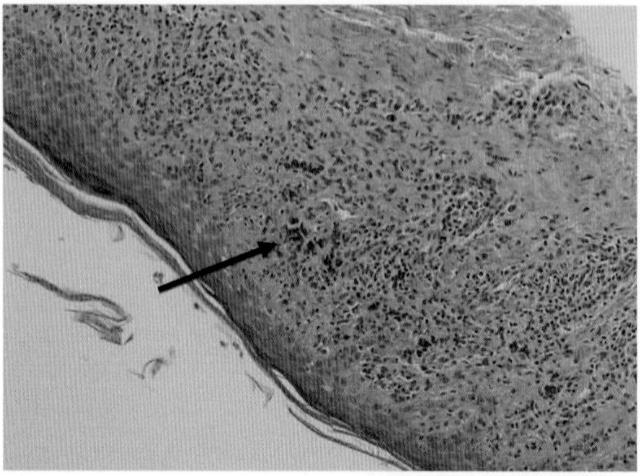

Fig. 39.10 Shave biopsy with focal pigment incontinence (black arrow) (H&E 100x).

CLINICAL PEARL

The five "P's" of lichen planus are pruritic, purplish, planar (flat), polygonal, and papules. The papules may have overlying fine reticulated white scales known as *Wickham striae*.

Many commonly prescribed medications, including antibiotics, ace inhibitors, beta blockers, thiazide diuretics, sulfonylureas, nonsteroidal antiinflammatory drugs, proton pump inhibitors, and statins, may result in lichenoid drug eruptions. The reaction may manifest shortly after the introduction of a new drug or up to a year later, making an accurate and thorough medical history extremely important (Fig. 39.3). Removing the offending drug is critical for resolution, although the lesions may persist months later. Reintroduction of the drug results in the eruption of new lesions.

Other entities with a lichenoid dermatitis pattern include lupus erythematosus, lichenoid keratosis, and acute graft-versus-host disease (GvHD). Regressing melanoma may show a lichenoid reaction. In addition, a lichenoid reaction may be present overlying a dermatofibroma.

CLINICAL PEARL

Lupus erythematosus is an autoimmune disorder that primarily affects women in their 20s and 30s. There are several variants with some affecting the skin alone and others involving multiple organs including kidneys. Patients may present with fever, fatigue, weight loss, myalgias, and lymphadenopathy as well as a pruritic rash primarily in sun-exposed areas. The malar (butterfly-shaped) facial rash is characteristic. Serologic testing may reveal antinuclear antibodies in up to 95% of patients or anti-double-stranded DNA, anti-Smith, antinuclear ribonucleic acid protein, anti-La antibody, anti-Ro antibody, anti-single-stranded DNA antibody, or antiphospholipid antibodies.

CLINICAL PEARL

Lichenoid keratosis, also known as solitary lichen planus, is very similar to lichen planus histologically; however, orthokeratosis or parakeratosis may be seen focally (Fig. 39.11). Clinically, only a single lesion is apparent.

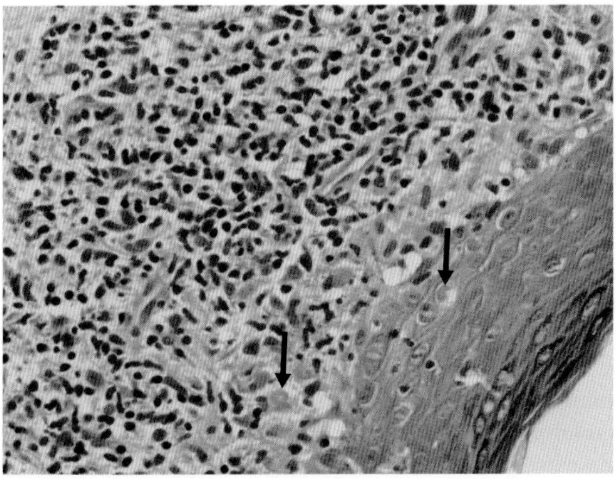

Fig. 39.11 Lichen keratosis with interface lymphoplasmacytic infiltrate and multiple Civatte bodies (black arrows) (H&E, 400x).

History of an allogenic bone marrow transplant would render GvHD in the differential. Histologically, interface dermatitis is a common feature. Hypergranulosis and irregular acanthosis with Civatte bodies are also typically present. However, GvHD may have less inflammation. Also, satellite cell necrosis and parakeratosis are seen more often in GvHD than in lichen planus.

CLINICAL PEARL

GvHD may affect multiple systems, particularly integument and gastrointestinal tract, and is most commonly seen in immunocompromised patients who receive allogenic bone marrow transplants. Donor T lymphocytes attack the recipient tissue due to incompatible major histocompatibility complex antigens.

Case Point 39.6

The patient denies any recent new medications or changes in medication. She has no history of malignancy or transplants. A diagnosis of lichen planus is rendered.

Lichen planus is an inflammatory dermatosis with etiology that is poorly understood. Less than 10% of cases may be associated with hepatitis C, which prompts testing for hepatitis C. Lichen planus is seen in middle-aged adults, with a slight predominance in women. The pruritic rash may be present for months but usually resolves in less than 2 years. Many sites may be affected, including the scalp, nails, and mucous membranes.

CLINICAL PEARL

Lichen planopilaris is a lichen planus variant on the scalp. It presents with scarring alopecia and follicular keratotic papules. The lymphocytes are predominantly found around plugged follicles and may spare the epidermis.

The histologic features of lichen planus are characteristic but may also be seen in other lichenoid dermatoses. The stratum corneum typically exhibits compact hyperkeratosis without parakeratosis (keratinocytes with retained nuclei). The underlying hypergranulosis is often wedge shaped. The rete ridges are "saw-toothed" due to irregular acanthosis. There is basal keratinocyte degeneration and liquefaction with the presence of colloid bodies (also known as Civatte bodies), which are degenerated keratinocytes, in the deep epidermis or superficial dermis. Pigmentation from melanin incontinence may be noted in long-standing lesions.

If untreated, lichen planus usually resolves on its own within 1 or 2 years; however, the pruritus may often be significantly disruptive for patients. The first-line treatment for lichen planus includes topical corticosteroids. Clobetasol propionate is a very-high-potency corticosteroid; betamethasone dipropionate is another corticosteroid in this class. Although they are considered relatively safe, there is risk of cutaneous atrophy, particularly if used on the face. Systemic glucocorticoids, oral acitretin, and phototherapy are second-line therapies with limited clinical data on efficacy. As lesions resolve, postinflammatory hyperpigmentation may persist.

Case Point 39.7

The patient is treated with clobetasol propionate ointment twice daily with instructions to taper its use as symptoms improve.

BEYOND THE PEARLS

- Squamous cell carcinoma may arise in ulcerative lichen planus, a rare variant. It is most commonly seen in chronic, traumatized oral lesions, particularly on the tongue. Biopsy is indicated in persistent ulcerative lesions of lichen planus to assess for malignancy.
- Lichen planus involves the oral mucosa 60%–70% of the time and may be the earliest or only site. Involvement of other mucosal sites, including penis, vagina, and anus, is less common.
- Besides oral lichen planus, other variants include actinic, atrophic, hypertrophic, annular, linear, bullous, and ulcerative lichen planus.
- The inflammatory infiltrate consists primarily of CD4+ T cells in early lesions. Bcl-2 is a proto-oncogene that prevents cellular apoptosis; its expression is increased in the infiltrating inflammatory cells of lichen planus.
- Immunofluorescence of lichen planus shows irregular deposition of complement and predominantly IgM in the papillary dermis. In addition, fibrin deposition is seen as an irregular band along the basal layer and papillary dermis.
- A familial predisposition to lichen planus is unlikely; there are rare familial cases. An association with HLA-D7 has been seen in these rare cases, and sporadic cases may be associated with HLA-DR1.

References

Collins G, Susa J, Cockerell C. *Contact Dermatitis*. ExpertPath. https://app.expertpath.com/document/contact-dermatitis. Accessed August 27, 2019.

Goldblum J, Lamps L, McKenney J, Myers J. *Rosai and Ackerman's Surgical Pathology*. 11th ed. Philadelphia, PA: Elsevier; 2018.

Hall B, Hall J, Fraga G. *Urticaria and Variants*. ExpertPath. https://app.expertpath.com/document/urticaria-and-variants. Accessed August 27, 2019.

Hiatt KM, SMoller BR. *Inflammatory Dermatoses. The Basics*. New York, NY Springer; 2010.

Jessup C, Mihm M. *Lichen Planus*. ExpertPath. https://app.expertpath.com/document/lichen-planus. Accessed August 27, 2019.

Motaparthi K. *Lichenoid Drug Eruptions*. ExpertPath. https://app.expertpath.com/document/lichenoid-drug-eruptions. Accessed August 27, 2019.

Nguyen K, Jessup C, Mihm M. *Lichen Simplex Chronicus*. ExpertPath. https://app.expertpath.com/document/lichen-simplex-chronicus. Accessed August 27, 2019.

Rapini R. *Practical Dermatopathology*. 2nd ed. Philadelphia, PA: Elsevier; 2012.

Venus M, Waterman J, McNab I. Basic physiology of the skin. *Surgery (Oxford)*. 2011;29(10):471–474. doi:10.1016/j.mpsur.2011.06.010.

Weedon D. *Weedon's Skin Pathology*. 3rd ed. London, UK: Churchill Livingstone Elsevier; 2010.

Wolff K, Katz GS, Gilchrest B, Paller AS, Leffell D. *Fitzpatrick's Dermatology in General Medicine*. 7th ed. New York, NY: McGraw-Hill; 2008.

CASE 40

A 75-Year-Old Male with a Blistering Skin Rash

Cynthia Reyes Barron ■ Tatsiana Pukhalskaya

A 75-year-old male presents to his primary care doctor complaining of a widespread pruritic, blistering skin rash. He had seen his primary care doctor for a rash 8 months prior. At that time, he had pruritic urticarial-type plaques on his back and bilateral antecubital fossae. His doctor prescribed antihistamines with some relief of pruritus. After 4 months, the rash spread to his shoulders and thighs and his doctor prescribed a topical steroid ointment with slight improvement. However, the persistent rash intensified and the lesions are now accompanied by diffuse bullae, prompting a referral to a dermatologist.

What infectious entities may present with vesiculobullous disease?

Shingles, a reactivation of latent varicella-zoster virus, is a common infectious cause of vesicular eruptions, particularly in an older patient. The vesicles are grouped and erupt from an erythematous base preceded by a painful or tingling sensation. The lesions follow the distribution of a dermatome and usually do not cross midline. Histologically, the blisters are intraepidermal with acantholytic keratinocytes in the cavity. Microscopic findings are indistinguishable from herpes simplex virus infections, and there are viral cytopathic changes.

BASIC SCIENCE PEARL

Cytopathic changes of herpes viral infections include the 3M's: Multinucleation, Margination of the chromatin, and Molding of the nuclei. Also, Cowdry type A nuclear inclusions may be observed. These are small eosinophilic deposits surrounded by a clear halo.

Impetigo is an acute pyogenic cutaneous infection typically affecting children. It may be nonbullous with thin vesicles that erupt easily to form crusted lesions or bullous with flaccid blisters and erosions. *Staphylococcus aureus* is usually the pathogenic culprit. The separation is intraepidermal and subcorneal. A superficial neutrophilic infiltrate is usually present.

Staphylococcal scalded skin syndrome is also more commonly seen in infants and children. It is caused by *S. aureus* exfoliative toxins A and B that cleave desmoglein-1 and cause superficial blistering separation between the stratum granulosum and spinosum layers. The onset is precipitous and usually involves the face and trunk. The bullae are large and flaccid with desquamation that forms large erosions and a positive Nikolsky sign. Dermal inflammation is sparse.

CLINICAL PEARL

The Nikolsky sign is often associated with pemphigus vulgaris but may also be observed in other blistering disorders with superficial epidermal damage. It refers to the clinical observation of blister formation following gentle pressure or slight friction on the skin.

Case Point 40.1

The patient received a shingles vaccine 3 years prior and denies fever, chills, and other signs of infection.

What malignancies may be associated with paraneoplastic bullous disease?

Paraneoplastic pemphigus is a rare blistering disorder preceding or accompanying an underlying malignancy. The most commonly associated neoplasms are non-Hodgkin lymphoma, chronic lymphocytic leukemia, Castleman's disease, carcinoma, thymoma, and sarcoma with lymphoproliferative disease implicated in the majority of cases. Clinically, the lesions may be bullous, lichenoid, or resemble erythema multiforme. Invariably, painful erosive stomatitis accompanies the cutaneous lesions. Serologically, testing reveals polyclonal IgG antibodies against plakin proteins and often desmogleins 1 and 3. Histologic findings vary because the lesions are generally polymorphous. Findings may include acantholysis, interface and lichenoid dermatitis, and vacuolar interface change. Blisters have an intraepidermal separation. Immunofluorescence studies will show characteristic deposition of IgG and complement on basilar and suprabasilar keratinocytes as well as basement membrane. However, false negatives are common. Paraneoplastic pemphigus has high mortality with few effective treatments available, and death often occurs due to sepsis and underlying complications of treatment or underlying malignancy.

Case Point 40.2

The patient has a history of basal cell carcinoma on the nose that was resected 10 years ago and no other history of malignancy. Additional medical history includes hypertension, hypercholesterolemia, and benign prostatic hyperplasia.

What medications may increase the risk of a bullous drug reaction?

Many drugs may induce skin eruptions that may be exanthematous, urticarial, lichenoid, pustular, or blistering. Blistering reactions may be severe, widespread/localized, and transient. Stevens–Johnson syndrome (SJS) and toxic epidermal necrolysis (TEN) are severe blistering disorders resulting in loss of skin and high mortality if untreated. Anticonvulsants such as phenytoin, carbamazepine, phenobarbital, and oxcarbazepine have been implicated as well as sulfonamide antibiotics, aminopenicillins, cephalosporins, quinolones, allopurinol, piroxicam, and dapsone.

CLINICAL PEARL

SJS and TEN are severe blistering disorders on a continuous spectrum. SJS involves less than 10% of the skin surface, and TEN involves greater than 30% with overlap between 10%–30%. There is high mortality if left untreated. Treatment consists of intravenous immunoglobulin, cyclosporine, and supportive care. Histologically, there is separation at the DE junction, mild inflammation, dyskeratosis, and full-thickness epidermal necrosis.

Other blistering drug eruptions may manifest as pseudoporphyria, a disorder that clinically and histologically resembles porphyria cutanea tarda (PCT) with normal urinary porphyrin levels. It has been associated with tetracycline, naproxen, and furosemide.

Linear IgA bullous dermatosis in adults is usually drug-induced and has been linked particularly to vancomycin as well as lithium, diclofenac, piroxicam, and amiodarone. The eruption consists of tense bullae and vesicles, erythematous patches, and erosions classically on the trunk and extremities. The bullae may form rings. Histologically, the blisters are large and subepidermal with collections of neutrophils and possibly eosinophils at the basement membrane and papillary tips, but the findings are not specific. A sharp linear band of IgA at the epidermal basement membrane zone identified by immunofluorescence is characteristic.

Drug-induced pemphigus may be seen with use of penicillamine, captopril, piroxicam, penicillin, rifampin, and propranolol. Finally, drug-induced bullous pemphigoid may develop with use of furosemide, penicillin, sulfasalazine, and angiotensin-converting enzyme inhibitors such as captopril.

A drug reaction may manifest as early as 1 day after initiating treatment or up to 1 year later. Therefore, efforts should be made to obtain a thorough patient history. Symptoms may resolve soon after discontinuation of the offending agent with supportive care only. However, drug-induced disease may also trigger persistent disease such as bullous pemphigoid by poorly understood immune-mediated mechanisms.

Case Point 40.4

The patient takes a calcium channel blocker and a statin as well as tamsulosin for urinary symptoms. He recalls no recent changes in medication and denies use of over-the-counter drugs other than occasional multivitamins and ibuprofen.

What inherited diseases may manifest with cutaneous blisters?

Porphyrias are a group of diseases caused by metabolic derangements in the biochemical synthesis of heme. PCT is the most common of these and may be familial, sporadic, or toxic. Patients have a defect in liver uroporphyrinogen decarboxylase function leading to accumulation of porphyrinogens that are transported to the skin and cause tissue damage when activated by light. The photosensitive cutaneous manifestations include vesicles and bullae with erosions and ulcers, alterations in skin pigmentation, sclerodermoid changes, scarring alopecia, onycholysis, and hypertrichosis of temples and cheeks (Fig. 40.1). Histologically, PCT has subepidermal blisters

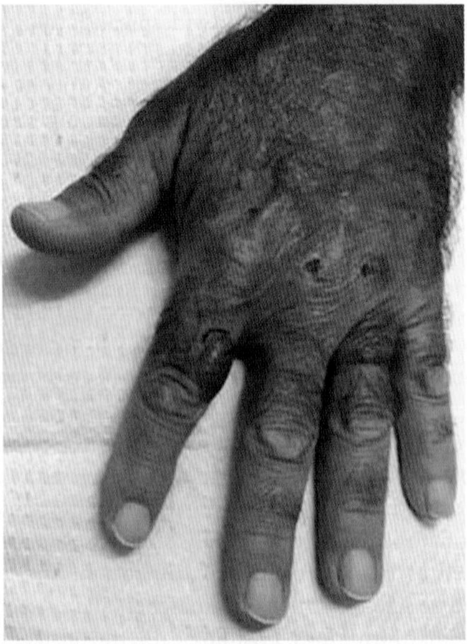

Fig. 40.1 Bullae of porphyria cutanea tarda on the dorsum of hand.

with scant inflammation and milia. Dermal vessels are hyalinized and thickened, with dermal festooning (projection of dermal papillae into blister cavity). Caterpillar bodies, which consist of type IV collagen, may be seen at the roof of the blister with erythrocytes inside the blister.

CLINICAL PEARL

In PCT, the cutaneous deposits of uroporphyrinogen decarboxylase react with ultraviolet light to produce reactive oxygen species with subsequent tissue damage manifested as vesicles and bullae. Other factors that exacerbate the condition include alcohol, oral contraceptives, hepatitis C, HIV, and hepatotoxins.

Darier disease, also known as keratosis follicularis, is an autosomal dominant disease caused by mutations in the ATP2A2 gene. Clinically, the lesions are verrucous and greasy plaques, papules or vesicles, and bullae. They may be extensive and foul smelling, and are commonly distributed in seborrheic areas such as the scalp, forehead, upper chest, and back. Histologically, there is marked hyperkeratosis and dyskeratosis in spinous and granular layers and acantholytic parakeratotic cells. Acantholysis is suprabasilar with cleft formation. There is usually a mild lymphocytic infiltrate.

Hailey–Hailey disease, also known as familial benign chronic pemphigus, is an autosomal dominant disease caused by mutations in the ATP2C1 gene. The lesions consist of small vesicles that are flaccid and have an erythematous base located mainly in the axillae and groin. Often, painful fissures form along flexural sites, and nails may display longitudinal white lines. Histologically, the roof of the blister has been described as a dilapidated brick wall because there is extensive loss of intercellular adhesion in the epidermis. There is a mixed inflammatory infiltrate and prominent spongiosis.

Epidermolysis bullosa is a group of inherited disorders that predispose patients to blistering or erosions with minor trauma. There is a spectrum of severity, and inheritance may be autosomal dominant or recessive depending on the specific etiology. Patients inherit mutations in proteins, including the basal cell cytoskeleton, anchoring filaments, and collagen fibrils, which are critical for the integrity of the basement membrane zone. Most cases are caused by mutations in cytokeratins 5 and 14. Bullae usually appear at acral sites and in areas prone to trauma such as the hands, feet, elbows, and knees. They may be present at birth or appear during childhood. Depending on the severity, some heal with scarring leading to alopecia and deformities including the mitten deformity caused by fusion of fingers or toes. The disease may affect eyelids and esophageal epithelium. Histologically, the bullae are subepidermal and have minimal inflammation.

CLINICAL PEARL

Acquired epidermolysis bullosa (epidermolysis bullosa acquisita) is an autoimmune disease with similar clinical presentation to the inherited forms. It is associated with hepatitis C as well as autoimmune or inflammatory diseases, such as inflammatory bowel disease, systemic lupus erythematosus, diabetes, and rheumatoid arthritis. It is also associated with certain malignancies including ovarian, cervical, uterine, gastric, and pancreatic cancers as well as multiple myeloma.

Case Point 40.5

There is no family or personal history of bullous cutaneous disease. The patient cannot recall a similar bullous eruption in the past.

What features should be noted on physical examination when evaluating a cutaneous bullous disorder?
As with other skin lesions, the location and extent of involvement is very important. For example, SJS has characteristic, exudative erosions of the oral mucosa. Pemphigus vulgaris commonly involves the scalp. Friction blisters, as the name implies, occur on the sites of friction such as palms and soles; pressure blisters may be seen in comatose patients on dependent surfaces including heels and upper extremities. PCT occurs on sun-exposed skin, and herpes zoster follows a dermatome. The bullous eruptions of dermatitis herpetiformis usually occur on the elbows and knees.

As the name implies, dermatitis herpetiformis manifests with small, grouped, erythematous lesions reminiscent of herpetic eruptions. The lesions consist of small vesicles which are rarely observed intact because they are intensely pruritic. Dermatitis herpetiformis is associated with gluten-sensitive enteropathy with circulating autoantibodies against epidermal transglutaminase and improves with a gluten-free diet.

The quality of the blisters themselves is important. In bullous pemphigoid and epidermolysis bullosa, two diseases with subepidermal separation, the blisters are tense, while pemphigus with intraepidermal separation manifests with flaccid bullae. Vesicles are defined as fluid-filled raised lesions measuring less than 5 mm in diameter, whereas bullae are large vesicles measuring greater than 5 mm in diameter. Many blistering diseases are vesiculobullous with lesions in a range of sizes. Some, like dermatitis herpetiformis, are classically vesicular, whereas others, like SJS, are classically bullous and present with large coalescing lesions. Pustules are vesicles or bullae that contain abundant neutrophils in the fluid.

BASIC SCIENCE PEARL

Many adhesion proteins play an important role in maintaining the integrity of the skin. Blistering occurs when this integrity is disrupted. Desmogleins are the most prominent adhesion molecules in the epidermis and are part of the cadherin family of proteins. Desmogleins 1 and 3 are targeted by autoantibodies in various disease entities. The hemidesmosomes that anchor basal keratinocytes to the basement membrane rely on integrin proteins.

Case Point 40.6

On physical examination, a full survey of the patient's skin is conducted revealing numerous blisters on the back, shoulders, arms, axillae, thighs, and inguinal region. The bullae are tense and measure approximately 1–4 cm in diameter. Some of the blisters are associated with urticarial plaques, others have erythematous bases. There are numerous ruptured bullae with different stages of erosion and crusting. There is no mucosal involvement.

What histologic features aid in the classification of a cutaneous bullous disease?
The histologic findings narrow the differential. The first feature to note is the anatomic level of the separation within the epidermis or subepidermis. Bullae are divided into two major categories: intraepidermal and subepidermal. The intraepidermal category is further subdivided into suprabasal, spinous, and subcorneal (Table 40.1). The quality of the blister depends on the level of the separation and the epidermal adhesion molecule that has been damaged. Suprabasilar separation occurs within the epidermis and is characteristic of disorders with acantholysis and autoantibodies against cell-cell adhesion proteins, desmogleins. In contrast, subepidermal separation, which occurs at the level of the dermal–epidermal (DE) junction, is characteristic of disease with autoantibodies directed against hemidesmosome proteins anchoring the keratinocytes to the basement membrane, such as bullous pemphigoid.

Additional histologic findings will help determine the mechanisms involved in the disruption of the skin's integrity. Spongiosis refers to intercellular edema. Marked spongiosis disrupts cell-cell adhesion leading to formation of vesicles. Viral infection may lead to swelling of keratinocytes and

TABLE 40.1 ■ **Selected Vesiculobullous Diseases With Histologic and Immunofluorescence Findings**

Location of Vesiculobullous Separation	Diagnosis	Histology	Immunofluorescence Findings
Intraepidermal - subcorneal	Pemphigus foliaceus	Mild acantholysis, cleft in granular layer, eosinophilic spongiosis and scattered eosinophils in dermis	IgG and C3 intercellular epidermal net-like deposits (Fig. 40.2)
	Staphylococcal scalded skin syndrome	Sparse mixed inflammatory infiltrate	Negative
	Bullous impetigo	Mild acantholysis, superficial neutrophilic infiltrate, superficial perivascular lymphocytic infiltrate	Negative
Intraepidermal - spinous	Hailey–Hailey disease	Extensive epidermal acantholysis resulting in "dilapidated brick wall" appearance; mixed inflammatory infiltrate	Negative
	Friction blister	Keratinocyte necrosis deep to stratum granulosum with degenerated keratinocytes on blister floor, scant inflammation	Negative
Intraepidermal - suprabasal	Pemphigus vulgaris	Acantholysis, "tombstoning" of basal keratinocytes, eosinophils	IgG and C3 intercellular epidermal net-like deposits
	Paraneoplastic pemphigus	Acantholysis, variable interface dermatitis with scattered dying keratinocytes, eosinophils in superficial dermis	IgG and C3 intercellular epidermal net-like deposits
	Darier disease	Acantholysis, hyperkeratosis, dyskeratosis, mild lymphoid infiltrate	Negative
Subepidermal	Porphyria cutanea tarda	Scant inflammation, festooning of dermal papillae	IgG and C3 around papillary dermal vessels with less staining at dermal–epidermal junction in lamina lucida
	Bullous pemphigoid	Eosinophils and lymphocytes in blister cavity and superficial dermis, abundant spongiosis without necrosis	IgG and C3 linear deposits at epidermal basement membrane zone
	Dermatitis herpetiformis	Small blisters, dermal papillary neutrophilic abscesses, superficial perivascular lymphocytes	IgA granular deposits in the epidermal basement membrane zone (Fig. 40.3)
	Linear IgA dermatosis	Abundant neutrophils at basement membrane and dermal papillary tips with scattered eosinophils	IgA linear deposits at epidermal basement membrane zone
	Epidermolysis bullosa acquisita	Scant inflammation	IgG and C3 linear deposits at epidermal basement membrane zone

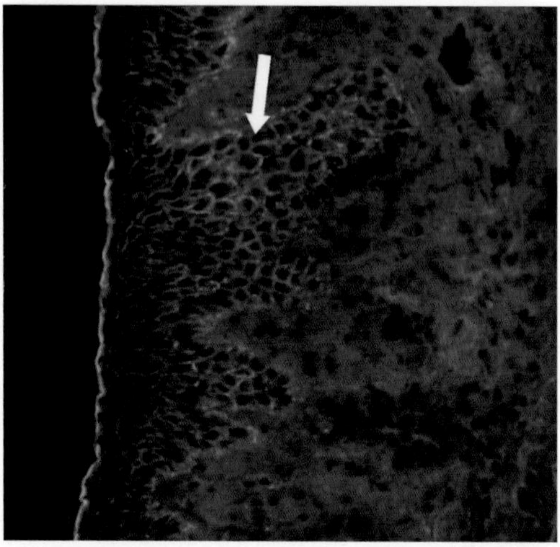

Fig. 40.2 Pemphigus foliaceus net-like C3 intercellular deposition on direct immunofluorescence of skin biopsy (white arrow); IgG showed a similar pattern.

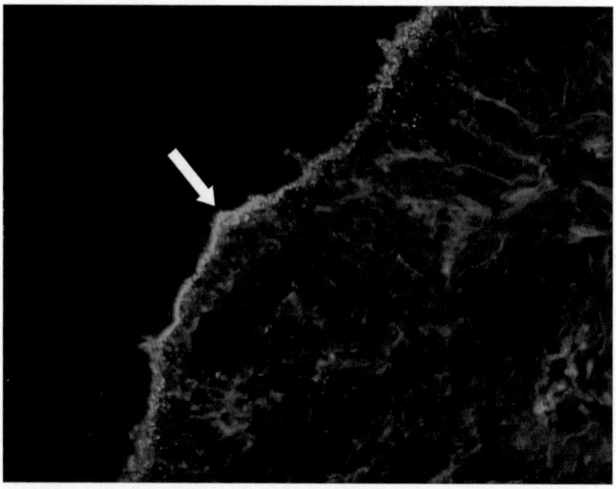

Fig. 40.3 Dermatitis herpetiformis granular IgA deposition in dermal papillae on direct immunofluorescence of skin biopsy (white arrow).

ballooning degeneration, thereby also disrupting cell-cell adhesion. Full-thickness necrosis is characteristic of TEN. Abnormalities in the keratinocytes such as dyskeratosis should also be noted. Acantholysis is the loss of cell-cell adhesion within the epidermis resulting in detached keratinocytes that appear to be floating among the others, and often accompanies a suprabasilar split.

BASIC SCIENCE PEARL

When the blistering separation is suprabasilar, basal keratinocytes may remain attached to the basement membrane, resulting in the "tombstone" effect, commonly used to describe the histologic findings of pemphigus vulgaris (Fig. 40.4).

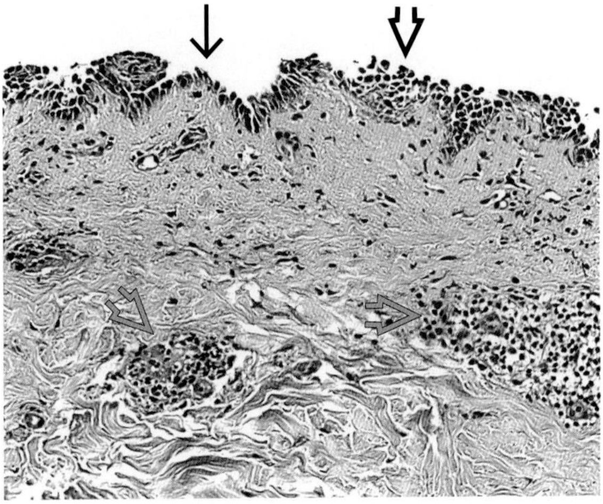

Fig. 40.4 Pemphigus vulgaris skin biopsy showing suprabasilar acantholysis (black open arrow) and characteristic tombstoning of the papillary dermis with basal keratinocytes (black solid arrow). Note the associated dermal perivascular infiltrate (cyan open arrows). (From *ExpertPath*. Copyright Elsevier).

Acantholysis is present in many bullous disorders, in particular those belonging to the pemphigus group. Pemphigus vulgaris is the most common variant. Autoantibodies against epithelial adhesion protein desmoglein 3 result in the damage of intercellular attachments in the epidermis and a suprabasilar intraepidermal separation. Eosinophils may be found within the blister cavity or superficial dermis. The mucosal epithelium is also affected, and oral blisters are often the initial manifestation, followed by blisters commonly on the trunk, groin, axillae, scalp, and face. The Nikolsky sign and the Asboe–Hansen sign (lateral blister extension with gentle pressure) are present. Mortality due to infection and sepsis has decreased with prompt diagnosis and appropriate treatment.

CLINICAL PEARL

Pemphigus vegetans is a variant of pemphigus vulgaris with localized manifestations that presents with verrucous, vegetating plaques surfaced by scattered pustules on the groin, axillae, and flexural surfaces. Autoantibodies against desmoglein 3, among others, are typically present.

Pemphigus foliaceus is a superficial variant that results from autoantibodies against desmoglein 1, and the oral mucosa is usually spared (Fig. 40.5). It is endemic in Brazil.

Pemphigus erythematosus results from autoantibodies to intercellular and basement membrane antigens. It may present with crusted plaques in the malar distribution, typical of lupus erythematosus.

Finally, the features of the inflammatory cell component, if present, are important in arriving at a diagnosis. The presence of neutrophils and eosinophils within the blister and in the dermis provides clues to the etiology of blister formation, particularly in the subepidermal category. Abundant neutrophils can be found at the basement membrane of linear IgA dermatosis, whereas lesions in PCT have no inflammatory infiltrate.

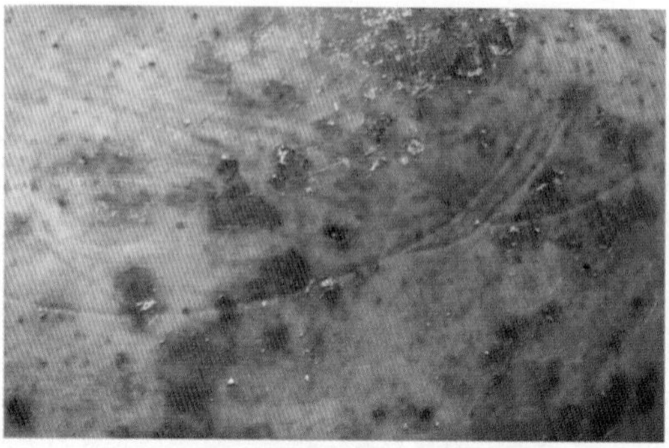

Fig. 40.5 Superficial lesions of pemphigus foliaceus on patient's back.

Case Point 40.7

A punch biopsy is taken from the edge of a newly formed blister. Sections show dermal–epidermal separation at the level of the junction (Fig. 40.6). Scattered eosinophils are identified within the blister cavity and in the superficial dermis (Fig. 40.7).

How is direct immunofluorescence performed on cutaneous biopsy specimens?

Direct immunofluorescence is a valuable tool for the diagnosis of cutaneous vesiculobullous disorders. Biopsy specimens are not placed in formalin for fixation, as done for usual histologic studies. Instead, they are placed in special media such as Michel's media or processed from frozen tissue sections. Slides are prepared from cut sections, typically 5 microns in thickness, and stained with antigens against immunoglobulins IgG, IgA, and IgM as well as complement factor C3 and fibrinogen. The antigens are conjugated to a fluorescent dye. Examination under a fluorescence microscope reveals characteristic patterns for multiple entities (Table 40.1).

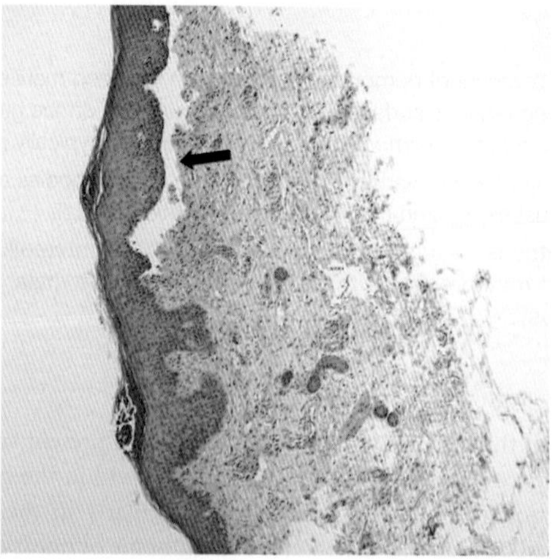

Fig. 40.6 Bulla with subepidermal separation (black arrow) on patient's skin biopsy (H&E, 40x).

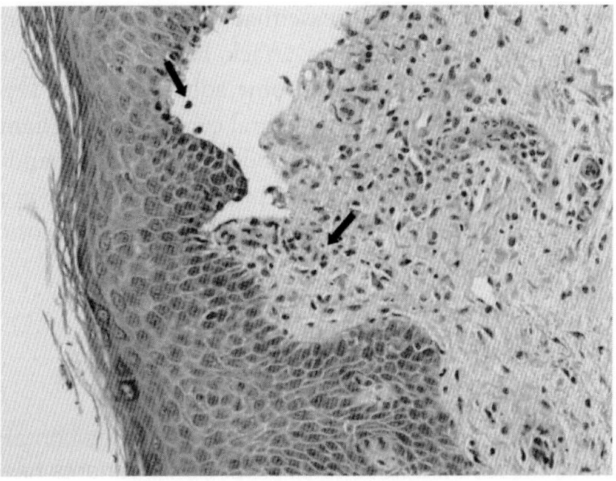

Fig. 40.7 Bullous pemphigoid with eosinophils in the blister cavity and superficial dermis (black arrow) on patient's skin biopsy (H&E, 200x).

Case Point 40.8

Direct immunofluorescence studies are conducted on the frozen tissue. Sections are cut 5 microns in thickness and stained with antibodies against human proteins: IgG, IgA, IgM, C3, and fibrinogen. Sharp, bright, linear staining with IgG and C3 is noted along the basement membrane in the tissue adjacent to the blister (Fig. 40.8). IgA and IgM are negative, fibrinogen has high background staining.

The clinical, histologic, and immunofluorescence studies are consistent with a diagnosis of bullous pemphigoid.

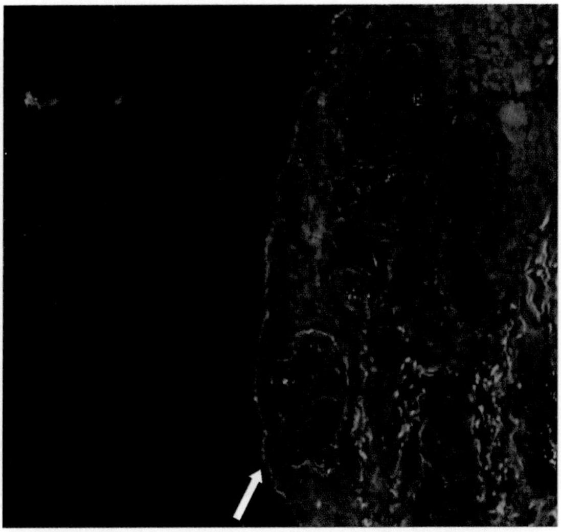

Fig. 40.8 Bullous pemphigoid linear IgG deposition at basement membrane zone (white arrow) on immunofluorescence of patient's skin biopsy.

Bullous pemphigoid is an autoimmune disease that usually affects older adults, with a slightly higher incidence in men. IgG autoantibodies attack bullous pemphigoid antigens 1 and 2 (BPAG1 and BPAG2) at the site of hemidesmosome adhesion in the DE junction. The bullae are tense and range in size from 1 centimeter to several centimeters in diameter (Fig. 40.9). They are commonly symmetrically spread through the abdomen, forearms, and thighs with very rare involvement of the mucosa. The bullae are severely pruritic and may be preceded by an urticarial prodrome. Histologically, the subepidermal cleft may contain numerous eosinophils. A perivascular lymphocytic infiltrate often affects superficial dermal vessels.

CLINICAL PEARL

Like bullous pemphigoid, cicatricial pemphigoid has linear deposition of IgG at the basement membrane zone and autoantibodies to BPAG2. Some variants have antibodies against antilaminin 332 or beta-4 integrin. Unlike bullous pemphigoid, there is atrophy and scarring of tissue, and 85% of cases present with oral lesions. An ocular variant may lead to blindness.

What is the treatment and prognosis of bullous pemphigoid?

Bullous pemphigoid is a chronic disease with remissions and exacerbations. The manifestation of bullous pemphigoid may be self-limited and resolve without treatment in months to a year. The lesions heal without scarring. The goal of treatment is to improve quality of life and manage symptoms. High-potency topical steroids or systemic glucocorticoids are first-line treatments. Other options include immunomodulatory agents such as mycophenolate mofetil, azathioprine, and methotrexate. High-dose intravenous immunoglobulin and plasmapheresis are options for refractory disease.

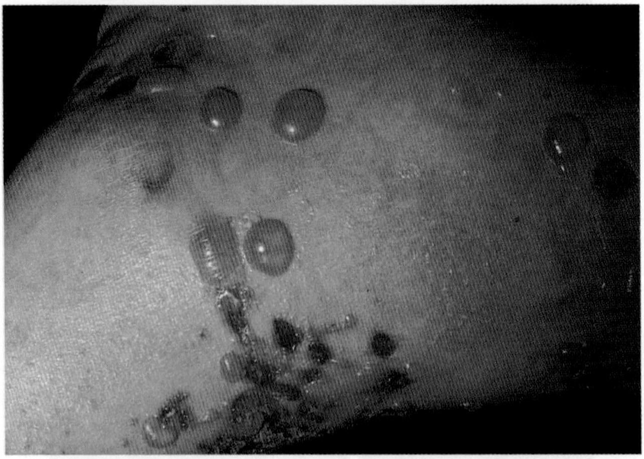

Fig. 40.9 Large bullae of bullous pemphigoid. (From Goldblum J, Lamps L, McKenney J, Myers J. *Rosai and Ackerman's Surgical Pathology*. 11th ed. Philadelphia, PA: Elsevier; 2018. Figure 2.46.)

Case Point 40.9

The patient is treated with oral prednisone with rapid improvement of pruritus and resolution of bullous eruptions.

Complaint/History: A 75-year-old man presents with a pruritic blistering rash affecting the trunk and upper and lower extremities.

Findings: Examination reveals widespread tense bullae with various stages of erosion and association with urticarial plaques.

Labs/Tests: No serologic laboratory tests are conducted, but a biopsy and direct immunofluorescence studies combined with clinical history and physical examination findings are diagnostic for bullous pemphigoid.

Diagnosis: Bullous pemphigoid.

Treatment: Oral prednisone.

BEYOND THE PEARLS

- Many factors may predispose individuals to develop adverse cutaneous drug reactions including HLA genotype, pharmacogenetic variations, and concurrent use of multiple medications as well as age and medical comorbidities.
- Bullous systemic lupus erythematosus presents in patients with severe inflammation, more commonly in acute or subacute cutaneous lupus erythematosus.
- ATP2A2, mutated in Darier disease, and ATP2C1, mutated in Hailey–Hailey disease, code for calcium pump proteins. Defects in these calcium pumps result in defective keratinocyte structure and function.
- The best place to see the IgG/C3 deposits by direct immunofluorescence in a biopsy specimen is at the DE junction adjacent to a blister. The disrupted nature of the blister itself obscures the deposits.
- A bullous lesion that was originally subepidermal may become intraepidermal due to re-epithelialization in the natural healing process. The best lesions to biopsy are new lesions, less than 24 hours old.
- Indirect immunofluorescence can be performed by taking serum from the patient and testing on normal human skin. If present, antibodies against desmosome and hemidesmosome antigens will bind on the cell surface in recognizable patterns.
- IgG autoantibodies in bullous pemphigoid are capable of activating complement by the classical pathway, leading to blister formation.
- Laboratory studies of patients with bullous pemphigoid often show eosinophilia in the peripheral blood and elevated IgE.

References

Elston D, Ferringer T, Ko C, et al. *Dermatopathology*. 3rd ed. Philadelphia, PA: Elsevier; 2018.

Goldblum J, Lamps L, McKenney J, Myers J. *Rosai and Ackerman's Surgical Pathology*. 11th ed. Philadelphia, PA: Elsevier; 2018.

Hiatt KM, Smoller BR. *Inflammatory Dermatoses: The Basics*. New York, NY: Springer; 2010.

Rapini R. *Practical Dermatopathology*. 2nd ed. Philadelphia, PA: Elsevier; 2012.

Taylor, E. *Pemphigus and Variants*. ExpertPath. https://app.expertpath.com/document/pemphigus-and-variants. Accessed August 23, 2019.

Weedon D. *Weedon's Skin Pathology*. 3rd ed. London, UK: Churchill Livingstone Elsevier; 2010

Wolff K, Katz GS, Gilchrest B, Paller AS, Leffell D. *Fitzpatrick's Dermatology in General Medicine*. 7th ed. New York, NY: McGraw-Hill; 2008.

CASE 41

A 65-Year-Old Female with a Pre-Auricular Skin Lesion

Tatsiana Pukhalskaya ■ Cynthia Reyes Barron ■ Julia Stiegler

A 65-year-old Caucasian female presents to her dermatologist for her annual skin examination. She noticed a new small lesion on her right ear that is not healing for several months. She has lived in Florida her entire life. She states that in her 20s, she used to be addicted to the sun and applied iodine and baby oil to her skin to tan faster. She is healthy overall and sees her primary care physician on an annual basis. She has never smoked and consumes alcohol socially. On full body skin examination, she has found to have a new, solitary, pink, well-circumscribed nodule measuring 0.5 cm with pearly elevated borders and mild telangiectasia on the anterior helix of the right ear (Fig. 41.1). In the office, the dermatologist performed a shave biopsy.

What is the differential diagnosis for nonhealing skin lesions with a history of long-term sun exposure?

This patient is an elderly woman with long-term skin exposure to ultraviolet (UV) radiation. Such a scenario is very common in the dermatological practice and should prompt high clinical

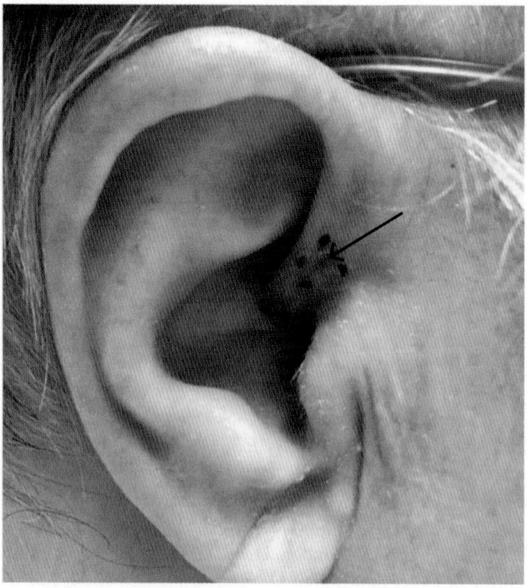

Fig. 41.1 Patient with lesion (arrow) on right pre-auricular area.

suspicion for skin malignancy. Overall, malignancies of the skin are the most commonly diagnosed cancers in the United States, with over a million new cases diagnosed annually and more than 10,000 deaths/year. They are commonly divided into two main categories, melanoma and non-melanoma skin cancers (NMSCs). Malignant melanoma accounts for roughly 4% of skin neoplasms but is the deadliest form. Conversely, NMSCs, derived from epidermal keratinocytes, are much more frequently diagnosed but cause fewer deaths. Basal cell carcinoma (BCC) and squamous cell carcinoma (SCC) together make up NMSC tumors, with BCC being the most common skin malignancy overall. Among Caucasians, the estimated lifetime risk for BCC is roughly 35% for men and 25% for women.

CLINICAL PEARL

Skin malignancies occur most commonly on the sun-exposed skin of the face, scalp, ears, and neck, and less often on the trunk and extremities. BCC tends to occur above the lip, whereas SCC occurs below the lip.

What are the major risk factors in the development of skin malignancy?

Although keratinocyte malignancies and melanomas display markedly different clinical characteristics, they share many common risk factors. Intensity of skin pigmentation correlates with the development of both melanoma and non-melanoma skin cancers, and in general, Caucasians are at much higher risk of skin malignancies than people of African, Asian, or Latino descent. As a rule, exposure to UV radiation is the main risk factor for the development of skin malignancy. UV radiation in the form of ambient sunlight or artificial tanning beds is a clear risk factor for BCC, SCC, and melanoma. Because more UV radiation can penetrate under non-melanized skin, fair-skinned individuals accrue more cancer-causing UV-induced mutations than highly pigmented individuals. Each of the skin malignancies is clearly linked to UV radiation, with chronic cumulative UV exposure being most relevant for BCC and SCC and intense, blistering sunburns most relevant for melanoma. Additionally, patient's age is a significant factor to consider, because the incidence of skin malignancy markedly increases with age. For BCC, the incidence doubles every 25 years and is very rarely diagnosed in patients aged below 40 years. The reason skin cancer incidence increases with age is not clearly understood, but may reflect the typical long latency required for the accumulation of sufficient mutations to result in carcinogenesis. Another significant risk factor in the development of skin malignancy is immunosuppression. Individuals with defective immunity, particularly T-cell immunity, are at increased risk for skin cancer. Thus, patients with inherited or acquired immune defects or those receiving immunosuppressive therapies (e.g., transplant recipients or cancer patients) all have a much higher risk of melanoma, BCC, and SCC than do other patients. Other risk factors include heavy metal exposure (e.g., chromium and cobalt) and defective DNA repair, particularly nucleotide excision repair (NER). NER is the major DNA repair pathway that reverses UV-induced photolesions (e.g., cyclobutane dimers, [6,4]-photoproducts).

What is the mechanism of skin carcinogenesis due to sunlight exposure?

UV radiation can promote carcinogenesis in multiple ways. First, UV energy can directly affect nucleotides in the double helix of genomic DNA, particularly the cleavage of the 5,6-double bond of pyrimidines. When two adjacent pyrimidines undergo this change, a covalent ring structure referred to as a cyclobutane pyrimidine (thymine) dimer can be formed. These molecular lesions can alter DNA structure, cause misreading during transcription or replication, or lead to arrest of replication. It is known that both BCC and SCC exhibit mutation of tumor suppressor p53 by formation of pyrimidine dimers. Second, UV radiation can damage cells by free radical formation and oxidative stress. Oxidative DNA lesions are also mutagenic and form after UV-induced free radical attack. Consequently, damaged keratinocytes trigger a cutaneous inflammatory response. As an attempt to avoid malignant transformation, they activate their surface death receptors (e.g., Fas), which leads to apoptosis. It is also essential to mention melanin (epidermal pigment) as the most important defense mechanism against UV damage. Melanin is a UV-absorbing pigment that dissipates UV radiation as heat. Therefore, UV-induced tan acts as a photo protection by providing a sun protection factor.

Case Point 41.1

The patient's shave biopsy was submitted for microscopic evaluation and demonstrates a neoplasm that histologically comprises several well-defined dermal nodules surrounded by mild chronic inflammation. Nodules are composed of small basaloid cells with large, elongated nuclei and scant pink cytoplasm. There is a notable palisading at the periphery of the nodules and several areas of separation between the nodule and surrounding stroma (clefting) (Fig. 41.2). The patient was diagnosed with a nodular BCC.

What are common dermoscopic features of BCC?

Our patient's skin lesion demonstrates all characteristic dermoscopic features of BCC. Usually it is a pink, violaceous or pearly-white, sometimes translucent appearing papule or nodule. Lesions may have a smooth surface with overlying telangiectasia. These tumors frequently bleed, become erosive, crusted, and ulcerate in the center. BCC may contain melanin that appears speckled brown, black, or blue.

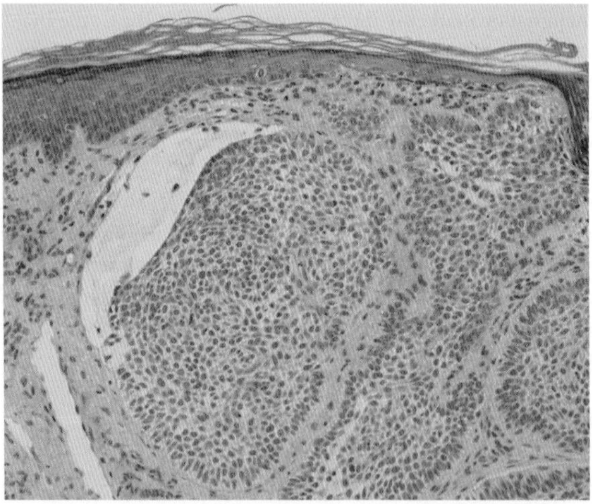

Fig. 41.2 Patient's skin biopsy demonstrating nodular variant of basal cell carcinoma. There are several well-defined dermal nodules composed of small dark basaloid cells with surrounding chronic inflammatory response. There is a notable palisading at the periphery of the nodules and several areas of separation between the nodule and surrounding stroma (clefting) (H&E, 40x).

What are common histologic features of BCC?

BCC displays a variety of growth patterns and even pattern combinations. Despite its histological diversity, this tumor tends to exhibit a hallmark blend of easily recognizable features highlighted below.

CLINICAL PEARL

Common histologic features of BCC:

- Cells with large, elongated nuclei that display variably prominent palisading at the edge of tumor nodules.
- Cytoplasm may be inconspicuous, pale, or lightly eosinophilic.
- Mitoses and single-cell apoptoses are usually present and may be prominent.
- Intratumoral mucin may form large pools or cystic spaces.
- Presence of characteristic clefting between the stroma and edges of tumor nodules, which may be extensive or focal.

What are the common immunostains used for BCC?

In majority of cases, BCC is easily recognizable and does not require additional studies. When it presents in its uncommon form, it might need to be distinguished from architecturally similar lesions by means of immunohistochemistry. BCC expresses cytokeratin CK5/6 and CK14 and is negative for cytokeratin CK20. Ber-EP4 typically shows strong expression. There is also diffuse nuclear expression of p63.

What are behavioral features of different histologic patterns of BCC?

Histologic patterns of BCC represent a major predictor of tumor behavior. They are broadly divided into nonaggressive (indolent) and aggressive types. Indolent BCC variants include superficial and nodular variants, where as aggressive growth variants are micronodular, infiltrative, morpheaform, and metatypical (Table 41.1). The latter demonstrate higher rates of recurrence and metastasis (although metastasis is rare for BCC of any growth pattern).

What is an "alternative differentiation pattern" and how does it relate to BCC?

The term "alternative differentiation" applies when histologic features of one tumor resemble those of tumors of different origin. For example, nodular BCC in particular may resemble adnexal tumors or, in some regions, SCC. These tumors are described as BCC with basosquamous, cystic, adenoid, pigmented, and infundibulocystic differentiation (Fig. 41.3A–E). The diversity in the phenotypic appearance of BCCs indicates that the cell of origin may be a stem or progenitor cell.

TABLE 41.1 ■ **Common Histologic Patterns of Basal Cell Carcinoma (BCC)**

Histologic Pattern	Histologic Picture
Superficial and nodular patterns	Small lobules extending into the papillary dermis from the basal layer of the epidermis or large nodules in the papillary and reticular dermis, respectively Cleft retraction, peripheral palisading, and stromal mucin are often prominent
Infiltrating pattern	Angulated nests and strands of tumor cells in a prominent, fibroblastic stroma
Micronodular pattern	Round to oval tumor nests, but unlike nodular BCC, the nests are smaller and widely dispersed
Pigmented pattern	Increased number of intratumoral melanocytes in scattered array
Morpheaform pattern	Thin columns and small nodules associated with intensely collagenized stroma
Metatypical pattern	BCC has a component of squamous differentiation within angulated nests of tumor cells, imparting morphologic overlap with squamous cell carcinoma

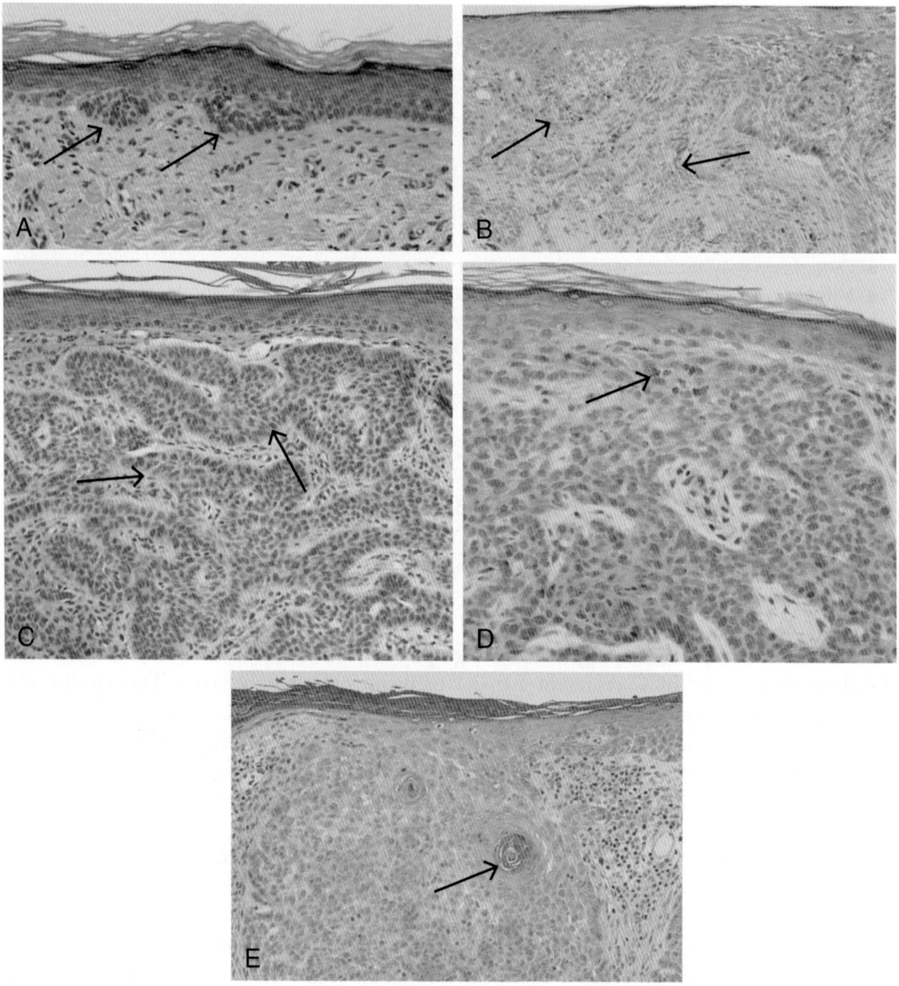

Fig. 41.3 Basal cell carcinoma: (A) Superficial variant. Biopsy demonstrates small lobules of darker cells extending into the papillary dermis from the basal layer of the epidermis (arrows) (H&E stain, 100x). (B) Infiltrating variant. Biopsy demonstrates angulated nests and strands of tumor cells (arrow) in a prominent, fibroblastic stroma (H&E stain, 100x). (C) Micronodular variant. Biopsy demonstrates widely dispersed oval tumor nests (arrows) (H&E stain, 40x). (D) Nodular pigmented variant. Biopsy demonstrates dermal nodules composed of basaloid cells with focal pigment deposition (arrow) (H&E stain, 40x). (E) With focal squamous differentiation. Biopsy demonstrates dermal nodule with focal formation of pink globules (keratin pearl; arrow) (H&E stain, 40x).

What genetic syndromes are associated with increased risk of BCC?

Increased risk of BCC may occur in the setting of certain inherited syndromes. The key role for the sonic hedgehog signaling pathway in BCC is highlighted by Gorlin–Goltz syndrome (basal cell nevus syndrome), which is an autosomal dominant condition related to germline patched 1(PTCH1) mutation. Other tumor syndromes that predispose patients to BCC are associated with decreased skin pigmentation or epidermal genomic instability, including xeroderma pigmentosum (XP), Rombo syndrome, and Bazex–Dupré–Christol syndrome.

CLINICAL PEARL

Gorlin–Goltz syndrome: multiple BCCs with a young age of onset, keratocystic odontogenic tumors, medulloblastoma, cardiac and ovarian fibromas, and other skeletal anomalies

XP: a clinical condition of homozygous deficiency of NER pathway. Patients with XP suffer lifelong extreme sensitivity to UV radiation with the highest risk for all types of UV-induced skin cancers (including melanoma). Thus, these individuals suffer severe and disfiguring UV-induced skin changes, and have a greatly increased (>1000-fold) incidence of skin cancers, often with their first skin cancer arising during childhood.

Bazex–Dupré–Christol syndrome: manifests during the neonatal period or during infancy. It is characterized by hypotrichosis, hypohidrosis, milia, and BCCs of early onset.

Rombo syndrome: characterized by vermiculate atrophoderma, milia, hypotrichosis, tricho-epitheliomas, peripheral vasodilation with cyanosis, and BCCs. The skin lesions become visible between 7 and 10 years of age and are most pronounced on the face. BCCs are frequent and develop at around 35 years of age.

Case Point 41.2

Two weeks after the biopsy, our patient is back to the office for the treatment. Her best options include an excision versus a Mohs surgery. As the lesion is located on the face, the dermatologist advocates proceeding with a Mohs procedure, which will assure the patient's best cosmetic result.

What are common treatment options for BCC?

The goal of the treatment is eradication of the tumor and return of normal anatomic form and function. Treatment of BCC is determined by the size and location of the tumor, the histologic variant, and the patient's concern (Table 41.2). Without treatment, BCC persists, enlarges, ulcerates, and invades and destroys the surrounding structures. Inadequately treated BCCs can recur, often underneath areas of scarring, which may lead to delay in detection.

Case Point 41.3

The patient is successfully treated with Mohs surgery and given recommendations to avoid sunlight exposure and usage of tanning beds. Recommendations also include the use of sunblock daily and to see a dermatologist every 6–12 months for full-body skin examination. Before leaving the office, she is confident that she is able to recognize the first signs of BCC but is curious to know about other skin lesions and malignancies that might develop due to her history of extensive sun exposure.

What is a common non-malignancy related to long-term sun exposure?

Years of cumulative sun exposure and keratinocyte damage lead to the formation of actinic keratosis (AK). These lesions are considered an intraepidermal precursor or early lesion of SCC. Individual lesions become progressively more common after the age of 40 years. Spontaneous regression and progression to SCC can occur. It initially presents as a poorly defined area of redness or telangiectasia. Over time, the lesion becomes more defined and develops a thin, adherent, yellowish or transparent scale. Biopsy is helpful to distinguish advanced AK from invasive SCC. The histologic marker of AK is a disordered epidermis with intraepidermal keratinocyte atypia (Fig. 41.4A and B).

TABLE 41.2 ■ **Treatment Options of Basal Cell Carcinoma (BCC)**

Treatment Option	Characteristic
Topical chemotherapy and immunotherapy	Imiquimod (an immune response modifier) and fluorouracil (topical chemotherapeutic agent) are used to treat superficial BCC
Photodynamic therapy	Includes topical application of photosensitizing agent with subsequent exposure to a light source. Light converts the agent into an oxidant that is damaging to most cancerous cells. Used for superficial BCC
Cryotherapy	By means of liquid nitrogen; used mainly for thin superficial BCC
Curettage	Physical "scraping-off" of the tumor with the curette; used for small, nodular-type BCC
Electrosurgery	Involves alternation curettage with the use of electrosurgical devise (electrodessication); used for superficial and small nodular BCC
Excision	Preferred method of removal for nonfacial BCC; allows conformation of surgical margins
Mohs surgery	Highly specialized, tissue-sparing method of tumor excision; used for recurrent BCC, histologically aggressive forms of BCC, tumors in anatomically important locations where tissue sparing is required (face), and tumors with a high risk of recurrence
	Excision is guided by sequential frozen-section mapping in three dimensions; this allows histologically confirmed removal of the tumor with the smallest of surgical margin and surgical defect
Radiation therapy	May be used for tumors at difficult sites to treat surgically (eyelids) and for patients who are unwilling or unable to tolerate surgery
Inhibition of hedgehog signaling pathway	Vismodegib is an oral inhibitor of the hedgehog pathway used for metastatic or advanced BCC.

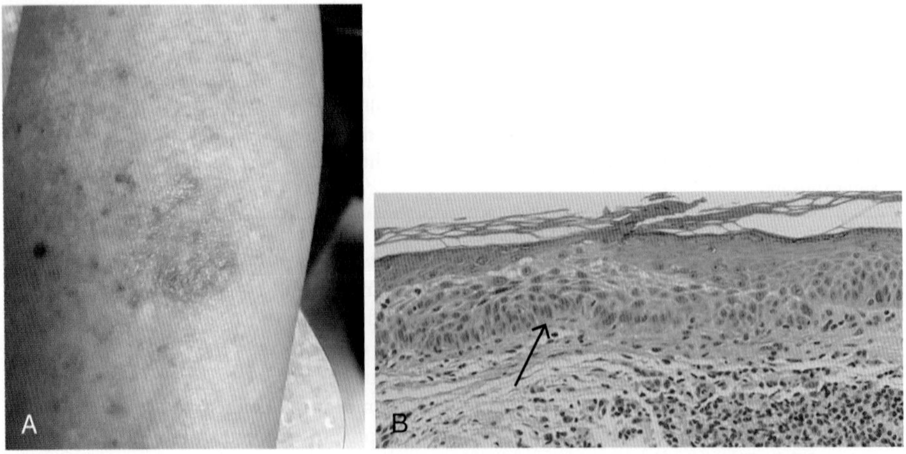

Fig. 41.4 (A) Patient with an actinic keratosis (AK) on their forearm. (B) Skin biopsy with cells demonstrating significant atypia at the basal layer of the epidermis (arrow) that is consistent with AK (H&E stain, 40x).

CLINICAL PEARL

Approximately 10% of AK progress to invasive SCC over several years.

What are the risk factors for development of SCC?

SCC is a low-grade tumor with a metastatic rate of less than 1%. Although the majority of SCCs are caused by UV light exposure, other extrinsic factors also play a causal role.

CLINICAL PEARL

Known risk factors of SCC include other form of radiation, chemicals (hydrocarbons and arsenic), tobacco, chronic infections (i.e., osteomyelitis), chronic inflammation, burns (Marjolin's ulcer), scars, and human papilloma virus.

What are common dermoscopic features of SCC?

SCC are found within a background of sun-damaged skin with atrophy, telangiectasias, and blotchy hyperpigmentation. Atypical lesions can have a pink to dull red, firm, poorly defined dome-shaped nodule with an adherent yellow-white scale. Untreated lesions becomes larger and more raised, developing into a firm red nodule with a necrotic crusted center (Fig. 41.5).

What are histologic variants of noninvasive SCC?

"Noninvasive" or "in situ" reflects inability of the tumor to spread/metastasize. In case of SCC, it indicates that tumor does not cross the basement membrane. Fortunately, many SCCs move through multiple stages before reaching the invasive presentation. If these precursors are identified, more conservative treatments can be utilized.

Bowen's disease is a full-thickness SCC in situ. It usually presents as flat, slow-expanding, psoriasiform, sharply bordered red or pink patch or plaque most frequently located on the trunk, but also can occur at any other site of the body. Histologically, there is a full-thickness epidermal dysplasia without evidence of invasion of basement membrane.

What are the most common histologic features of SCC?

SCC represents proliferation of epithelial tumor cells, corresponding to the keratinocytes of the spinous layer of the epidermis. Tumor cells are usually large with abundant eosinophilic (pink)

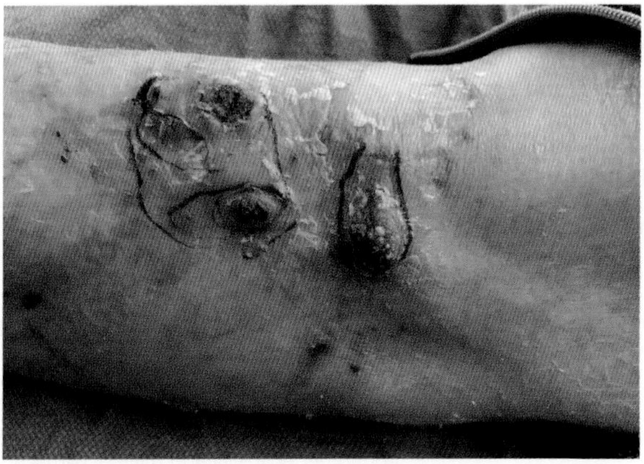

Fig. 41.5 Patient's lower leg demonstrated a raised and ulcerated squamous cell carcinoma.

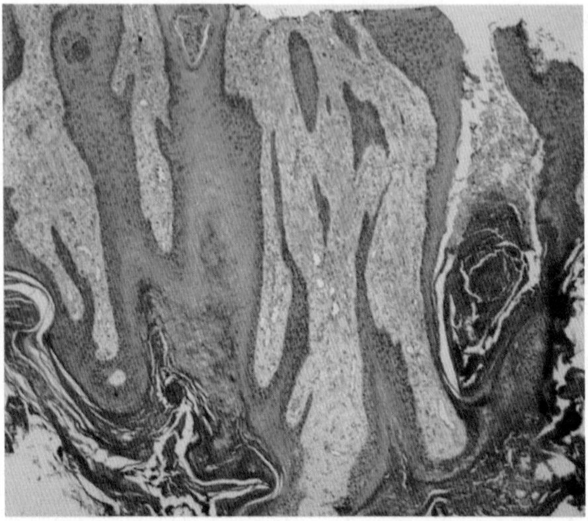

Fig. 41.6 Skin biopsy demonstrates proliferation of atypical keratinocytes with abundant eosinophilic cytoplasm, keratin pearls, and infiltrating pattern of growth, consistent with the common histologic findings in squamous cell carcinoma (H&E stain, 40x).

cytoplasm. Presence of mitotic figures, infiltrating pattern of growth, focal necrosis, and keratinization (horn pearls) are common histologic features (Fig. 41.6).

What are three histologic grades of SCC?

SCC can be subdivided into three broad histologic grades based on their associated degree of nuclear atypia and keratinization. The majority of SCC arising from AK are well differentiated, with tumor cells containing only slightly enlarged, hyperchromatic nuclei with abundant amounts of cytoplasm. They often produce large amounts of keratin, resulting in the formation of extracellular keratin pearls. In contrast, SCC can also present as a poorly differentiated tumor with greatly enlarged, pleomorphic nuclei demonstrating a high degree of atypia and frequent mitoses. Keratin production in these cells will be markedly reduced. This subtype of SCC occurs less commonly and shows more aggressive clinical behavior. A third, moderately differentiated subtype shares features of both well-differentiated and poorly differentiated tumors.

What are rare histologic variants of SCC?

There are several known histological variants of SCC. These variants are relatively rare but have more aggressive behavior and significant potential to locally reoccur and metastasize (Table 41.3).

TABLE 41.3 ■ **Histologic Variants of Squamous Cell Carcinoma**

Histologic Variant of Squamous Cell Carcinoma	Most Prominent Histologic Feature
Acantholytic	A poorly differentiated variant with free-floating keratinocytes Intracellular adhesions have been lost through the entire tumor (tumoral acantholysis)
Spindle cell	May be almost entirely composed of atypical spindle cells arranged in a whorled pattern This variant should be immunohistochemically differentiated from other epithelial and mesenchymal spindle cell tumors

What are treatment options for SCC?

Similarly to BCC, treatment of SCC involves wide local excision with histologic conformation of negative margins. Mohs microscopic surgery may be useful for specific sites where tissue sparing is of importance (face), and radiation therapy may be considered when surgical resection is not feasible.

CLINICAL PEARL

Keratoacanthoma: large, nodular, crateriform, fast-growing nodule with central necrosis. It should be considered a low-grade variant of invasive SCC.

Erythroplasia of Queyrat (squamous carcinoma in situ of the penis): pink, smooth patch, erosion or ulcer and may also become invasive.

SCC of the oral mucosa: particularly worrisome and prone to metastasis, especially of the lower lip.

Bowen's disease: SCC in situ.

BEYOND THE PEARLS

- The regular use of sunscreens prevents the development of new AK as well as hastening the resolution of those that already exist.
- SCC arising in AK has a low metastatic potential.
- Trichoepithelioma is a benign tumor of the hair follicle that may clinically resemble BCC.
- Shave biopsies of BCC have a 50% recurrence rate, but complete excision is usually curative.
- Keratoacanthoma is a well-differentiated SCC, which is rapidly growing with dome-shaped nodules and a central keratin-filled crater; they may also regress spontaneously.

References

Goldblum J, Lamps L, McKenney J, Myers J. *Rosai and Ackerman's Surgical Pathology*. 11th ed. Philadelphia, PA: Elsevier; 2018.

Patterson JW, Hosler GA. *Weedon's Skin Pathology*. 4th ed. Philadelphia, PA: Elsevier; 2016.

Rapini R. *Practical Dermatopathology*. 2nd ed. Philadelphia, PA: Saunders; 2012.

Wolff K, Katz GS, Gilchrest B, Paller AS, Leffell D. *Fitzpatrick's Dermatology in General Medicine*. 7th ed. New York, NY: McGraw-Hill; 2008.

CASE 42

A 32-Year-Old Female with a Mole

Tatsiana Pukhalskaya ■ Cynthia Reyes Barron ■ Julia Stiegler

A 32-year-old Caucasian female presents to her dermatologist for her annual skin examination. She has a fair complexion with blue eyes and blonde hair. Her skin burns easily. She does not have any concerns except an old mole on the right thigh that is getting bigger and darker. She noticed the mole several years ago; it was always stable in size and color. However, 2 weeks ago the mole became intermittently itchy and changed in appearance. She has never had similar lesions in the past but admits to being addicted to tanning since it helps to cope with her seasonal affective disorder. The patient's mother had several moles biopsied, but otherwise there is no history of melanoma in the family. The patient is healthy overall and yearly sees her primary care physician. She has never smoked and occasionally drinks one glass of wine. Her skin examination revealed a 0.3-cm dark brown, sharply demarcated macule (Fig. 42.1). The lesion grossly appears to be symmetrical and uniform. Upon dermoscopy, there is a diffuse reticular pattern of pigmentation at the periphery of the lesion surrounding a central amorphous area. In the office, the dermatologist performed a shave biopsy.

What are the types, pathophysiology, and epidemiology of benign melanocytic nevi?

Benign melanocytic nevi (or "moles") can be present at birth (congenital), but most arise during adolescence or early adulthood (acquired). Acquired nevi are more prevalent in boys than in girls. The number of nevi in young adults varies from approximately 15 to 40 and progressively decreases in number after the age of 50. Commonly acquired nevi include junctional (Fig. 42.2), compound, and dermal nevi (Fig. 42.3), which are all considered benign. These distinctions are based upon the location of melanocytic nests in the epidermis, dermis, or both, respectively. This is a result of a progressive maturation (or melanocyte differentiation pathway) with increasing age of the lesion. Initially, the acquired melanocytic nevus is a flat macular lesion (junctional nevus) in which nests of proliferating melanocytes are confined to the dermoepidermal junction. The lesion becomes progressively more elevated as nests of nevus cells extend ("drop off") into the underlying dermis (compound nevus). With further maturation, junctional activity ceases and the lesion is composed only of dermal nevus cells (intradermal nevus). Compound nevi are more common in individuals with lighter skin photo types. Other forms of nevi (those on palms, soles, conjunctiva, and in the nail bed) are more common in individuals of African and Asian descent. It appears that the emergence of nevi in adolescents is under strong genetic control, whereas environmental exposures affect the mean number of nevi. For example, sun exposure in childhood predisposes to the development of more nevi in the future, some of which may be larger than usual or have atypical features. Although the BRAF V600E mutation is common in melanoma, it is also found in the significant number of benign nevi. This finding suggests that BRAF mutations may be early events in melanoma development. Microsatellite instability, loss of heterozygosity, and other markers of malignancy could be infrequently found in benign nevi, suggesting that some are precursors of melanoma.

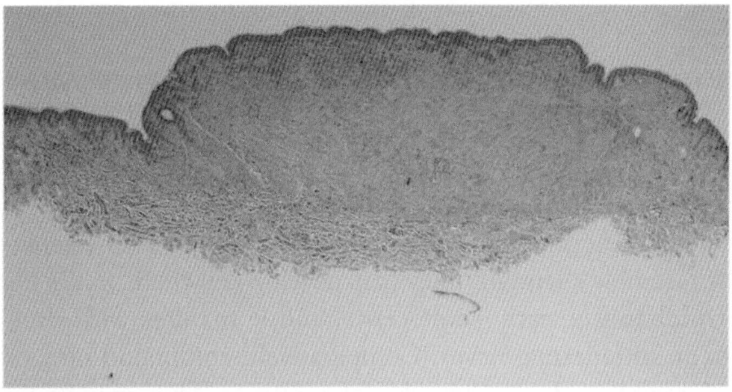

Fig. 42.1 Compound nevus composed of nests of nevus cells within the epidermis as well as nevus cells within the dermis (H&E stain, 20x).

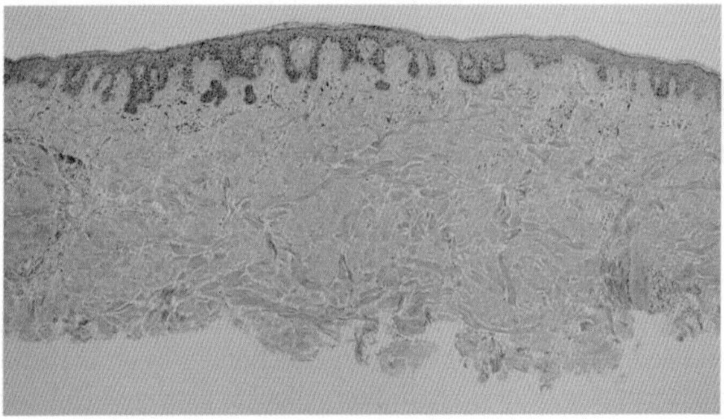

Fig. 42.2 Junctional nevus composed of discrete nests of nevus cells at the dermoepidermal junction (H&E stain, 40x).

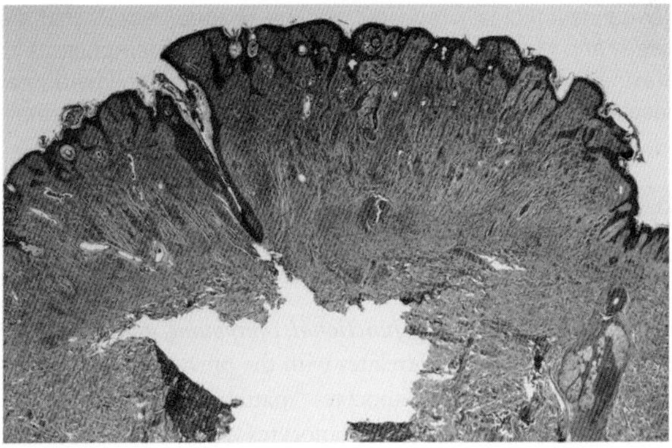

Fig. 42.3 Intradermal nevus displaying nests of nevus cells within the dermis (H&E stain, 40x).

CLINICAL PEARL

The presence of large numbers of nevi is a risk factor for the development of malignant melanoma.

CLINICAL PEARL

The use of a sunscreen reduces the development of new nevi on intermittently sun-exposed body sites.

What are the clinical characteristics of acquired melanocytic nevi?

The junctional melanocytic nevi are flat (macular), well-circumscribed, deeply pigmented lesions, which may clinically resemble a lentigo. They may develop anywhere on the body surface. Usually, it appears during childhood or early adolescence, and it matures with time into a compound nevus and later into an intradermal nevus. Comparatively, compound nevi vary from minimally elevated lesions to dome-shaped or polypoid configurations. They may be tan or dark brown in color. Rarely, compound nevi might present with multiple, tiny, dark brown to black dots on the skin-colored background. Dermal nevi are the most common type of melanocytic nevi. They are nodular or polypoid in shape and commonly lose their pigment, appearing flesh-colored or only lightly pigmented.

CLINICAL PEARL

Nevi are frequently cosmetically removed. Shave excision is a method of choice with excellent cosmetic results.

What could be observed upon dermoscopy of acquired melanocytic nevi?

Dermoscopy is a valuable noninvasive method of distinguishing benign and malignant lesions. It can also be used on fixed specimens to guide tissue sectioning in gross pathology. Examples of most common benign patterns of nevi are diffuse reticular, patchy reticular, peripheral reticular with central hypopigmentation, and peripheral reticular with hyperpigmentation (blotch).

CLINICAL PEARL

Dermoscopy of dermal nevi typically revealed comma-shaped vessels that are not sharply in focus, hairpin vessels, and blue-brown globules. They will also demonstrate the "wobble sign," where the nevi will move freely with the dermatoscope when lateral pressure is applied, in contrast to a basal cell carcinoma, for example, where the lesion will remain fixed in place.

CLINICAL PEARL

The dermoscopic appearance of nevi may change after tanning or ultraviolet B therapy.

What are the common histologic features of junctional, compound, and dermal nevi?

Histology of acquired melanocytic nevi correlates with the previously mentioned theory of progressive maturation (Table 42.1). Dermal melanocytes "mature" (get smaller) when descending from upper dermal levels to deeper layers. Large melanocytes eventually may evolve into smaller cells with roundish or epithelioid, sometimes even neuroid cell-like morphology (type C melanocytes).

CLINICAL PEARL

Benign melanocytic nevi in certain anatomical sites may show unusual histological features. The best known of these are nevi of the vulva and acral region. Some vulvar nevi in premenoposal women show atypical histologic features characterized by enlargement of junctional melanocytic nests, with variability in the size, shape, and position of the nests. Melanocytic lesions of the palms and soles may also cause diagnostic difficulties.

TABLE 42.1 ■ **Common Histologic Features of Acquired Melanocytic Nevi**

Melanocytic Nevus	Histologic Description
Junctional nevus	Clusters and nests of melanocytes at the dermoepidermal junction. The cells are oval to cuboidal in shape with clear cytoplasm and variable amount of pigment (melanin). No atypia or mitoses can be seen. Melanophages and slight lymphocytic infiltrate may be present.
Compound nevus	• Junctional part: intraepidermal nests of melanocytes • Dermal part: dermal nests of melanocytes Cells in the upper dermis are usually cuboidal, with melanin pigment in the cytoplasm; deeper cells are often smaller and contain less melanin. Apoptosis is sometimes seen in the deeper cells. Rete ridges are commonly elongated. Single melanocytes above the basal layer ("pagetoid" cells) may occur secondary to trauma in childhood and in acral sites, but should not be abundant.
Dermal nevus	Nests and sheets of densely packed melanocytes within the dermis. Melanocytes show well-defined cytoplasm, roundish or oval nuclei with fine chromatin. Multinuclear melanocytes are sometimes found. The amount of melanin is variable.

Case Point 42.1

Our patient is reassured upon biopsy results, and no further treatment is required. She is recommended to limit skin exposure to the ultraviolet light and to use sunblock with minimum SPF 30 when such exposure is unavoidable. The patient agrees to the plan but inquires about the difference in doctor's strategy if her mole appeared to be "cancerous."

What are the risks behind dysplastic nevi?

Dysplastic nevi (nevi with architectural disorder) are pigmented lesions with some clinical and histologic features of melanoma but with still undetermined biologic behavior. Individuals with these nevi have an increased risk of developing melanoma. Dysplastic nevus syndrome refers to the familial or sporadic occurrence of multiple dysplastic nevi in one individual. The cumulative lifetime risk of developing melanoma in such individuals approaches 100%.

What are the common characteristics of dysplastic nevi (nevi with architectural disorder)?

Clinically, dysplastic nevi are usually larger than ordinary nevi (>5 mm in diameter), and often show irregular borders and variegated pigmentation (a mixture of tan, dark brown, and pink areas). Nonpigmented variants are rare. Dysplastic nevi predominate on the trunk. In females, there may be considerable numbers on the legs as well. A rare clinical presentation of dysplastic nevi is an eruptive form (it has been reported in a patient with AIDS). Dysplastic nevi in pregnancy may undergo a change in appearance. In patients with the dysplastic nevus syndrome, the number of nevi is large (up to ≥80).

CLINICAL PEARL

There are currently no dermoscopic criteria that can clearly distinguish dysplastic nevi from in situ melanoma.

What are the known genetic abnormalities seen in dysplastic nevi (nevi with architectural disorder)?

Molecular data show that dysplastic nevi frequently have BRAF mutations similar to common nevi, and some of them have alterations in p16 or p53 expression. In familial cases, the dysplastic nevus trait has a complicated inheritance with dominant inheritance being the most frequent.

The dysplastic nevus syndrome has also been associated with partial deletion of chromosome 11 and with deletion of 17p13 (p53).

What are common histologic features of dysplastic nevi (nevi with architectural disorder)?

The best approach in diagnosing dysplastic nevi is to perceive them as compound nevi with peripheral lentiginous and junctional activity and random cytological atypia in the epidermal component.

Dysplastic nevi have three characteristic histologic features (Table 42.2; Fig. 42.4). Atypia may also be present in nevi that do not otherwise fulfill the criteria for the diagnosis of a dysplastic nevus.

A dermal nevus cell component is usually present in the central part of the lesion, consisting of small cells or epithelioid cells but showing only slight evidence of maturation and with impairment of pigment synthesis.

TABLE 42.2 ■ **Common Histologic Features of Dysplastic Nevi**

Feature	Description
1. Intraepidermal lentiginous hyperplasia of melanocytes	• Proliferation of melanocytes singly but also in nests along the basal layer • "Bridging": anastomoses between nests of melanocytes • Irregular distribution of junctional nests along rete ridges • Increased numbers of single melanocytes present along elongated rete ridges
2. Cytological atypia of melanocytes	• Melanocytes with enlarged hyperchromatic nuclei, increased cytoplasm, and prominent nucleoli (variable)
3. Stromal response	• Lamellar and concentric fibroplasia of the papillary dermis • Lymphocytic infiltrate
4. Architectural atypia	• Extension of junctional component of nevus beyond dermal component: "shouldering"

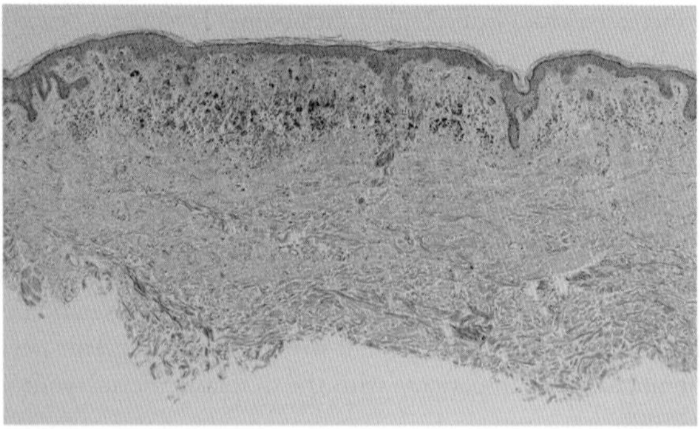

Fig. 42.4 Dysplastic nevus composed of basilar nests of atypical melanocytes (H&E stain, 40x).

Case Point 42.2

Three years after the last visit, the patient presents to her dermatologist with a new concerning lesion. She was not able to schedule her visit earlier due to lack of health insurance. She regularly checks her skin and has taken pictures of all her moles. Two weeks ago, she noticed a new pigmented lesion on the shoulder that is growing and changing in color. Examination revealed an irregularly pigmented nodule, measuring 0.7 cm, on the right upper shoulder. The dermatologist performed shave biopsy of the lesions and requested the pathology laboratory to rush the case.

During self-evaluation of pigmented lesion, presence of which features is suspicious for melanoma?
Catching melanoma early could mean the difference between life and a life-threatening cancer. Knowing what to look for and performing regular skin self-examinations may help patients to be more aware of unusual spots.

CLINICAL PEARL

The ABCDEs of melanoma are potential worrisome features:

A—Asymmetry: one half of the lesion does not mirror the other half.
B—Border: the borders are irregular or indistinct.
C—Color: the color is variegated and the pigmentation is not uniform, or there are varying shades and/or hues.
D—Diameter: the lesion is > 6 mm in diameter.
E—Evolving: changes in appearance or new symptoms in a lesion over time.

Biopsy can be considered for any new, changing, or atypical-appearing melanocytic lesion to rule out melanoma.

What is the gender difference in the incidence of melanoma in the United States?
The incidence of cutaneous melanoma has significantly increased since 1970. Overall, it varies by age, sex, ethnicity, and histologic subtype. Before the age of 40 years, the incidence is higher in women, with most melanomas occurring on the lower extremities and exhibiting the superficial spreading histology. After the age of 40 years, the incidence is much higher in men, with most melanomas presenting on the head and neck. The largest increase in incidence during the past several decades is among elderly white men, and this increase is mirrored by the relative rise in the frequency of lentigo maligna and lentigo maligna melanoma histologic subtypes. The gender incidence difference and histologic subtypes of melanoma are likely attributed in part to patterns of ultraviolet light exposure (including tanning salon use). The difference does not appear to be related to hormones. Notably, although the incidence of cutaneous melanoma clearly has increased, mortality curves have largely remained flat.

What are the known risk factors for developing melanoma?
Genetic and environmental factors play a role in the epidemiology of any disease, including melanoma. The most important environmental factor is ultraviolet light exposure (natural and artificial), especially intermittent sun exposure and history of sunburns in childhood. Individuals with pale skin, blond and red hair, and poor tanning ability are particularly at risk. Patients who have received multiple psoralen and ultraviolet A light exposures in the treatment of psoriasis and other conditions appear to have an increased risk of melanoma. Other known environmental exposures include exposure to the polyvinyl chloride, insecticides, chemical solvents, arsenic-polluted water, electron beam radiation therapy, and voriconazole therapy. Melanomas occur more frequently in organ transplant recipients and immunosuppressed individuals.

Approximately 10% of melanomas are familial (hereditary) with melanoma-related germline mutation. The majority of familial melanomas are inherited in autosomal dominant manner. A positive family history equals to approximately a twofold risk in developing a melanoma.

What is the genetic base and pathogenesis of melanoma?
Melanoma is a genetically heterogeneous group of tumors, which are tied together only by the common bond of originating within a melanocyte. Melanoma susceptibility genes play roles in cell cycling, melanocyte development, and melanin biosynthesis. They can be subdivided into high-, intermediate-, and low-risk genes (Table 42.3). Genetic alterations lead to formation of signaling molecules and pathways within the melanocyte that are involved in melanomagenesis.

TABLE 42.3 ■ **Genes Associated With Melanoma**

Gene	Characteristic
CDKN2A	High-risk gene, located on chromosome 9p21. Mutations result in familial melanoma syndrome.
MC1R	Intermediate-risk locus involved in melanin synthesis. Mutation of this gene can increase the risk for developing melanoma up to 2.7-fold.
CDK4	Germline mutations result in familial melanoma.

CLINICAL PEARL

Examples of signaling pathways involved in melanomagenesis:

- **CDKN2A(p16)/CDK4/Rb:** results in inactivation of tumor suppressor gene p16.
- **MAP kinase (RS/RAF/MEK/ERK):** one of the main conduits for transmitting signals from the cell surface to the nucleus. NRAS is more frequently observed in nodular melanoma. BRAF is one of the most commonly somatically mutated proto-oncogenes in melanoma, observed in approximately half of all melanomas.
- **PI3K/Akt/mTOR/PTEN:** an activation pathway running parallel to the MAP kinase pathway. Similar to MAP kinase pathway, it leads to cellular growth, proliferation, and survival of the cell.

What is the classification and histologic features of melanoma subtypes?

The clinicopathologic classification of melanoma consists of six groups. Subtypes (groups) of melanoma mostly differ in their pattern of growth and clinical presentation (Table 42.4). The relative incidence of each type varies considerably in different geographical areas as well. Importantly, there is a variation between experts in the diagnosis of melanocytic neoplasms, but errors in diagnosis leading to litigation are not common. Histologic criteria for the diagnosis of malignant melanoma in general include asymmetry, poor circumcision, consumption (presence of atypical cells) of epidermis, architecture of melanocytic nests and solitary epidermal melanocytes, presence of melanocytes in lymphovascular spaces, and degree of cytologic atypia (Figs. 42.5 and 42.6).

TABLE 42.4 ■ **Types of Melanoma and Their Characteristics**

Lentigo maligna melanoma	• Occurs most frequently on the face and sun-exposed upper extremities in the elderly • Lentigo maligna: the precursor lesion. It is an irregularly pigmented macule that expands slowly. • Associated with BRAF V600K mutation	• Atypical melanocytes, singly and in nests, usually confined to the basal layer and with little pagetoid (migration of melanocytes into epidermis) invasion of the epidermis
Superficial spreading melanoma	• May develop on any part of the body at any age • BRAF mutation is less common	• Proliferation of atypical melanocytes, singly and in nests, at all levels within the epidermis
Nodular melanoma	• Nodular, polypoid, or pedunculated • Dark brown or blue-black lesions occurring anywhere on the body	• Has no adjacent intraepidermal component of atypical melanocytes, although there is usually epidermal invasion by malignant cells directly overlying the dermal mass • The dermal component is usually composed of oval to round epithelioid cells

Continued on following page

TABLE 42.4 ■ **Types of Melanoma and Their Characteristics** (continued)

Acral lentiginous melanoma	• Develop on palmar, plantar, or subungual skin • Particularly common in black people and Japanese • Alteration in RAS pathways are present in more than 87% of acral lentiginous melanomas	• The epidermal component might look misleadingly benign
Desmoplastic melanoma	• Usually found on the head and neck regions as a spreading indurated plaque • Male predominance	• Islands of elongated cells (spindle cells) surrounded by mature collagen bundles
Miscellaneous	• Melanomas arising in blue nevi • Spitzoid melanomas • Primary dermal melanomas • BAP-1 mutated melanomas	

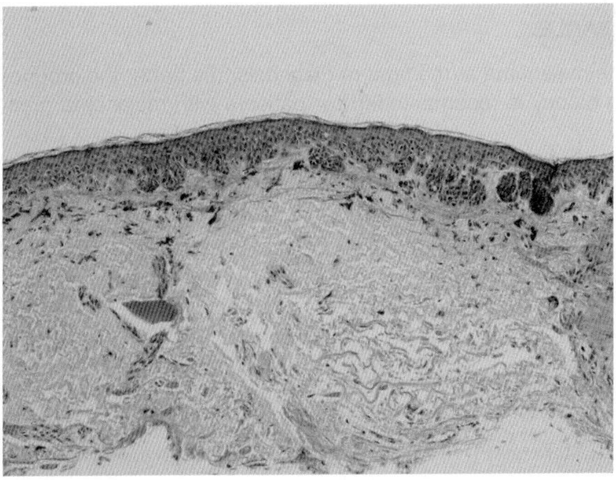

Fig. 42.5 Melanoma in situ displaying atypical melanocytes in the epidermis with no dermal invasion (H&E stain, 100x).

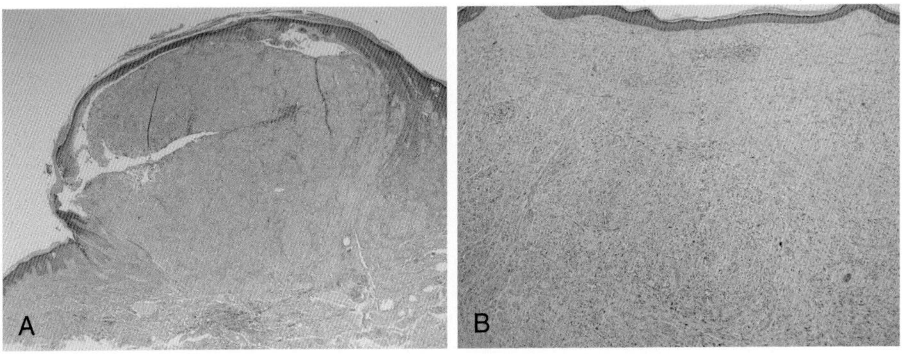

Fig. 42.6 (A) Malignant melanoma displaying dermal involvement of atypical melanocytes with cytologic atypia and no maturation (H&E stain, 20x). (B) Melanoma composed of atypical melanocytes and sclerotic stroma (H&E stain, 40x).

Case Point 42.3

The patient is diagnosed with malignant melanoma and is back to the office for further management. She inquires about different options of treatment.

What are the options of managing melanoma after confirming the diagnosis on biopsy?

Melanoma is primary a surgically treated disease, and surgery remains virtually the only necessary treatment modality for thin melanomas. Treatment for the advanced melanoma patient recently has become more complex. In addition to the palliative surgery, patients with the metastatic melanoma could be offered cytotoxic chemotherapeutic agents (dacarbazine, temozolomide), interferon-alpha, high-dose interleukin-2, and radiation, targeted therapy directed against known oncogenes (vemurafenib: a selective BRAF inhibitor; trametinib: allosteric MEK1/2 inhibitor). Simultaneous targeting of multiple checkpoints may provide a greater initial tumor response and may minimize resistance.

BEYOND THE PEARLS

- The thinner the melanoma at the time of diagnosis, the better the prognosis.
- Sentinel node biopsy is recommended for patients with melanoma greater than 1 mm in depth.
- Pigmented basal cell carcinoma contains melanin and could mimic melanoma.
- If lesion is clinically suspicious for melanoma, excisional biopsy is the best next step.
- If biopsy showed mildly dysplastic nevus, patient is usually observed; if moderately dysplastic nevus, patient might be observed or lesion re-excised; if severely dysplastic nevus, re-excision is recommended.

References

Goldblum J, Lamps L, McKenney J, Myers J. *Rosai and Ackerman's Surgical Pathology*. 11th ed. Philadelphia, PA: Elsevier; 2018.

Patterson JW, Hosler GA. *Weedon's Skin Pathology*. 4th ed. Philadelphia, PA: Elsevier; 2016.

Rapini R. *Practical Dermatopathology*. 2nd ed. Philadelphia, PA: Saunders; 2012.

Wolff K, Katz GS, Gilchrest B, Paller AS, Leffell D. *Fitzpatrick's Dermatology in General Medicine*. 7th ed. New York, NY: McGraw-Hill; 2008.

Nervous System

CASE 43

A 70-Year-Old Male with a Brain Mass

Lanisha Denise Fuller

A 70-year-old male presents to his primary care physician with his wife. The wife describes the patient as being more forgetful than usual and veering to the side of the road while driving, having led to him running over a street sign. He also complains of "feeling sick a lot for no reason" and having to vomit "even though he has not eaten anything before that." His other medical history is only significant for long-standing hypertension, which is successfully treated with an angiotensin-converting enzyme inhibitor and a sodium-restricted diet. He does not drink alcohol, does not smoke, and does not take illicit drugs. He is up to date with the recommended screening tests and immunizations. His physical and neurologic examinations are within normal limits. His primary care physician refers him to a neurologist.

What are the differential diagnoses for an elderly patient presenting with new-onset nausea, vomiting, and cognitive changes?

This patient's clinical presentation is highly suspicious for an increase in the intracranial pressure, which can have multiple causes. A common approach to generate differential diagnoses is by categorizing symptoms according to their root problem. The underlying causes of a symptom can be genetic, vascular, traumatic, infectious, immunologic, metabolic, degenerative, or neoplastic. Vascular conditions, such as ischemia, intracranial hemorrhage, and hypertension, are a possibility in this patient because of his age and comorbidity. However, vascular conditions commonly present as acute events. A neoplasm certainly can be responsible for his symptoms. They can cause an increase in the intracranial pressure through blocking cerebrospinal fluid outflow or simply through mass effect and edema. Infectious causes include meningitis, encephalitis, or abscesses. Central nervous system (CNS) infections should always be in the differential, as many can be cured without persistent neurologic damage if identified and treated early on. Increased intracranial pressure can be observed in some immunologic conditions like Guillain–Barré syndrome; however, this would be an unusual presentation and other symptoms are more likely (extremity weakness and paralysis). Metabolic derangements like hypoxia and hypercapnia can cause increased intracranial pressure through cerebral vascular dilatation. This is usually seen in more acute situations like trauma. Nevertheless, the more likely derangements are quickly ruled out by pulse oximetry or arterial blood gases. The less likely etiologies in this patient are genetic (wrong age; it is unlikely for a genetic condition to manifest the first time in late adulthood) as well as traumatic because the patient did not report any trauma.

Case Point 43.1

The neurologist orders a brain magnetic resonance imaging (Fig. 43.1) that demonstrates a heterogeneously enhancing mass, measuring 5 × 4 × 3.5 cm, within the right frontoparietal region and posterior right temporal lobe with extensive surrounding vasogenic edema and mass effect.

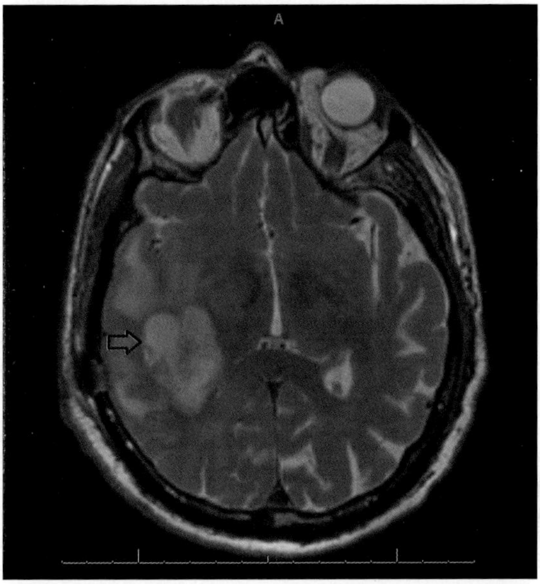

Fig. 43.1 Magnetic resonance imaging scan of the brain demonstrates a heterogeneously enhancing mass (arrow) within the right frontoparietal and posterior right temporal lobe with surrounding vasogenic edema.

What are the symptoms that can occur with an intracranial neoplasm?

Apart from nausea, vomiting, and cognitive changes, other common presentations are seizures and headache. Symptoms that are tumor location–dependent present as focal neurologic deficits and include but are not limited to acoustic, visual, or other sensory changes, motoric deficits, or changes in personality.

Case Point 43.2

The patient is admitted to the hospital where he is evaluated by neurosurgery and started on glucocorticoids in order to decrease his edema as well as an anticonvulsant to prevent seizures. His symptoms improve thereafter. A brain biopsy is scheduled and demonstrates a glial neoplasm.

What are the differential diagnoses of glial neoplasms and what are their different histologic features?

Although the pathology report describes the neoplasm as glial, the first neoplasms that come to mind are metastases. The most common sources are the lung, breast, kidney, and skin (melanoma). On imaging, they usually present as multiple lesions that are located at the junction of gray and white matter (Table 43.1).

Glial neoplasms resemble glial cells morphologically, which are astrocytes, oligodendrocytes, and ependymal cells. They are not staged via the TNM classification but graded using the World Health Organization's (WHO) guidelines into prognostic groups ranging from grade I to grade IV. They rarely metastasize outside of the CNS. Gliomas in adults usually occur above the tentorium, while in children they mostly are located infratentorial.

CLINICAL PEARL

Eighty percent of adult gliomas are astrocytomas, the majority of which are glioblastomas.

TABLE 43.1 ■ **Metastasis Versus Central Nervous System (CNS) Primary**

Metastasis	Brain Primary
Multiple lesions	Solitary lesion
Circumscribed	Ill-defined
At gray and white matter junction	Anywhere in the CNS

Astrocytomas are neoplasms of star-shaped cells called astrocytes. The cell processes of astrocytes as well as astrocytic tumor cells usually stain for glial fibrillary acidic protein (Fig. 43.2). Astrocytomas exist in two broad categories: diffuse astrocytic tumors and tumors that do not fall under the "diffuse astrocytic tumor" category. The difference between the two is the range of infiltration. While diffuse astrocytic tumors broadly and widely infiltrate the brain parenchyma, the other category is more circumscribed and less infiltrative. Diffuse astrocytic tumors include diffuse astrocytomas (WHO grade II), anaplastic astrocytomas (WHO grade III), and glioblastomas (WHO grade IV). A diffuse astrocytoma shows increased cellularity compared with normal brain tissue and nuclear atypia (hyperchromatic, variably shaped nuclei). Adding mitoses to the picture of a diffuse astrocytoma upgrades it to an anaplastic astrocytoma. If necrosis and/or microvascular proliferation (thick-walled vessels with more than one layer of endothelial cells) are identified, a glioblastoma can be diagnosed (Figs. 43.3 and 43.4). Defining characteristics of diffuse astrocytomas are summarized in Table 43.2. The most well-known nondiffuse astrocytoma is a pilocytic astrocytoma, which is considered WHO grade I and usually occurs in children. Histology shows astrocytic cells with long hair-like processes. Other frequently seen features are Rosenthal fibers, thick eosinophilic processes that are sometimes described as "worm-like," and eosinophilic granular bodies, pink and granular, vaguely round structures located in the neuropil.

CLINICAL PEARL

On imaging, pilocytic astrocytomas often present as cystic lesions with a solid component that are located in the cerebellum.

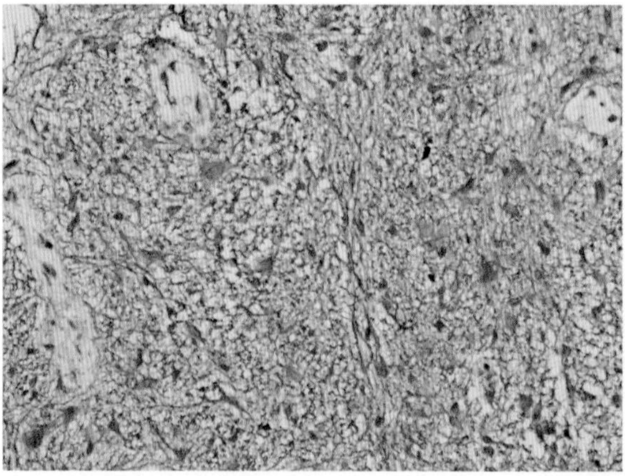

Fig. 43.2 Neoplastic astrocytes and their processes stain brown for glial fibrillary acidic protein (GFAP; GFAP stain, 10x).

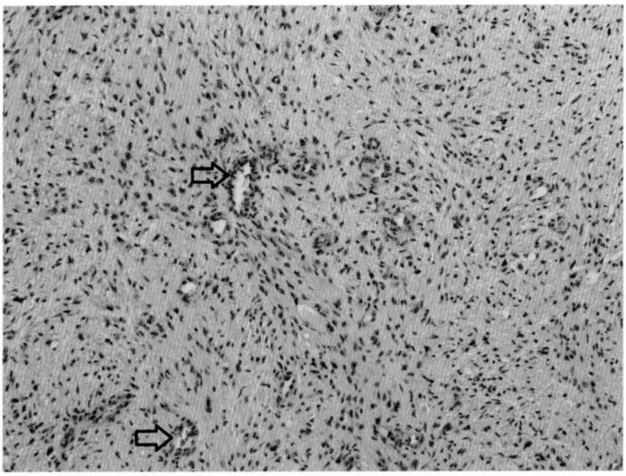

Fig. 43.3 High-power view of a glioblastoma demonstrating increased cellularity, atypical nuclei, high pleomorphism, and microvascular proliferation (arrow). The cells are embedded in a neurofibrillary background characteristic of the central nervous system tissue (H&E 10x).

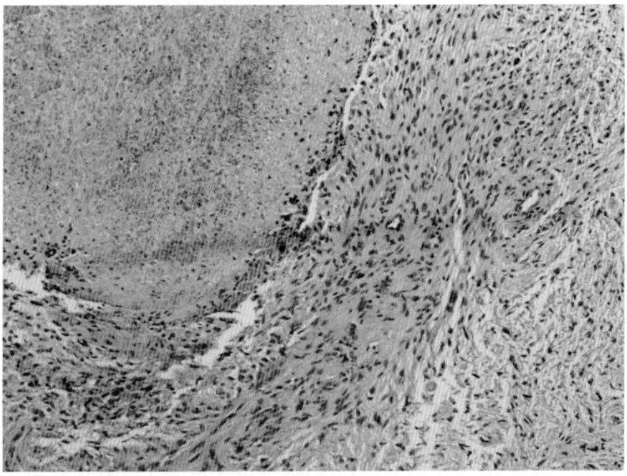

Fig. 43.4 Glioblastoma with large area of necrosis. While palisading of tumor cells around areas of necrosis is a feature commonly seen in glioblastoma, simple necrosis is sufficient for diagnosis (H&E 10x).

TABLE 43.2 ■ **Grading of Diffuse Astrocytomas (Defining Histologic Features are Underlined)**

WHO grade II diffuse astrocytoma	Moderately increased cellularity with nuclear atypia compared with normal brain
WHO grade III anaplastic astrocytoma	Increased cellularity and nuclear atypia compared with WHO grade II; significant proliferative activity (mitotic activity)
WHO grade IV glioblastoma	Nuclear atypia, cellular pleomorphism, mitotic activity, necrosis, and/or microvascular proliferation

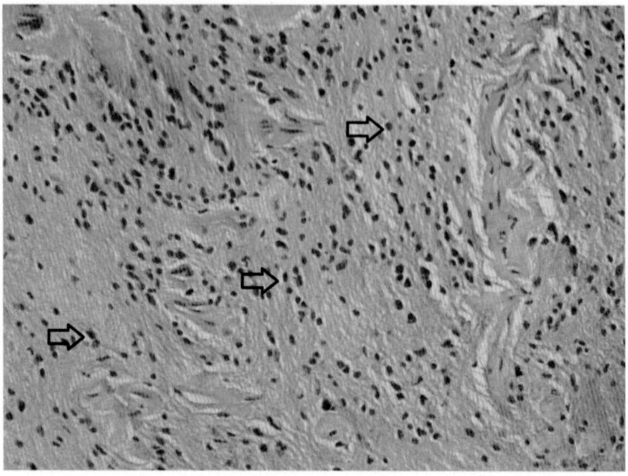

Fig. 43.5 Oligodendroglioma with relatively round, monomorphic cells having a "fried egg" appearance (arrows; H&E 10x).

Oligodendrogliomas are tumors of oligodenroglial-looking cells that only exist in diffuse variants. As per definition, they are isocitrate dehydrogenase (IDH) mutant and show 1p19q codeletion. Oligodendrogliomas WHO grade II are slow-growing tumors; their histology classically shows moderately increased cellularity of monomorphous cells with a "fried-egg" appearance—a round, central nucleus and a perinuclear halo (Fig. 43.5). The cells are embedded in a network of fine, branching capillaries creating a "chicken-wire" appearance. They are frequently calcified, which is also evident on imaging. In anaplastic oligodendroglioma WHO grade III, the tumor shows features of anaplasia with prominent mitotic activity, necrosis, and microvascular proliferation histologically resembling glioblastoma. However, 1p19q codeletion together with IDH mutation classify the tumor as an oligodendroglioma.

CLINICAL PEARL

A glioma showing IDH mutation together with 1p19q codeletion as per definition is an oligodendroglioma regardless of its histology.

Ependymomas are malignant neoplasms that resemble ependymal cells and occur usually in children. They range in grade from I to III. The most common location is at the fourth ventricle. Histology shows uniform small cells that form characteristic perivascular pseudorosettes around the blood vessels (Fig. 43.6).

Tumors that are of nonglial origin should also be considered, as they are more common than glial neoplasms. Meningiomas are extraaxial tumors (in the skull, but outside of the brain parenchyma) that are dural based and arise from arachnoid cells, also called meningothelial cells. They are usually benign and correspond to WHO grade I; however, there are more aggressive variants that show poorer treatment response and, therefore, are of a higher WHO grade. The typical histology shows whorled growth patterns and psammoma bodies (Fig. 43.7).

CLINICAL PEARL

Meningiomas usually do not invade the brain parenchyma. They push and compress it causing symptoms like seizures.

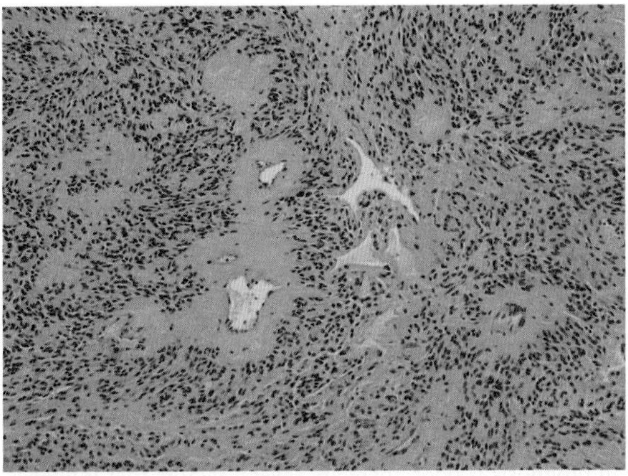

Fig. 43.6 Perivascular pseudorosettes in an ependymoma (H&E 10x).

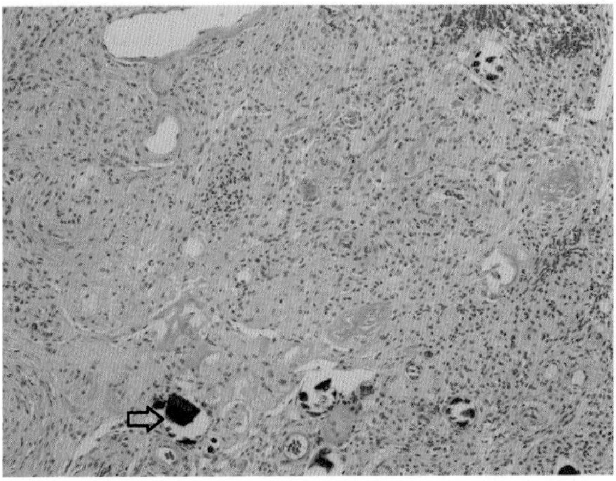

Fig. 43.7 Meningioma demonstrating a whorled pattern and psammoma bodies (arrow; H&E 10x).

Case Point 43.3

A craniotomy is performed and a variegated tumor with central necrosis and irregular borders is identified. The obtained specimens are submitted for pathology and reveal the tumor to be a glioblastoma, WHO grade IV.

CLINICAL PEARL

Glioblastomas can cross the midline via the corpus callosum and create nearly symmetrical lesions. Therefore, it is sometimes referred to as "butterfly glioma."

What is the treatment of glioblastomas?

The current treatment consists of a multimodal approach of a combination of surgery, radiation, and chemotherapy. Usually, a debulking surgery is followed by adjuvant radiation and chemotherapy. Unfortunately, therapy is rarely curative owing to the tumor being highly and rapidly infiltrative. At surgery, most of the evident tumor mass is resected. However, single cells not visible to the naked eye escape resection and are thought to be a source of recurrent disease.

Case Point 43.4

After surgery, the patient is started on chemotherapy and radiation. He is followed up by his neurooncological team regularly.

What is the prognosis for glioblastomas?

Although the overall prognosis is poor, there are several factors that influence the length of survival. The patient's age and frailty correlate negatively with length of survival. If the tumor is located in an area that makes resection impossible, this also has a negative impact on survival. Finally, certain mutations are linked to better or poorer prognoses. Whether a tumor is IDH wildtype or mutant is the single most important genetic information that influences prognosis. IDH wildtype glioblastomas are thought to arise de novo and generally follow a more aggressive course than do IDH mutant tumors. In treated IDH wildtype glioblastomas, the median overall survival is about 15 months, whereas patients with treated IDH mutant glioblastomas have a median overall survival of 31 months. An important genetic alteration is O6-methylguanine-DNA-methyltransferase, short MGMT, promoter methylation status. If the promoter is methylated and the gene is hence silenced, the tumor is susceptible to an alkylating chemotherapeutic drug called temozolomide. However, if the promoter is not methylated and the gene is active, the tumor is usually resistant to the drug.

BEYOND THE PEARLS

- 5-aminolevulinic acid is used during surgery of diffuse gliomas to better visualize the tumor. After uptake of 5-ALA by a cell, it is converted into a fluorescent chemical.
- Loss of ATRX and TP53 mutations are characteristic of astrocytomas; however, they are not required to make the diagnosis.
- Tumor syndromes associated with an increased risk of glioblastoma are neurofibromatosis type 1, Li-Fraumeni, Ollier/Maffucci, and Turcot syndrome
- Most cases of glioblastomas are primary, which means that they do not arise out of lower-grade lesions. They are IDH wildtype.
- Medulloblastomas are the most common malignant primary CNS tumors of children. They are located in the cerebellum. Histology exhibits a small, round, blue cell tumor that may form Homer Wright rosettes. They have the tendency to metastasize via cerebrospinal fluid causing "drop metastasis."
- Remnants of Rathke's pouch, which form the adenohypophysis during embryogenesis, can become neoplastic and form craniopharyngiomas. They are benign tumors of children that cause symptoms usually via compression of the optic chiasm.

References

Kumar V, Abbas AK, Aster JC, Perkins JA. *Robbins Basic Pathology*. Philadelphia PA: Elsevier; 2018.

Louis DN, Perry A, Reifenberger G, et al. *WHO Classification of Tumours of the Central Nervous System*. Lyon, France: International Agency for Research on Cancer, 2016.

An 8-Year-Old Female with Brown Macules and Soft Papules

Lanisha Denise Fuller

An 8-year-old female presents with her parents to a pediatrician for a well-child assessment prior to enrolling in a sports team at her new school. They recently moved to the area from out of the country. According to her parents, she has always been a healthy and active girl. Her immunizations are up to date. She takes no medications and has no known allergies. Her developmental assessment is within normal limits. The physical examination is notable for multiple, uniformly pigmented, light-brown macules ranging in size from 0.5 cm to 4.5 cm on her right flank. Furthermore, there are a few soft papules ranging in size from 0.2 cm to 0.4 cm in the same area. Further questioning of the parents reveals that the macules have appeared shortly after her birth slowly increasing in size, and the papules have developed recently. They did not seek medical attention, as they thought they would disappear over time. These findings prompt the pediatrician to do an eye examination that turns out to be unremarkable.

What condition is the pediatrician suspecting? Why did the pediatrician do an eye exam?
The patient's presentation with relatively large brown macules as well as soft skin papules raises the concern for neurofibromatosis type 1 (NF1), which is a tumor syndrome that is part of the neurofibromatosis disorders.

CLINICAL PEARL

The incidence for NF1 is about 1 per 3000 births.

The macules most likely are café-au-lait macules that clinically present as uniformly pigmented, brown lesions present at birth or developing in the first few years of life. They can range in size from very small punctate lesions to large patches. One or two café-au-lait macules occur in about 10% of the population that are not affected by NF1. The differential for soft skin papules is broad. However, given the combination with café-au-lait macules, they most likely are neurofibromas, which can be confirmed histologically. The pediatrician probably suspected NF1 and was looking for iris hamartomas (Lisch nodules). These raised, pigmented aggregates of melanocytes of the iris are fairly specific to NF1. Café-au-lait macules, axillary and inguinal freckling, multiple neurofibromas, and Lisch nodules are the most common clinical manifestations of NF1. Each of them is present in over 80% of NF1 patients and usually starts to manifest in childhood.

CLINICAL PEARL

The pattern of inheritance for NF1 is autosomal dominant. Fifty percent of NF1 patients inherited the mutation, whereas the other 50% developed a sporadic mutation.

Which other syndromes are considered part of the neurofibromatosis disorders?

Other neurofibromatoses are neurofibromatosis type 2 (NF2) and schwannomatosis. While manifestations of NF1 typically are peripheral, NF2 is characterized mainly by central lesions. Essentially, anyone can have a schwannoma, but having schwannomas of both the vestibulocochlear nerves (eighth cranial nerve) is nearly exclusively found in NF2. Other neoplasms that more frequently occur in NF2 are astrocytomas, meningiomas, and ependymomas. Less frequent are non-neoplastic manifestations including cataracts.

CLINICAL PEARL

Cause of NF2 is a mutation in the merlin gene on chromosome 22. Like NF1, it has an autosomal dominant inheritance.

The diagnosis of schwannomatosis should be considered in individuals with multifocal, non-vestibular schwannomas and chronic pain without other neurofibromatosis signs. So far, no single causative mutation has been discovered for this disorder. Additionally, there is segmental NF1. Segmental NF1 is not a separate entity per se. It is caused by the same mutation as NF1.

CLINICAL PEARL

Cause of NF1 is a mutation in the neurofibromin 1 gene on chromosome 17.

Instead of it being a germline mutation, it arises through a somatic mutation acquired in early development and therefore only affects the body parts that arise out of the mutated cell. This patient presents with a localized process (right flank), raising the concern for segmental NF1.

What are the clinical criteria for the diagnosis of NF1?

The National Institute of Health (NIH) Consensus Development Conference has compiled seven diagnostic features of which at least two need to be present in order to clinically diagnose NF1. The diagnostic criteria are summarized in Box 44.1. Genetic testing is not necessary to establish the diagnosis.

Are there other manifestations of NF1?

Manifestations of NF1 are not restricted to one organ system. The peripheral organ systems including the peripheral nervous system, as well as the skin and bones, are most prominently involved. However, central nervous system involvement is also frequent. Abnormalities of melanocytes lead to café-au-lait macules, axillary and inguinal freckling, and Lisch nodules. Histologically, café-au-lait macules and axillary and inguinal freckling in NF1 show as an increased number of

BOX 44.1 ■ National Institute of Health Diagnostic Criteria for Neurofibromatosis Type 1 (NF1; (≥ 2 Features are Diagnostic)

History of NF1 in a first-degree relative
Optic nerve glioma
≥2 neurofibromas or ≥1 plexiform neurofibroma
≥2 iris hamartomas
≥6 café-au-lait macules (≥5 mm prepubertal; ≥15 mm postpubertal)
Axillary or inguinal freckling
A distinctive bony lesion

melanocytes and melanin pigment. As mentioned earlier, Lisch nodules are aggregates of melanocytes of the iris. Bone abnormalities include scoliosis and sphenoid dysplasia. Patients can have thinned cortices of long bones, predisposing them to fractures with dysfunctional healing, which in turn can cause pseudarthroses. Nervous system involvement includes neoplastic as well as non-neoplastic conditions, with the neoplastic conditions being far more frequent than the latter. Seizures with or without lesions and hydrocephalus are non-neoplastic manifestations. Gliomas, especially of the optic pathway, occur more frequently in patients with NF1 than in the general population. Gliomas of the optic pathway are usually pilocytic astrocytomas and classically occur bilaterally. They affect younger patients; however, most are indolent, and only few require intervention. All three WHO grades of diffuse astrocytic tumors are more common in patients with NF1 compared to unaffected individuals. Neurofibromas, one of the most frequent manifestations of NF1, are benign tumors of the nerve sheath. On the other hand, malignant peripheral nerve sheath tumors (MPNSTs) are, as the name indicates, malignant. They occur less frequently than benign tumors, but the overall risk is increased in NF1 patients. In contrast to the general population where MPNSTs usually develop without a precursor lesion, in NF1 patients they most commonly arise from neurofibromas.

CLINICAL PEARL

Fifty percent of MPNSTs are associated with NF1. NF1-associated MPNSTs present more frequently in younger patients than sporadic cases.

Case Point 44.1

The pediatrician biopsies one of the nodules, which is then evaluated by pathology. The patient and her parents come back to the office for follow-up 3 weeks later, during which the pathology report is ready. Histologic findings are depicted in Figs. 44.1 and 44.2. The pathology report reveals a neurofibroma. The patient fulfills two of the NIH diagnostic criteria for NF1 and, therefore, can clinically be diagnosed with NF1. Given the localized presentation, it is likely the segmental variant.

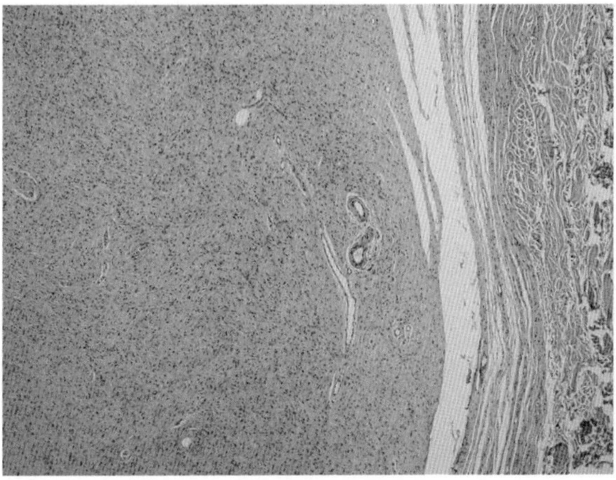

Fig. 44.1 Low-power view of a well-circumscribed cutaneous neurofibroma with dense, collagenous stroma (H&E x4).

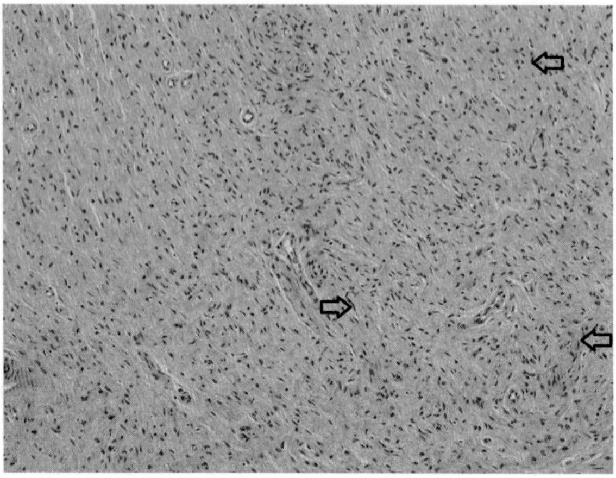

Fig. 44.2 High-power view of Fig. 44.1 reveals characteristic wavy nuclei (arrows; H&E 10x).

What are histologic features of neurofibromas?

Neurofibromas are benign tumors of the nerve sheath that consist of well-differentiated neoplastic Schwann cells mixed with non-neoplastic cells such as fibroblasts. They grow inside of the nerve. The Schwann cells have long, thin, wavy nuclei and little cytoplasm. The matrix ranges from myxoid and loose to collagenous and dense. Since the tumor arises from the nerve sheath, residual nerve elements such as ganglion cells and axons might still be evident. Plexiform neurofibromas are a variant of neurofibromas that involve multiple fascicles of a nerve (Fig. 44.3). They are strongly associated with NF1.

What are histologic differential diagnoses of neurofibromas?

Other tumors of the peripheral nervous system as well as soft tissue tumors should be considered as differentials. The following differentials will only include tumors of the peripheral nervous system. Schwannomas are relatively more common neoplasms of the peripheral

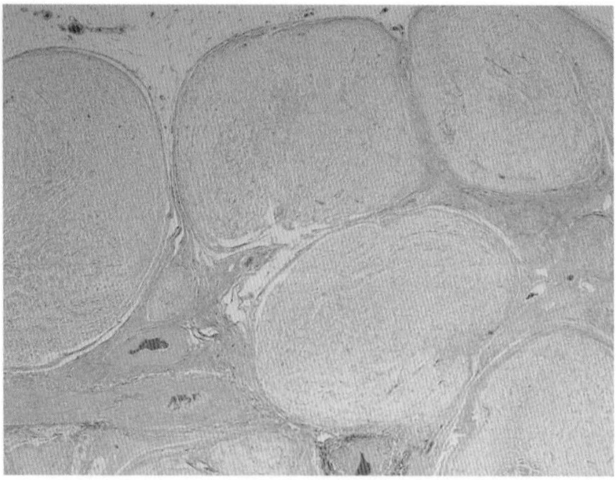

Fig. 44.3 Plexiform neurofibroma displaying a nodular architecture. This example displays loose, edematous stroma (H&E x2).

nervous system. They are benign, encapsulated lesions of well-differentiated Schwann cells. In contrast to neurofibromas, the entire lesion is composed of neoplastic cells. Schwannomas show characteristic growth patterns of areas with high cell density and areas with low cell density. Antoni A pattern describes areas of high cell density, whereas Antoni B pattern describes areas of low cell density (Fig. 44.4). Some areas might show nuclear palisading around an anucleate zone. This complex is referred to as a Verocay body. Antibodies to S100 highlight Schwann cells and can be used in the diagnosis of neurofibromas and schwannomas. Both tumors stain with S100. However, as schwannomas are composed entirely of Schwann cells, they show near-complete staining of the entire lesion (Fig. 44.5), whereas neurofibromas have intervening S100-negative cells (Fig. 44.6).

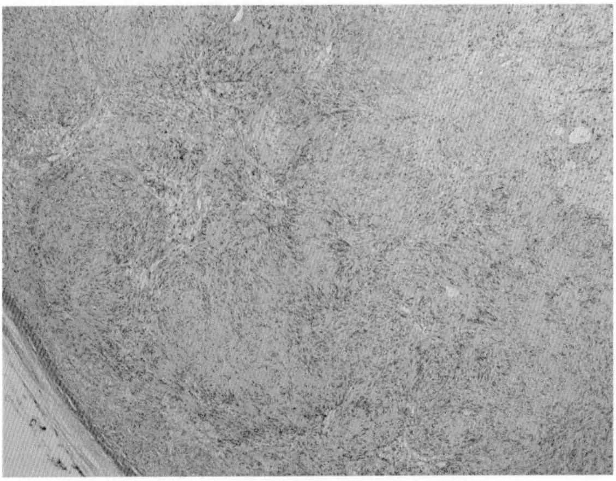

Fig. 44.4 Schwannoma. Mainly Antoni A pattern with hypocellular Antoni B in top right corner. Alternating palisading nuclei and anucleate zones begin to form Verocay bodies (H&E x4).

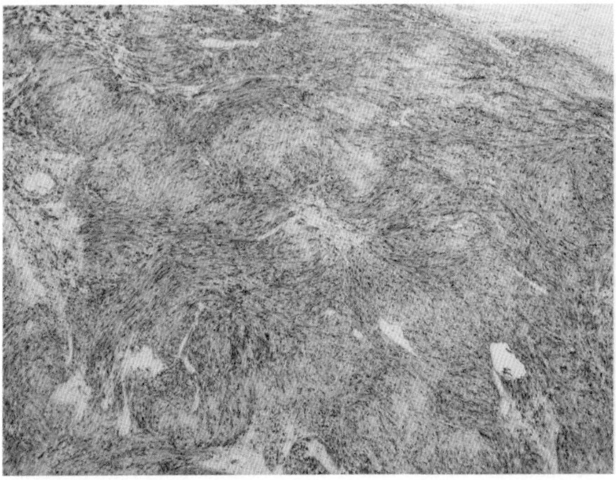

Fig. 44.5 Schwannoma with sheets of S100-positive cells (S100 x4).

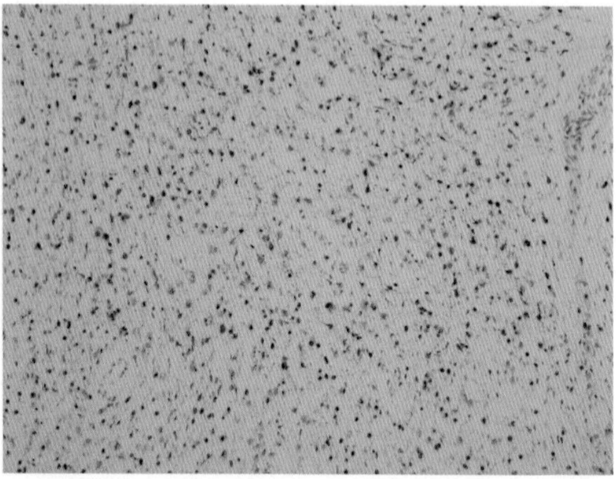

Fig. 44.6 Neurofibroma with diffusely distributed S100-positive cells (S100 10x).

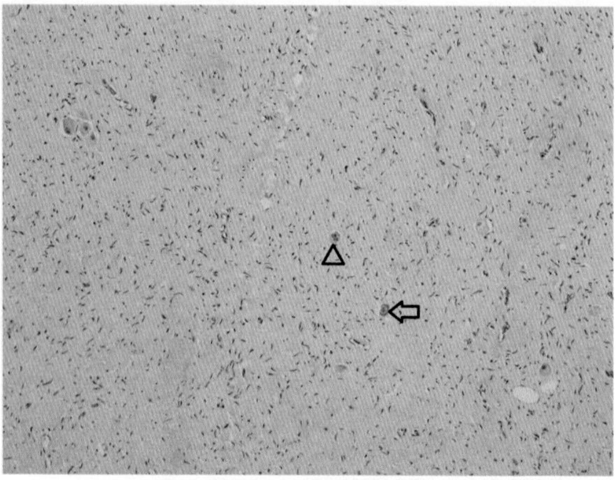

Fig. 44.7 Ganglioneuroma. Embedded within schwannian stroma are variably sized ganglion cells. A binucleated ganglion cell (arrowhead) and accumulated neuromelanin pigment (arrow) are present (H&E 10x).

CLINICAL PEARL

Schwann cells stain with S100, which causes both schwannomas and neurofibromas to be positive for S100. However, since schwannomas are entirely composed of neoplastic Schwann cells, the whole lesion stains uniformly. Neurofibromas are a mixed tumor with non-neoplastic cells. Only the neoplastic Schwann cells stain with S100.

Ganglioneuromas are benign tumors that occur mostly in young patients. Since they arise in sympathetic ganglia, they are usually found along the sympathetic axis. They consist of neoplastic, well-differentiated ganglion cells in a mature schwannian stroma. Even though the ganglion cells are well differentiated, they can vary in size and show vacuolization, pigment accumulation, inclusions, and even multinucleation (Fig. 44.7).

MPNSTs are a group of malignant neoplasms that usually arise in the large nerves. Also included are malignant neoplasms that show schwannian or perineurial cell differentiation even when they are not associated with a peripheral nerve. Histologically, MPNSTs can look quite variable. They are proliferations of elongated cells that often grow in fascicles. Since they are malignant, they infiltrate adjacent structures such as the nerve they originated in or the adjacent bone (Fig. 44.8). Additionally, most are high-grade neoplasms and show features including high cellularity, high mitotic activity, and necrosis (Fig. 44.9). It might be challenging to diagnose MPNST if it is not associated with a nerve, and ancillary studies might be necessary. The ancillary studies, however, are mostly useful for excluding other differentials because many high-grade MPNSTs even lose expression of S100.

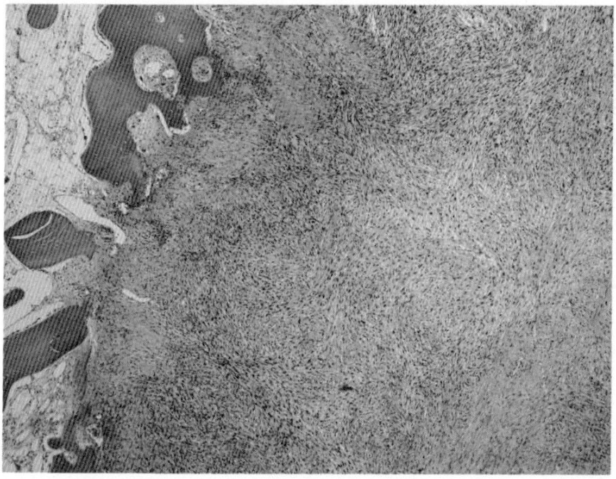

Fig. 44.8 Malignant peripheral nerve sheath tumor showing invasion of the bone (H&E x4).

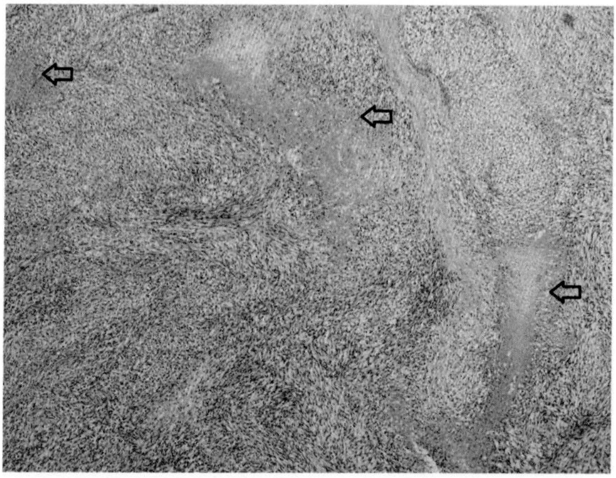

Fig. 44.9 Necrotic areas (arrows) in malignant peripheral nerve sheath tumor (H&E x4).

How is NF1 managed?

To this day, NF1 is incurable. However, yearly follow-up visits are recommended to note complications such as malignant transformation of a neurofibroma in an early stage. Patients should be assessed for skeletal abnormalities and, especially children, learning disabilities. If neurofibromas cause pain, they can be excised. Patients might elect cosmetic surgery to remove disfiguring neurofibromas. Genetic counseling should be offered to patients of childbearing age and the parents to inform them of the probability of passing on the mutated gene.

Case Point 44.2

The pediatrician explains the diagnosis to the parents and the patient and the need for annual follow-up visits. Psychological and social support is offered. Since NF1 is not a contraindication to physical activity, there are no medical reasons to deny access to a sports team.

BEYOND THE PEARLS

- Usually MPNSTs have a combined inactivation of the genes NF1 (hence, the more frequent incidence in NF1 patients) and cyclin-dependent kinase inhibitor 2A (CDKN2A), which, among other codes for p16, is a tumor suppressor protein.
- Even most sporadic schwannomas show inactivating mutations of the NF2 gene.
- Other neoplasms that occur more frequently in NF1 patients are gastrointestinal stromal tumors (GISTs) of the small bowel, rhabdomyosarcoma, various neuroendocrine tumors, juvenile xanthogranuloma, and juvenile chronic myeloid leukemia.
- GISTs in NF1 patients are c-kit and PDGRFA wildtype.

References

Goldblum J, Lamps L, McKenney J, Myers J. *Rosai and Ackerman's Surgical Pathology*. Philadelphia, PA: Elsevier; 2018.

Louis DN, Perry A, Reifenberger G, et al. *WHO Classification of Tumours of the Central Nervous System*. Lyon, France: International Agency for Research on Cancer. 2016.

Perry A, Brat J. *Practical Surgical Neuropathology: A Volume in the Pattern Recognition Series*. Philadelphia, PA: Elsevier; 2010.

CASE 45

An 85-Year-Old Female with Progressive Dementia

Lanisha Denise Fuller

An 85-year-old right-handed female presents to her primary care physician with her granddaughter. The granddaughter reports that her grandmother seems to have changed over the past 2 years. She repeats information multiple times, sometimes even in the same sentence. This has gradually become worse. Additionally, she now needs help dressing herself and cooking after multiple times of leaving the house wearing her sweater inside out and not turning off the stove. She has always been very active before doing charity work and going out with friends, but now she mostly avoids leaving the house. The patient denies this and states that she is doing fine and just prefers a quieter life at the moment. She currently lives alone, but her family members check on her regularly and help her with daily activities like taking her medication. Her past medical history is significant for hypertension and hypercholesterolemia, for which she takes ramipril and atorvastatin daily. She had a minor stroke 5 years ago but does not suffer any sequelae. Physical examination reveals a slenderly built, well-groomed woman. Her blood pressure is 125/70 mm Hg, pulse rate is 80 beats per minute, respiration rate is 14 breaths per minute, and oxygen saturation is 95% on room air. The remainder of the examination is normal. The physician suspects the patient has dementia.

What is dementia?

The granddaughter describes symptoms that should alert you to dementia. According to the WHO ICD-10, dementia is "a syndrome due to disease of the brain, usually of a chronic or progressive nature, in which there is disturbance of multiple higher cortical functions, including memory, thinking, orientation, comprehension, calculation, learning capacity, language, and judgement. Consciousness is not clouded. The impairments of cognitive function are commonly accompanied, and occasionally preceded, by deterioration in emotional control, social behavior, or motivation."

What are some common causes of dementia?

There are various common and rare, reversible as well as irreversible causes of dementia, which are summarized along with some examples in Table 45.1. The prevalence of dementia in general increases in older age groups. Of all causes, Alzheimer's disease, a neurodegenerative process, is by far the most common. Its most striking clinical feature is gradually progressive memory loss. Hypertension can lead to vascular dementia by eliciting multiple small strokes, especially if occurring in deeper brain structures. The clinical picture shows a stepwise decline in cognitive functions. Other etiologies are relatively rare but include reversible causes, such as hypothyroidism, vitamin B12 deficiency, and normal pressure hydrocephalus; these should be excluded as they can be treated.

TABLE 45.1 ■ **Causes of Dementia**

Cause	Example
Neurodegenerative	Alzheimer's dementia, most common form of neurodegenerative disease
Vascular	Strokes due to hypertension, shared risk factors for atherosclerosis
Toxic/Drugs	Anticholinergics
Psychiatric	Depression
Endocrine	Hypothyroidism
Metabolic	Vitamin B12 deficiency
Infectious	Syphilis
Genetic	Cerebral autosomal dominant arteriopathy with subcortical infarcts and leukoencephalopathy (CADASIL)
Autoimmune	Autoimmune encephalitis
Neoplastic	Really any neoplasm in the right location can cause dementia symptoms

CLINICAL PEARL

The symptom triad of normal pressure hydrocephalus is gait deviation, dementia, and urinary incontinence.

What is the best way to determine the cause of this patient's dementia?

The initial step is to determine if the patient actually shows signs of dementia via careful history taking and physical examination. If suspicious, one should assess the degree of cognitive impairment with the Mini-Mental State Examination (MMSE), a quick screening tool widely used in practice. If the exam indicates cognitive impairment, reversible causes should be ruled out. This is done by assessment for depression and laboratory testing for vitamin B12 levels and thyroid function. Imaging studies might be helpful if one suspects a process like normal pressure hydrocephalus or stroke. The patient's history often helps to narrow down the differential diagnosis significantly. Are they also presenting with other symptoms, such as hallucinations, or movement disorders? Do they have hypertension and is it well controlled? However, even if you can narrow down the diffevrentials using the clinical history, certain diseases might only be definitively diagnosed postmortem as a combination of clinical presentation and autopsy findings.

Case Point 45.1

The family physician performs MMSE on the patient. Her score is 19. The physician orders the appropriate laboratory tests and a computed tomography (CT) scan of the head. The patient and her granddaughter come back to the office 2 weeks later. The results of the laboratory tests are within normal limits. A CT scan of the head demonstrates a small remote infarct in the right frontal lobe. There is minimal overall volume loss consistent with age-related changes. No additional infarcts or other lesions are identified.

CLINICAL PEARL

The MMSE has a maximum score of 30. Scores equal or greater than 24 are considered normal. Scores below that indicate mental impairment.

What are the top differential diagnoses?

This is an 85-year-old woman who presents with progressive dementia without significant laboratory and imaging abnormalities. Neurodegenerative diseases are the top differential diagnoses at this point, as they do not have to show imaging or laboratory abnormalities, especially in early stages. Also, they represent the most common causes of dementia in the elderly. Given her history of hypertension and a prior stroke, vascular causes of her dementia also seem plausible. Symptoms depend upon localization of the strokes. They can also impair memory and cognition. These, however, usually present as a stepwise decline of function and not a gradually progressive downward trend.

Which diseases are considered neurodegenerative diseases? What would be their clinical presentations and radiologic features?

Neurodegenerative diseases encompass a heterogeneous group of progressive and currently incurable diseases that lead to neuronal dysfunction and loss. Many are associated with accumulation of abnormal proteins. The clinical picture of many overlaps; however, there are some symptoms that occur more often as well as earlier in certain diseases.

Alzheimer's disease, the most common cause of dementia overall, typically presents with memory loss. At first, short-term memory is most prominently affected. As the disease progresses, other brain functions, including motor control, start to deteriorate as well. Early in the disease, brain imaging might not show any changes. However, gradual cortical atrophy, most pronounced in the mesial temporal lobe structures, will become evident over time.

CLINICAL PEARL

Mesial temporal lobe structures: amygdala, hippocampus, uncus, dentate gyrus, parahippocampal gyrus

The classical triad of Parkinson's disease is akinesia, (resting) tremor, and rigor. The first symptom frequently is unilateral tremor of an extremity. No specific imaging abnormalities are evident on regular CT or magnetic resonance imaging.

Dementia with Lewy bodies' most striking clinical presentation is fluctuating cognitive impairment—alternating periods of cognitive impairment being more and less severe. Additionally, most patients have visual hallucinations and Parkinsonism.

Pick's disease belongs to a group of neurodegenerative diseases with primarily frontotemporal lobar degeneration. The classical triad is change in personality, semantic dementia (loss of word meaning), and progressive nonfluent aphasia (speech production difficulty). Early in the disease, patients present with changes in personality rather than with memory loss. Imaging shows marked atrophy of the frontal and temporal lobes.

Multiple system atrophy (MSA) causes autonomic dysfunction. Depending on the additional presentation of the patient, it can be subclassified into MSA-P or MSA-C. MSA-P presents with Parkinsonism, whereas MSA-C presents with cerebellar symptoms, especially with ataxia. Imaging shows atrophy of the caudate, putamen, cerebellum (especially in MSA-C), and the pons. Additionally, MSA-C can show the "hot cross bun sign," seen as a cross-shaped T2 hyperintense signal in the pons on transverse sections.

Amyotrophic lateral sclerosis (ALS) destroys upper and lower motoneurons, which is why patients present with a combination of upper and lower motoneuron signs. Upper motor neuron signs are hyperreflexia, spastic paralysis, and pathologic reflexes. Lower motor neuron signs are hyporeflexia, flaccid paralysis, and fasciculations. Imaging can show T2 hyperintensity of the corticospinal tracts. Patients with ALS can show a spectrum from ALS only to ALS with frontotemporal dementia to pure frontotemporal dementia.

CLINICAL PEARL

Cu/Zn superoxide dismutase 1 (SOD1) gene mutations are associated with familial forms of ALS.

What are the gross and histologic hallmarks of Alzheimer's?

The diagnosis of Alzheimer's is a combination of the clinical picture as well as neuropathologic examination of the brain. When examining the brain grossly at autopsy, there are no specific findings that would establish the diagnosis. Alzheimer's mostly affects but is not exclusive to the medial temporal lobe, which is also where one would expect most pronounced widening of the sulci and gyral atrophy. Loss of brain substance usually also goes hand in hand with lateral ventricular dilatation, especially in the temporal lobe region. Apart from neuronal loss, you see extracellular neuritic plaques and intracytoplasmic neurofibrillary tangles on microscopic sections (Figs. 45.1 and 45.2).

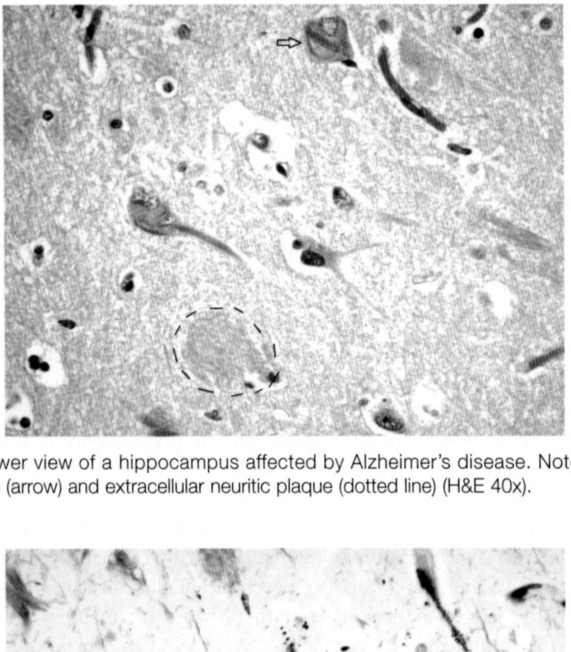

Fig. 45.1 High-power view of a hippocampus affected by Alzheimer's disease. Note the intraneuronal neurofibrillary tangle (arrow) and extracellular neuritic plaque (dotted line) (H&E 40x).

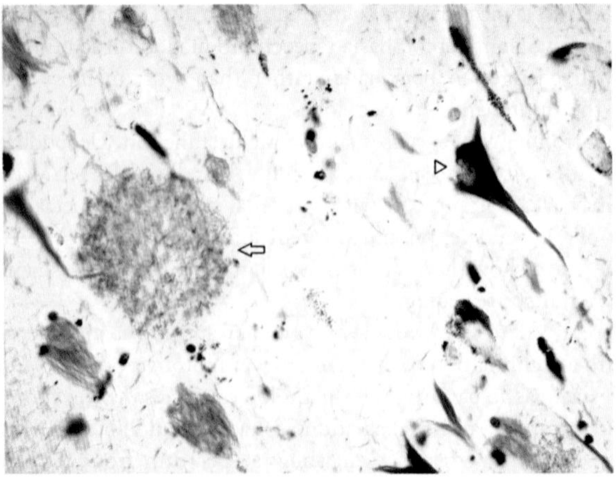

Fig. 45.2 Hippocampus affected by Alzheimer's disease. Note the intraneuronal neurofibrillary tangle (arrowhead) and extracellular plaque (arrow) highlighted by silver stain (Bielschowsky 40x).

CLINICAL PEARL

Neuritic plaques (highlighted by Congo red or anti-Aβ immunohistochemistry) consist of extracellular Aβ peptide aggregates associated with thickened neuritic processes. Aβ peptide is derived from amyloid precursor protein (gene located on chromosome 21). Neurofibrillary tangles (highlighted by a silver stain) consist of intracellular abnormally phosphorylated tau protein aggregates.

What are the gross and/or histologic findings of the other neurodegenerative diseases?

At autopsy, Parkinson's disease shows pallor of the substantia nigra. Histologically, this correlates with loss of neurons in the substantia nigra and gliosis. The pigment of the dead neurons then gets phagocytosed by macrophages. However, this alone is not enough to make the diagnosis of Parkinson's. The presence of Lewy bodies, round intracytoplasmic inclusions, which can be found throughout the brain, is necessary for the pathologic diagnosis (Fig. 45.3). Lewy bodies of the substantia nigra additionally have a clear halo around them, which is not usually found in cortical Lewy bodies.

CLINICAL PEARL

Lewy bodies are neuronal, intracytoplasmic, eosinophilic inclusions. They consist of alpha synuclein, neurofilament, and ubiquitin.

Dementia with Lewy bodies cannot histologically be differentiated from Parkinson's, as both show Lewy bodies throughout the brain. Correlation with the clinical history is necessary to distinguish between these entities.

Both types of MSA show overlapping features like pallor of the substantia nigra. Depending on the clinical picture, each feature is either more or less pronounced. MSA-C shows more cerebellar atrophy, whereas MSA-P usually shows a discolored, atrophic putamen. Histologically, the presence of glial cytoplasmic inclusions in areas of neuronal loss is necessary to diagnose MSA. Neuronal loss of the striatonigral system is more severe in MSA-P, whereas neuronal loss of the olivopontocerebellar system is usually associated with MSA-C.

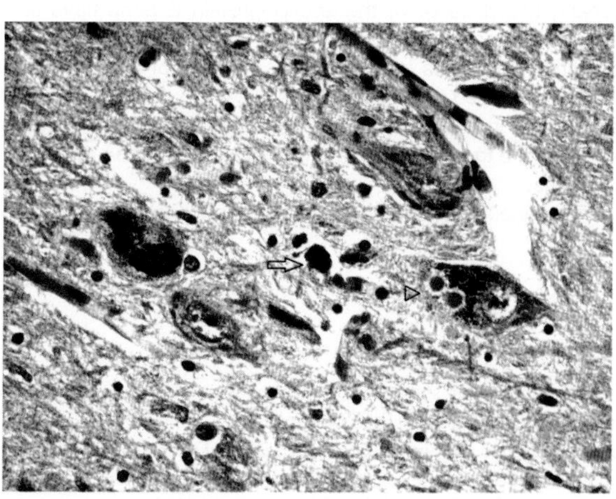

Fig. 45.3 High-power view of a midbrain affected by Parkinson's disease. A neuron shows two Lewy bodies (arrowhead). Note pigment phagocytosed by macrophages (arrow) (H&E 40x).

Pick's disease grossly impresses mostly with severe atrophy of the frontal and temporal lobes. On microscopic sections, there is marked neuronal loss and gliosis as well as spongy changes of the superficial cortex. A hallmark is the presence of Pick bodies, neuronal intracytoplasmic inclusions, in the frontal and temporal lobes.

ALS grossly impresses with severe, diffuse muscle atrophy and thinned anterior roots of the spinal nerves. Histologically, there is loss of upper and lower motor neurons. Small, eosinophilic, intraneuronal cytoplasmic inclusions (Bunina bodies) can be found in anterior horn cells.

How is Alzheimer's disease treated? What is the prognosis?

Neurodegenerative diseases including Alzheimer's are incurable to this day. These diseases result in progressive impairment of function with eventual increasing needs for supportive care. The average duration of Alzheimer's is 7 years. However, the length of survival is highly variable among individuals. Pharmacologic therapy aims at reducing cognitive as well as behavioral symptoms. Cholinesterase inhibitors and memantine are used to control cognitive symptoms. Other psychiatric medications such as antidepressants are used to treat behavioral symptoms. An important nonpharmacological component of therapy is creating a safe and stable environment. Due to progressive decreasing immobility, patient's extrapyramidal symptoms are prone to increasing weakness, thereby decreasing nutritional intake and falls. Aspiration pneumonia and respiratory infections are a common cause of death for these patients.

Case Point 45.2

The physician explains that the diagnosis is likely Alzheimer's disease. Therapy with donepezil is initiated and psychological as well as social support is offered. Hereupon, the patient's mental impairment lessens in severity; however, it starts progressing again after a few months. This is when the patient accepts the offer of her family to move into their home where she spends the remainder of her life.

BEYOND THE PEARLS

- Most Alzheimer's disease cases are sporadic. However, there is an inherited form called familial Alzheimer's disease that is caused by a mutation of preseniline-1 gene on chromosome 14. It has an autosomal dominant pattern of inheritance.
- Individuals carrying the allele $\epsilon 4$ of the apolipoprotein E gene have an increased risk of developing Alzheimer's and developing it earlier.
- The glial cytoplasmic inclusions in MSA are composed of alpha-synuclein and ubiquitin. They can be better visualized with silver stains.
- Pick bodies are intraneuronal, cytoplasmic inclusions composed of tau protein, neurofilament, and ubiquitin. Like the glial cytoplasmic inclusions in MSA, they can be better visualized with silver stains.
- Bunina bodies are intraneuronal, cytoplasmic eosinophilic inclusions that consist of cystatin C.

References

Falk N, Meredith TJ. Evaluation of suspected dementia. *American Family Physician*. March 15, 2018. Available at: www.aafp.org/afp/2018/0315/p398.html.

World Health Organization. (2015). *International statistical classification of diseases and related health problems*, 10th revision, Fifth edition, 2016. Geneva: World Health Organization.

Prayson RA. *Neuropathology*. 2nd ed. Philadelphia, PA: Saunders; 2012.

Hematopoietic System

CASE 46

A 16-Year-Old Female with Fatigue, Breathlessness, and Pallor

Mushal Noor

A 16-year-old female presents to her primary care physician with a 1-month history of progressive fatigue, breathlessness, and pallor. She reports episodes of dizziness and lightheadedness, especially after climbing stairs. Her menstrual cycle is regular, with moderately heavy bleeding for 4 days, and her last period ended 3 days prior. She eats a balanced diet and has no dietary restrictions. She denies fever, night sweats, weight loss, abnormal bleeding or bruising, rashes, diarrhea, constipation, or melena. She reports no significant past surgical history; however, she reports a severe urinary tract infection 5 weeks ago, which required hospital admission and intravenous antibiotics. She denies any illicit drug use and does not drink alcohol.

Case Point 46.1

On physical examination, her temperature is 37°C (98.6°F), blood pressure is 120/75 mm Hg, pulse rate is 93 beats per minute, respiration rate is 18 breaths per minute, and oxygen saturation is 99% on room air. Her body mass index is 22. She has marked pallor of the conjunctivae but is non-jaundiced, well nourished, and well developed with normal heart and lung sounds. Her thyroid is not palpable. Her abdomen is soft, nontender, and nondistended with no hepatosplenomegaly. No lymphadenopathy is appreciated.

Case Point 46.2

The primary care physician orders labs that demonstrate a normal chemistry panel, normal thyroid panel, and negative urine pregnancy test. A complete blood count (CBC) shows: white blood cell count 6.4×10^9/L, red blood cell (RBC) count 5.2×10^9/L, hemoglobin (Hb) concentration 6.7 g/dL, platelet count 293×10^9/L, and mean corpuscular volume (MCV) of 70 fL.

What are the pathologic causes of anemia and how do you work it up?

The normal Hb concentration is 13.5–17.5 g/dL in males and 12–15.5 g/dL in females. Anemia is defined as Hb concentration of less than 13.5 g/dL in males and less than 12 g/dL in females. Patients may present with fatigue, lethargy, breathlessness, pallor of skin, nails, and conjunctiva, dizziness and lightheadedness, palpitations, and even angina. In cases of suspected anemia, RBC indices, especially the MCV, can provide useful information to help classify anemia and determine the pathogenesis.

CLINICAL PEARL

RBC indices

- *MCV*
  The average volume or size of RBCs. Based on MCV, anemias can be classified as microcytic (MCV <80 fL), normocytic (MCV 80–100 fL), or macrocytic (MCV > 100 fL).
- *MCH*
  The average Hb content in an RBC. A low MCH may be seen as hypochromia on peripheral blood smear and may be a feature of iron deficiency anemia and thalassemia.
- *MCHC*
  The average Hb concentration per RBC. Very low MCHC values are seen in iron deficiency anemia, and very high MCHC values may indicate spherocytosis.
- *Red cell distribution width (RDW)*
  A measure of the variation in RBC size, i.e., anisocytosis. A high RDW reflects a large variation in RBC sizes, whereas a low RDW reflects a more homogeneous population of RBCs. A high RDW can be seen in iron deficiency anemia, MDS, and hemoglobinopathies. Patients with anemia who have received a blood transfusion may have a higher RDW.

Based on the MCV, anemias can be classified as microcytic, normocytic, or macrocytic. In the evaluation of a microcytic anemia, the next step in determining the etiology is to perform iron studies.

Case Point 46.3

The patient is diagnosed with microcytic anemia. The physician orders a peripheral smear, reticulocyte count, and iron studies. The peripheral smear shows hypochromia, microcytosis, few target cells, and some basophilic stippling (Fig. 46.1). The reticulocyte count is 2%. Iron studies show serum iron and serum ferritin are mildly increased, whereas the total iron-binding capacity (TIBC) and % saturation are within normal range.

What is microcytic anemia and what is your differential diagnosis?

Microcytic anemia (MCV < 80 fL) is caused by decreased Hb production. This may be due to decrease in either the iron or protoporphyrin needed to produce heme or due to a deficiency in globin chain production. Microcytic anemias include iron deficiency anemia, anemia of chronic disease (ACD), sideroblastic anemia, and thalassemia.

Iron deficiency anemia is the most common type of anemia. Iron is required for heme production and is absorbed in the duodenum. In the blood, iron is transported by transferrin, whereas the storage form of iron in the tissues is ferritin. Iron deficiency is caused by either decreased intake/absorption of dietary iron or due to blood loss. Breastfed infants are at risk of iron deficiency anemia as breast milk is low in iron. Malnutrition, malabsorption, and resection of the stomach or small bowel may result in decreased iron absorption. Gastrointestinal blood loss (ulcers, adenoma/carcinoma, and hookworm) in adult males and menstrual blood loss in females may also result in iron deficiency. In addition to anemia, patients may have spoon-shaped nails (koilonychia), pica, or Plummer–Vinson syndrome (atrophic glossitis and esophageal webs). Laboratory finding are helpful in the diagnosis (Table 46.1). Peripheral smear shows hypochromic, microcytic anemia with marked anisopoikilocytosis, frequent elliptocytes, and target cells (Fig. 46.2)

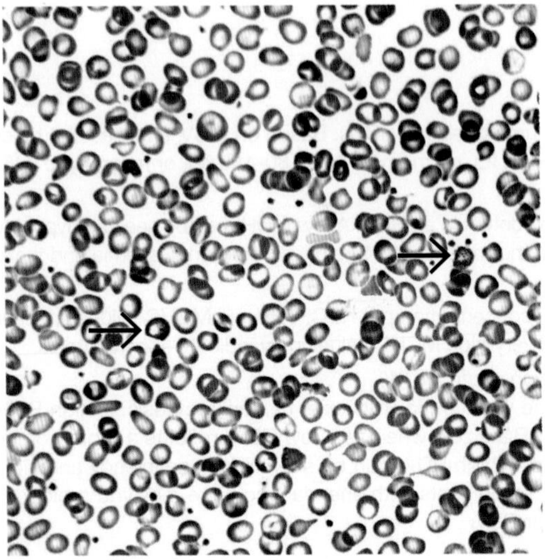

Fig. 46.1 Patient's peripheral smear shows hypochromic microcytic red blood cell population, which in this case exhibits more elliptocytes and hypochromic cells than target cells. Some basophilic stippling (black solid arrow) is seen. (From *ExpertPath*. Copyright Elsevier.)

TABLE 46.1 ■ **Iron Studies in Microcytic Anemia**

	Iron Deficiency	Thalassemia	ACD	Sideroblastic
Serum iron	↓	↔/↑	↓	↑
Serum ferritin	↓	↔/↑	↑	↑
TIBC	↑	↔	↓	↓
% saturation	↓	↔/↑	↓	↑
RBC count	↓	↔/↑	↔/↓	↔/↓
RDW	↑	↔	↔	↔

ACD, anemia of chronic disease; *RBC*, red blood cell, *RDW*, red cell distribution width; *TIBC*, total iron-binding capacity.

ACD or anemia of inflammation is the commonest anemia in hospitalized patients. Inflammatory cytokines suppress the renal production of erythropoietin, resulting in decreased RBC production. In addition, the acute-phase reactant hepcidin, which is produced by the liver, decreases iron absorption in the small intestine and reduces release of iron from body stores. This lack of iron availability leads to microcytosis and anemia. Laboratory studies show decreased serum iron in the presence of increased serum ferritin (Table 46.1).

Sideroblastic anemia is a heterogeneous group of microcytic anemias of varying severity, which may be congenital or acquired, and are characterized by the presence of ring sideroblasts in the bone marrow. Ring sideroblasts are RBC precursors, or erythroblasts, which contain iron-laden mitochondria that are seen on Prussian blue staining as a ring of blue granules around the nucleus (Fig. 46.3). Sideroblastic anemia is due to defective protoporphyrin synthesis; despite adequate iron stores, the body is unable to use iron to produce protoporphyrin, and consequently,

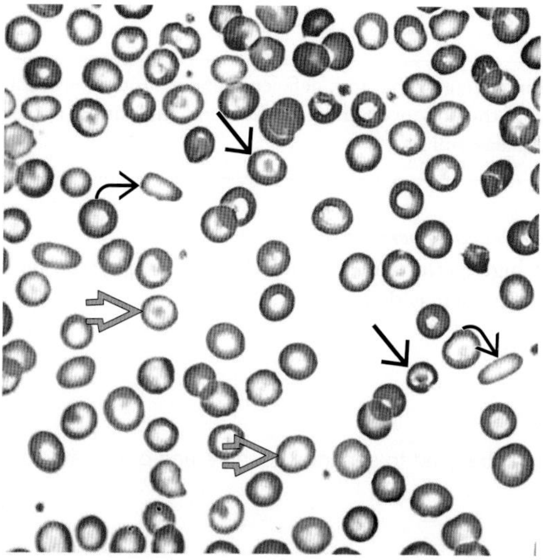

Fig.46.2 Peripheral blood smear of a marked iron deficiency anemia (hemoglobin 7.7 g/dL) exhibits marked anisopoikilocytosis. There are frequent hypochromic red blood cells (cyan open arrow), elliptocytes (black curved arrow), and target cells (black solid arrow). (From *ExpertPath*. Copyright Elsevier.)

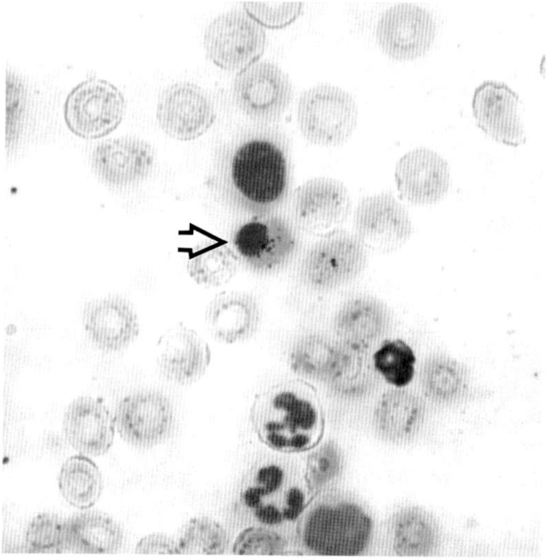

Fig. 46.3 Prussian blue iron stain of a bone marrow aspirate smear reveals a classic ring sideroblast (black open arrow). The granules encircle at least one-third of the red cell nucleus and are often larger. Ring sideroblasts are a hallmark of sideroblastic anemias. (From *ExpertPath*. Copyright Elsevier.)

heme. Congenital causes include enzyme defects in the heme synthesis pathway. Acquired causes include alcoholism, lead poisoning, and deficiency of pyridoxine (vitamin B6), which may occur as a side effect of isoniazid therapy. Certain types of myelodysplastic syndrome (MDS) can also present with a sideroblastic anemia. Lab studies will show an increased serum iron and ferritin, with a decreased TIBC (Table 46.1).

Case Point 46.4

The patient's lab findings suggest that iron deficiency anemia is unlikely (Table 46.1). Microcytic, hypochromic anemia, in the presence of high RBC count, and normal to elevated serum iron and ferritin may indicate thalassemia.

What additional testing should be performed?

Hb electrophoresis or high-performance liquid chromatography can be performed to demonstrate hemoglobinopathies such as thalassemia.

CLINICAL PEARL

Hb Electrophoresis

Hb electrophoresis may be used to separate, identify, and quantitate normal and abnormal Hbs.

Normal Hbs

Dominant Hb in adults is HbA (approximately 96%), while minor forms of Hb are HbA_2 and HbF (approximately 3% and 1%, respectively).

- HbA: two α chains and two β chains
- HbA_2 two α chains and two δ chains
- HbF two α chains and two γ chains

The presence of abnormal Hbs, such as Hb Barts (gamma chain tetramers) or HbH (beta chain tetramers), is consistent with alpha thalassemia. Absence of fetal Hb (HbF) and the adult Hbs, HbA and HbA_2, suggests alpha thalassemia major. Increases in HbF or HbA_2, with decreased HbA, are consistent with a beta thalassemia syndrome. The diagnosis of a thalassemia is best confirmed by globin gene testing.

Case Point 46.5

The patient's Hb electrophoresis shows an elevated HbA2 of 8.5%, elevated HbF of 30%, and decreased HbA of 61.5%.

What is thalassemia and what are the different types?

Thalassemia is a quantitative Hb defect characterized by decreased production of structurally normal Hbs. Alpha thalassemia is characterized by decreased production of α-globin chains, whereas beta thalassemia has decreased production of β-globin chains. The continued synthesis of the unaffected chains results in a relative excess, and they are precipitated, leading to RBC damage and shortened life span. Thalassemia is more prevalent in the Mediterranean, Africa, and Southeast Asia.

There are four α-globin genes on chromosome 16; alpha thalassemia results from gene deletion, and the severity of disease depends on the number of α-globin genes deleted. In **silent carriers**, one gene is deleted (–α/αα). Such individuals are completely asymptomatic with normal CBC and Hb electrophoresis. In **alpha thalassemia trait,** two genes are deleted. The cis genotype has deletions on the same chromosome (– –/αα) and is seen in Asians, whereas the trans genotype has one deletion on each chromosome (–α/–α) and is seen in African-Americans.

The implication of a trans genotype is that offspring would not develop the more severe forms of thalassemia such as HbH disease or hydrops fetalis. **HbH disease** results from three gene deletions (– –/–α) with the excess β-globin chains forming tetramers called HbH. HbH can be detected on Hb electrophoresis and may be seen as Heinz bodies on crystal blue stains. Deletion of all four globin genes is incompatible with life and results in **hydrops fetalis**. The excess γ chains form tetramers called Hb Barts.

There are two β-globin genes on chromosome 11; beta thalassemia results from point mutations resulting in decreased (β^+) or absent (β^0) production of β-globin chains. As β chains are expressed only in adult Hbs, the disease manifests later in life. **Beta thalassemia minor** (β/β^+) is asymptomatic; however, lab studies reveal an increased RBC count, microcytic and hypochromic RBCs on peripheral smear, as well as increased HbA2 (5%–8%) and HbF (2%) on electrophoresis. **Beta thalassemia major** (β^0/β^0) is the most severe form of the disease. At birth, high levels of HbF prevent symptoms; however, as HbF declines around 6–9 months, patients present with severe hemolytic anemia. Hb electrophoresis shows increased HbF (50%–90%), normal to elevated HbA_2, and little or no HbA. Additional features are erythroid hyperplasia in the bone marrow leading to "crewcut" appearance of the skull on x-ray, increased size of the maxilla or "chipmunk facies," hepatosplenomegaly, and lifelong transfusion dependence. **Beta thalassemia intermedia** presents with varying degrees of anemia; however, despite lab findings that may be similar to those of beta thalassemia major, it does not require regular transfusions. Patients usually present in late childhood or even adulthood with mild to moderate anemia and an Hb concentration between 7 g/dL and 10 g/dL. However, many patients may require intermittent RBC transfusions in the setting of infection or pregnancy.

Case Point 46.6

The patient is diagnosed with beta thalassemia intermedia and is transfused with one unit of packed RBCs for her anemia. She is counselled that she may have become acutely anemic following her urinary tract infection; however, it is unlikely that she will require regular transfusions. Outpatient follow-up is advised.

What is the treatment for thalassemia?

Recent clinical trials have reported successful use of gene therapy for the treatment of beta thalassemia. For most patients with thalassemia major, transfusion therapy with iron chelation is the mainstay of treatment. HbF induction with hydroxyurea may increase total Hb levels and decrease the need for transfusions.

What are the types of macrocytic anemia?

Macrocytic anemia (MCV >100 fL) may be megaloblastic or nonmegaloblastic. Megaloblastic anemia is caused by a deficiency of vitamin B12 or folate, which is required for normal DNA synthesis. In B12 or folate deficiency, impaired DNA synthesis leads to nuclear-cytoplasmic asynchrony, and large macro-ovalocytes and hypersegmented neutrophils are seen in the peripheral blood (Fig. 46.4). The bone marrow is usually hypercellular with megaloblastic changes, and ineffective erythropoiesis leads to hemolysis and anemia. Nonmegaloblastic anemia may be caused by liver disease, alcoholism, hypothyroidism, and certain drugs.

Vitamin B12 deficiency due to dietary insufficiency is uncommon and is generally seen only in strict vegetarians or vegans. B12 is stored in the liver, and it takes years to develop a dietary deficiency. B12 binds to intrinsic factor (IF) produced by the parietal cells of the stomach, and this B12-IF complex is then absorbed in the ileum. The more common cause of B12 deficiency is decreased B12 absorption due to autoimmune destruction of stomach parietal cells leading to IF deficiency (pernicious anemia). Pancreatic insufficiency, diseases of the ileum such as bacterial

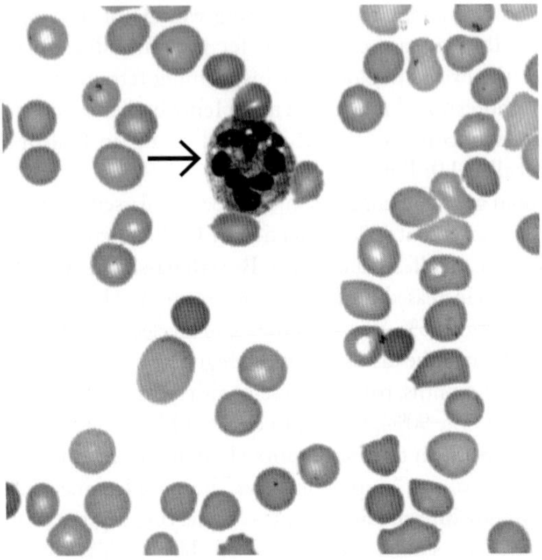

Fig. 46.4 Peripheral blood smear demonstrates macrocytic red blood cells. A hypersegmented neutrophil (black solid arrow) is pathognomonic for megaloblastic anemia, but does not indicate the underlying cause. (Photo credit: John R. Hess, MD, MPH. From *ExpertPath*. Copyright Elsevier.)

overgrowth or Crohn's disease, and parasites such as fish tapeworm (*Diphyllobothrium latum)* may also cause decreased B12 absorption. In addition to megaloblastic anemia, other features seen in B12 deficiency include glossitis and subacute combined degeneration of the spinal cord. Lab tests show decreased serum B12, increased serum homocysteine, and increased serum methylmalonic acid (which helps distinguish from folate deficiency).

Folate deficiency produces a megaloblastic anemia without neurologic deficits. Green leafy vegetables are a good source of folate; however, body stores are minimal. Consequently, a deficiency can develop within months, especially in the elderly, infants, and alcoholics, or in cases of increased requirement, such as pregnancy, hemolytic anemia, or cancer. Folate antagonists such as methotrexate may also result in deficiency and anemia. Lab results are essentially similar to those seen in B12 deficiency; however, serum methylmalonic acid is normal.

What are the types of normocytic anemia?

Normocytic anemia (MCV 80–100 fL) can be further classified based on reticulocyte count into those characterized by increased peripheral destruction (high reticulocyte count) or decreased production (low or normal reticulocyte count).

CLINICAL PEARL

Reticulocytes

Reticulocytes are immature RBCs seen as larger, polychromatic (bluish) cells on peripheral smear. Normal reticulocyte count is 1%–2%. Appropriate response to anemia is increased production of reticulocytes by the marrow.

Corrected reticulocyte count: % reticulocytes × hematocrit/45

A corrected count >3% indicates a good marrow response, i.e., the cause of anemia is increased peripheral destruction. On the other hand, a corrected count <3% indicates decreased production by the marrow.

Anemia with a high reticulocyte count indicates increased destruction, i.e., hemolytic anemia. This includes various intrinsic RBC disorders with defects of red cell membrane, enzymes, and Hb. Other causes of hemolytic anemia may be extrinsic to RBCs (Table 46.2).

Sickle cell anemia is an autosomal recessive Hb disorder characterized by a single amino acid change at position 6 of the β-globin change, which replaces glutamic acid with valine. The resulting defective Hb is called HbS, which has a propensity to polymerize when deoxygenated, resulting in sickled RBCs that can occlude small vessels (Fig. 46.5). Homozygous individuals (SS) have sickle cell disease and Hb electrophoresis shows >80% HbS, 1%–20% HbF, 1%–4% HbA_2, and

TABLE 46.2 ■ **Classification of Normocytic Anemia**

Normocytic Anemia (MCV 80–100 fL)		
High reticulocyte count, i.e., hemolytic anemia	Intrinsic RBC defects	Sickle cell anemia Hemoglobin C disease Hereditary spherocytosis Hereditary elliptocytosis Glucose-6-phosphate dehydrogenase (G6PD) deficiency Pyruvate kinase deficiency Paroxysmal nocturnal hemoglobinuria
	Extrinsic RBC defects	Autoimmune hemolytic anemia (warm and cold) Microangiopathic hemolytic anemia Parasitic hemolysis
Low reticulocyte count, i.e., decreased production	Aplastic anemia Parvovirus B19 Myelofibrosis Renal failure Anemia of chronic disease Marrow infiltration by leukemia/metastasis	

MCV, mean corpuscular volume; *RBC,* red blood cell.

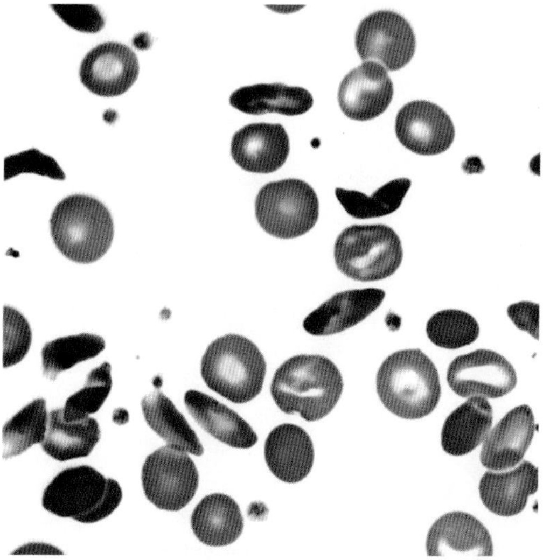

Fig. 46.5 HbS is less soluble in deoxygenated conditions, such as during infection or at high altitude. Rigid polymers form and distort the erythrocytes into the characteristic sickled shape. (From *ExpertPath*. Copyright Elsevier.)

no HbA. The sickled RBCs have a shortened life span of about 17 days and undergo both intravascular and extravascular hemolysis, accompanied by erythroid hyperplasia. The sickled RBCs may block small vessels, resulting in painful vaso-occlusive crises, hand-foot syndrome, or acute chest syndrome. HbF prevents HbS polymerization; therefore, treatment with hydroxyurea is utilized to increase HbF levels.

Heterozygous individuals (AS) have sickle cell trait, and Hb electrophoresis shows 35%–45% HbS, 50%–65% HbA, and <3% HbA_2. They are generally asymptomatic, but may have an increased incidence of hematuria, isosthenuria (inability to concentrate urine), renal papillary necrosis, and medullary carcinoma. They also have resistance to *Plasmodium falciparum* infection, which may explain the persistence of the HbS gene in African populations.

Hereditary spherocytosis is an autosomal dominant RBC membrane disorder caused by a defect in the cytoskeletal proteins spectrin, ankyrin, or band 3. This results in a loss of RBC membrane, and the cells become spherical instead of the usual biconcave disc (Fig. 46.6). The spherocytes are more fragile and are destroyed by the splenic macrophages, resulting in extravascular hemolysis. Splenomegaly, jaundice, and bilirubin gallstones are possible complications. Lab tests show normal mean corpuscular hemoglobin (MCH), increased mean corpuscular hemoglobin concentration (MCHC), and increased osmotic fragility. The treatment is splenectomy.

Glucose-6-phosphate dehydrogenase (G6PD) deficiency is an X-linked recessive RBC enzyme disorder where RBCs are susceptible to oxidative stress as a result of decreased G6PD enzyme. Acute oxidative stress such as drugs (sulfa drugs, primaquine), infection, or fava beans may precipitate Hb as Heinz bodies, which are removed by splenic macrophages ("bite" or "blister" cells) resulting in episodic intravascular hemolysis (Fig. 46.7). Enzyme studies for G6PD activity should be performed when the patient is not actively hemolyzing.

Paroxysmal nocturnal hemoglobinuria results from an acquired mutation in hematopoietic stem cells in the gene required to produce glucose-6-phosphate isomerase (GPI). GPI is necessary to anchor the membrane proteins CD55 (decay accelerating factor or DAF) and CD59 to the cell surface; its absence, with a resulting lack of CD55 and CD59 on the cell membrane, leads

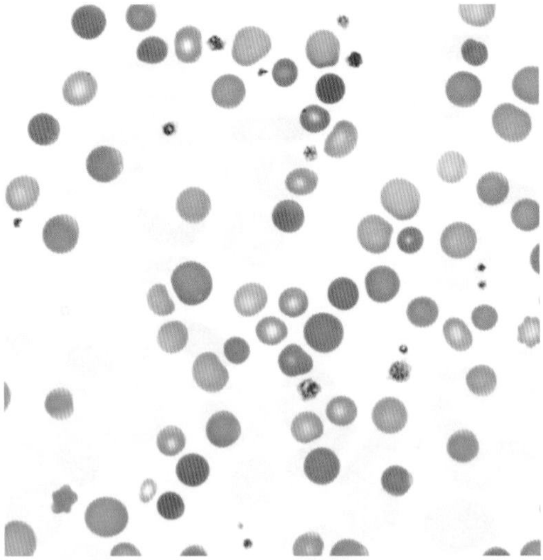

Fig. 46.6 Spherocytes are nearly perfectly round in shape and are smaller than normal red cells; they lack central pallor (hyperchromic). (From *ExpertPath*. Copyright Elsevier.)

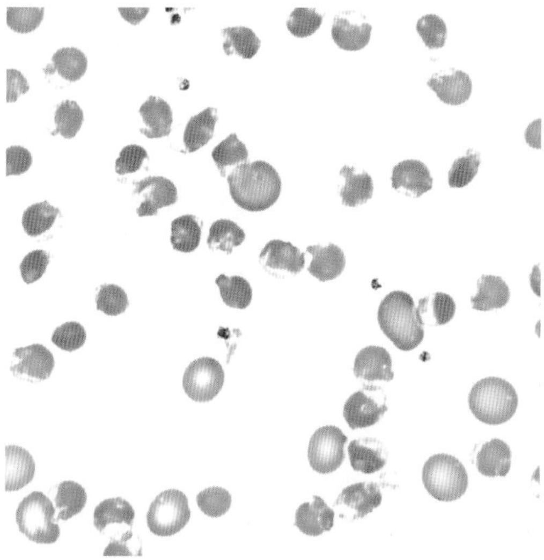

Fig. 46.7 Numerous blister cells in a patient with G6PD and acute hemolytic episode related to a recent viral infection. (From *ExpertPath*. Copyright Elsevier.)

to complement-mediated hemolysis of RBCs and complement activation of platelets. This results in episodic intravascular hemolysis, especially at night or during exercise, due to acidosis. Venous thrombosis can be a fatal complication. There is a small risk of evolution to acute leukemia. Flow cytometry can be used to detect the presence of DAF/CD55 on blood cells.

Autoimmune hemolytic anemias (AIHA) may be warm or cold. Warm AIHA is more common and usually caused by IgG antibodies, which are most active at 37°C. The peripheral smear may show spherocytosis. The direct antiglobulin test (DAT or direct Coomb's test) will be positive; IgG, complement, or both may be detectable on RBCs. Common causes include autoimmune disorders, lymphoproliferative disorders, and drugs.

Cold AIHA is usually caused by IgM antibodies, which fix complement at colder temperatures. The peripheral smear may show agglutination; the DAT will be positive, with complement detectable on RBCs. Common causes include mycoplasma or Epstein–Barr virus infection, chronic lymphocytic leukemia, and Waldenstrom macroglobulinemia. Both warm and cold AIHA may also be primary or idiopathic.

Microangiopathic hemolytic anemias (MAHA) occur due to mechanical disruption and fragmentation of RBCs as a result of microvascular pathology. Diseases such as thrombotic thrombocytopenic purpura, hemolytic uremic syndrome, and disseminated intravascular coagulation may all result in MAHA. Shear stress from prosthetic heart valves or conditions such as aortic stenosis may also damage RBCs. Peripheral smear shows fragmented RBCs in the form of schistocytes and helmet cells (Fig. 46.8).

On the other hand, anemia with a low reticulocyte count indicates decreased production of RBCs by the bone marrow. This includes conditions such a aplastic anemia, myelofibrosis, and marrow infiltration or replacement by leukemia or other malignancies (Table 46.2).

Aplastic anemia is marrow failure resulting in pancytopenia. Around 70% of cases are idiopathic and likely autoimmune mediated; however, drugs and chemicals such as benzene, insecticides, chloramphenicol, and chemotherapeutic agents, as well as radiation and certain viruses may

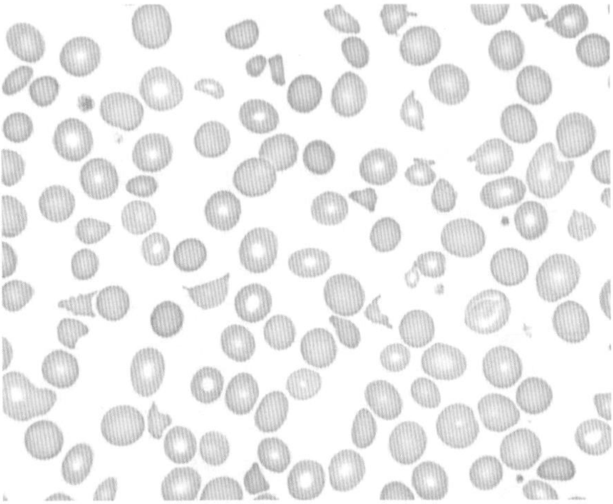

Fig. 46.8 Schistocytes/red cell fragmentation in a patient with a defective cardiac valve. The morphologic features are similar to those seen in microangiopathic hemolytic anemia. (From Hsi E. *Hematopathology*. 2nd ed. Philadelphia: Saunders. 48, 2012. FIG 1.42)

cause damage to the hematopoietic cells. The bone marrow is profoundly hypocellular with decrease in all cell lines and extensive marrow fat replacement.

Myelofibrosis is a myeloproliferative neoplasm characterized by proliferation of megakaryocytic and granulocytic lineages, with progressive marrow fibrosis. Patients can present with a modest to severe anemia, with many teardrop-shaped RBCs (dacryocytes). In marrow infiltration by **leukemia/metastasis,** the normal hematopoietic precursors are crowded out, resulting in pancytopenia.

CLINICAL PEARL

- *Hypochromia:* increase in the size of central pallor of RBC
- *Anisocytosis:* variation in cell size
- *Poikilocytosis:* variation in cell shape
- *Spherocytes:* result from decreased RBC membrane; seen in hereditary spherocytosis and immune hemolytic anemia
- *Elliptocytes:* seen in hereditary elliptocytosis
- *Target cells:* result from increased RBC membrane; seen in thalassemia and hemoglobinopathies
- *Acanthocytes/Spur cells:* RBCs have spicules on the surface; seen in abetalipoproteinemia and liver disease
- *Echinocytes/Burr cells:* seen in uremia; RBCs have short, blunt projections
- *Schistocytes:* RBC fragments; seen in MAHA
- *Dacrocytes:* "teardrop cells"; seen in myelofibrosis and occasionally in thalassemia
- *Sickle cells:* Seen in sickle cell anemia
- *Rouleaux:* coin-like stacking of RBCs; seen in multiple myeloma
- *Reticulocytes:* immature larger RBCs with polychromasia

BEYOND THE PEARLS

- Patients with sickle cell disease may undergo autosplenectomy due to repeated splenic infarcts, which predisposes them to infections by encapsulated organisms.
- Intravascular hemolysis is RBC destruction within the blood vessels and is characterized by hemoglobinemia, hemoglobinuria, hemosiderinuria, and decreased serum haptoglobin. Splenomegaly is generally not seen.
- Extravascular hemolysis is RBC destruction by the reticuloendothelial system in the spleen or liver. There is splenomegaly, and serum unconjugated bilirubin may be increased with a decrease in haptoglobin.
- Parvovirus B19 infects and is cytotoxic to RBC precursors. This may result in transient aplastic crises, especially in patients with other hemolytic disorders, such as thalassemia or sickle cell anemia.
- Parasitic infection such as malaria or babesiosis may rarely result in a hemolytic anemia.

References

Cazzola M, Invernizzi R. Ring sideroblasts and sideroblastic anemias. *Haematologica.* 2011;96(6):789-792. doi:10.3324/haematol.2011.044628.

DeLoughery TG. Microcytic anemia. *N Engl J Med.* 2014;371(14):1324-1331.

Gardner RV. Sickle cell disease: advances in treatment. *Ochsner J.* 2018;18(4):377-389. doi:10.31486/toj.18.0076.

Hsi E. *Hematopathology.* 2nd ed. Philadelphia, PA: Elsevier; 2012.

Louderback AL, Shanbrom E. Hemoglobin electrophoresis. *JAMA.* 1967;202(8):718-719. doi:10.1001/jama.1967.03130210092016.

Musallam KM, Taher AT, Rachmilewitz EA. β-thalassemia intermedia: a clinical perspective. *Cold Spring Harb Perspect Med.* 2012;2(7):a013482. doi:10.1101/cshperspect.a013482.

Nagao T, Hirokawa M. Diagnosis and treatment of macrocytic anemias in adults. *J Gen Fam Med.* 2017;18(5):200-204. doi:10.1002/jgf2.31.

Thompson AA, Walters MC, Kwiatkowski J, et al. Gene therapy in patients with transfusion-dependent β-thalassemia. *N Engl J Med.* 2018;378(16):1479-1493.

CASE 47

A 62-Year-Old Male with Fatigue and Weight Loss

Mushal Noor

A 62-year-old male presents to his primary care doctor with a 3-month history of fatigue, loss of appetite, and vague fullness in the left upper abdomen. He also reports a 12-pound weight loss during this period. He denies fever, night sweats, abnormal bleeding or bruising, rashes, shortness of breath, diarrhea, constipation, melena, or joint swelling.

He has no significant past medical or surgical history, but he does take nonsteroidal anti-inflammatory drugs (ibuprofen) frequently for chronic low back pain. He denies any illicit drug use but reports alcohol use on the weekends. On physical examination, his temperature is 37°C (98.6°F), blood pressure is 138/88 mm Hg, pulse rate is 87 beats per minute, respiration rate is 13 breaths per minute, and oxygen saturation is 99% on room air. His body mass index is 27. He has mild pallor of the conjunctiva but is nonjaundiced, well nourished, and well developed with normal heart and lung sounds. His abdomen is soft, mildly tender to deep palpation, with palpable splenomegaly but no hepatomegaly. No cervical, axillary, or inguinal lymphadenopathy is appreciated. The primary care physician orders a complete blood count that shows: white blood cell (WBC) count $89.2 \times 10^9/L$, hemoglobin 11 g/dL, and platelet count $137 \times 10^9/L$.

What are the pathologic causes of leukocytosis and how do you work it up?

The normal circulating WBC count is $4–11 \times 10^9/L$. Leukocytosis refers to an increase in the number of WBCs in the circulation and can be caused by a variety of reactive or neoplastic processes (Table 47.1).

In determining whether the underlying cause of leukocytosis is reactive or neoplastic, the next step is establishing which types of WBCs comprise the excess.

CLINICAL PEARL

- Neutrophilia: absolute neutrophil count $>7.0 \times 10^9/L$ in adults
- Monocytosis: absolute blood monocyte count $>0.8 \times 10^9/L$ in adults
- Eosinophilia: absolute eosinophil count $>0.5 \times 10^9/L$, independent of age
- Basophilia: absolute basophil count $>0.2 \times 10^9/L$
- Lymphocytosis: absolute blood lymphocyte count $>4.0 \times 10^9/L$

CLINICAL PEARL

Leukemoid reaction

- Exaggerated leukocytosis usually $>50 \times 10^9/L$
- Predominantly neutrophilia with left shift
- May be mistaken for leukemia, especially CML
  - Leukocyte alkaline phosphatase activity is high in leukemoid reaction but low in CML.
- Causes: severe infection, glucocorticoids, stress

TABLE 47.1 ■ **Causes of Leukocytosis**

Type of Leukocytosis	Causes
Neutrophilia	Acute bacterial infections; inflammatory/metabolic disorders (burns, trauma, infarction, inflammatory bowel disease, collagen vascular diseases); medications (G-CSF, chemokines, epinephrine, corticosteroids, lithium); malignancies
Eosinophilia	Allergic disorders; parasitic infections; medications; collagen vascular disorders; malignancies
Basophilia	Myeloproliferative diseases; secondary basophilia in allergic disorders and chronic inflammation
Monocytosis	Chronic infections (tuberculosis, syphilis, subacute bacterial endocarditis); inflammatory/immune-mediated disorders (collagen vascular diseases, e.g. SLE, RA); inflammatory bowel diseases; malignancies
Lymphocytosis	Viral infections (infectious mononucleosis); *Bordetella pertussis* infection; transient stress lymphocytosis; malignancies

G-CSF, granulocyte-colony stimulating factor; *RA,* rheumatoid arthritis; *SLE,* systemic lupus erythematosus.

Case Point 47.1

The patient's peripheral blood differential count shows neutrophilia ($67.3 \times 10^9/L$), eosinophilia ($10.1 \times 10^9/L$), basophilia ($4.2 \times 10^9/L$), and monocytosis ($4.1 \times 10^9/L$). The lymphocyte count is within normal limits ($3.5\times 10^9/L$).

What additional testing should be performed?

In addition to blood counts, the morphology of blood cells is also an important key to the nature of the underlying disease process. Peripheral smears stained with Wright–Giemsa stain are examined for WBC, red blood cell (RBC), and platelet abnormalities. Evaluation of neutrophil granularity, RBC shape, size, and color, and platelet size and granularity should be taken into account.

Bone marrow aspirate smears are stained with Wright–Giemsa or May–Grünwald–Giemsa for optimal examination of cytoplasmic granules and nuclear chromatin. The features best seen under a microscope are the presence of dysplasia in one or more cell lineages, an increased or decreased bone marrow cellularity, and presence of increased blasts.

Bone marrow trephine biopsy stained with hematoxylin and eosin provides important information about overall cellularity (age-matched), proportion and maturation of hematopoietic cells, and bone marrow stromal fibrosis. Immunohistochemical stains can be performed on the biopsy to help further characterize cell types and markers for diagnostic and prognostic purposes. Flow cytometry is another essential tool for immunophenotypic analysis of hematological neoplasms.

CLINICAL PEARL

Flow Cytometry:

Flow cytometry measures multiple characteristics of individual particles flowing in single file in a stream of fluid. Specimens that can be examined include whole blood, bone marrow, serous cavity fluids, cerebrospinal fluid, urine, as well as solid tissues.

Light scattering at different angles can distinguish differences in size and internal complexity, whereas light emitted from fluorescently labeled antibodies can identify a wide array of cell surface and cytoplasmic antigens. Characteristics that can be measured include cell size, cytoplasmic complexity, DNA or RNA content, and a wide range of membrane-bound and intracellular proteins.

CLINICAL PEARL

Ancillary Tests to Evaluate Bone Marrow:

- Immunohistochemistry
  - CD34/CD117: assess for number of blasts
  - Myeloperoxidase: assess for myeloid differentiation
  - CD71/glycophorin A: assess erythroid precursors/erythroblasts
  - CD42b/CD31/CD61: assess for immature megakaryocytes
  - CD3/CD20: assess for T and B cells, respectively.
  - Reticulin stain: to assess for fibrosis
  - Iron: to assess iron stores and sideroblasts
- Flow cytometric immunophenotyping
  - Essential for blast lineage determination
  - Useful for aberrant antigen detection in myeloid neoplasms
  - Useful in disease monitoring
- Cytogenetics/FISH
  - Essential for subclassification, especially myeloid neoplasms
  - Delineation of structural and numerical abnormalities that define neoplastic clones
  - Essential in disease monitoring

Case Point 47.2

The patient's peripheral smear shows markedly increased mature granulocytes with left shift (immature forms such as myelocytes and metamyelocytes in the circulation), and increased circulating basophils and eosinophils. However, all cells are morphologically normal; no dysplasia is seen. There are no circulating blasts (Fig. 47.1).

Bone marrow aspirate and core biopsy show a hypercellular marrow (90% cellularity), with 4% blasts. Granulocytic lineage predominates with a myeloid-to-erythroid ratio of 14:1 (normal 2:1 to 4:1; Figs. 47.2, 47.3A and B).

What are the diseases caused by increased WBCs?

Malignancies composed of increased WBCs in the marrow, tissues, or circulation include acute leukemias, mature B- and T-cell neoplasms, and myeloproliferative disorders.

Acute leukemias are neoplastic proliferations of immature hematopoietic cells called blast cells, and are characterized by greater than 25% blasts in the bone marrow. Blasts are large cells, with very fine chromatin, prominent nucleoli, and scant cytoplasm. Acute leukemias usually present with symptoms caused by replacement of normal functioning marrow by malignant blasts: anemia (fatigue), leukopenia (infections), and thrombocytopenia (bleeding). They arise more commonly in children and young adults and may often involve the central nervous system and testes.

Acute leukemias can be of lymphoid origin (acute lymphoblastic leukemia [ALL]) arising from precursor B or T cells (Fig. 47.4) or they can be of myeloid origin (acute myeloid leukemia,

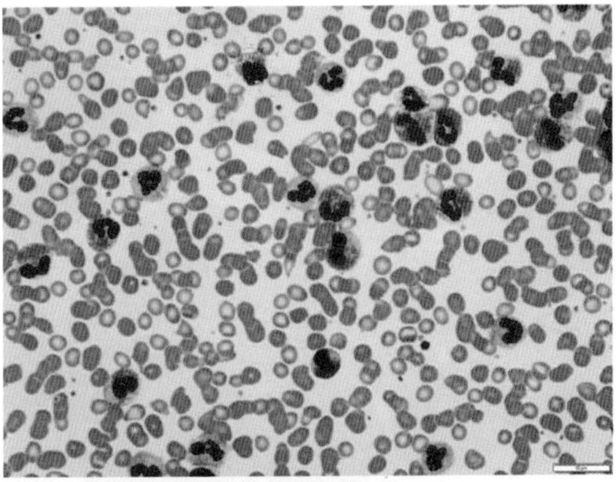

Fig. 47.1 Patient's peripheral blood smear showing numerous neutrophils, bands, and eosinophils (H&E).

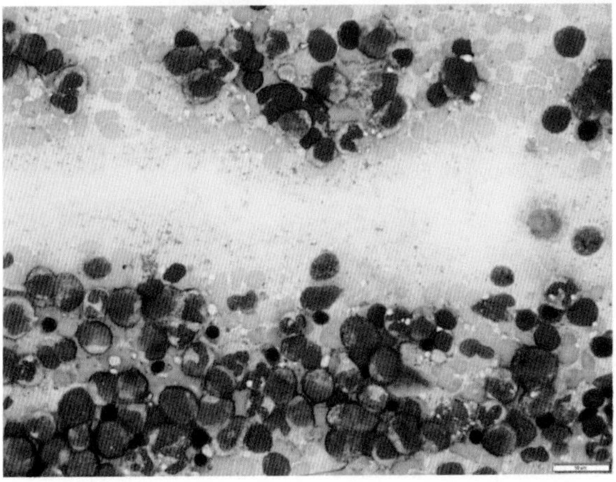

Fig. 47.2 Patient's bone marrow aspirate showing increased myeloid precursors.

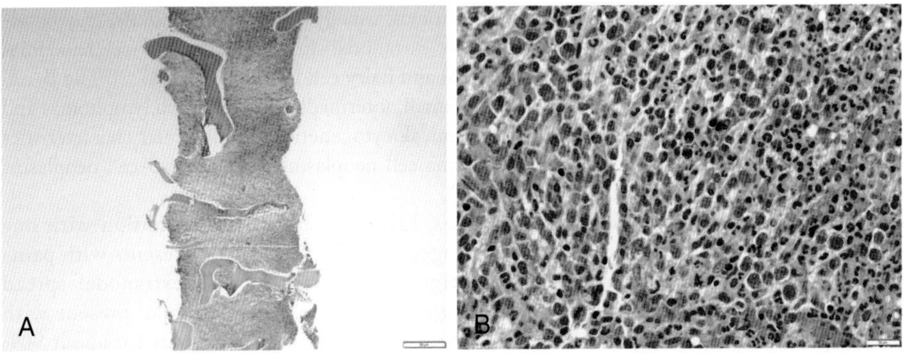

Fig. 47.3 (A and B) Patient's bone marrow core biopsy showing markedly hypercellular marrow with increased myeloid precursors.

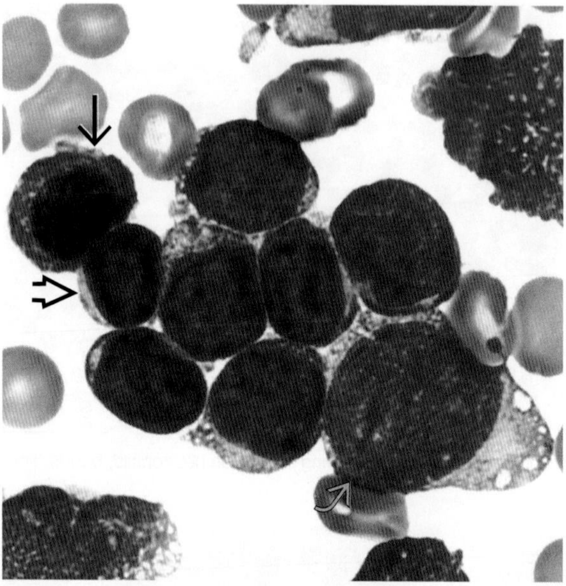

Fig. 47.4 Typical small uniform lymphoblasts (L1 blasts) are seen in this bone marrow smear from a 3-year-old boy with a new diagnosis of B-cell acute lymphoblastic leukemia. Rare L2 blast (cyan curved arrow), erythroid precursor (black solid arrow), and mature lymphocyte (black open arrow) are seen next to the lymphoblasts. (From *ExpertPath*. Copyright Elsevier.)

AML) arising from immature myeloid precursors, such as myeloblasts, erythroblasts, promyelocytes, or even megakaryocytes (Fig. 47.5A and B). These myeloid leukemias have been classified in various ways including the French–American–British classification; however, the eighth edition of World Health Organization (WHO) classifies myeloid leukemias primarily on the basis of genetics (Table 47.2).

Mature B- and T-cell neoplasms include both leukemias and lymphomas. Leukemias are increased neoplastic lymphoid cells in the marrow and/or circulation. Lymphomas are neoplastic proliferations of lymphoid cells in the lymph nodes and/or extranodal tissues.

B-cell neoplasms can be divided into non-Hodgkin lymphoma (NHL) and Hodgkin lymphoma (HL). NHLs comprise about 60% lymphomas, usually occur in older adults, may be associated with a leukemic phase, and often involve extranodal sites. The mature B-cell leukemias include chronic lymphocytic leukemia (Fig. 47.6) and hairy cell leukemia (Fig. 47.7). The B-cell lymphomas can be morphologically classified as small, intermediate, or large cell lymphomas and are further classified based on immunohistochemical, cytogenetic, and molecular characteristics (Table 47.3) (Figs. 47.8, 47.9, and 47.10). Plasma cell neoplasms are mature B-cell neoplasms composed of neoplastic plasma cells (Fig. 47.11).

HL comprises about 40% lymphoma cases. HL has a bimodal distribution with one peak in late 20s and the other peak in adults aged over 50. HL usually presents with painless lymphadenopathy that spreads to contiguous nodal sites, with extranodal spread being uncommon. Staging is important in guiding therapy. Patients may present with "B symptoms" of fever, night sweats, and weight loss. Classic HL accounts for about 90% of the cases, whereas nodular lymphocyte predominant HL accounts for 10% of the cases (Table 47.4; Fig. 47.12).

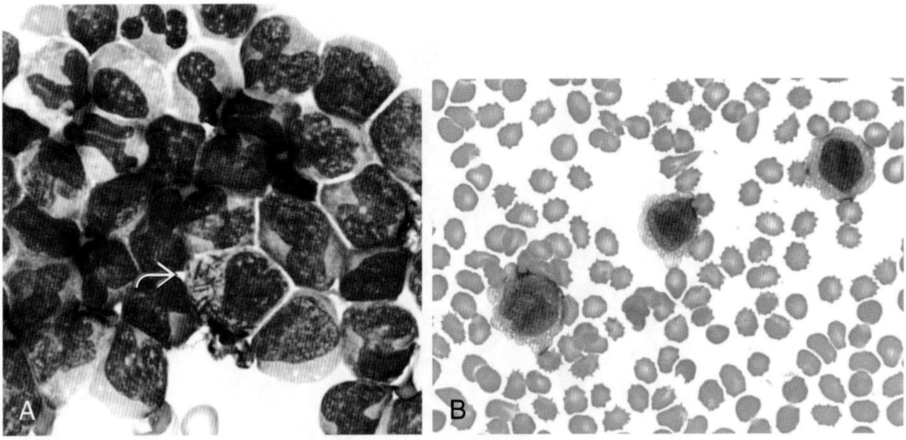

Fig. 47.5 (A) Acute promyelocytic leukemia showing frequent bilobed to multilobated blasts and a rare blast with numerous Auer rods (white curved arrow). (From *ExpertPath*. Copyright Elsevier.) (B) Acute monoblastic leukemia showing cells with large nuclei, fine chromatin, prominent nucleoli, and a moderate amount of pale cytoplasm with fine vacuoles; some have slight nuclear convolutions consistent with immature monocytes. (Courtesy Cynthia Reyes-Barron, MD. Used with permission).

TABLE 47.2 ■ **Acute Leukemias**

Diagnosis		**Salient Features**
Acute lymphoblastic leukemia (ALL)	B-cell ALL	Most common childhood neoplasm; expresses TdT and CD34 (markers of immaturity) and B-cell markers CD10, CD19, CD79a, subset CD20
	T-cell ALL	More common in adolescents; CNS and extranodal involvement common, may present with mediastinal mass; expresses TdT, CD2, CD3, CD5, CD7
Acute myeloid leukemia (AML)	With recurrent genetic abnormalities	Acute promyelocytic leukemia with t(15;17); *PML-RARA* AML with t(8;21); *RUNX1-RUNX1T1* AML with inv(16) AML with t(9;11); *KMT2A-MLLT3*
	With myelodysplasia related changes	History of MDS or presence of MDS-related cytogenetic abnormalities
	Not otherwise specified	AML with minimal differentiation AML without maturation AML with maturation Acute myelomonocytic leukemia Acute monoblastic and monocytic leukemia Pure erythroid leukemia Acute megakaryoblastic leukemia

CNS, central nervous system; *MDS*, myelodysplastic syndrome.

CLINICAL PEARL

Reed–Sternberg (RS) Cells and Hodgkin cells

HL is characterized by a paucity of neoplastic cells and a rich inflammatory background of non-neoplastic cells including T cells, eosinophils, plasma cells, histiocytes, and neutrophils.

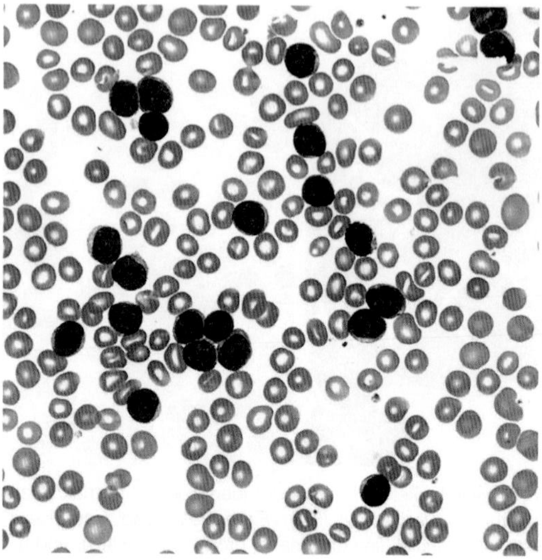

Fig. 47.6 Wright–Giemsa shows chronic lymphocytic leukemia/small lymphocytic lymphoma involving the peripheral blood. There is marked lymphocytosis, and most lymphocytes have sparse cytoplasm, round to oval nuclei, and no evident nucleoli. (From *ExpertPath*. Copyright Elsevier.)

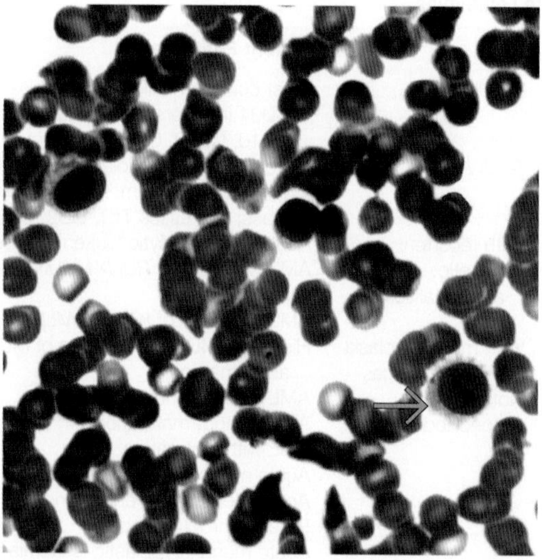

Fig. 47.7 Wright–Giemsa stain of hairy cell leukemia demonstrating one of the cells (cyan solid arrow) clearly shows cytoplasmic projections "hairs." (From *ExpertPath*. Copyright Elsevier.)

RS cells and Hodgkin cells are the malignant cells in HL. RS cells are large, binucleate or multinucleated B cells with abundant amphophilic cytoplasm, with prominent eosinophilic "owl-eye" nucleoli (Fig. 47.12), whereas Hodgkin cells are mononuclear RS cells. RS cells are positive for CD30, with dot-like (Golgi zone) positivity for CD15. They are usually negative for CD45, and stain dimly with PAX5.

TABLE 47.3 ■ **Mature B-Cell Neoplasms**

Diagnosis	Salient Features
Leukemias	
Chronic lymphocytic leukemia (CLL)/ small lymphocytic lymphoma (SLL)	Indolent; increased neoplastic small mature B cells in circulation, which co-express CD5 and CD23 in addition to B-cell markers CD19 and CD20 (dim). "Smudge cells" on blood smear. Involvement of lymph nodes leads to lymphadenopathy and is called SLL.
Hairy cell leukemia	Rare, indolent. Presents with pancytopenia and splenomegaly; usually no lymphadenopathy. Mature B cells with circumferential hairy cytoplasmic processes. Positive for CD103, CD25, CD11c, CD22, and TRAP. BRAF V600E mutation in all cases.
Lymphomas/Non-Hodgkin Lymphomas	
Diffuse large B-cell lymphoma (DLBCL)	High-grade, aggressive. Most common lymphoma worldwide. Sheets of large CD20+ B cells. ABC (activated B-cell) subtype: MUM1/IRF4+, BCL2+. The GCB (germinal center B-cell) subtype: CD10+, BCL6+. May arise sporadically, or from transformation of a low-grade lymphoma (i.e., Richter's syndrome: CLL to DLBCL).
Follicular lymphoma (FL)	Second commonest lymphoma worldwide. Small CD20+ B cells forming numerous back-to-back neoplastic follicles that express aberrant BCL2, with attenuated mantle zones and no tingible body macrophages. Grade 1–3 based on number of centroblasts (larger cells)/high-power field. BCL2 on chromosome 18 translocates to IgH on chromosome 14: t(14;18). Pediatric-type FL may lack t(14;18).
Burkitt lymphoma (BL)	High-grade, aggressive. More common in children and young adults. Intermediate-sized B cells with "starry sky" appearance due to numerous tingible body macrophages. Characteristic MYC-IgH translocation t(8;14). • African (endemic) type: maxilla, mandible involvement; associated with Epstein–Barr virus • American (sporadic) type: abdominal involvement
Mantle cell lymphoma	Rare; moderately aggressive. Older adults with painless lymphadenopathy, extranodal involvement common. Small CD5+, CD23-negative lymphocytes with characteristic translocation t(11;14); cyclin D1 on chromosome 11 translocates to IgH locus on chromosome 14.
Marginal zone lymphoma	Diverse group of B-cell neoplasms with no characteristic translocation. Can involve lymph nodes, spleen, and extranodal sites. Includes MALTomas. Gastric MALTomas are associated with *Helicobacter pylori* and can regress after treatment of infection.
Plasma Cell Neoplasms	
Plasma cell myeloma/ multiple myeloma	Most common primary malignancy of bone. Neoplastic proliferation of plasma cells with >10% clonal plasma cells in bone marrow *AND* end-organ damage due to plasma cell disorder *OR* one of the following: >60% plasma cells, free light chain ratio >100, >1 focal lytic bone lesion on magnetic resonance imaging. End-organ damage (CRAB: hypercalcemia, renal insufficiency, anemia, bone lesions) Rouleax formation of RBCs, Bence Jones urinary proteins, amyloidosis, elevated serum proteins, and increased risk of infections may be seen. Positive staining for CD138, CD79a, kappa, and lambda immunohistochemistry aid the diagnosis.
Monoclonal gammopathy of uncertain significance	Increased serum proteins with an M spike on SPEP. Clonal plasma cells <10%, no CRAB. 1% to 2% annual risk of progressing to multiple myeloma
Lymphoplasmacytic lymphoma (LPL)	Neoplasm of small B lymphocytes, plasmacytoid lymphocytes, and plasma cells. Often associated with paraproteins. LPL in marrow with IgM paraprotein is called Waldenstrom macroglobulinemia (WM), which can have a hyperviscosity syndrome. MYD88 mutation seen in 90%–100% of WM patients.

MALTomas, mucosa-associated lymphoid tissue lymphomas; *SPEP,* serum protein electrophoresis; *TRAP,* tartrate resistant acid phosphatase.

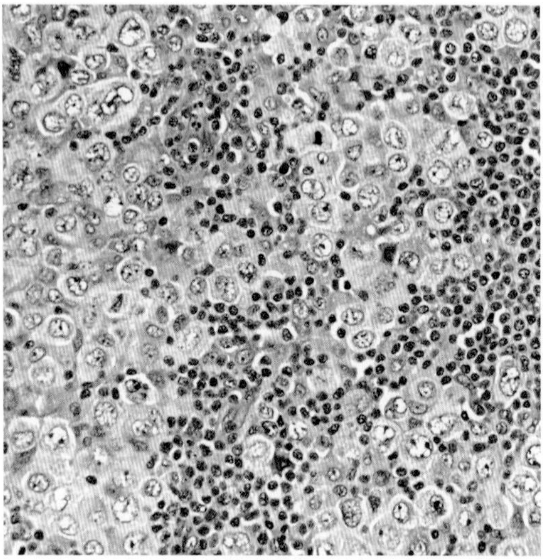

Fig. 47.8 Diffuse large B-cell lymphoma. The lymphoma cells are large (compared with reactive lymphocytes) and have vesicular chromatin, two to three small nucleoli, and moderate to abundant eosinophilic cytoplasm. (From *ExpertPath*. Copyright Elsevier.)

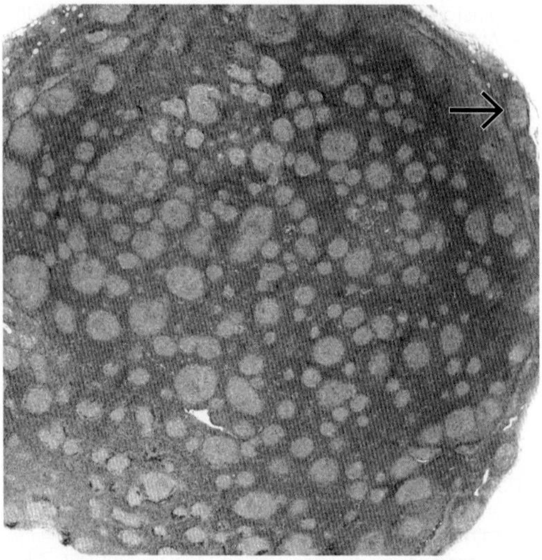

Fig. 47.9 Follicular lymphoma involving a lymph node shows numerous follicles throughout the cortex and medulla, extending beyond the capsule (black solid arrow). The large number and random distribution of follicles supports lymphoma. (From *ExpertPath*. Copyright Elsevier.)

T-cell and natural killer (NK)-cell neoplasms are rare and phenotypically resemble mature T cells and NK cells. They can present primarily as leukemias or lymphomas (Table 47.5). There are many NK-/T-cell neoplasms, but the more common ones include adult T-cell leukemia/lymphoma, mycosis fungoides/Sézary syndrome (Fig. 47.13A and B), anaplastic large cell lymphoma (Fig. 47.14), and extranodal NK-/T-cell lymphoma.

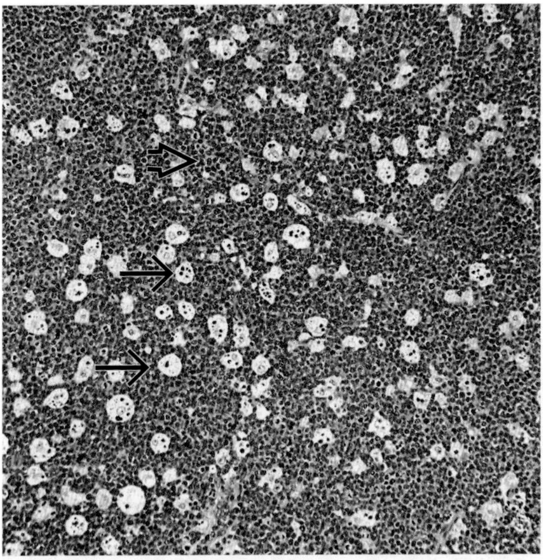

Fig. 47.10 A prominent starry sky pattern is characteristic of Burkitt lymphoma. Sheets of intermediate-sized lymphocytes represent the "dark sky" (black open arrow), whereas the histiocytes with abundant cytoplasmic debris (tingible body macrophages) represent the "stars" (black solid arrow). (From *ExpertPath*. Copyright Elsevier.)

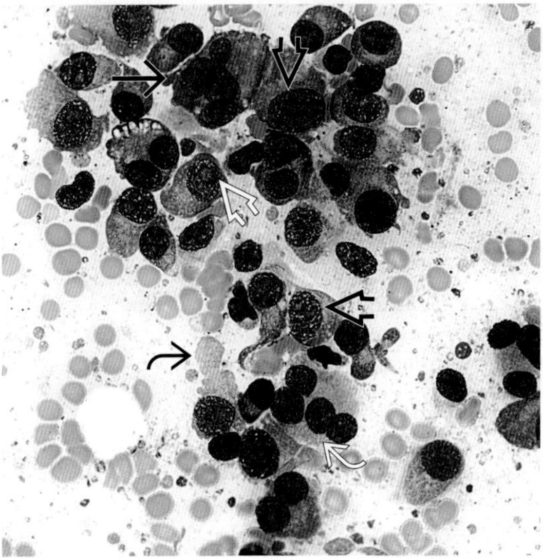

Fig. 47.11 Plasma cell myeloma. Features of plasma cell atypia are illustrated in this aspirate, including cellular and nuclear enlargement, nuclear pleomorphism (black solid arrow), multinucleation (white curved arrow), dispersed nuclear chromatin (black open arrow), prominent nucleoli (white open arrow), and cytoplasmic fraying or shedding (black curved arrow). (From *ExpertPath*. Copyright Elsevier.)

TABLE 47.4 ■ **Hodgkin Lymphoma**

Diagnosis	Salient Features
Hodgkin Lymphomas	
Nodular lymphocyte-predominant HL	Eosinophils and plasma cells are scant; abundant lymphocytes surrounding lymphocytic and histiocytic (L&H) cells with multilobed nuclei "popcorn cell." L&H cells have a distinct staining profile compared with Reed–Sternberg (RS) cells: negative for CD30 and CD15, while positive for CD20.
Classic Hodgkin Lymphoma	
Nodular sclerosis	Most common subtype; broad collagen bands separating nodules of inflammatory cells with scattered lacunar and diagnostic RS cells
Mixed cellularity	Abundant eosinophils due to interleukin-5 produced by RS cells. Esptein–Barr virus positive (EBV) in 70%. Often presents at higher stage.
Lymphocyte rich	Uncommon type, older males. Best prognosis; EBV+ in 40%.
Lymphocyte depleted	Uncommon, older males, HIV-infected individuals. Most aggressive subtype; often EBV+.

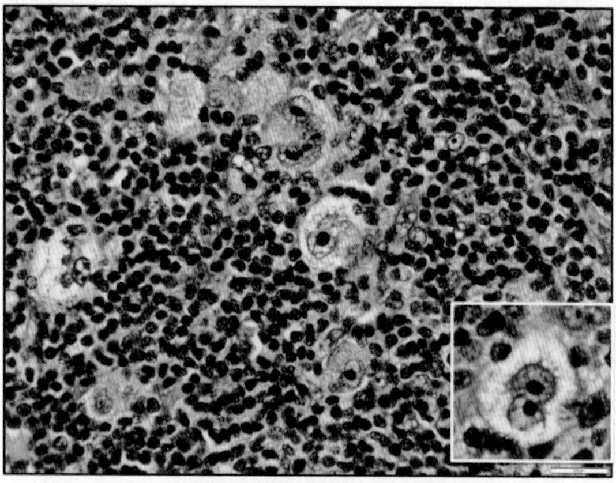

Fig. 47.12 Hodgkin lymphoma with large binucleate and multinucleate Reed–Sternberg cells with prominent "owl-eye" nucleoli (Courtesy Cynthia Reyes-Barron MD. Used with permission.)

Case Point 47.3

The patient's blood is sent for cytogenetics and is found to have the characteristic t(9;22) reciprocal translocation that results in the Philadelphia (Ph) chromosome.

This translocation fuses the BCR gene on chromosome 22 with the ABL1 gene on chromosome 9. This chromosomal translocation is seen in 90% to 95% cases of chronic myeloid leukemia (CML), a myeloproliferative neoplasm. The Ph chromosome can be detected by karyotyping, fluorescence in situ hybridization (FISH), or reverse transcriptase–polymerase chain reaction (Fig. 47.15).

CLINICAL PEARL

Diseases with Ph Chromosome

All cases of CML have t(9;22); however, the Ph chromosome is not specific for CML. It may also be seen in cases of ALL in up to 25% of adult cases and 5% of pediatric cases.

TABLE 47.5 ■ **Mature T-Cell Neoplasms**

Diagnosis	Salient Features
Adult T-cell leukemia/ lymphoma	Neoplasm of malignant CD4+ T cells infected by human T-cell leukemia virus type 1. Multilobated "cloverleaf" or "flower" cells in peripheral blood. Seen in Japan and the Caribbean.
Mycosis fungoides (MF)/ Sézary syndrome	MF: Cerebriform neoplastic CD4+ T-cells in the skin resulting in a pruritic erythematous rash, which can progress to patch, plaque, or nodule/ tumor stage. Sézary syndrome characterized by erythroderma and cerebriform Sézary cells in the circulation.
Anaplastic large cell lymphoma (ALCL)	Characteristic ALK gene rearrangement. Large CD30+ T cells with eccentric horseshoe-/kidney-shaped nuclei. ALK-negative ALCL also exists.
Extranodal natural killer-/ T-cell lymphoma	Highly aggressive; associated with Epstein–Barr virus. Commonly presents as destructive nasopharyngeal mass. Tumor cells often surround and invade blood vessels.

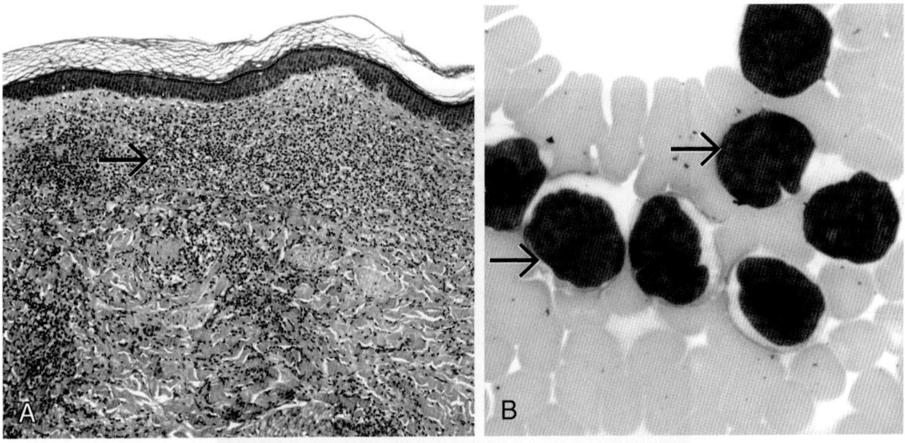

Fig. 47.13 Mycosis fungoides: (A) Histologic section of skin of the buttock in a pediatric patient shows a dense dermal (black solid arrow) infiltrate consistent with a patch lesion (From *ExpertPath*. Copyright Elsevier.) (B) Peripheral blood smear from a patient with Sézary syndrome shows intermediate-sized Sézary cells (black solid arrow) with folded cerebriform nuclei and scant to moderate cytoplasm. To fulfill the criterion of peripheral blood involvement in Sézary syndrome, at least 1 × 10^9/L of these cells are required. (From *ExpertPath*. Copyright Elsevier.)

What are other myeloproliferative diseases?

Myeloproliferative neoplasms (MPN) are clonal hematopoietic stem cell disorders characterized by proliferation of one or more cell types in the myeloid lineage. They mainly occur in adults and are characterized by increased numbers of granulocytes, RBCs, and/or platelets in the peripheral blood. The marrow is usually hypercellular, but the cells mature normally. Massive splenomegaly and hepatomegaly are commonly seen. Most MPNs have mutations in tyrosine kinase genes (Table 47.6). It may be difficult to distinguish between the various MPNs, such as polycythemia vera (Fig. 47.16), essential thrombocythemia (Fig. 47.17A and B), and primary myelofibrosis

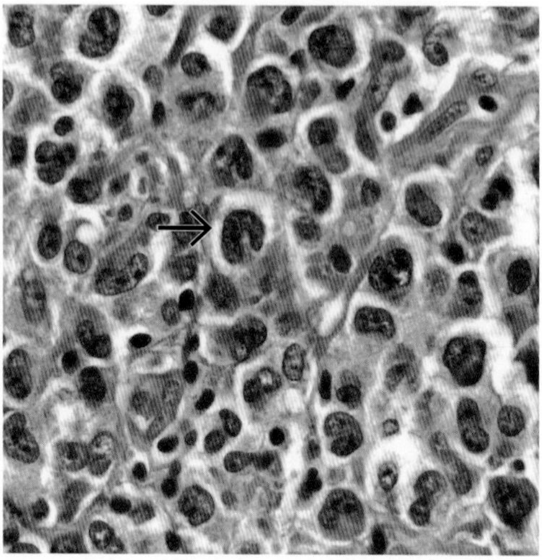

Fig. 47.14 Under oil magnification, a number of hallmark cells with horseshoe-shaped nuclei are seen (black solid arrow). Hallmark cells are characteristic but not specific for anaplastic large cell lymphoma. (From *ExpertPath*. Copyright Elsevier.)

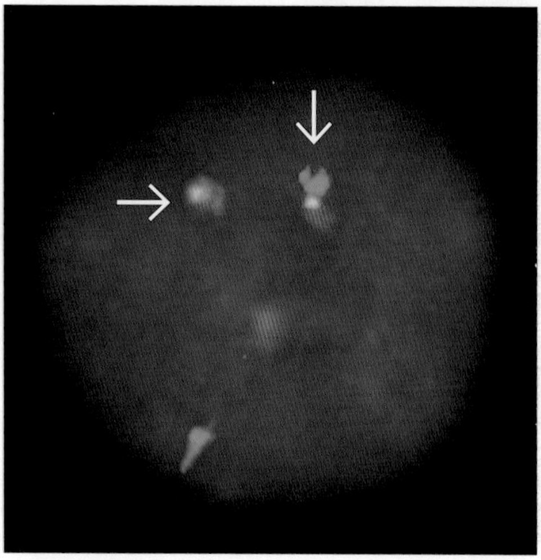

Fig. 47.15 Using a dual-color, dual-fusion probe strategy, fluorescence in situ hybridization shows a classic abnormal cell in chronic myeloid leukemia demonstrating the presence of a BCR–ABL1 gene fusion. The abnormal fusion signals confirming the positive result are seen as fusion of the orange and green signals (yellow) (white solid arrow). (From *ExpertPath*. Copyright Elsevier.)

(Fig. 47.18); however, the clinical, morphologic, and genetic findings in conjunction with WHO criteria can help establish a diagnosis.

What is the treatment and prognosis of CML?

CML is one of the few hematological malignancies for which successful targeted therapy is available in the form of tyrosine kinase inhibitor (TKI) therapy.

TABLE 47.6 ■ **Myeloproliferative Neoplasms**

Malignancy	Salient Features	Mutations
Chronic myeloid leukemia	Granulocytic leukocytosis with left shift and <5% blasts; basophilia is seen. May progress to a blast phase with ≥20% blasts in the marrow.	BCR–ABL1 (Philadelphia chromosome)
Polycythemia vera	Increased red blood cell production; hemoglobin >16.5 g/dL in men and >16 g/dL in women; decreased serum erythropoietin.	JAK2 V617F kinase
Essential thrombocythemia	Sustained thrombocytosis (platelets >450 × 10^9/L), increased large mature megakaryocytes in marrow.	JAK2 V617F, MPL, CALR
Primary myelofibrosis	Proliferation of abnormal megakaryocytes and granulocytes in the marrow, with marrow fibrosis	JAK2 V617F, CALR, MPL

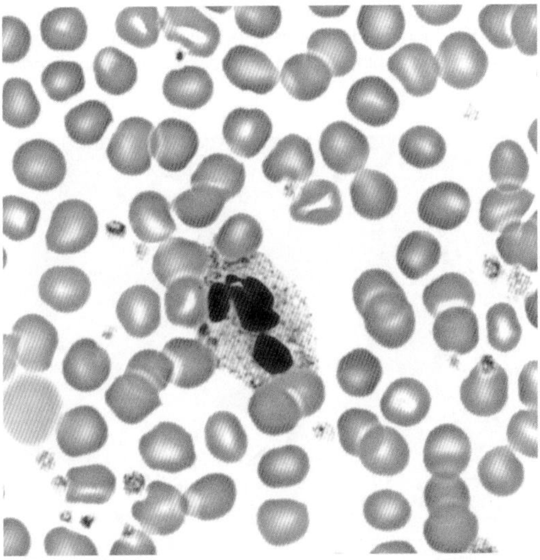

Fig. 47.16 Peripheral blood smear from an elderly woman shows polycythemic phase of polycythemia vera. Note normocytic, normochromic erythrocytosis, and thrombocytosis. Additional workup showed a low serum erythropoietin level and a JAK2 mutation. (From *ExpertPath*. Copyright Elsevier.)

CLINICAL PEARL

TKIs

In CML, the BCR–ABL fusion protein has increased tyrosine kinase activity. TKIs block the tyrosine kinase enzyme. Imatinib was the first TKI approved by the Food and Drug Administration in 2001. Resistance to imatinib may develop, which prompted the development of other TKIs such as such as nilotinib and dasatinib. TKI therapy may lead to 5-year progression-free and overall survival rates of 80%–95%.

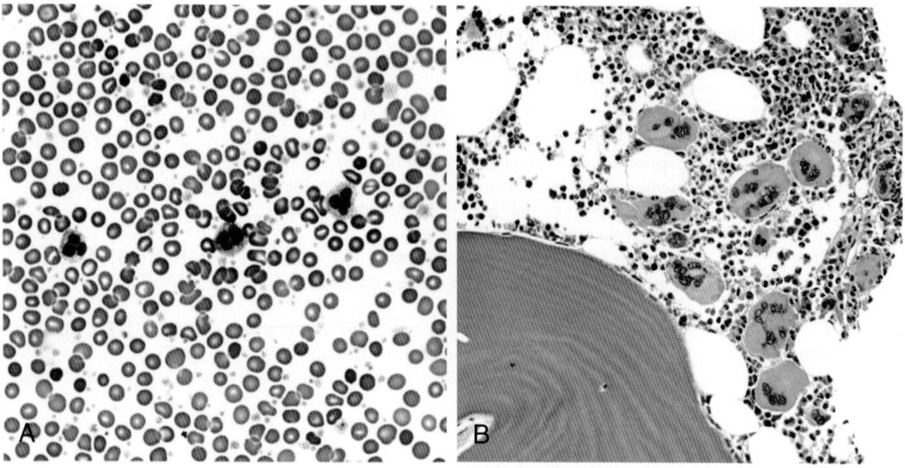

Fig. 47.17 (A) Essential thrombocytosis (ET) with peripheral thrombocytosis and normal white blood cell and red blood cell numbers and morphology. (From *ExpertPath*. Copyright Elsevier.) (B) Bone marrow core biopsy shows typical appearance of ET: increased, enlarged, hyperlobulated megakaryocytes in loose clusters. There is no significant proliferation of granulocytic and erythroid series. (From *ExpertPath*. Copyright Elsevier.)

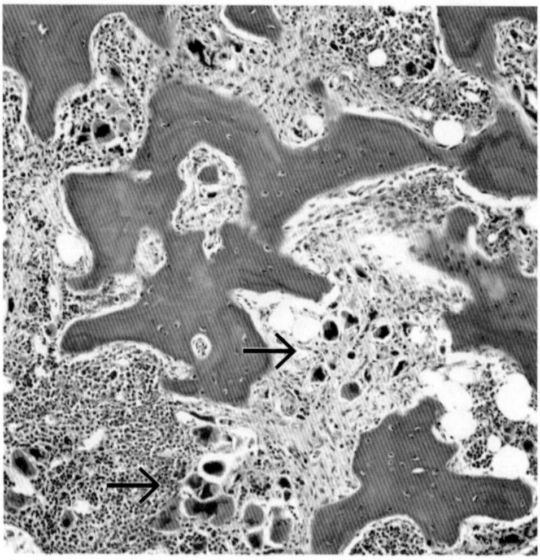

Fig. 47.18 Marked osteosclerosis, myelofibrosis, and megakaryocytic pleomorphism are hallmark histologic features of primary myelofibrosis. Megakaryocytes range from small to large and are hyperchromatic and clustered (black solid arrow). (From *ExpertPath*. Copyright Elsevier.)

Case Point 47.4

The patient is started on a TKI imatinib. His symptoms improve and blood counts normalize within a few months. For the next 3 years, his blood counts remain normal, and minimal residual disease monitoring using quantitative PCR for BCR–ABL1 transcript levels shows undetectable levels. However, at his next check-up a year later, his peripheral blood has 25% blasts, with markedly depressed platelet and white cell count. Bone marrow core biopsy shows replacement of marrow by sheets of blasts (Fig. 47.19).

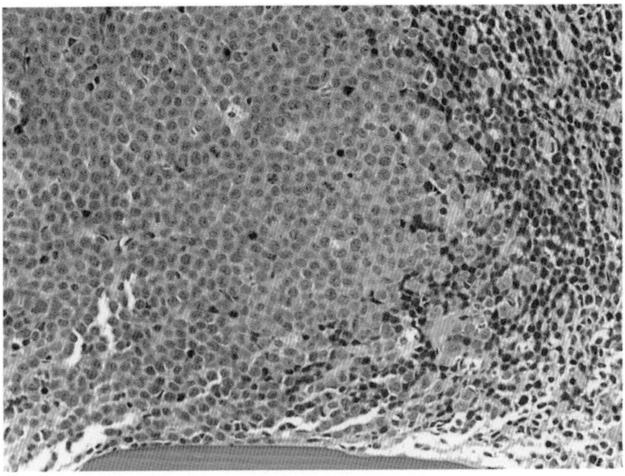

Fig. 47.19 Patients' bone marrow biopsy showing involvement by sheets of blasts, consistent with a blast crisis.

What is a blast crisis in CML?

CML has three classic phases: chronic, accelerated, and blast. The chronic phase is characterized by stable disease and <5% blasts. Accelerated phase indicates disease progression and has 10%–19% blasts in the marrow. Blast phase indicates aggressive disease, which is usually refractory to therapy and is characterized by ≥20% blasts in the marrow. These blasts are usually myeloid in 70%–80% cases, but may be lymphoid in 20%–30% cases.

TKI therapy has greatly improved overall survival in patients with CML; however, some patients still undergo transformation to the blast phase for unknown reasons. With TKIs, progression to blast phase is around 1%–3% per year compared with >20% per year in the pre-TKI era. The average survival for blast crisis patients ranges from 7 to 11 months.

Case Point 47.5

The patient was administered a different TKI with the goal of resolving the blast phase and proceeding to allogeneic stem cell transplantation. Unfortunately, the patient died shortly afterwards due to pneumonia and sepsis as a complication of blast crisis and the resulting cytopenias.

BEYOND THE PEARLS

- Infectious mononucleosis "kissing disease" caused by Epstein–Barr virus is a common cause of lymphocytosis in adolescents. It is characterized by fever, sore throat, and lymphadenitis, with frequent splenomegaly. Atypical lymphocytes may be seen in the blood.
- Acute promyelocytic leukemia (APL) is a hematological emergency; prompt diagnosis followed by immediate initiation of treatment with all-trans retinoic acid (ATRA) is essential. Disseminated intravascular coagulation is a common complication.
- APL has the translocation t(15;17) PML–RARA, which makes it sensitive to treatment by ATRA.
- Auer rods are needle-like condensations of cytoplasmic granules and are characteristic of AML.
- "Starry sky" pattern is not exclusive to Burkitt lymphoma and may also be seen in ALL.
- CML is defined by the presence of t(9;22) ABL–BCR, which can be targeted by TKIs such as imatinib.
- Leukoerythroblastosis (immature WBCs and nucleated RBCs in the circulation) along with teardrop RBCs can be seen in primary myelofibrosis.

- Tumor lysis syndrome is a serious complication of cancer therapy and is characterized by hyperuricemia, hyperkalemia, hyperphosphatemia, and hypocalcemia due to lysis of tumor cells.
- Post-transplant lymphoproliferative disorders may occur in the setting of bone marrow or solid organ transplants.
- Rituximab is an anti-CD20 monoclonal antibody, which can be used in the treatment of many B-cell malignancies.
- Programmed cell death-1 (PD-1 or CD279) is a cell surface protein that binds to its ligand PD-L1. Inhibiting the interaction of PD-1 and PD-L1 is the basis for newer cancer therapies known as immune checkpoint blockade, for which the 2018 Nobel Prize in medicine/physiology was awarded.
- Chimeric antigen receptor T-cell (CAR-T cell) therapy is the newest frontier in the treatment of hematological malignancies. T cells are genetically engineered to recognize cancer cells; these CAR-T cells are subsequently infused into the patient where they can destroy the cancer cells.

References

Brown M, Wittwer C. Flow cytometry. Principles and clinical applications in hematology. *Clin Chem.* 2000;46(8 Pt 2):1221-1229.

Hsi E. *Hematopathology.* 2nd ed. Philadelphia, PA: Elsevier; 2012.

Shi Y, Rand RJ, Crow JH, Moore JO, Lagoo AS. Blast phase in chronic myelogenous leukemia is skewed toward unusual blast types in patients treated with tyrosine kinase inhibitors: a comparative study of 67 cases. *Am J Clin Pathol.* 2015;143(1):105-119. doi:10.1309/AJCPWEX5YY4PHSCN.

Swerdlow SH, Campo E, Harris NL, et al. *World Health Organization Classification of Tumours of Hematopoietic and Lymphoid Tissue.* Revised 4th ed. Lyon, France: IARC Press; 2017.

Endocrine System

CASE 48

A 35-Year-Old Female with a Midline Neck Mass and No Other Symptoms

Hasan Khatib

A 35-year-old female presents to her primary physician with a main complaint of feeling a nodule in her neck for several weeks. Her past medical and surgical history is unremarkable aside from appendectomy at the age of 20. The patient works as a waitress in a local restaurant, she is a nonsmoker, and drinks socially. Medications include only multivitamins. Upon physical examination, the patient demonstrates vital signs within normal range, blood pressure of 110/80 mm Hg, pulse rate of 82 beats per minute, and respiratory rate of 16 breaths per minute. The patient is slightly pale but not in any distress. She denies chest pain, headache, and vision changes. Her menstrual periods are regular. Physical examination of patient's neck reveals a nodule of approximately 2 cm at the area of thyroid with no overlying skin changes or lymphadenopathy. She also denies any hoarseness, dysphagia, neck pain, and hemoptysis. The patient denies any history of radiation exposure, and her aunt has a history of thyroid cancer.

What is the medical definition of thyroid nodule? And what are the risk factors for thyroid cancer?
A thyroid nodule is a discrete lesion within the thyroid gland that is radiologically distinct from the surrounding thyroid parenchyma. Epidemiology speaking, thyroid nodules are seen in 5% of women and 1% of men. The clinical importance of thyroid nodules is to exclude thyroid cancer. Generally, most thyroid nodules are benign, and only 5% to 10% of thyroid nodules are malignant.

CLINICAL PEARLS

The risk factors of thyroid cancers are:

- Age and gender
- Familial thyroid carcinoma
- Radiation exposure history

Patients with familial thyroid cancer should have a careful history and neck examination as a part of routine health examination. Syndromes associated with thyroid cancer are:

- Multiple endocrine neoplasia (MEN syndrome)
- PTEN hamartoma tumor syndrome (Cowden's disease)
- FAP
- Carney complex

Clinically, all patients with a thyroid nodule should undergo a physical examination focusing on the thyroid gland and adjacent lymph nodes. In addition, a complete history should be obtained. Radiation exposure should be noted.

CLINICAL PEARLS

Vocal cord paralyses, cervical lymphadenopathy, adherent nodule to surrounding tissue, dysphagia, hemoptysis, and airway symptoms are very worrisome symptoms of thyroid malignancy.

What are the initial and subsequent steps for a patient with a thyroid nodule?

Serum thyroid-stimulating hormone (TSH) is the initial evaluation of a patient with a thyroid nodule.

- If the serum TSH is low, then radionuclide thyroid scan should be obtained.
- If the serum TSH is normal or elevated, then neck ultrasound should be obtained.

Case Point 48.1

The Patient's\Serum TSH Was 1.3 mIU/L (Normal Range: 0.4–4.0 mIU/L).

What Is the Next Step with This Patient?

Thyroid/neck ultrasound is the second step in evaluating all patients with a detected thyroid nodule and normal or elevated serum TSH.

Case Point 48.2

Patient undergoes an ultrasound, which confirms a thyroid hypoechoic nodule that measures 0.8 × 0.7 cm in the right thyroid lobe. The nodule is taller than wider, solid with central cystic changes, and with lobulated margins (Fig. 48.1).

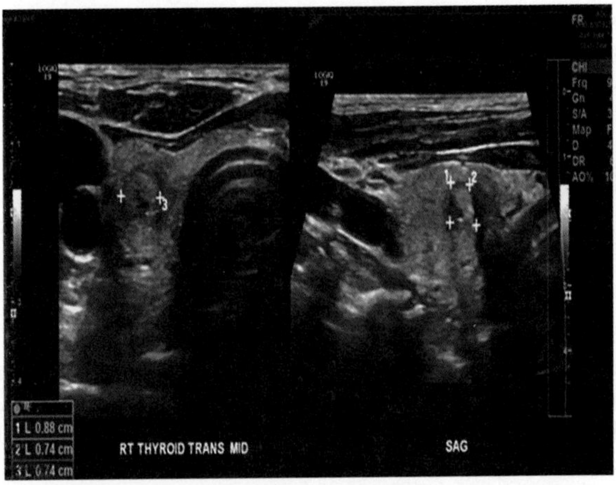

Fig. 48.1 Ultrasound thyroid/neck displays hypoechoic thyroid nodule measures 0.8 × 0.7 cm in the right thyroid lobe. The nodule is taller than wider, solid with central cystic changes, and with lobulated margins.

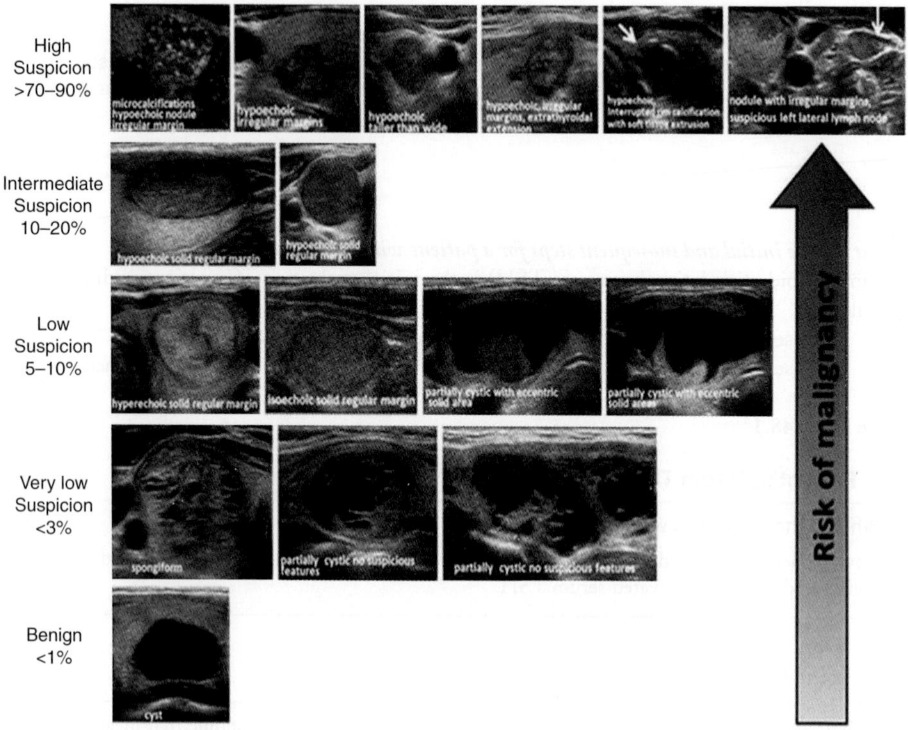

Fig. 48.2 Illustration of nodule sonographic patterns and risk of malignancy according to American Thyroid Association management guidelines.

Thyroid ultrasound can yield the following information (Fig. 48.2 and Table 48.1):

- Thyroid parenchyma echogenicity (heterogeneous or homogenous)
- Thyroid nodule size in three dimensions, location (right, left, upper, lower, posterior, or isthmus), the nodule echogenicity, the nodule margin (ill-defined versus well-defined margin), and the shape of the nodule (taller than wider)
- Presence and type of calcifications
- Suspicious cervical lymphadenopathy

CLINICAL PEARLS

Thyroid nodules with microcalcifications, hypoechogenicity, irregular margins, and taller shape have a higher rate of malignancy

What is the procedure of choice for the ultrasound suspicious thyroid nodules?

Fine-needle aspiration (FNA) is the most accurate, safe, cost-effective, and minimally invasive method for evaluating thyroid nodules. Generally, thyroid nodules with a size more than 1 cm should be sampled by FNA. The ultrasound features of the thyroid nodule combined with nodule size, along with clinical symptoms, are the major factors to decide whether the patient needs thyroid FNA or not.

Thyroid FNA procedures can be performed using palpation or employing ultrasound guidance, which is preferred for deep and posteriorly located thyroid nodules.

TABLE 48.1 ■ **Ultrasound Features of Thyroid Nodule and Associated Estimated Risk of Malignancy, Along with Fine-Needle Aspiration (FNA) Aspiration Guidance, According to 2015 American Thyroid Association (ATA) Management Guidelines**

Sonographic Pattern	Ultrasound Features	Estimated Risk of Malignany	FNa Size Cutoff (Largest Dimension)
High suspicion	Solid hypoechoic nodule or parially cystic nodule **with** one or more of the following features: • Irregular margins • Microcalicfications • Taller than wide shape • Rim calcifications with small • Extrusive soft tissue component • Evidence of extrathyroidal • Extension (ETE)	>70%–90%	Recommended FNA at ≥1 cm
Intermediate suspicion	Hypechoic solid nodule with smooth margins **without** microcalcifications, ETE, or taller than wide shape.	10%–20%	Recommended FNA at ≥1 cm
Low suspicion	Isoechoic or hyperechoic solid nodule, or partially cystic nodule with eccentric solid areas, **without** microcalcifications, ETE, or taller than wide shape.	5%–10%	Recommended FNA at ≥1.5 cm
Very low suspicion	Spongiform or partially cystic nodule **without** any of the sonographic features described in low, intermediate, or high suspicion patterns.	<3%	Consider FNA at ≥2 cm. Observation without FNA is also a resonable option
Benign	Purely cystic nodules (no solid component)	<1%	No biopsy

CLINICAL PEARLS

Bleeding, bruising, pain, infection (rare), and damaging surrounding organs (rare) are the most common thyroid FNA complications.

What is the role of thyroid nodule FNA cytology?

The main purpose of performing thyroid FNA is to obtain adequate sample of few follicular groups for microscopic evaluation. The results of microscopic examination will effectively aid in triage each patient case (clinical follow-up, molecular studies, or surgical treatment).

Generally, three passes with a 25- or 27-gauge needle is the preferred method in sampling thyroid nodule. An adequate (quantity) and well-preserved specimen (quality, staining, and sample media) is essential for rendering accurate cytologic interpretation.

CLINICAL PEARLS

Criteria for specimen adequacy are six groups of well-preserved follicular cells with at least 10 cells in each group. The rapid on-site evaluation of thyroid FNA passes by doing rapid Diff-Quick stain aids in obtaining adequate sample and lessening the nondiagnostic samples rates.

An exception of adequacy is made for colloid nodule upon obtaining abundant thick colloid without adequate follicular groups.

Thyroid FNA cytology should be reported using the Bethesda system for reporting thyroid cytopathology that recognizes six diagnostic categories:

- Category I: Nondiagnostic/unsatisfactory
- Category II: Benign
- Category III: Atypia of undetermined significance/follicular lesion of undetermined significance
- Category IV: Follicular neoplasm/suspicious for follicular neoplasm, a category that also encompasses the diagnosis of Hürthle cell neoplasm/suspicious for Hürthle cell neoplasm
- Category V: Suspicious for malignancy
- Category VI: Malignant

Each of these categories carries an estimated risk of malignancy and the follow-up management (Table 48.2).

What is the classification of thyroid tumors?

Thyroid tumors can be categorized into malignant and benign, and epithelial, nonepithelial tumors, in addition to secondary tumors (metastasis). The epithelial tumors can be categorized into follicular and parafollicular tumors. The most common benign epithelial follicular thyroid tumor is follicular adenoma. The most common epithelial follicular thyroid malignant tumor is papillary thyroid carcinoma (PTC; 80%).

The modified version of World Health Organization classification of nonthyroid tumors has a large differential diagnosis which can be broadly categorized as:

- Epithelial/follicular tumors
- Benign: follicular adenoma, hyalinizing trabecular tumor, Hürthle cell adenoma
- Carcinoma: papillary, follicular, Hürthle cell, poorly differentiated, anaplastic carcinoma
- Parafollicular tumor: medullary carcinoma
- Nonepithelial tumors
- Paraganglioma
- Peripheral nerve sheath tumors: Schwannoma, malignant peripheral nerve sheath tumor
- Vascular tumors: hemangioma, lymphangioma, angiosarcoma
- Smooth muscle tumors: leiomyoma, leiomyosarcoma.
- Histiocytic tumors: Langerhans cell histiocytosis, Rosai–Dorfman disease.
- Lymphoma
- Teratoma
- Solitary fibrous tumor
- Secondary tumors (metastases)

TABLE 48.2 ■ **Bethesda System Categories (Assigned Estimated Malignancy Risk and Usual Management)**

Diagnostic Category	Estimated Risk of Malignancy (%)	Usual Management
Nondiagnostic/unsatisfactory	1–4	Repeat FNA with ultrasound guidance
Benign	0–3	Clinical follow-up
AUS/FLUS	5–15	Molecular studies
FN/SFN	15–30	Molecular studies
Suspicious for malignancy	60–75	Subtotal thyroidectomy surgical lobectomy
Malignant	97–99	Thyroidectomy

AUS, atypia of undetermined significance; *FNA*, fine-needle aspiration; *FUN*, follicular neoplasm; *FUS*, follicular lesion of undetermined significance; *SFN*, suspicious for follicular neoplasm.

Case Point 48.3

Patient underwent thyroid FNA, and the cytology preparations reveal flat monolayered fragments with cellular crowding, chromatin clearing, oval nuclei, nuclear grooves, and intranuclear inclusion (Fig. 48.3). The cytological evaluation of thyroid nodule confirms the diagnosis of PTC.

PTC is the most common type of thyroid cancer, accounting for approximately 80% to 85% of cases. PTC is a malignant epithelial neoplasm showing follicular cell differentiation characterized by distinctive nuclear features. Papillary architecture is not essential for PTC diagnosis.

PTC diagnosis depends on nuclear features which includes:

- Enlarged oval or irregular nuclei
- Powdery, ground-glass chromatin ("orphan Annie") nuclei
- Abundant nuclear longitudinal grooves (coffee beans)
- Marginal micronucleoli
- Nuclear pseudoinclusions are usually present in few tumor cells
- Psammoma bodies are sometimes present
- Multinucleated giant cells are common.

PTC has several histopathological variants (Fig. 48.4A–H).

- Columnar cell: aggressive tumor, widespread dissemination (lung, brain, bone), fatal outcome
- Cribriform morular: patients with Gardner syndrome or familial adenomatous polyposis (FAP)
- Diffuse sclerosing: sclerotic stroma, abundant psammoma bodies, extensive lymphatic invasion
- Follicular: second most common variant of PTC (30%)
- Macrofollicular: rare variant, large dilated follicles
- Microcarcinoma PTC: carcinoma is 1 cm or less in size, multifocal in familial form
- Oncocytic: Hürthle cell-like cytoplasm but nuclear features of PTC
- Solid: rare type, more than 50% of tumor with solid growth pattern, higher risk of relapse
- Tall cell: aggressive variant with poor prognosis

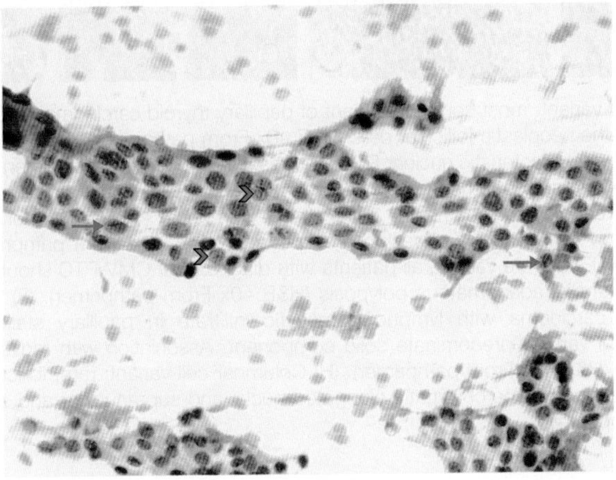

Fig. 48.3 Thyroid right lobe nodule fine-needle aspiration: flat monolayered fragment with cellular crowding, oval nuclei, nuclear grooves (arrows), and intranuclear inclusion (arrow heads). (Liquid-based preparation, Papanicolaou stains 40x).

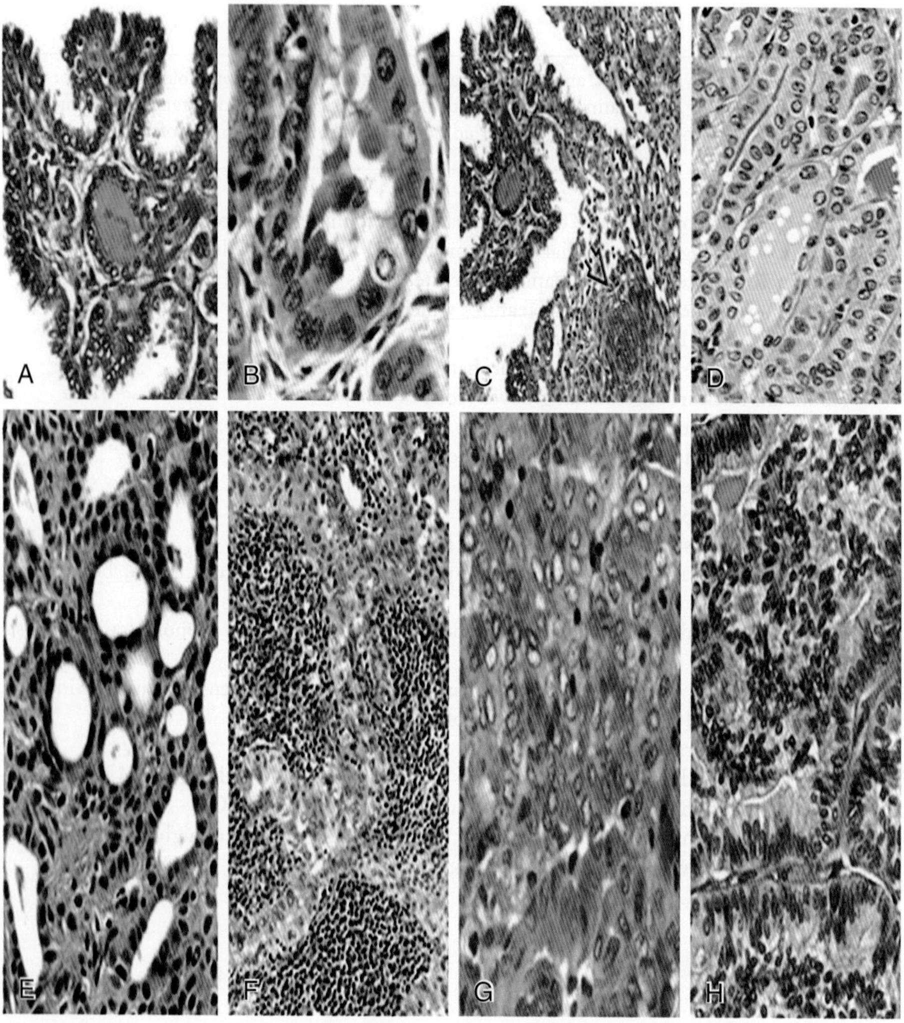

Fig. 48.4 (A) Classic variant: most common variant of papillary thyroid carcinoma (PTC), thin fibrovascular core surrounded by the neoplastic follicular cells (H&E 40x From pathprimer). (B) Follicular variant: various sized follicles that have characteristic nuclear PTC features (H&E 40x From pathprimer). (C) Diffuse sclerosing variant: fibrosis/sclerosis, squamoid morules (arrow), innumerable Psammoma bodies (H&E 40x From pathprimer). (D) Tall cell variant: cell height 2–3 x width, comprise >50% of tumor cells for diagnosis. Extrathyroid extension lymphvascular invasion are common (H&E 40x From pathprimer). (E) Cribriform morular variant (CMV-PTC): rare variant, all patients with diagnosis of CMV-PTC should undergo colonoscopy to screen for familial adenomatous polyposis (H&E 40x From pathprimer). (F) Warthin-like variant: oncocytic papillary carcinoma with lymphoplasmacytic infiltrate in papillary stalks (H&E 40c From pathprimer). (G) Solid variant: predominate solid component. Association with radiation-associated and pediatric population (H&E 40x From pathprimer). (H) Columnar cell variant: rare, follicular cells with stratified, tall epithelial cells with hyperchromatic elongated nuclei and supranuclear and subnuclear vacuoles (H&E 40x From pathprimer).

- Warthin-like: resembles Warthin tumors of salivary glands; coexisting with Hashimoto thyroiditis
- Hobnail features: aggressive variant with poor prognosis.

What is the prognosis of PTC?

The prognosis of PTC is excellent with a 10-year survival of >90%. Patients with BRAF mutation have more aggressive tumors. Vascular invasion and nuclear atypia are poor prognostic signs (Fig. 48.5).

What are other tumors that can occur in the thyroid gland?

Follicular thyroid carcinoma (FTC) is a malignant epithelial tumor with follicular cell differentiation but lacking diagnostic features of PTC. FTC relies on these two histological features: (1) capsular invasion: neoplastic cells penetrate the entire thickness of tumor capsule; (2) vascular invasion: intravascular tumor cells should be adherent to vascular wall, covered by endothelium, or in context of thrombus or fibrin. Many histopathological variants of FTC exist: clear cell, signet-ring cell type, glomeruloid pattern, and spindle cell type. The prognosis of FTC is good with excellent cure rate if disease is confined to thyroid.

Poorly differentiated thyroid carcinoma (PDTC) is a follicular cell-derived carcinoma with limited structural follicular or papillary features. PDTC clinical behavior intermediates between well-differentiated (papillary and follicular) and undifferentiated (anaplastic)

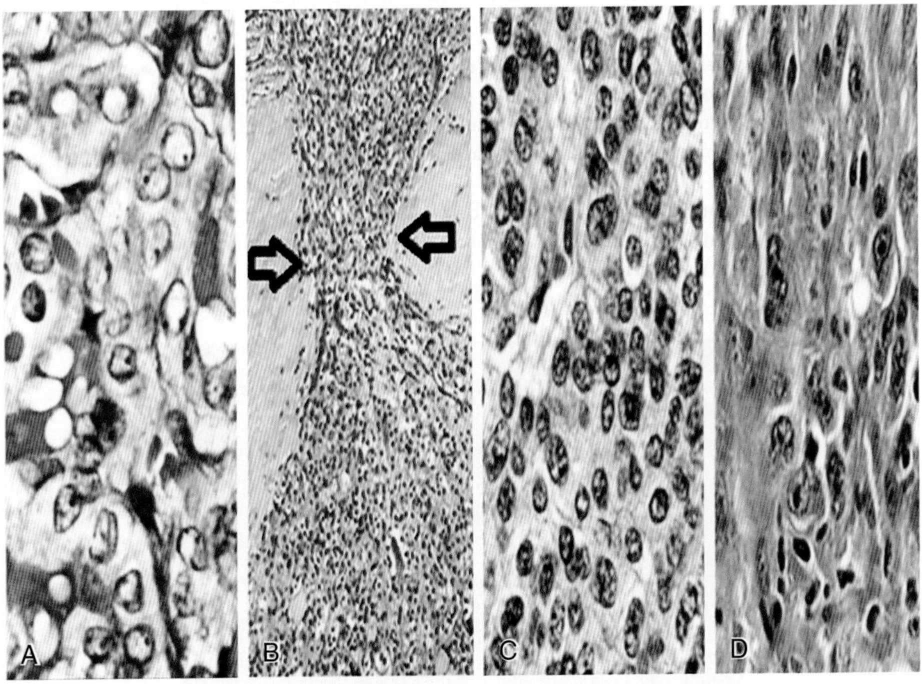

Fig. 48.5 (A) Papillary thyroid carcinoma with characteristic nuclear features (H&E 40x From pathprimer). (B) Follicular thyroid carcinoma, tumor cells penetrate the entire thickness of tumor capsule (arrows) (H&E 40x From pathprimer). (C) Poorly differentiated thyroid carcinoma, solid growth pattern with no conventional nuclear PTC features (H&E 40x From pathprimer). (D) Anaplastic thyroid carcinoma, malignant squamoid tumor nests (H&E 40x From pathprimer).

carcinomas. The diagnostic criteria of PDTC include: presence of solid, trabecular, or insular growth pattern; absence of conventional nuclear features of PTC; and presence of at least one of following: convoluted nuclei, mitotic activity ≥3/10 HPF, and tumor necrosis. The poorly differentiated component should be mentioned in pathology report even if it is present focally.

Anaplastic thyroid carcinoma (ATC) is a follicular cell-derived carcinoma with aggressive behavior, rapid expanding growth, widely adjacent organs invasion, and high 1-year mortality rate. Histologically, ATC presents with tumor necrosis, vascular invasion, and high mitotic activity along with one or more of these three patterns: (1) sarcomatoid: malignant spindle cells resemble high-grade pleomorphic sarcoma; (2) giant cell: highly pleomorphic malignant cells with giant cells; and (3) epithelial: squamous and/or squamoid tumor nests with regional and occasional keratinization. ATC prognosis is poor with mortality rate of more than 90% within 6 months.

Case Point 48.4

At a follow-up visit, the patient was scheduled for total thyroidectomy surgery. The patient tolerates the surgery without any complications. The gross examination reveals a thyroid gland with a total weight of 29 grams. The left lobe is sectioned from superior to inferior to reveal an ill-defined, 0.9 × 0.7 × 0.7-cm, gray-white, firm mass. The final histopathology confirms a diagnosis of multifocal PTC of follicular variant; the largest tumor foci size is 0.9 cm (Fig. 48.6). No lymphatic invasion or extrathyroidal extension is identified. The surgical margins are negative.

What are the principles of the molecular testing of FNA samples?

There have been major advances in molecular pathological techniques in the last few years, particularly with the introduction of next-generation sequencing for DNA and RNA. Molecular studies can be used for differential diagnosis, patient prognostication, and as a marker for targeted therapy.

Putative molecular pathogenic pathway for classical type papillary carcinoma is typically BRAF V600E driven, and some cases with RET/PTC, whereas follicular adenoma, FTC is RAS- and PAX8/PPARγ-driven lesions.

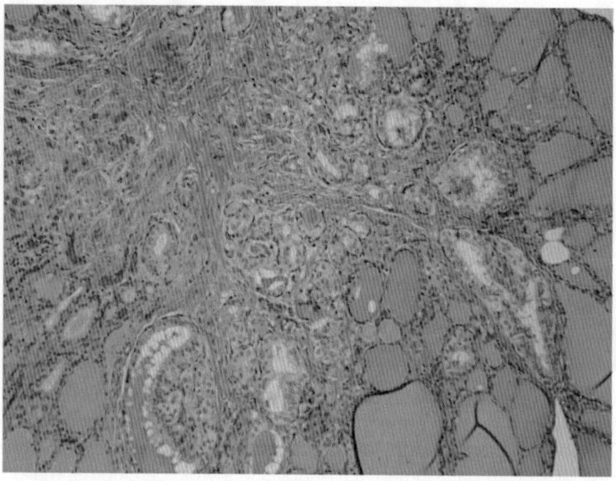

Fig. 48.6 Papillary thyroid carcinoma of follicular variant, size is 0.9 cm (H&E, 200x).

TABLE 48.3 ■ **Average Prevalence of Mutations in Follicular Cell-derived Thyroid Cancer**

Altered gene	PDTC	PTC	FTC	ATC
RET/PTC	0%	20%	0%	0%
BRAF	15-20%	45%	0%	20%
RAS	30-35%	10%	45%	50-55%
PAX8/PPARγ	0%	0%	35%	0%

ATC, anaplastic thyroid carcinoma; *FTC,* follicular thyroid carcinoma; *PDTC,* poorly differentiated thyroid carcinoma; *PTC,* papillary thyroid carcinoma.

Molecular methods have become important diagnostic and developmental tools in thyroid disease, in the understanding of the pathogenesis of thyroid cancer, and in diagnosis, prognosis, and treatment. Many of these methods can be used preoperatively on small samples of DNA or RNA or micro-RNAs from thyroid FNA aspirates (Table 48.3).

BEYOND THE PEARLS

- Renal cell carcinoma is the most common metastatic carcinoma to thyroid glands. Melanoma and mammary lobular carcinoma are other malignancies that metastasize to thyroid gland.
- Multinodular goiter (nontoxic goiter) is an enlarged thyroid gland with multiple benign nodules.
- Hashimoto's thyroiditis is an autoimmune disease with destruction of the thyroid gland and resultant hypothyroidism; it may be associated with other autoimmune diseases.
- De Quervain thyroiditis is the second most common form of thyroiditis and is typically preceded by a viral illness that produces an enlarged thyroid gland with transient hyperparathyroidism.
- Medullary thyroid carcinoma accounts for 5% of malignant thyroid tumors and arises from the parafollicular (C cells) and secretes calcitonin; some can be associated with MENII and MENIII syndromes.

References

Ali SZ, Cibas ES. The Bethesda system for reporting thyroid cytopathology II. *Acta Cytol.* 2016;60(5):397–398.

Ali SZ, MD, Krane JF, Nayar R, Westra WH. *Atlas of Thyroid Cytopathology.* Springer; 2013.

Haugen BR, Alexander EK, Bible KC, et al. 2015 American Thyroid Association Management Guidelines for Adult Patients with Thyroid Nodules and Differentiated Thyroid Cancer. The American Thyroid Association Guidelines Task Force on Thyroid Nodules and Differentiated Thyroid Cancer. *Thyroid.* 2016;26(1):1–133.

Lam AKY. Pathology of Endocrine Tumors Update: World Health Organization New Classification 2017-Other Thyroid Tumors. *AJSP Rev Rep.* 2017;22(4):209–216.

Nosé V, Kovacs CM. Thyroid neoplasms. 2019. Elsevier Expertpath pathprimer.

Poller DN, Glaysher S. Molecular pathology and thyroid FNA. *Cytopathology.* 2017;28(6):475–281.

CASE 49

A 69-Year-Old Female with Weakness, Shortness of Breath, and Syncopal Episodes

Jennifer J. Prutsman-Pfeiffer

A 69-year-old female is evaluated in the emergency department with weakness, shortness of breath, and several near-syncopal episodes. The patient had surgery for total hip replacement 4 days prior and was discharged home on a prophylactic dose of rivaroxaban for prevention of deep vein thrombosis. Past medical history is significant for chronic obstructive pulmonary disease, type 2 diabetes mellitus, anemia, depression, gastroesophageal reflux disease, hyperlipidemia, hypertension, obesity, remote history of previous deep vein thrombosis (15 years prior), right mastectomy for breast cancer, right knee arthroscopy, right knee arthroplasty, and left total hip replacement for degenerative joint disease. She is retired, drinks socially, and quit smoking 25 years ago. Medications include amitriptyline, atorvastatin, escitalopram, gabapentin, tramadol, lansoprazole, metformin, multivitamin, and rivaroxaban.

Case Point 49.1

Upon physical examination at triage, the patient demonstrates blood pressure of 84/63 mm Hg (hypotensive), pulse rate of 117 beats per minute (tachycardic), respiratory rate of 32 breaths per minute (tachypneic), and she is hypoxic. The patient is pale and diaphoretic, but not in respiratory distress. There is a clean, dressed surgical wound of the lower extremity as well as superficial hematomas on the anterior and lateral aspects of the left leg. The diameter of the left leg is larger than that of the right. Arterial blood gases show pH 7.59, pCO_2 of 23 mm Hg, pO_2 of 74.7 mm Hg on 2–3 L oxygen. There is no chest pain, and troponin levels are within normal limits. Her complete blood count is unremarkable, except for elevated white cell count of 13.7 Th/mm^3 (reference range 4.0–10.0 Th/mm^3). A chest computerized tomography angiography (CTA) scan reveals small filling defects of the right anterior and right apical subsegmental pulmonary arteries, compatible with acute pulmonary embolism. A 2.8-cm heterogeneous mass-like density in the right upper abdomen is incidentally discovered. The mass was not seen on a previous positron emission tomography (PET) scan from 10 years ago. Venous Doppler ultrasound is negative for deep vein thrombosis. An echocardiogram shows an ejection fraction of 60% with poor acoustic window, normal left ventricular size and function, no valve abnormalities, and normal right heart function.

What is an incidentaloma?

The prevalence of advanced medical imaging since the 1980s has resulted in a new clinical category known as the incidentaloma. Incidentalomas are also known as “clinically inapparent” masses, which tend to be less than 3 cm in size.

Case Point 49.2

The patient had a chest CTA scan, which confirmed a pulmonary embolism and incidentally found a right adrenal mass (Fig. 49.1). This finding is fortuitous, as typical anatomical boundaries for chest CT scans to diagnose pulmonary embolism are top of lung apices to the lung base. This patient's CT scan reports the "visualized abdomen" and the chest findings.

The most important aspect of management of incidentalomas is to assess the clinical impact the mass will have on the patient. In patients who have a history of malignancy and where there is a suspicion for metastasis, the lesions are more often bilateral. In patients without a history of malignancy, the majority of incidentalomas will turn out as benign lesions. Adrenal incidentalomas have a wide differential to include secreting and nonsecreting neoplasms (Fig. 49.2).

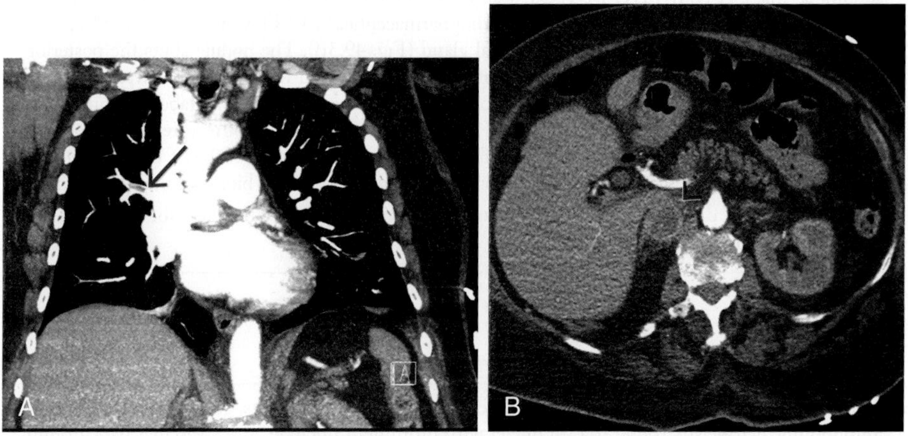

Fig. 49.1 Chest computerized tomography angiography scan showing (A) acute pulmonary embolism in the right upper lobe of lung, subsegmental branch (arrow) and (B) incidental mass in right upper abdomen (arrow).

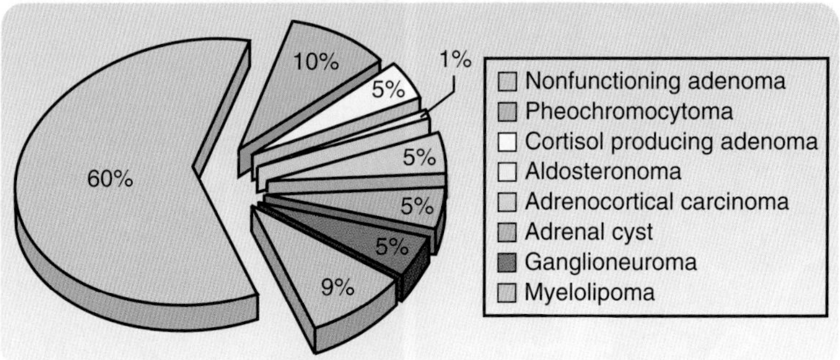

Fig. 49.2 Differential diagnosis of adrenal incidentaloma in patients without a history of malignant disease. Approximate proportions of the various pathologic processes are shown. (From Yeh, MW, Livhits, MJ and Duh, Q-Y. The Adrenal Glands, Chapter 39 in *Sabiston Textbook of Surgery*, 20th edition, 2017:963-995. Figure 39-20.)

CLINICAL PEARL

Incidentalomas are unexpected findings discovered when imaging of the body is performed for some other reason. Some of the more common incidentalomas are found in the pituitary gland, thyroid, lungs, liver, pancreas, adrenal glands, kidneys, and ovaries.

What additional testing should be performed for the incidental right upper abdomen mass?

In a patient with history of previous malignancy, a PET scan might be useful. This is an imaging test that helps reveal how tissues and organs are functioning by using a radioactive drug (tracer), typically fludeoxyglucose F18 (F18 FDG) to show activity. In some instances, this scan can detect disease before it shows up on other imaging tests.

Case Point 49.3

A CT scan of the abdomen and pelvis with contrast is performed (Fig. 49.3A) to verify the upper abdominal mass. A body FDG PET/CT scan is performed and reveals a 3.8 × 2.6-cm upper abdominal mass with increased uptake of the radiopharmaceutical F18 FDG with a standard uptake value (SUV) of 8, adjacent to the right adrenal gland (Fig. 49.3B). The nodule abuts the posterior aspect of the inferior vena cava and the crus of the hemidiaphragm without visible invasion. There are prominent retroperitoneal, iliac, and periaortic lymph nodes and a hypermetabolic lymph node anterior to the left psoas muscle with an SUV of 8. There is no evidence of recurrence of the right breast cancer. There are additional findings of increased uptake in the left lobe of the thyroid and isthmus (SUV 4). Recommendation is made for Interventional Radiology biopsy of the adrenal mass.

The patient is discharged home and returns approximately 2 months later for a CT-guided retroperitoneal biopsy.

Case Point 49.4

The CT-guided biopsy demonstrated a core composed of small nests of polygonal cells with amphophilic cytoplasm, round to oval nuclei with prominent nucleoli, and a vascular background (Fig. 49.4). Immunostains were performed in addition to the H&E section for further evaluation.

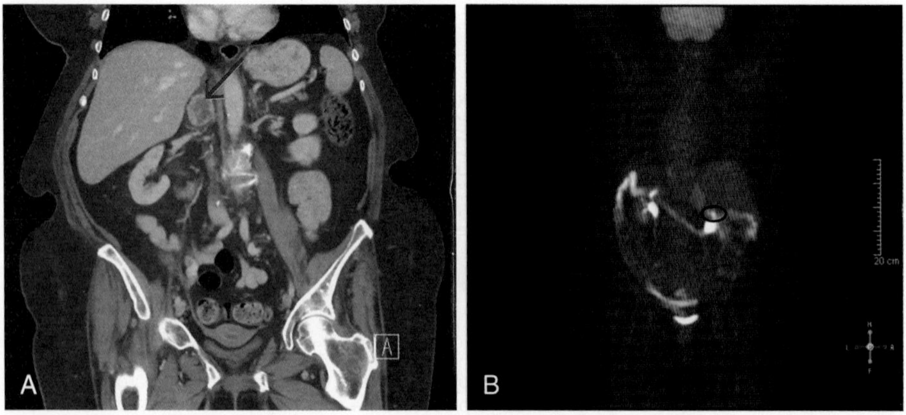

Fig. 49.3 Right upper abdominal mass: (A) Computed tomography scan of the abdomen and pelvis with contrast showing right upper abdominal mass (arrow); (B) Positron emission tomography scan with increased uptake of right upper abdomen nodule (circle). Bright areas indicate fluid collections.

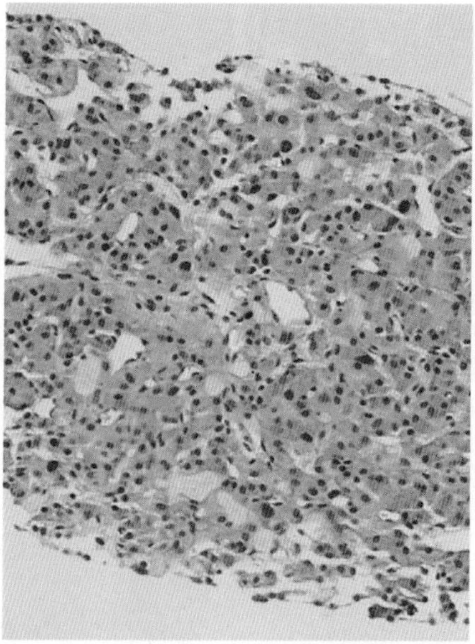

Fig. 49.4 Core biopsy of right adrenal mass, small nests of polygonal cells with amphophilic cytoplasm, round to oval nuclei with prominent nucleoli, and a vascular background (H&E stain 200x).

Immunostains were positive in the lesional cells for chromogranin and synaptophysin (Fig. 49.5A and B) and negative for pankeratin and inhibin; the sustentacular cells were highlighted with S100 (Fig. 49.5C). The histopathologic evaluation of the mass confirmed a pheochromocytoma.

What are the histologic features of a pheochromocytoma?

Histologically, pheochromocytomas are usually well-circumscribed masses, with sheets of neoplastic polygonal or rounded cells with nested architecture. Markedly amphophilic cytoplasm and a vascular background may be additional features identified. Immunohistochemical staining shows tumor cells to be positive for chromogranin and synaptophysin; S100 stain can highlight sustentacular cells within the tumor. Negative stains of pancytokeratin, inhibin, GCDFP 15, and estrogen receptor put together with the above findings favor the diagnosis of pheochromocytoma. Spindle cell morphology, increased mitotic rate, and invasion of the adrenal capsule are indicative of aggressive tumor growth.

CLINICAL PEARL

Histologic and microscopic features of pheochromocytoma:

- Zellballen (small nests or alveolar pattern), trabecular or solid patterns of polygonal/spindle-shaped cells in rich vascular network
- Finely granular basophilic or amphophilic cytoplasm
- Intracytoplasmic hyaline globules
- Round/oval nuclei with prominent nucleolus and variable inclusion-like structures
- Marked pleomorphism
- Capsular and vascular invasion common in benign-behaving tumors
- Nests outlined by sustentacular cells (cannot see in H&E but S100+)

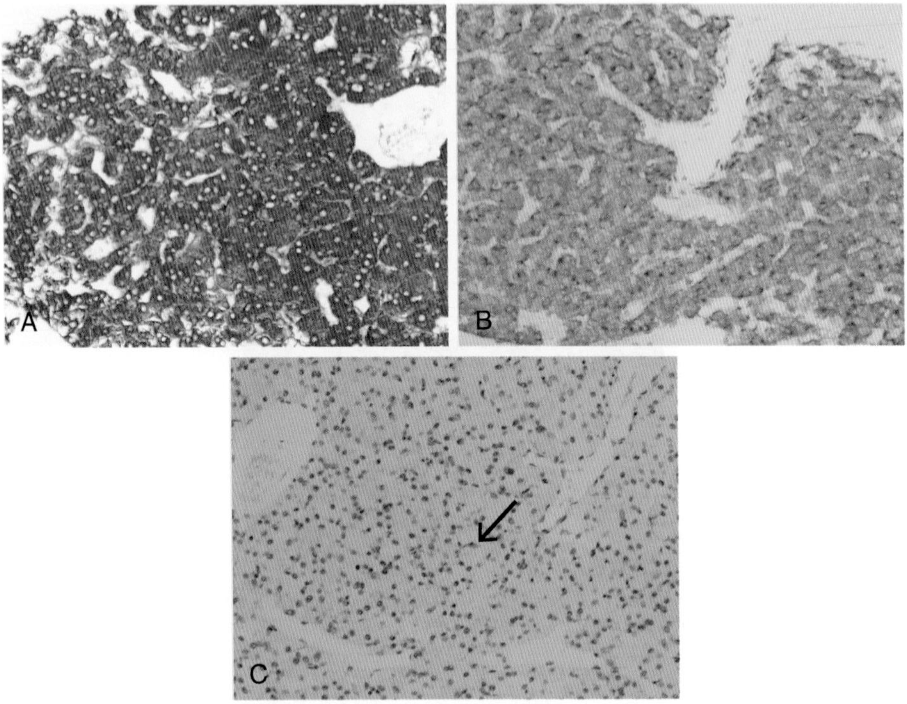

Fig. 49.5 Immunostains: (A) Chromogranin demonstrates diffusely positive tumor cells and is present in the secretory granules (200x). (B) Synaptophysin demonstrates diffuse cytoplasmic staining in the tumor cells (200x). (C) S100 highlights the sustentacular cells (arrow) in the tumor (200x).

- Amyloid common
- Rare/no mitotic figures
- May be mixed with neuroblastoma, ganglioneuroma, ganglioneuroblastoma, cortical adenoma, spindle cell sarcoma
- Unusual morphological features: Coexisting cortical hyperplasia, vacuolar degeneration of tumor cells, presence of pheochromoblasts (small cells), ganglion-like cells, calcospherites, melanin pigmentation insular growth pattern, and brown fat

Case Point 49.5

At a follow-up visit, the patient recalls having very high blood pressure around the time of her previous surgeries and reveals that she often has spells where she gets dizzy that require her to sit and rest. She does not monitor her blood pressure at home. She is prescribed terazosin, which blocks adrenaline's action on alpha-1 adrenergic receptors and helps control hypertension.

Plasma serum and 24-hour urine metanephrines were ordered, and results were elevated (Table 49.1). This test measures metanephrine and normetanephrine in the blood and urine, which are catecholamines that result when adrenaline breaks down. Significant elevation of one or both metanephrines (three or more times the upper reference limit) is associated with an increased probability of a neuroendocrine tumor.

TABLE 49.1 ■ **Blood Plasma and 24-Hour Urine Metanephrine Results**

	Reference Range	3 Months Ago	8 Months Ago
Metanephrine, plasma	0.00–0.49 nmol/L	<0.10	0.15
Normetanephrine, plasma	0.00–0.89 nmol/L	6.32*	3.55*
Metanephrines, urine	39–143 ug/d	–	99
Normetanephrine, urine	109–393 ug/d	–	2172*

*Indicates elevated values.

What are the classic symptoms of pheochromocytoma?

Symptoms include chest and abdominal pains, palpitations, diaphoresis, and headache; patients are also found to be hypertensive. These "episodes" typically wax and wane and are not always persistent. The symptoms are related to the extra catecholamines produced by the pheochromocytoma.

CLINICAL PEARL

The triad of symptoms for pheochromocytoma includes sweating attacks, tachycardia, and headaches that are related to catecholamine hypersecretion.

What lesions occur in the adrenal gland?

The adrenal gland (Fig. 49.6) is composed of a medulla, which resides in the middle of the gland, surrounded by a cortex of three zones: glomerulosa, fasciculata, and reticularis. Each layer secretes predominately one class of hormones: glomerulosa produces mineralocorticoids (aldosterone); fasciculate produces glucocorticoids (cortisol), and reticularis produces weak androgens (dehydroepiandrosterone or DHEA). Adrenal cortical adenomas arise from the zona fasciculata; however, benign or malignant tumors can originate from any of the zones. Distinguishing an adrenal cortical adenoma from an adrenal cortical carcinoma can be challenging. The gross appearance of the lesion is helpful in making a diagnosis. Adrenal cortical adenomas are benign and tend to be under 3 cm and less than 50 g. Adrenal cortical carcinomas are larger in size, over 100 g, show necrosis, have mitotic figures and atypical mitoses, invasive growth, and high nuclear grade. Ultrastructural studies may be employed that show features including abundant smooth endoplasmic reticulum and mitochondria with prominent tubular or vesicular cristae. The variants of adrenal cortical tumors include oncocytic tumors and the myxoid variant. Pheochromocytomas are lesions of the medullary adrenal gland.

CLINICAL PEARL

Cortical Tumors:

Adrenal cortical adenoma (benign, 50 g or less)
Adrenal cortical carcinoma (malignant, 100 g or more, necrosis, variegated appearance with nodularity and intersecting fibrous bands)

Medullary Tumors:

Pheochromocytoma (benign or malignant/metastatic)
Paraganglioma (tumors arising in the organ of Zuckerkandl at the root of the inferior mesenteric artery of the inferior aorta have the highest incidence of malignancy)

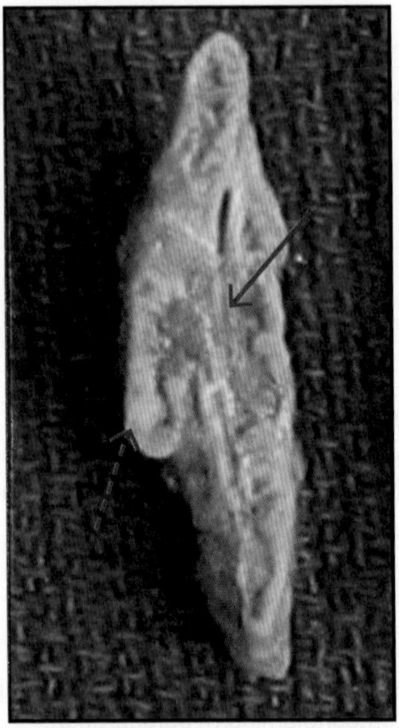

Fig. 49.6 Adrenal gland anatomy demonstrating maroon medulla (solid arrow) and golden yellow cortex (dashed arrow).

What are the characteristics of pheochromocytoma?

The term *pheochromocytoma* is reserved for intra-adrenal tumors. Most neural crest-derived chromaffin cells degenerate after the fetal stage of development; however, some residual chromaffin cells reside within the adrenal medulla. Extra-adrenal chromaffin tissue that persists after the fetal period can occur anywhere along the sympathetic nervous system chain (adrenal medulla and organ of Zuckerkandl) and the supradiaphragmatic branches of the parasympathetic nervous system (vagus and glossopharyngeal nerves as well as carotid body). When tumors occur outside of the medulla of the adrenal gland, they are known as extra-adrenal paragangliomas (Fig. 49.7). About 98% of pheochromocytomas are located in the abdomen, and 90% are found within the adrenal medulla. The term is derived from a description by Poll in 1905 as the cut surface having a dusky (pheo) color (chromo).

Pheochromocytomas are catecholamine-secreting tumors and are also known as the "10% tumor." Hypertension is surgically correctable by removal of the tumor.

CLINICAL PEARL

10% Rule of Pheochromocytomas:

10% are extra-adrenal
10% are malignant
10% are bilateral
10% are familial (MEN 2A and 2B)
10% occur in children
10% are found incidentally

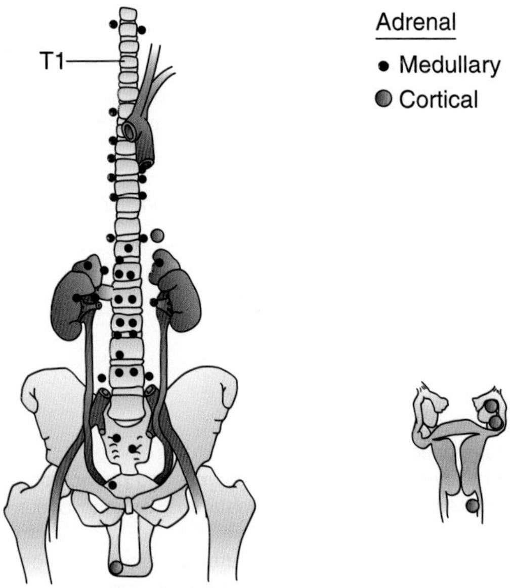

Fig. 49.7 Sites of extra-adrenal cortical and medullary tissue. Larger figure shows male reproductive organs; T1 indicates the first thoracic vertebra. Smaller figure shows female reproductive organs. (From Yeh, MW, Livhits, MJ and Duh, Q-Y. The Adrenal Glands, Chapter 39 in *Sabiston Textbook of Surgery*, 20th edition, 2017:963-995. Figure 39-2.)

Tumors are generally sporadic and benign, with the most common occurrence during the fourth and fifth decades of life. Malignant tumors comprise 10% of all pheochromocytomas. The symptoms are the same as in benign cases; catecholamine production may be increased due to multiple sites with metastatic disease. Metastatic disease is the most reliable indicator of malignancy.

What syndromes can pheochromocytomas occur in?

There are five genetic syndromes associated with pheochromocytoma: von Hippel–Lindau (vHL) syndrome, multiple endocrine neoplasia type 2A and 2B (MEN 2A and 2B), neurofibromatosis type 1 (NF1), and familial paraganglioma syndrome.

CLINICAL PEARL

vHL

10%–30% of patients have pheochromocytomas and restricted to patients with type 2 vHL, also cysts of kidney, liver, and epididymis; patients with type 1 vHL develop renal cell carcinoma (clear cell type), retinal angiomas, and cerebellar hemangioblastoma and do not usually develop pheochromocytomas.

CLINICAL PEARL

MEN 1 (Werner syndrome):

Pituitary tumors, parathyroid hyperplasia or adenoma, pancreatic hyperplasia or adenoma and carcinoid tumors

CLINICAL PEARL

MEN 2A (Sipple syndrome):
Autosomal dominant with high penetrance, 30%–50% develop pheochromocytomas, all have familial medullary thyroid carcinoma, and 10%–15% have parathyroid hyperplasia
Due to mutation in RET proto-oncogene
MEN 2B
MEN 2A signs/symptoms plus mucosal neuromas and ganglioneuromas
Autosomal dominant or sporadic
May lack parathyroid hyperplasia

CLINICAL PEARL

NF1 (von Recklinghausen):
1%–5% of patients have pheochromocytomas
Neurofibromatosis, schwannoma, meningioma, glioma, and pheochromocytoma
Composite tumors with neuroblastoma, ganglioneuroma, or ganglioneuroblastoma may be associated with NF1
NF1 carries 100% disease penetrance within families; pheochromocytoma has greater incidence in patients with NF1 than in general population

CLINICAL PEARL

Hereditary paraganglioma-pheochromocytoma syndromes
Autosomal dominant inheritance
Paragangliomas (tumors from neuroendocrine tissue along paravertebral axis from skull base to pelvis) and pheochromocytomas (confined to adrenal medulla)
Sympathetic paragangliomas cause catecholamine excess; parasympathetic paragangliomas are most often nonsecretory
Extra-adrenal parasympathetic paragangliomas are confined to skull base and neck and upper mediastinum, 95% are nonsecretory
Extra-adrenal sympathetic paragangliomas are confined to lower mediastinum, abdomen, pelvis, and are secretory; they have greater risk of developing metastatic disease than pheochromocytoma

What are the features for malignancy?

Malignant (metastatic) pheochromocytoma is diagnosed based on local invasion of adjacent structures or the presence of multifocal disease. Localized tumors are considered benign, whereas multiple tumors are considered malignant (metastatic). A definition of malignancy requires that metastasis occurs in a location where paraganglionic tissue is not typically present (e.g., liver, lung, bone, lymph node). The choice of treatment, whether benign or malignant, is surgical resection. Larger tumors tend to be malignant and tend to be infiltrative, lobulated, and nodular with areas of necrosis. Histologic features of malignancy include capsular invasion, vascular invasion, diffuse growth and extension into the periadrenal adipose tissue, necrosis, increased cellularity and tumor cell spindling, marked nuclear pleomorphism and macronuclei, and increased mitosis and atypical mitosis. The Pheochromocytomas of the Adrenal gland Scaled Score (PASS) is a method to distinguish benign from malignant pheochromocytomas based on the aforementioned histologic features.

CLINICAL PEARL

The PASS method uses features of growth pattern, necrosis, cellularity, cellular monotony, tumor cell spindling, mitotic count, atypical mitosis, invasion, nuclear pleomorphism, and hyperchromasia to separate benign from malignant tumors (score of 4 or higher is associated with higher probability of malignancy)

0–3 points: benign

1 point: vascular invasion, capsular invasion, profound nuclear pleomorphism, or hyperchromasia

2 points: invasion of periadrenal adipose tissue, large nests or diffuse growth, focal or confluent necrosis, high cellularity, tumor cell spindling, cellular monotony, 4+ mitotic figures per 10 HPF, atypical mitotic figures

What additional testing should be performed for the pheochromocytoma and the related hypermetabolic areas?

A nuclear medicine scan using radioactive iodine, called a meta-iodo-benzylguanidine (MIBG) scan, can be used to further characterize the nature of the multifocal hypermetabolic areas discovered on PET scan. This radioactive iodine is attached to the MIBG molecule, which is structurally similar to noradrenaline. The tracer is administered through a vein, and the patient returns for the scan the following day; the delay allows the MIBG compound to concentrate in any tumor cells, and the radioactivity allows visualization during the scan. The radioactive part of the compound allows these areas of tumor to be visualized on the scan.

Case Point 49.6

An MIBG scan is performed, and findings are consistent with neuroendocrine tumor of the right adrenal gland without scintigraphic evidence of metastases.

A fine-needle aspiration (FNA) of hypermetabolic sites may further diagnose the nature of those areas histologically.

Surgical resection is the treatment of choice for the diagnosed pheochromocytoma of the adrenal gland.

A conservative approach is taken for the ancillary sites. If there is a family history of neuroendocrine tumors, genetic testing should be performed.

Case Point 49.7

The patient underwent a right adrenalectomy and recovered on postoperative day 2. The physical symptoms of episodic hypertension, palpitations, tachycardia, diaphoresis, and syncope are attributable to pheochromocytoma. The 48-g adrenal gland specimen demonstrates a 3 × 2.8 × 2.5-cm golden yellow, well-circumscribed mass in the adrenal medulla (Fig. 49.8). The final histopathology is similar to the core biopsy and demonstrated a nested tumor, well circumscribed and encapsulated with zellballen, no capsular invasion, no vascular invasion, necrosis, or spindle cells noted (Fig. 49.9). Rare mitosis 1/30 HPF and rare Ki67-positive cells (<1%) are noted. Immunostains showed the same profile demonstrating positive chromogranin and synaptophysin (Fig. 49.10). The immunostain profile and morphology are consistent with pheochromocytoma. Two additional sites were biopsied to exclude metastatic disease. The left groin lymph node FNA reveals cellular evidence of a lymph node and no malignancy. The thyroid FNA is benign and consistent with a nodular goiter.

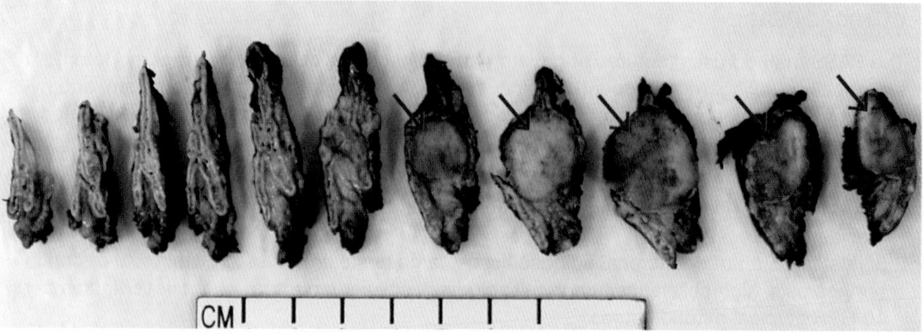

Fig. 49.8 Gross photograph of the right adrenal gland inked and serially sectioned with well-circumscribed, 3-cm golden mass in the adrenal medulla (arrow, gross photograph).

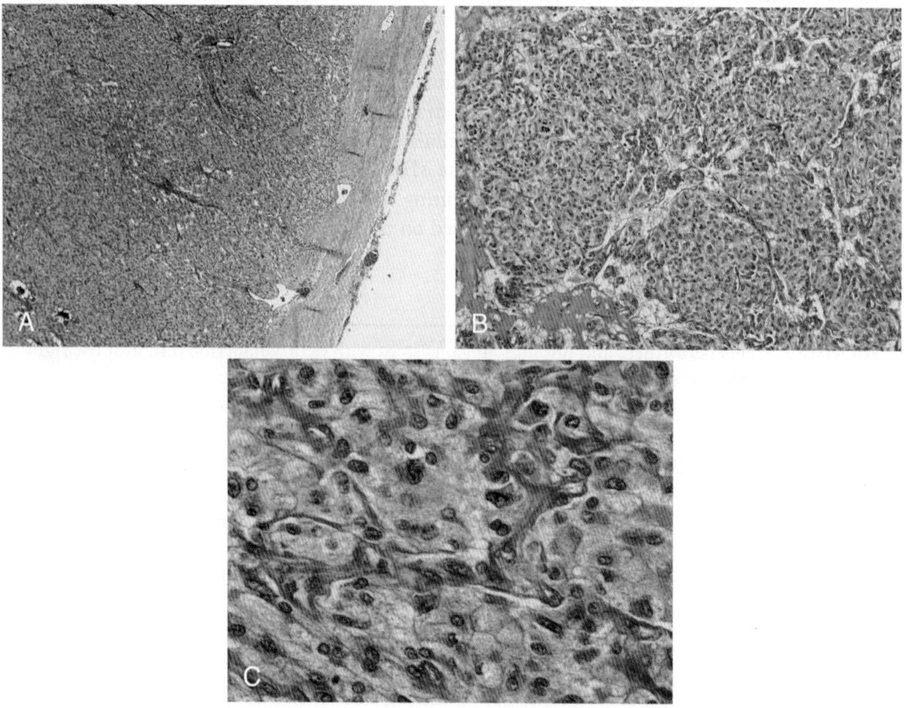

Fig. 49.9 Histologic sections of the mass at (A) low, (B) medium, and (C) high power showing a well-circumscribed tumor composed of nested cells. No capsular invasion, vascular invasion, or necrosis was noted. (B) demonstrates zellballen (H&E stain, A 40x, B 100x, C 400x).

How are these patients followed?

A conservative approach is taken for cases of metastatic pheochromocytoma after the main adrenal lesion is surgically removed. If the patient does not experience continued symptoms of paroxysmal hypertension, tachycardia, headaches, and diaphoresis, the disease is considered indolent and no further treatment is necessary. Patients with a higher risk of malignancy (age 40 or younger, tumor size greater than 5 cm and secreting norepinephrine) should undergo biochemical screening every 6 months and imaging on a yearly basis.

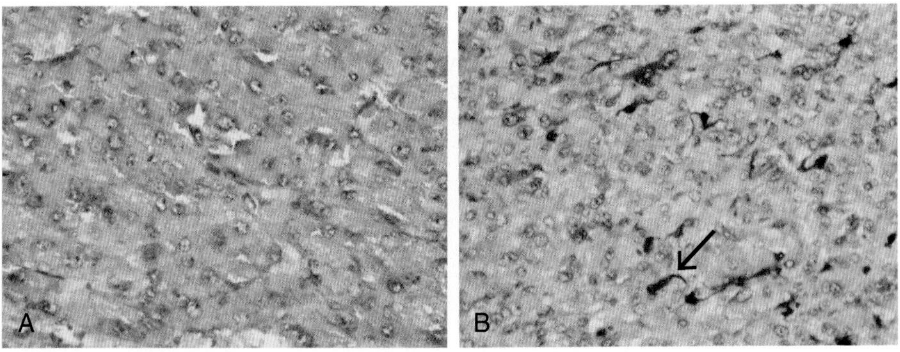

Fig. 49.10 Immunostains: (A) Synaptophysin demonstrates diffuse cytoplasmic staining in the tumor cells (400x). (B) S100 highlights the sustentacular cells in the tumor (arrow) (200x).

BEYOND THE PEARLS

- Sturge–Weber syndrome: Cavernous hemangiomas (port-wine spots) of trigeminal nerve (cranial nerve V), pheochromocytoma
- Cushing syndrome: Hyperadrenalism, increase in levels of glucocorticoids, most commonly administration of exogenous glucocorticoids; endogenous causes include: Cushing disease (hypersecretion of adrenocorticotropic hormone (ACTH) due to pituitary microadenoma)
  ACTH stimulates cortisol production
  ACTH secretion from nonpituitary tumors (small cell lung cancer)
  ACTH-independent Cushing syndrome due to adrenal neoplasia
- Addison's disease: chronic adrenocortical insufficiency caused by destruction of the renal cortex; most common cause is autoimmune adrenalitis.
- Hyperaldosteronism:
  Primary – adrenocortical neoplasm (adenoma) or bilateral nodular hyperplasia of the adrenal
  Secondary – increased plasma renin due to renal artery stenosis
- Adrenogenital syndrome: excess production of androgens and virilization, caused by adrenocortical adenoma or adrenocortical carcinoma or congenital adrenal hyperplasia (cluster of autosomal recessive enzyme defects, most common 21-hydroxylase deficiency)
- Waterhouse–Friderichsen syndrome: acute adrenal insufficiency, bilateral hemorrhagic infarct in of adrenal glands associated with sepsis

References

Beard CM, Sheps SG, Kurland LT, Carney JA, Lie JT. Occurrence of pheochromocytoma in Rochester, Minnesota, 1950 through 1979. *Mayo Clin Proc*. 1983;58:802-804.

Johnson MH, Cavallo JA, Figenshau RS. Malignant and metastatic pheochromocytoma: case report and review of the literature. *Urol Case Rep*. 2014;2(4):139-141.

Liao EA, Quint LE, Goodsitt MM, Francis IR, Khalatbari S, Myles JD. Extra Z-axis coverage at CT imaging resulting in excess radiation dose: frequency, degree and contributory factors. *J Comput Assist Tomogr*. 2011;35(1):50-56.

Lloyd RV. Adrenal cortical tumors, pheochromocytomas and paragangliomas. *Mod Pathol*. 2011;24: S48-S65.

Tischler AS. Pheochromocytoma and extra-adrenal paraganglioma: updates. *Arch Pathol Lab Med.* 2008;132:1272-1284.

Yeh MW, Livhits, MJ, Duh, QY. Chapter 39 - The Adrenal Glands. In: Townsend JR, Courtney M, Beauchamp RD, et al, eds. *Sabiston Textbook of Surgery.* 20th ed. Philadelphia, PA: Elsevier; 2017:963-995.

Zelinka T, Musil Z, Dušková J, et al. Metastatic pheochromocytoma: clinical, genetic, and histopathologic characteristics. *Eur J Clin Invest.* 2011;41(10):1121-1128.

INDEX

Page numbers followed by '*f*' indicate figures, '*t*' indicate tables, and '*b*' indicate boxes.

C

D

H

M

N

Q

R

S

T